Landmark Studies in Critical Care

Jose Chacko • Donald B. Chalfin
Ian Seppelt • Swapnil Pawar • Gagan Brar

Landmark Studies in Critical Care

The Evidence Base of Contemporary Practice

Springer

Jose Chacko
Department of Critical Care
Narayana Health
Bangalore, Karnataka, India

Ian Seppelt
Department of Intensive Care Medicine
Nepean Hospital
Sydney, NSW, Australia

Gagan Brar
Department of Critical Care Medicine
Aster RV Hospital
Bangalore, Karnataka, India

Donald B. Chalfin
Department of Epidemiology
and Biostatistics
University of California
Berkeley, CA, USA

Swapnil Pawar
Department of Intensive Care Medicine
St George Hospital
Sydney, NSW, Australia

ISBN 978-981-95-0672-9 ISBN 978-981-95-0673-6 (eBook)
https://doi.org/10.1007/978-981-95-0673-6

This Springer imprint is published by the registered company Springer Nature Singapore Pte Ltd.
The registered company address is: 152 Beach Road, #21-01/04 Gateway East, Singapore 189721, Singapore

Foreword

Over the last 75 years, Intensive Care Medicine has evolved to become keystone in the pantheon of hospital medicine across the world.

From origins as a specific facility for prolonged mechanical ventilation of patients during the Copenhagen polio epidemic in 1952; the evolution into surgical Intensive Care Units (ICUs) in the 1970s for the management of complex post-operative patients; the development of multidisciplinary ICUs for adults and children in the 1980s and the expansion of ICUs for the management of acute admissions to hospitals requiring intensive nursing, monitoring and vital organ support and an increasing role in medical emergency teams and end-of-life management.

Most of this evolution has been driven by technological advances, life-prolonging therapies, and increased demand due to extended life-expectancy and complex multimorbidity.

Over the formative years, educational programs developed in parallel with the establishment of international learned societies and colleges, albeit with limited research outside small unit-based research programs and pharmaceutical trials.

The establishment of national critical care clinical trial networks in Canada, Australia, New Zealand, Scandinavia, and the United Kingdom in the 1990s, all underpinned by universal access public healthcare systems, resulted in the completion and publication of landmark clinical trials published in the highest impact international journals over the last 25 years.

These trials have primarily focused determining the comparative effectiveness of standard therapies, addressing long-standing clinician uncertainty and assessing the impact of these interventions on patient-centered outcomes.

This has been a unique aspect of Intensive Care Medicine that has surpassed other clinical areas of medicine.

In this context, the authors of this book have selected a collection of landmark, high-impact clinical trials published by Intensive Care clinician-researchers over the last 25 years.

The book is divided into 20 parts focused on fundamental clinical areas of Intensive Care Medicine.

A total of 76 papers are presented, each with a summary or “quick take” and accompanied by a visual abstract. The reports are concise and readable highlighting clinically relevant background in informing the hypothesis and key clinical question. Each paper is summarized in terms of the internal validity, statistical analysis plan with presentation of the primary, and key secondary outcomes and subgroup analyses. A critique on the relevant strengths and weaknesses is followed by a concise executive summary and impact through subsequent evidence and the impact on clinicians.

Some of the landmark trials include the Saline vs. Albumin Fluid Evaluation Study (SAFE) that heralded the impact and success of the Australian and New Zealand Intensive Care Society Clinical Trials Group and the subsequent fluid resuscitation research programs that have emanated from Canada, Scandinavia, Brazil, and Kenya—all of which changed clinical practice worldwide.

Other high impact trials include those directed at aspects of glycemic control, transfusion thresholds, intracranial hypertension, corticosteroids and resuscitation in septic shock and mechanically ventilation.

The remarkable outputs by clinician-researchers in the United Kingdom during the COVID-19 pandemic informing clinicians about effective therapies in a time-critical fashion through innovative trial design is a particular highlight that portends well for the future of Intensive Care Medical research into the next 25 years.

This book is an important contribution to the literature.

Not only as an archive of a remarkable period in the history of the specialty, but also as an important, highly readable and referable resource for clinicians regardless of the phase of career – whether this be a vocational trainee or established Intensive Care Physician.

Professor of Intensive Care Medicine
University of New South Wales
Sydney, NSW, Australia
The George Institute for Global Health
Sydney, Australia

John Myburgh AO

Preface

A systematic approach to the critical appraisal of medical literature took root in the early 1980s, thanks to clinical epidemiologists led by David Sackett at McMaster University in Ontario, Canada. In 1991, Gordon Guyatt, his protégé, coined the term "evidence-based medicine," ushering in a new era of scientific inquiry and clinical decision-making. Although critical care medicine is a relatively new area of specialization, it has rapidly evolved over the past more than five decades. During this period, there has been a steady influx of literature with many landmark clinical trials that left a lasting impact on the way we practice. It may be a daunting task for trainees in the field and perhaps seasoned practitioners, too, to keep themselves abreast of the way evidence has emerged and influenced practice over time. Considering the dynamic nature of science, the passage of time and the advent of new research may have diminished the relevance of some of these seminal papers; however, they remain beacons that guided and shaped practice.

In *Landmark Studies in Critical Care: The Evidence Base of Contemporary Practice*, we attempt to focus on clinical trials that left an indelible impression on the practice of critical care medicine. We present each study in a standard, easy-to-assimilate format, highlighting the background, methodology, key findings, clinical implications, and the emergence of later evidence that reflects current practice. We have divided the papers into sections based on organ systems that they pertain to. The studies were chosen through consensus after extensive discussion among the authors. We acknowledge that our choice of papers may be subject to bias; indeed, some of the impactful literature may have been left out, albeit inadvertently.

We have designed the book to guide trainees as they navigate the complexities of this challenging area of specialization and to inspire seasoned practitioners to revisit the enduring evidence that has shaped contemporary practice. We hope our endeavor serves as a valuable resource for understanding the evidence base of critical care medicine and its evolution.

Bangalore, Karnataka, India	Jose Chacko
Berkeley, CA, USA	Donald B. Chalfin
Sydney, NSW, Australia	Ian Seppelt
Sydney, NSW, Australia	Swapnil Pawar
Bangalore, Karnataka, India	Gagan Brar

Contents

Part III Cardiopulmonary Resuscitation

Part IV Neurosciences

Part XIV Therapeutic Hypothermia

Part XVII Glucose Control

Part I

Mechanical Ventilation and Respiratory Failure

Neuromuscular Blockade in ARDS: The ACURASYS Trial

1

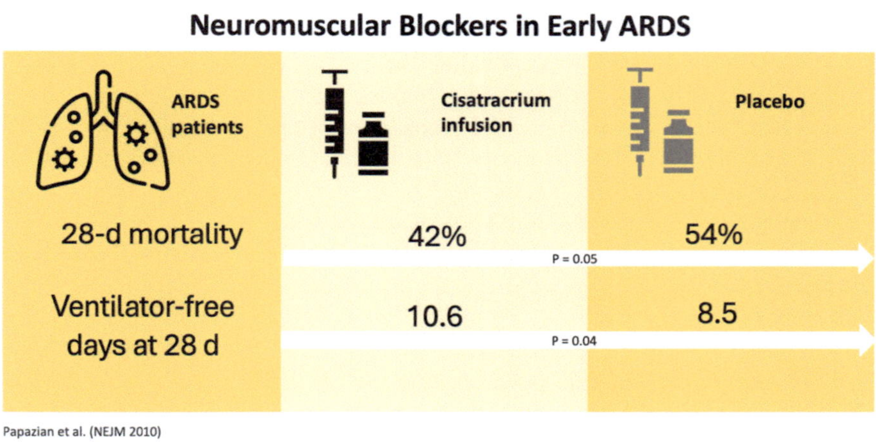

Quick Take

Could muscle relaxants be life-saving in acute respiratory distress syndrome (ARDS)? The ACURASYS trial unveils how cisatracurium, used early in severe ARDS, improved survival, reshaping ventilatory management strategies.

The ACURASYS trial investigated the effects of early administration of a 48-h infusion of cisatracurium, a neuromuscular blocking agent, in patients with severe

Papazian L, Forel JM, Gacouin A, et al. Neuromuscular blockers in early acute respiratory distress syndrome. N Engl J Med. 2010;363(12):1107–1116.

J. Chacko et al., *Landmark Studies in Critical Care*,
https://doi.org/10.1007/978-981-95-0673-6_1

ARDS. This randomized controlled trial included 340 patients with a PaO_2/FiO_2 ratio of less than 150. The cisatracurium group showed significantly lower 90-day mortality (31.6% vs. 40.7%) compared to the placebo group, despite similar rates of adverse events, including ICU-acquired weakness. The study highlighted the role of early neuromuscular blockade in improving oxygenation and outcomes when combined with lung-protective ventilation strategies.

1.1 Introduction

Neuromuscular blockade has been in routine practice in anesthesia and critical care for more than half a century. Claude Bernard, one of the pioneer researchers on neuromuscular blocking agents, conducted groundbreaking animal experiments on the effect of curare in the nineteenth century. He watched with interest and intrigue as curare administration instantly abolished convulsions arising from strychnine poisoning. By 1857, he had established the neuromuscular junction as the site of action of curare [1]. Early preparations of curare were crude extracts from *Chondrodendron tomentosum*, a woody climbing plant native to the rainforests of South America. The first commercial preparation of curare, branded Intocostrin, was introduced in 1938. On 23 January 1942, Harold Griffith, an anesthetist, and his resident, Enid Johnson, used curare in a young man who underwent appendicectomy, heralding the modern-day use of neuromuscular blockade. In those early days, they confined curare administration mainly towards the end of the surgery; within a minute, the abdomen turned "soft as dough," enabling peritoneal closure with effortless ease [2].

The administration of neuromuscular blocking agents in the ICU took it roots from contemporary anesthetic practice. Widespread, often indiscriminate use followed, and by the early 1980s, most ventilated ICU patients routinely received neuromuscular blockade. Although generally considered safe, especially with the introduction of several newer agents with fewer adverse effects, concerns arose from persisting neuromuscular weakness after prolonged administration [3]. Thomas Petty, who, along with his colleagues, first reported acute respiratory distress syndrome (ARDS), lamented in an editorial in the *Chest* journal of August 1998: "What I see these days are paralyzed, sedated patients, lying without motion, appearing to be dead, except for the monitors that tell me otherwise. Why this syndrome of sedation and paralysis has emerged baffles me, because this was not the case in the past" [4].

1.2 Background to the ACURASYS Trial

Neuromuscular blocking agents had been widely used in mechanically ventilated patients with ARDS to enable patient-ventilator synchrony and improved gas exchange. A four-center randomized controlled trial (RCT) had previously been conducted to evaluate the impact of 48 h of neuromuscular blockade with cisatracurium on the gas exchange over a 5-day period among patients with ARDS [5]. The control group received conventional care, without neuromuscular blockade. Both groups of patients were ventilated on the assist-control mode with a tidal volume of 6–8 m/kg ideal body weight. Patients who received neuromuscular blockade with cisatracurium revealed significantly higher PaO_2/FiO_2 ratios compared to the conventional arm after 48 h, 96 h, and 5 days after randomization. The improved PaO_2/FiO_2 ratio enabled a reduction of the PEEP level among patients who received neuromuscular blockade. A trend towards improved ICU survival was also noted in patients who received continuous neuromuscular blockade for 48 h. However, this RCT was not powered to evaluate clinical outcomes.

Considering the relative lack of robust evidence regarding the beneficial impact of neuromuscular blockade on clinical outcomes among patients with severe ARDS from available studies, the *ARDS et Curarisation Systematique* (ACURASYS) trial investigators embarked upon a large RCT using cisatracurium infusion early in the course of the disease [6].

1.3 Population and Design

The study was conducted during a 2-year period between 2006 and 2008 across 20 ICUs in France. Patients with severe ARDS, with a PaO_2/FiO_2 ratio of <150 mm Hg, while being ventilated with a tidal volume of 6–8 ml/kg predicted body weight and a PEEP level ≥5 cm H_2O were included within the first 48 h of meeting the above criteria. Those suspected to have cardiogenic pulmonary edema were excluded. Patients were randomly assigned to receive a continuous infusion of cisatracurium besylate or a matching placebo for 48 h.

1.4 Sample Size Calculation

The authors calculated the sample size based on a 90-day mortality of 50% based on previous studies of ARDS. They assumed a 15% absolute reduction in mortality with the use of cisatracurium infusion. A sample size of 340 patients was calculated, providing an 80% statistical power with a two-sided alpha value of 0.05.

1.5 Intervention and Control groups

After administration of sedative agents to attain a target Ramsay sedation score of 6 (no response to glabellar tap), and adjustment of ventilator settings, a rapid infusion of cisatracurium besylate, 15 mg, followed by a continuous infusion of 37.5 mg/h was commenced and maintained for 48 h. In the control group, identical volumes of placebo were administered.

1.6 Management of Mechanical Ventilation

A tidal volume of 6–8 ml/kg of predicted body weight was employed, with titration of the PEEP level based on the ARDSNet table. A plateau pressure of ≤32 cm H_2O was targeted, aiming for a SaO_2 of 88–95%. A dose of 20 mg of cisatracurium was allowed as a rescue measure to both groups of patients if the plateau pressure remained >32 cm H_2O, despite adequate use of sedative agents.

1.7 Results

The study included 340 patients—178 were randomized to receive cisatracurium and 162 to placebo. The time from ARDS onset to study inclusion was 16 (6–29) hours in the study cohort and was similar between the two groups. The duration of mechanical ventilation before inclusion was also similar between groups. However, the mean PaO_2/FiO_2 ratio was significantly lower in the cisatracurium group at study onset (106 vs. 115 mm Hg).

1.7.1 The Primary Outcome: 90-Day Mortality

The unadjusted 90-day mortality was lower in the cisatracurium 31.6% (95% CI, 25.2–38.8), compared to the placebo group 40.7% (95% CI, 33.5–48.4), but fell short of statistical significance ($P = 0.08$). After adjustment for the baseline PaO_2/FiO_2 ratio, the SAPS II score, and plateau pressure, the 90-day mortality was lower with cisatracurium infusion (hazard ratio: 0.68; 95% CI, 0.48–0.98; $P = 0.04$). Improved 90-day survival among patients who received cisatracurium was confined to those who were severely hypoxic, with a PaO_2/FiO_2 ratio of <120 mm Hg.

1.7.2 Secondary Outcomes

The ICU and hospital mortality were lower with cisatracurium, but the difference was not significantly different between groups. The 28-day mortality was also lower in the cisatracurium group ($p = 0.05$). The cisatracurium group had significantly more ventilator-free days at 28 and 90 days compared to the placebo group. The probability of weaning from mechanical ventilation by 90 days was significantly greater in the cisatracurium group (adjusted hazard ratio: 1.41; 95% CI, 1.08–1.83; $p = 0.01$). Cisatracurium-treated patients also experienced more organ failure-free days at 28 days (15.8 ± 9.9 days, vs. 12.2 ± 11.1 days; $p = 0.01$). ICU-free days at day 90 were also significantly higher in the cisatracurium group. Among the adverse events, pneumothorax occurred more often in the placebo group (11.7% vs. 4%). The incidence of ICU-acquired weakness did not differ between groups on day 28 and at ICU discharge. On day 7, the cisatracurium group experienced a higher PaO_2/FiO_2 ratio and a lower $PaCO_2$. Rescue interventions, including prone positioning,

Table 1.1 Main study outcomes

Outcome	Cisatracurium (177 patients)	Placebo (162 patients)	Significance
Crude 90-day mortality	31.6%	40.7%	$P = 0.08$
90-day mortality on adjusted analysis			0.68 (95% CI: 0.48–0.98; $P = 0.04$ (significantly lower with cisatracurium)
28-day mortality	23.7%	33.3%	$P = 0.05$
Ventilator-free days at 90 day	53.1 ± 35.8 days	44.6 ± 37.5 days	$P = 0.03$
Organ failure-free days at 28 day	15.8 ± 9.9 days	12.2 ± 11.1 days	$P = 0.01$
Patients free of ICU-acquired paresis at 28 day	70.8%	67.5%	$P = 0.64$

nitric oxide, or almitrine use either solely or in combination, were similar in both groups.

The ACURASYS trial showed that continuous neuromuscular blockade for 48 h in early ARDS resulted in improved survival, reduced the duration of mechanical ventilation, and ICU stay. The main results of the study are summarized in Table 1.1.

1.8 Strengths of the Study

At the time of its publication, the ACURASYS trial was the largest RCT that evaluated the efficacy of continuous neuromuscular blockade among patients with ARDS. The strong points of the study included its double-blinded and multicentric design, although clinicians may have been able to identify patients who received neuromuscular blockade. A protocolized ventilation strategy was followed, and analysis was by intention to treat. Patients were included from 20 ICUs that followed international standard of care, thus enhancing the external validity of the study. Although persisting neuromuscular weakness is considered to be a significant adverse effect with neuromuscular blockade, the ACURASYS trial did not identify this as a significant disadvantage.

1.9 Limitations

The sample size was calculated based on an expected 90-day mortality of 50% based on previous studies. However, the mortality in the placebo group was lower than expected (40.7%), thus rendering the study underpowered. According to the authors themselves, a sample size of 885 patients was required for 80% power and a two-sided alpha level of 0.05 (in contrast to the 339 patients included in the final analysis). The question remained whether neuromuscular blockade would be beneficial to patients with early, less severe, ARDS. This is especially relevant considering that on post-hoc analysis, improved survival was confined to the most severely hypoxic patients with a PaO_2/FiO_2 ratio of <120 mm Hg. According to the trial protocol published earlier, the primary outcome was "Reduction of the mortality rate of ARDS patients at d-90"; however, the study reported the primary outcome as the 90-day mortality based on adjusted analysis using the Cox regression model. A substantial number of patients were excluded (986/1325), which may limit the generalizability of the study. Whether the beneficial effects observed with cisatracurium would apply to other muscle relaxants also remained unanswered.

1.10 A Decade Later—The ROSE Trial

Although the results of the ACURASYS trial supported the use of early neuromuscular blockade in mechanically ventilated patients with severe ARDS, it did not result in a widespread change of practice, with many guidelines continuing to proffer a weak recommendation [7]. The ROSE trial followed nearly a decade later, conducted by The National Heart, Lung, and Blood Institute PETAL Clinical Trials Network, and was published in 2019 [8]. The study aimed to compare the safety and efficacy of neuromuscular blockade combined with deep sedation with usual care, using lighter levels of sedation among patients with moderate to severe ARDS. The study included patients with moderate to severe ARDS with a PaO_2/FiO_2 ratio of <150 mm Hg and a PEEP level of ≥8 cm H_2O, across 48 ICUs in the US. They randomized patients to receive a 48-h continuous infusion of cisatracurium with deep sedation or a usual care strategy with lighter levels of sedation. Light sedation was titrated based on pre-defined targets. Patients in both groups were treated with a low-tidal volume, high-PEEP strategy. Open label cisatracurium in 20 mg boluses was allowed in both groups based on pre-defined criteria.

The trial was stopped for futility after enrolment of 1006 patients. During the 48-h period after randomization, 97.4% of patients (488/501) in the cisatracurium group received the infusion, while 17% (86/505) of patients in the light sedation group received a neuromuscular blocking agent. Hospital mortality at 90 days, the primary endpoint, was similar in both groups (cisatracurium infusion vs. control, 42.5% vs. 42.8%, $p = 0.93$). The secondary endpoints, including hospital mortality at 28 days, ventilation-free days, and the number of days of ICU and hospital stay were not significantly different between the two groups. ICU-acquired weakness was marginally higher with cisatracurium infusion, although the difference was not statistically significant.

These results contrasted with the findings of the ACURASYS trial which had revealed improved survival at 90 days with atracurium infusion compared with placebo. However, there were differences between the two trials that may have led to the disparate findings. Unlike ACURASYS, the ROSE trial was unblinded, which may have led to bias and confounded the findings. The ACURASYS trial employed deep sedation in both groups, unlike the ROSE trial which used light sedation in the control group. The PEEP levels used were higher in the ROSE trial. In the ROSE trial, a large number of patients were excluded (3840/4848) during the initial screening; 655 among them were already on a cisatracurium infusion. The ROSE trial was stopped prematurely and hence, resulted in an underpowered trial. No pre-defined criteria were set for prone ventilation in both trials; however, far fewer patients were ventilated in the prone position in the ROSE trial (16% vs. 50%).

1.11 Summary

Neuromuscular blockade permeated into the ICU following its introduction and experience in anesthetic practice. By the 1980s, it was employed fairly routinely among critically ill patients on mechanical ventilation. However, there was growing concern regarding adverse effects from long-term use of muscle relaxants, including persisting neuromuscular weakness, deep vein thrombosis, and pressure ulcers. In patients with severe ARDS, the putative benefits of neuromuscular blockade were recognized from early studies, including improved patient-ventilator synchrony, optimization of PEEP, and improved gas exchange. A previous underpowered RCT had also revealed a trend towards improved survival with the short-term use of neuromuscular blockade in ARDS. Against this background, the ACURASYS trial investigators evaluated the impact of a 48-h infusion of cisatracurium in patients with severe ARDS with a PaO_2/FiO_2 ratio of <150 mm Hg. The authors noted a reduction in the 90-day mortality with the use of cisatracurium infusion for the first 48 h after randomization. The survival benefit was confined to patients with a PaO_2/FiO_2 ratio of <120 mm Hg, suggesting that patients with severe hypoxia are the most likely to benefit with neuromuscular blockade. Besides, cisatracurium use was associated with reduced organ failure, a higher likelihood of weaning, less time on mechanical ventilation and in the ICU. The incidence of neuromuscular weakness was no higher compared to the placebo group. Thus, the ACURASYS trial strongly suggested benefits with a 48-h duration of neuromuscular blockade in severe ARDS. Although the subsequent ROSE trial did not corroborate these findings, the ACURASYS trial triggered a change of practice in mechanically ventilated patients with severe ARDS.

References

1. Black J. Claude Bernard on the action of curare. BMJ. 1999;319(7210):622.
2. Ball C, Westhorpe R. Muscle relaxants—intocostrin. Anaesth Intensive Care. 2005;33(3):289.
3. Hansen-Flaschen J, Cowen J, Raps EC. Neuromuscular blockade in the intensive care unit. More than we bargained for. Am Rev Respir Dis. 1993;147(1):234–6.
4. Petty TL. Suspended life or extending death? Chest. 1998;114(2):360–1.

5. Gainnier M, Roch A, Forel JM, Thirion X, Arnal JM, Donati S, et al. Effect of neuromuscular blocking agents on gas exchange in patients presenting with acute respiratory distress syndrome. Crit Care Med. 2004;32(1):113–9.
6. Laurent P, Jean-Marie F, Arnaud G, Christine PR, Gilles P, Anderson L, et al. Neuromuscular blockers in early acute respiratory distress syndrome. N Engl J Med. 2010;363:1107.
7. Rhodes A, Evans LE, Alhazzani W, Levy MM, Antonelli M, Ferrer R, et al. Surviving sepsis campaign: international guidelines for management of sepsis and septic shock: 2016. Crit Care Med. 2017;45(3):486–552.
8. National Heart, Lung, and Blood Institute PETAL Clinical Trials Network, Moss M, Huang DT, Brower RG, Ferguson ND, Ginde AA, et al. Early neuromuscular blockade in the acute respiratory distress syndrome. N Engl J Med. 2019;380(21):1997–2008.

2 Ventilation with Lower Tidal Volumes in Acute Lung Injury and Acute Respiratory Distress Syndrome: The ARMA Trial

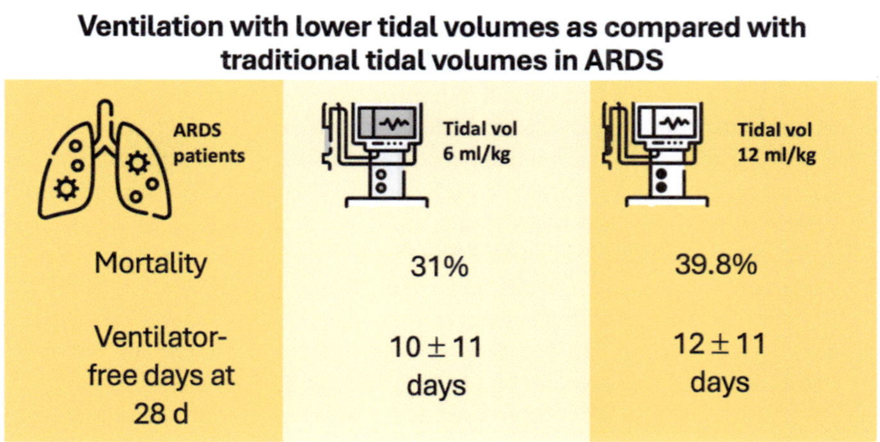

Acute Respiratory Distress Syndrome Network (NEJM, 2000)

Quick Take

Can smaller breaths save lives in ARDS?

The ARDSNet trial compared two different tidal volumes in patients with acute respiratory distress syndrome (ARDS): 6 ml/kg of predicted body weight vs. 12 ml/kg. This large, multicenter, randomized trial involved 861 patients and found that using a lower tidal volume (6 ml/kg) significantly reduced 28-day mortality

The Acute Respiratory Distress Syndrome Network. Ventilation with lower tidal volumes as compared with traditional tidal volumes for acute lung injury and the acute respiratory distress syndrome. N Engl J Med. 2000 May 4;342(18):1301–8.

J. Chacko et al., *Landmark Studies in Critical Care*,
https://doi.org/10.1007/978-981-95-0673-6_2

compared to the standard higher tidal volume (12 ml/kg). The study demonstrated that lower tidal volume ventilation was not only safer but also led to more favorable clinical outcomes, including improved survival and more ventilator-free days with a low tidal volume, lung-protective ventilation strategy. This landmark trial established low tidal volume ventilation as the standard of care for patients with ARDS.

2.1 Introduction

In the early days of mechanical ventilation, the primary aim was to normalize arterial blood gases. Little was known about the potential deleterious effects of positive pressure ventilation on the lung that could add insult to injury. Back in the 1990s, a tidal volume of 10–15 ml/kg was often employed to ensure adequate gas exchange [1]. Respiratory acidosis was considered detrimental; higher tidal volumes were often employed to target arterial pH levels. Animal studies had shown that high tidal volume ventilation was associated with the release of inflammatory mediators, culminating in damage to the alveolar epithelium and the capillary endothelium, leading to atelectasis and worsening hypoxemia [2]. Furthermore, the release of inflammatory mediators from the lung could result in multiorgan dysfunction [2]. While the use of lower tidal volumes appeared to offer putative benefits through lung protection and amelioration of the inflammatory response, this strategy carried the potential for harm from hypercapnia and acidemia. The evidence from early studies on animal models and clinical trials that followed was conflicting.

Nearly half a century ago, Webb and Tierney demonstrated in a rat model that ventilation with high positive pressures of 45 cm H_2O and zero PEEP led to rapid development of alveolar and perivascular edema, severe hypoxia, and decreased lung compliance. The application of a PEEP of 10 cm H_2O protected against high-inspiratory pressure-related lung injury [3]. In an observational study, Hickling et al., using a lung-protective strategy of low tidal volumes between 4 and 7 ml/kg and limiting the peak inspiratory pressure to 30–40 cm of H_2O, demonstrated lower mortality than predicted by the APACHE II score [4].

Amato et al. randomly assigned patients with early acute respiratory distress syndrome (ARDS) to a conventional or lung-protective ventilation strategy [5]. The conventional strategy included using tidal volumes of 12 ml/kg and the lowest level of PEEP to maintain oxygenation and normal carbon dioxide levels. The lung-protective strategy involved the application of PEEP above the lower inflection point on the static pressure-volume curve, tidal volumes of <6 ml/kg and driving pressures of <20 cm H_2O, allowing permissive hypercapnia. The lung-protective strategy was associated with improved 28-day survival, more rapid weaning from mechanical ventilation, and less barotrauma. However, contrasting findings emerged from other randomized controlled trials (RCTs).

Brochard et al. compared a tidal volume of 10 ml/kg, limiting plateau pressure to 25 cm H_2O, compared with tidal volumes of >10 ml/kg, aiming for normal PCO_2. A low tidal volume, limited Pplat strategy did not lead to improved survival, duration of mechanical ventilation, barotrauma, or multiorgan failure [6]. These findings were echoed by another RCT that compared tidal volumes of <8 ml/kg compared with 10–15 ml/kg in patients at high risk of ARDS [7]. Yet another study compared a lung-protective (tidal volume of 5–8 ml/kg ideal body weight, plateau pressure of <30 cm H_2O) vs. conventional strategy (tidal volume of 10–12 ml/kg ideal body weight, plateau pressure of <55 cm H_2O). Although a lung-protective strategy was found to be safe, there was no significant difference in important clinical outcomes, including the duration of ventilation or mortality [8].

The use of low tidal volumes offered potential clinical benefit by reducing injurious lung stretch. Considering the lack of robust evidence from available studies, the Acute Respiratory Distress Syndrome Network (ARDSNet) group of the National Heart, Lung, and Blood Institute in the US conceived an RCT that compared lower with traditional, high tidal volumes among patients with ARDS [9].

2.2 Population and Design

The ARDSNet trial was conducted between March 1996 and March 1999 and enrolled patients from 10 university centers of the network. The study enrolled adult patients with ARDS who underwent invasive mechanical ventilation, with a PaO_2/FiO_2 ratio of ≤300 mm Hg, bilateral infiltrates on the chest radiograph with no clinical evidence of left atrial hypertension, and a pulmonary artery wedge pressure, if measured, of ≤18 mm Hg. Enrolment in the study was based on the American-European Consensus Conference definitions of ARDS [10].

2.2.1 Exclusion

Patients were excluded if more than 36 h had elapsed after meeting the ARDS criteria. Patients with intracranial hypertension, neuromuscular disease, severe chronic respiratory disease, burns of >30% of body-surface area, and a body weight of >1 kg/cm of height were also excluded. Other exclusion criteria were the presence of chronic liver disease and those who had undergone bone marrow or lung transplantation.

2.3 Ventilation Strategy in Both Groups

Patients were ventilated in the volume-assist-control mode until weaning or for 28 days post-randomization. The predicted body weight was calculated as follows.

Male patients: 50 + 2.3 [height in inches – 60]
Female patients: 45.5 + 2.3 [height in inches – 60]

2.3.1 Traditional Tidal Volume Group

The initial tidal volume was set at 12 ml/kg of predicted body weight. The tidal volume was reduced by 1 ml/kg in a stepwise manner to maintain the plateau pressure (Pplat) ≤50 cm H_2O, down to a minimum tidal volume was 4 ml/kg. If the Pplat was <45 cm H_2O, the tidal volume was increased by 1 ml/kg at a time for a minimum Pplat of 45 cm H_2O. The maximum tidal volume used was 12 ml/kg. Thus, the Pplat was maintained between 45 and 50 cm H_2O, for a maximum tidal volume of 12 ml/kg.

2.3.2 Low Tidal Volume Group

The initial tidal volume was set at 6 ml/kg of predicted body weight. If the Pplat exceeded 30 cm H_2O, the tidal volume was reduced by 1 ml/kg at a time to maintain the Pplat below this level. If the Pplat was <25 cm H_2O, the tidal volume was increased in steps of 1 ml/kg until the Pplat rose to this level. The tidal volume could be increased to 7–8 ml/kg if considered appropriate, provided the Pplat remained ≤30 cm H_2O. The Pplat in this group was maintained between 25 and 30 cm H_2O.

2.3.3 Both Groups

The tidal volume was not allowed to drop below 4 ml/kg in either group. The Pplat limit of 30 cm H_2O in the low tidal volume group and 50 cm H_2O in the conventional tidal volume group could be exceeded to achieve a minimum tidal volume of 4 ml/kg, and an arterial pH of not less than 7.15. Other ventilation procedures, including the weaning protocol, were similar in both groups. If a patient required reinstitution of mechanical ventilation after being weaned off within the 28-day period, the same tidal volume protocol was followed.

2.4 Sample Size Calculation

Four interim analyses were planned after the recruitment of 200, 400, 600, and 800 patients. The trial was designed to detect a 10% difference in mortality in the low tidal volume group (from 50% to 40%) with 87% power at a two-sided significance level.

2.5 Results

The trial was stopped after the fourth planned interim analysis following the enrollment of 861 patients. At this stage, the low tidal volume strategy was found to be more efficacious compared with the use of traditional tidal volumes. Baseline characteristics were similar in both groups, except for higher minute ventilation in the low tidal volume group.

The tidal volume and Pplat were significantly lower on days 1, 3, and 7 in the low tidal volume group. Overall, there was a clear difference in the tidal volume between the two groups. The mean tidal volume on days 1–3 was 6.2 ± 0.8 ml/kg in the low tidal volume group compared with 11.8 ± 0.8 ml/kg in the traditional tidal volume group. The mean Pplat levels were also significantly lower in the low tidal volume group (25 ± 6 vs. 33 ± 8 cm H_2O). In the low tidal volume group, the $PaCO_2$ levels were significantly higher on days 1, 3, and 7; the arterial pH was significantly lower on days 1 and 3. The PaO_2/FiO_2 ratio was lower in the low tidal volume group on days 1 and 3.

2.6 Primary Outcomes

The first primary outcome, death before hospital discharge and before being able to breathe without assistance, was significantly lower in the low tidal volume group (31.0% vs. 39.8%, $p = 0.007$). The second primary outcome, the ability to breathe without assistance by day 28, was significantly higher in the low tidal volume group (65.7% vs. 55.0%, $p < 0.001$).

2.7 Other Outcomes

Among other outcomes, the number of ventilator-free days at 28 days was higher in the low tidal volume group (mean of 12 vs. 10 days). The number of days without non-pulmonary organ failure was also higher in the low tidal volume group. Specifically, the incidence of circulatory failure, renal failure, and coagulation failure was lower in the low tidal volume group. The incidence of barotrauma was similar in both groups. There was no significant difference in the use of neuromuscular blockers and sedatives between the two groups. On day 3, the decrease in the plasma interleukin-6 levels was greater in the low tidal volume group, suggesting a reduced inflammatory response. Table 2.1 represents the main trial outcomes.

Table 2.1 Main trial outcomes

Outcome	Low tidal volume	Traditional tidal volume	*p*-value
Death before discharge and before being able to breathe without assistance	31%	39.8%	0.007
Ability to breathe without assistance at day 28	65.7%	55%	<0.001
Ventilator-free days from day 1 to day 28	12 ± 11 days	10 ± 11 days	0.007
Barotrauma from day 1 to day 28	10%	11%	0.43
Non-pulmonary organ failure-free days from day 1 to day 28	15 ± 11 days	12 ± 11 days	0.006

2.8 Study Conclusions

The authors concluded that in patients with ARDS, mechanical ventilation with lower compared to traditionally used tidal volumes reduced mortality and the duration of mechanical ventilation. They suggested that prevention of lung stretch by reducing tidal volumes is a key strategy during mechanical ventilation in patients with ARDS.

2.9 Strengths

The results of the ARDSNet trial provided important insights into improving outcomes in patients with ARDS on mechanical ventilation. The trial design and methodology were robust and appropriate to address the comparison between low and higher tidal volumes and their impact on clinical outcomes. The trial was conducted across multiple centers in the USA, providing external validity. The large sample size provided adequate power to identify a difference between groups in the primary outcome. Interim analyses were performed meticulously, and the trial was ceased when the results favored the low tidal volume group. The investigators evaluated clinically relevant, objective outcomes, including mortality and the duration of ventilation.

2.10 Weaknesses

In the traditional tidal volume group, patients may have been exposed to relatively high tidal volumes compared to usual practice during the study period. The Pplat levels were also correspondingly higher compared to conventional practice. The mean tidal volume employed at baseline was approximately 10 ml/kg; this essentially meant that the tidal volume was increased in most patients in the traditional group to comply with the study protocol.

The authors did not provide information on the immediate cause of death; it is plausible that the impact on mortality may have been due to extra-pulmonary organ failure, and not primarily due to a lung-protective effect from the use of low tidal volumes.

Was a low tidal volume strategy associated with a more favorable hemodynamic status, and hence, improved outcomes? No information was available on the cardiovascular status or the use of vasopressors.

The study allowed the non-standardized use of intravenous sodium bicarbonate to combat hypercapnic acidosis. The authors contend that the buffering effect may have contributed to improved outcomes among hypercapnic patients in the low tidal volume group. This assertion is in contrast to available evidence suggesting that hypercapnia may not be harmful, and indeed, may have beneficial effects [11].

In the traditional tidal volume group, the Pplat was maintained between 45 and 50 cm H_2O; this was considerably higher than the recommendations in vogue during the study period [12]. Besides, in earlier studies that compared low vs. high tidal volumes that did not show a difference in outcomes, the mean Pplat levels in the higher tidal volume groups were much lower, at 29 ± 7 [7] and 31 ± 9 cm H_2O [6].

Although more than 6000 patients were screened, 2587 were considered ineligible due to technical reasons, although they had met the enrollment criteria. These patients received usual care; however, the mortality in this cohort was similar to the mortality of the low tidal volume group (31.7% vs. 31%). This finding suggests that conventional care was compared with higher than usual tidal volumes in the trial, and could perhaps have contributed to increased mortality [13].

Would tidal volume-related outcomes depend on lung compliance? Among patients with low lung compliance, higher tidal volumes appear to have increased mortality; in contrast, in patients with higher lung compliance, a higher tidal volume was associated with lower mortality [13]. This observation is particularly relevant considering the wide variability of lung involvement and compliance in ARDS. Anatomic studies have also revealed a poor correlation between the ideal body weight and the extent of lung involvement in ARDS [14].

2.11 Subsequent Evidence: Driving Pressure vs. Tidal Volumes

Is driving pressure (ΔP, Pplat – PEEP) an important determinant of survival in patients with ARDS who are mechanically ventilated? Amato et al. performed a multi-level mediation analysis of data from 3562 patients with ARDS from nine RCTs to answer this question [15]. They observed that ΔP was the most robust predictor of survival, even among patients who were being ventilated using a lung-protective strategy with low tidal volumes and Pplat. The tidal volume or PEEP levels were not independently associated with survival; low tidal volumes were associated with improved survival only if it resulted in a reduction in the ΔP.

2.12 Summary

The ARDSNet trial addressed an important, albeit contentious clinical question of the time by evaluating a lung-protective ventilation strategy that had been studied in previous clinical trials with no definitive answers. The trial focused on testing a lung protective ventilation strategy, which involved using lower tidal volumes and lower airway pressures. The investigators compared a low tidal volume of 6 ml/kg of predicted body weight compared to a more traditional tidal volume of 12 ml/kg. They observed improved survival and more ventilator-free days with the low tidal volume, lung-protective ventilation strategy. Although there were criticisms related to the use of a fixed tidal volume and a "one-size fits all" strategy, the findings appeared robust and applicable to a heterogeneous patient population with ARDS. This approach has since become the standard of care in managing patients with ARDS, as it has been shown to reduce ventilator-induced lung injury. The findings of this pivotal trial had a profound influence on the management of ARDS. It was widely accepted by the critical care fraternity, leading to perceptible changes in clinical practice, with the use of low tidal volumes as part of a lung-protective ventilation strategy.

References

1. Marini JJ. Evolving concepts in the ventilatory management of acute respiratory distress syndrome. Clin Chest Med. 1996;17(3):555–75.
2. Dreyfuss D, Basset G, Soler P, Saumon G. Intermittent positive-pressure hyperventilation with high inflation pressures produces pulmonary microvascular injury in rats. Am Rev Respir Dis. 1985;132(4):880–4.
3. Webb HH, Tierney DF. Experimental pulmonary edema due to intermittent positive pressure ventilation with high inflation pressures. Protection by positive end-expiratory pressure. Am Rev Respir Dis. 1974;110(5):556–65.
4. Hickling KG, Walsh J, Henderson S, Jackson R. Low mortality rate in adult respiratory distress syndrome using low-volume, pressure-limited ventilation with permissive hypercapnia: a prospective study. Crit Care Med. 1994;22(10):1568–78.
5. Amato MB, Barbas CS, Medeiros DM, Magaldi RB, Schettino GP, Lorenzi-Filho G, et al. Effect of a protective-ventilation strategy on mortality in the acute respiratory distress syndrome. N Engl J Med. 1998;338(6):347–54.
6. Brochard L, Roudot-Thoraval F, Roupie E, Delclaux C, Chastre J, Fernandez-Mondéjar E, et al. Tidal volume reduction for prevention of ventilator-induced lung injury in acute respiratory distress syndrome. The Multicenter Trail Group on Tidal Volume reduction in ARDS. Am J Respir Crit Care Med. 1998;158(6):1831–8.
7. Stewart TE, Meade MO, Cook DJ, Granton JT, Hodder RV, Lapinsky SE, et al. Evaluation of a ventilation strategy to prevent barotrauma in patients at high risk for acute respiratory distress syndrome. Pressure- and Volume-Limited Ventilation Strategy Group. N Engl J Med. 1998;338(6):355–61.
8. Brower RG, Shanholtz CB, Fessler HE, Shade DM, White P, Wiener CM, et al. Prospective, randomized, controlled clinical trial comparing traditional versus reduced tidal volume ventilation in acute respiratory distress syndrome patients. Crit Care Med. 1999;27(8):1492–8.
9. Acute Respiratory Distress Syndrome Network, Brower RG, Matthay MA, Morris A, Schoenfeld D, Thompson BT, et al. Ventilation with lower tidal volumes as compared with traditional tidal volumes for acute lung injury and the acute respiratory distress syndrome. N Engl J Med. 2000;342(18):1301–8.
10. Bernard GR, Artigas A, Brigham KL, Carlet J, Falke K, Hudson L, et al. The American-European Consensus Conference on ARDS. Definitions, mechanisms, relevant outcomes, and clinical trial coordination. Am J Respir Crit Care Med. 1994;149(3 Pt 1):818–24.
11. Laffey JG, O'Croinin D, McLoughlin P, Kavanagh BP. Permissive hypercapnia–role in protective lung ventilatory strategies. Intensive Care Med. 2004;30(3):347–56.

12. Mercat A, Graïni L, Teboul JL, Lenique F, Richard C. Cardiorespiratory effects of pressure-controlled ventilation with and without inverse ratio in the adult respiratory distress syndrome. Chest. 1993;104(3):871–5.
13. Deans KJ, Minneci PC, Cui X, Banks SM, Natanson C, Eichacker PQ. Mechanical ventilation in ARDS: one size does not fit all*. Crit Care Med. 2005;33(5):1141–3.
14. Chiumello D, Carlesso E, Cadringher P, Caironi P, Valenza F, Polli F, et al. Lung stress and strain during mechanical ventilation for acute respiratory distress syndrome. Am J Respir Crit Care Med. 2008;178(4):346–55.
15. Amato MBP, Meade MO, Slutsky AS, Brochard L, Costa ELV, Schoenfeld DA, et al. Driving pressure and survival in the acute respiratory distress syndrome. N Engl J Med. 2015;372(8):747–55.

Prone Ventilation in Acute Respiratory Distress Syndrome: The PROSEVA Trial

3

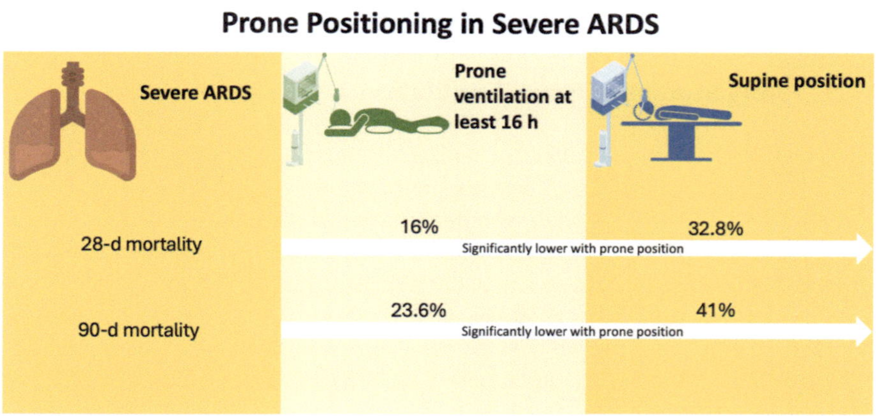

Guérin et al. (NEJM, 2013)

Quick Take

Can prone positioning improve outcomes in patients with severe ARDS?

The PROSEVA trial evaluated the efficacy of prone positioning in patients with severe acute respiratory distress syndrome (ARDS) who were receiving mechanical ventilation. This multicenter randomized controlled trial enrolled patients with PaO_2/FiO_2 ratios of 150 or less and compared the outcomes of patients placed in the prone position for at least 12 h per day with those maintained in the supine position. The study found that prone positioning significantly reduced 28-day mortality, with

---

Guérin C, Reignier J, Richard JC, Beuret P, Gacouin A, Boulain T, et al. Prone positioning in severe acute respiratory distress syndrome. N Engl J Med. 2013 Jun 6;368(23):2159–68.

J. Chacko et al., *Landmark Studies in Critical Care*,
https://doi.org/10.1007/978-981-95-0673-6_3

patients in the prone group experiencing improved oxygenation and lower incidence of ventilator-associated complications. These results support prone positioning as an effective and life-saving strategy for managing severe ARDS, providing a strong evidence base for its routine use in critical care settings.

3.1 Introduction

More than half a century ago, it was well-known that ventilation of the dependent lung might be impaired in mechanically ventilated patients. Children with cystic fibrosis could expectorate thick, tenacious secretions characteristic of the disease by positioning themselves on their hands and knees. Quite often, such positioning also enabled them to breathe easier [1]. Based on this observation, the prone position was proposed as a measure to recruit the dependent lung regions that are predominantly affected in acute respiratory distress syndrome (ARDS) [2].

3.1.1 Early Studies of Prone Ventilation

In the early 1970s, Margaret Piehl, a registered nurse, and Robert Brown, an ICU medical officer, noted improved oxygenation with prone ventilation among ARDS patients while working in a small community hospital in Midland, Michigan. They published their seminal paper on mechanical ventilation in the prone position titled "Use of extreme position changes in acute respiratory failure" in the *Critical Care Medicine* journal of January 1976 [3]. Their case series included five patients—three with polytrauma, and two postoperative cases, one following femoropopliteal bypass surgery and the other, after repair of an abdominal aortic aneurysm. All five patients developed severe acute respiratory distress syndrome (ARDS) and remained profoundly hypoxic despite optimization of ventilation, including increasing levels of PEEP. They used a novel rotating bed to turn their patients to the prone position. Assuming the prone position resulted in a remarkable improvement of PaO_2 levels by a mean of 47 mm Hg, while all ventilatory parameters were held constant. The prone position also enabled postural drainage and suctioning out of copious secretions. The authors hypothesized that improved ventilation-perfusion matching and enhanced clearance of secretions in the prone position could explain the striking effect on oxygenation.

In 1988, Langer et al. evaluated gas exchange and hemodynamic status on assuming the prone position in 13 patients with moderate to severe ARDS. Patients who showed improvement in the PaO_2 by at least 10 mm Hg were considered responders. Eight patients were considered responders and two, non-responders by this definition. In this pioneering study, the authors used CT scans of the chest to assess the impact of prone ventilation in two patients; as previously hypothesized, the posterobasal areas of the lungs revealed improved aeration with adoption of the prone position in these patients. The authors suggested a brief trial of prone ventilation in patients with severe ARDS to assess response [4].

3.1.2 The Gattinoni et al. Trial—The Turning Point

By the turn of the century, the salutary effect of prone ventilation on oxygenation in ARDS was fairly established, with 60–70% showing improved PaO_2 levels. However, the impact of prone position on clinical outcomes, including survival, was unknown. Gattinoni et al. sought to answer this question in a multicenter RCT conducted across 28 ICUs in Italy and two in Switzerland between 1996 and 1999 [5]. The study included mechanically ventilated patients with ARDS, with a PaO_2/FiO_2 ratio of <200 while on at least 5 cm H_2O PEEP, or a PaO_2/FiO_2 ratio of <300 with a PEEP of at least 10 cm H_2O. Patients were prone ventilated daily for 6 hours or more for a maximum duration of 10 days and compared with a control group who received conventional management in the supine position. There was no difference in mortality between the prone and supine groups during the ICU stay, at the end of the 10-day study period, or at 6 months.

Improved oxygenation was noted on assuming the prone position; the mean rise in the PaO_2/FiO_2 ratio during the study period in the prone group was 63.0 ± 66.8 compared with 44.6 ± 68.2 in the supine group ($P = 0.02$). The improvement in oxygenation was noted in more than 70% of patients on assuming the prone position; the effect was most pronounced in the first hour after turning prone. The incidence of non-pulmonary organ failure was similar between the two groups. Notably, on post-hoc analysis, the authors observed a significantly lower mortality with prone ventilation among patients with the lowest PaO_2/FiO_2 ratio, and the highest quartile of Simplified Acute Physiology Score (SAPS) scores.

The incidence of complications related to accidental removal of endotracheal tubes, lines, and intercostal drains was similar in both groups. Pressure-related injury related to the prone position was observed; however, the number of patients with new or worsening pressure sores was similar in both groups.

The Gattinoni et al. trial was the first large RCT that compared clinical outcomes with prone positioning in patients with ARDS. However, the study was limited by the relatively short duration of prone ventilation. Besides, the study included patients with mild ARDS, with a PaO_2/FiO_2 ratio of >300 mm Hg. The question remained whether prone positioning would improve survival in patients with more severe disease at baseline. A meta-analysis of four RCTs published later found mortality benefit in the most severely hypoxic patients at baseline, with a PaO_2/FiO_2 ratio of <100 mm Hg [6]. Based on this evidence, the stage was set for Guérin et al. to explore the impact of prone ventilation on clinical outcomes in patients with severe ARDS in a large RCT.

3.2 The PROSEVA Trial

The PROSEVA trial was conducted across 26 ICUs in France and one in Spain over a three-and-a-half-year period from 2008 to 2011 [7]. The study centers had more than 5 years of experience with prone ventilation. The study included patients with ARDS who were on mechanical ventilation for less than 36 h on FiO_2 more than

0.6, a PEEP level of at least 5 cm of water, and a PaO_2/FiO_2 ratio of less than 150 mm Hg. Mechanical ventilation was continued for a 12–24-h period, followed by confirmation of the inclusion criteria prior to randomization.

3.2.1 Study Groups

Prone ventilation was commenced within an hour of randomization and continued for at least 16 consecutive hours. In the supine group, a semi-recumbent position was maintained. In both groups of patients, volume-controlled mode of ventilation was employed, with a tidal volume of 6 ml/kg of predicted body weight. PEEP was applied according to a standard PEEP-FiO_2 table. A Pplat of 30 cm H_2O was targeted with the maintenance of pH between 7.20–7.45. A repeat session of prone ventilation could be carried out at any time while waiting for a 4-h assessment. Prone ventilation could be carried out daily for up to 28 days, based on clinician discretion. Crossover from the supine group was allowed only in the presence of life-threatening hypoxemia, based on predefined criteria. Sedative agents and neuromuscular blocking agents were administered to both groups of patients as appropriate. Weaning from mechanical ventilation was based on a standard protocol.

3.2.2 Sample Size

The sample size was calculated based on a 60% mortality at 28 days in the supine group. The authors assumed an absolute reduction in mortality of 15% with prone ventilation (60% mortality in the supine group and 45% mortality in the prone group). A sample size of 456 patients was required based on this assumption, providing 90% power and a type I error rate of 5%.

3.2.3 Baseline Characteristics

The underlying etiology was pneumonia in the majority of patients in both groups. The tidal volume, PEEP, and Pplat levels were similar at baseline. The mean PaO_2/FiO_2 ratio at the time of inclusion was 100 mm Hg in both groups. The $PaCO_2$ levels were also similar. The Sequential Organ Failure Assessment score (SOFA) score and vasopressor use were higher in the supine group, while the use of neuromuscular blocking agents was higher in the prone group.

3.2.3.1 Findings

Analysis was performed based on intention to treat, with 229 patients in the supine and 237 patients in the prone group.

Patients were placed in the prone position within a mean duration of 55 min after randomization. The prone position was maintained for 17 ± 3 h at a time. The $PaO_2/$

FiO_2 ratio rose with prone ventilation and was significantly higher compared to the supine group on days 3 and 5, while the PEEP was lower. The $PaCO_2$ levels were similar between the two groups.

3.2.4 The Primary Outcome

Mortality at 28 days, the primary outcome, was significantly lower in the prone group (16% vs. 32.8%, $p < 0.001$). The mortality difference was similar after adjusted analysis based on the SOFA score, use of vasopressors and neuromuscular blockers, which differed between the groups at baseline.

3.2.5 Secondary Outcomes

Mortality at 90 days was significantly lower in the prone group (23.6% vs. 41%, $p < 0.001$). Extubation by 90 days was higher, and the ICU length of stay was shorter among patients who were prone ventilated. Similarly, ventilation-free days were significantly higher at 28 and 90 days in the prone group. The main study outcomes are summarized in Table 3.1.

3.2.5.1 Complications

The incidence of cardiac arrests was higher in the supine group (31 vs. 16). Other adverse events, including accidental extubation, endobronchial intubation, and blocked endotracheal tube were similar between the two groups.

The PROSEVA trial marked a turning point in the history of ARDS, providing robust evidence for improved survival among patients with severe ARDS who were prone ventilated. The participating centers had long-standing experience with prone ventilation. An initial 12–24-h period of stabilization was followed, which enabled the selection of patients who were more likely to deteriorate and experience worse outcomes. Unlike previous trials, the prone position was maintained for a longer duration of 16 h per day. The duration of prone ventilation at the peak of illness was 73% compared with approximately 30% in previous trials. A lung-protective

Table 3.1 Main study outcomes

Outcomes	Prone ventilation	Supine ventilation	Significance
28-day mortality	16%	32.8%	$P < 0.001$
90-day mortality	23.6%	41%	$P < 0.001$
Successful extubation, 90 days	80.5%	65%	
Mean ICU LOS among survivors	24 ± 22 days	26 ± 27 days	$P = 0.05$
Mean ventilation-free days at 28 days	14 ± 9 days	10 ± 10 days	$P < 0.001$
Mean ventilation-free days at 90 days	57 ± 34 days	43 ± 38 days	$P < 0.001$

Abbreviation: *LOS*, length of stay

ventilation strategy was strictly adhered to; besides, prone ventilation was initiated expeditiously soon after randomization. The study chose the most severely hypoxic patients, with a PaO_2/FiO_2 ratio of >150 mm Hg, who were more likely to benefit, in contrast to the Gattinoni et al. trial of 2001 that included patients with PaO_2/FiO_2 ratio of <300 mm Hg.

3.2.5.2 Limitations

There were imbalances between the prone and supine groups at baseline. The SOFA score was lower among patients who underwent prone ventilation; besides, more patients received vasopressors in the supine group. This difference between groups may suggest a higher severity of illness in patients who were maintained supine. However, the improved survival with prone ventilation persisted after adjustment for baseline differences between the two groups. Only one-third of patients who were screened underwent randomization. Besides, a 12–24-h period of stabilization allowed the exclusion of patients who showed early improvement, allowing the inclusion of a highly selective patient population. Despite these limitations, the PROSEVA trial provided robust evidence with prone ventilation among the sickest of patients with ARDS.

3.3 Summary

ARDS had witnessed a track record of failed therapies, notably nitric oxide, prostacyclin, and high-frequency oscillation. The PROSEVA trial offered a fresh ray of hope for the most severely hypoxic patients with ARDS. Although previous studies had consistently revealed improved oxygenation, none had shown improved clinical outcomes. Maintenance of the prone position for more than 16 h at a time and inclusion of the most severely hypoxic patients at baseline were clearly important factors that led to improved outcomes in the PROSEVA trial. Besides, study centers had sufficient experience and expertise with prone ventilation, probably reducing the incidence of complications related to positioning. The PROSEVA trial remains a pioneering study that demonstrated improved survival and more ventilator-free days with prone ventilation besides improved oxygenation.

References

1. Mellins RB. Pulmonary physiotherapy in the pediatric age group. Am Rev Respir Dis. 1974;110(6 Pt 2):137–42.
2. Bryan AC. Conference on the scientific basis of respiratory therapy. Pulmonary physiotherapy in the pediatric age group. Comments of a devil's advocate. Am Rev Respir Dis. 1974;110(6 Pt 2):143–4.
3. Piehl MA, Brown RS. Use of extreme position changes in acute respiratory failure. Crit Care Med. 1976;4(1):13–4.

4. Langer M, Mascheroni D, Marcolin R, Gattinoni L. The prone position in ARDS patients. A clinical study. Chest. 1988;94(1):103–7.
5. Gattinoni L, Tognoni G, Pesenti A, Taccone P, Mascheroni D, Labarta V, et al. Effect of prone positioning on the survival of patients with acute respiratory failure. N Engl J Med. 2001;345(8):568–73.
6. Sud S, Friedrich JO, Taccone P, Polli F, Adhikari NKJ, Latini R, et al. Prone ventilation reduces mortality in patients with acute respiratory failure and severe hypoxemia: systematic review and meta-analysis. Intensive Care Med. 2010;36(4):585–99.
7. Guérin C, Reignier J, Richard JC, Beuret P, Gacouin A, Boulain T, et al. Prone positioning in severe acute respiratory distress syndrome. N Engl J Med. 2013;368(23):2159–68.

4 Early vs. Late Tracheostomy in Mechanically Ventilated Patients: The TRACMAN Trial

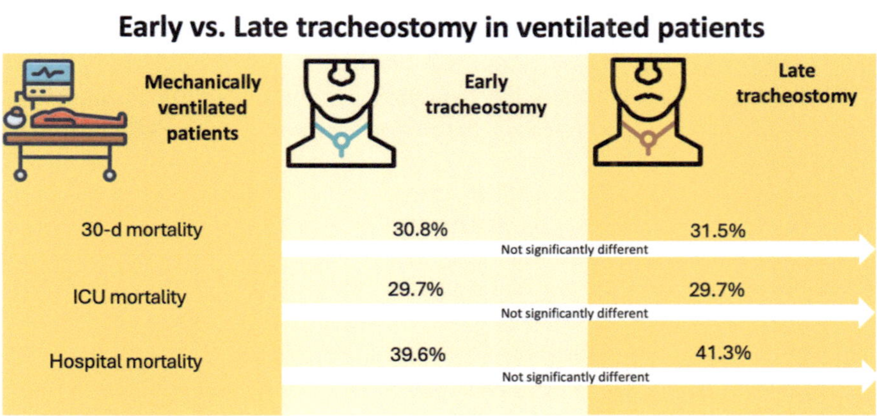

Young et al. (JAMA, 2013)

Quick Take

The TracMan trial compared early versus late tracheostomy placement in critically ill patients requiring prolonged mechanical ventilation. This multicenter randomized controlled trial (RCT) enrolled over 900 patients and assessed the impact of tracheostomy timing on survival and outcomes. The study found no significant difference in mortality between the early and late tracheostomy groups. The duration

---

Young D, Harrison DA, Cuthbertson BH, Rowan K, TracMan Collaborators. Effect of early vs late tracheostomy placement on survival in patients receiving mechanical ventilation: the TracMan randomized trial. JAMA. 2013 May 22;309(20):2121–9.

J. Chacko et al., *Landmark Studies in Critical Care*,
https://doi.org/10.1007/978-981-95-0673-6_4

of ICU stay and hospital stay were also similar. The TracMan trial provided robust evidence that tracheostomy within 4 days of ICU does not lead to improvement in key clinical outcomes.

4.1 Historical Background

Tracheostomy appears to have been in practice as a life-saving intervention to relieve upper airway obstruction for more than 2000 years. Descriptions of a throat incision, suggestive of tracheostomy, are found in the sacred Hindu text, the *Rig Veda,* that dates back to 1500 BCE [1]. Alexander the Great, the King of Macedonia who lived between 356 and 323 BCE, is believed to have used his sword to cut open the throat of one of his soldiers as he lay choking on a piece of meat, on the verge of death. Emergency tracheostomy was often resorted to during the diphtheria epidemics of the eighteenth and nineteenth centuries.

Chevalier Jackson introduced the present-day concept of tracheostomy in the early twentieth century. He proposed that "there are several classes of cases in which intubation does not meet the indication and there are frequent individual cases where, for some special reason, the cutting operation is easier, safer and more efficient" [2].

In 1943, Galloway first reported the performance of a tracheostomy for suctioning secretions from the airway in patients with bulbar poliomyelitis. In his paper published in the Journal of the American Medical Association [3], he reported that "The results with 3 patients seen in the past two months have convinced me that the operation may be a very important procedure in this disease. Two were undoubtedly saved by it, and the third might have been had intervention been done ten minutes earlier." The Scandinavian polio epidemic ushered in the era of ventilatory support through a tracheostomy, with Bjørn Ibsen pioneering the use of positive pressure ventilation, marking a paradigm shift from the technique of negative pressure ventilation that had largely been ineffective [4].

In 1984, Pasquale Ciaglia watched in awe as a urologist, ably assisted by his radiologist, removed a renal calculus with consummate ease using the Seldinger technique and a set of serial dilators [5]. Inspired by this technique, he performed cadaver dissections and designed a tracheostomy tube that could be introduced over a snugly fitting dilator and a "J"-shaped guidewire. His original technique involved a vertical incision from the lower border of the cricoid cartilage. The introducer needle and guidewire were inserted, by palpation, between the cricoid cartilage and the first tracheal ring, or between the first and second tracheal rings. This was followed by serial dilatation and insertion of a flanged tracheostomy tube.

Ciaglia et al. published their seminal paper in 1985. Their preliminary report included 26 procedures, including two patients who underwent repeat tracheostomy [6]. They proposed that the percutaneous procedure could be performed through the cricothyroid membrane, between the cricoid and the first tracheal cartilages, or between the first and second tracheal cartilages. The authors did not encounter any serious complications during the procedure. There was occasional difficulty in passing the tracheostomy tube, but this could be overcome by using larger dilators. With increasing experience, and realizing the simplicity of the technique, they began performing the procedure at the bedside in the ICU. Over the next decade, the bedside percutaneous technique was increasingly adopted as the preferred technique in ICU patients by many intensive care physicians.

Over the years, the percutaneous technique became increasingly popular among clinicians with the performance of a tracheostomy earlier in the course of illness [7]. An early tracheostomy was considered to improve patient comfort compared to an endotracheal tube and, thereby, had the potential to reduce the use of sedation. Besides, other perceived benefits included earlier weaning and a reduced incidence of ventilator-associated pneumonia (VAP) [8].

4.2 Background to the TracMan Trial

The availability of ICU beds in the UK is much lower compared to other high-income countries. In many centers, the prevailing trend favored early tracheostomy, with the presumed benefit of reducing the duration of mechanical ventilation and ICU stay. Surveys of UK practice reflected the practice of early tracheostomy; 50% of tracheostomies were carried out within a week of ICU admission while 21% were performed as early as within 5 days of admission [9, 10].

In 2004, an RCT of 120 patients from the US suggested that early tracheostomy with 48 h of intubation compared with later tracheostomy between 14 and 16 days of intubation resulted in a significantly reduced duration of mechanical ventilation and lower mortality [11]. A meta-analysis of 406 patients from five studies followed; early tracheostomy was found to reduce the duration of mechanical ventilation, although the mortality was similar [12]. The TracMan (Tracheostomy Management) trial was conceived in light of these findings, considering the potential benefit of early tracheostomy in a healthcare system with a constraint on ICU beds [13].

4.3 Population and Design

The TracMan trial was conducted during a 4-year period between November 2004 and November 2008 across 82 hospitals, including 70 general and two cardiothoracic surgical ICUs in the UK. The study included patients within the first 4 days of ICU admission who were on mechanical ventilation and likely to require continued ventilator support for at least 7 more days based on clinician judgment. The study excluded patients in whom an urgent life-saving tracheostomy was required and those with a contraindication to tracheostomy. Patients who were deemed to require early tracheostomy due to chronic neurological disease were also excluded. The study patients were randomly assigned in a 1:1 ratio to undergo an early tracheostomy or late tracheostomy. The planned sample size was 1692 patients, assuming a 6.3% absolute reduction in the 30-day all-cause mortality.

4.3.1 Early vs. Late Tracheostomy

In the early group, tracheostomy was planned to be carried out within 4 days of ICU admission. In the late group, tracheostomy was planned on day 10 or later of ICU admission if it was still considered appropriate by the treating clinician. The chosen technique, whether bedside percutaneous or open tracheostomy, was based on the practice at the participating unit.

4.4 Results

After 4 years of the commencement of the study, there was a gradual decline in patient recruitment with exhaustion of funds. Hence, the final sample included only 899 patients, compared with the calculated sample size of 1692 patients. The reduced sample had 80% power to detect an 8.3% reduction in the 30-day all-cause mortality in the early group with a significance level of 5%.

The intention-to-treat analysis included 451 patients in the early tracheostomy group and 448 patients in the late group. The baseline characteristics were similar between the two groups. A total of 622 tracheostomies were performed during the study, including 418 in the early and 204 in the late group. A bedside percutaneous tracheostomy was performed in 551 (88.7%) cases. Among 455 patients randomized to the early group, 385 (84.6%) underwent tracheostomy within 4 days of ICU admission as planned. Sixty-six patients randomized to the early group did not undergo early tracheostomy. Among them, 35 underwent a late tracheostomy, while 31 did not require a tracheostomy. In 33 patients (7.3%) assigned to the late group, tracheostomy was performed before day 10.

Among the 454 patients randomized to the late group, 244 (53.7%) did not undergo tracheostomy. The majority of patients who did not undergo tracheostomy included those who were discharged alive from the ICU (89 patients), weaned off ventilator support (78 patients), or died (54 patients). Eleven patients were too unstable to undergo the procedure, while two were offered end-of-life care. In 10 patients, no clear reason was discernible for not performing a tracheostomy.

4.4.1 Outcomes

The 30-day all-cause mortality, the primary outcome, was similar between the two groups. The mortality was 30.8% in the early compared with 31.5% in the late group. The ICU and hospital mortality and the mortality at 1 and 2 years were also not significantly different between the two groups. The duration of stay in the ICU and in hospital was also similar between the two groups. Among 30-day survivors, the median number of days on sedation was significantly lower with early tracheostomy (5 [IQR: 3–9] vs. 8 [IQR 4–12]) days. In contrast, among non-survivors at 30 days, there was no significant difference in the number of days on sedation.

Table 4.1 Main study outcomes

Outcomes	Early tracheostomy	Late tracheostomy	Significance
30-day mortality	30.8%	31.5%	$P = 0.89$
ICU mortality	29.7%	29.7%	$P > 0.99$
Hospital mortality	39.6%	41.3%	$P = 0.63$
1-year mortality	45.9%	49%	$P = 0.38$
2-year mortality	51%	53.7%	$P = 0.42$

The TracMan trial revealed no improvement in survival, ICU or hospital stay among general critically ill patients who underwent a tracheostomy within 4 days of ICU admission compared to a wait-and-watch policy until day 10. Among patients assigned to the late group, the majority did not undergo tracheostomy. Thus, the study revealed that a delayed approach could avert an unnecessary procedure in the majority of patients.

Clinically significant bleeding requiring intravenous fluids or other active intervention occurred in 7% of patients. In the early group, 11 (2.6%) patients experienced bleeding compared to eight patients in the late group (3.9%). The main study outcomes are summarized in Table 4.1.

4.5 Limitations

The TracMan trial could not attain the projected sample size as recruitment slowed down over time, leading to an underpowered study. The study centers, on average, recruited just two patients per year, suggesting a large number of exclusions for reasons that are largely unclear. Patients with respiratory failure due to chronic neurological disease were excluded, as the existing practice was to perform an early tracheostomy in these patients. The eligibility for inclusion in the study was based on clinician judgment regarding the requirement for prolonged ventilation; no validated tool was used to assist with the decision-making.

4.6 Comments

The TracMan trial was the largest RCT that addressed the timing of tracheostomy in ICU patients. The study employed a robust methodology and evaluated relevant clinical outcomes. Although the trial did not provide evidence regarding the optimal timing of tracheostomy in a heterogenous group of critically ill patients, it demonstrated that an early tracheostomy within the first 4 days does not improve clinical outcomes, compared to waiting for a minimum of 10 day after ICU admission.

The decision to perform a tracheostomy depends on clinical judgment regarding the need for prolonged mechanical ventilation. The TracMan trial clearly demonstrated that this is no easy task; 89/454 (19.6%) patients considered to require prolonged ventilation, and randomized to the late group, were weaned off ventilator support and discharged from the ICU by day 10. Clearly, an early tracheostomy within the first 4 days may involve performing an unnecessary and potentially risky procedure on a significant number of patients. The study highlights the need for a validated tool that may help clinicians predict the need for prolonged mechanical ventilation and tracheostomy. In the absence of objective guidance, it is probably appropriate to wait for 10 days or longer for a clearer picture to emerge regarding the trajectory of illness.

4.7 Summary

The timing of tracheostomy had long been the subject of debate among intensivists. Prior to the TracMan trial, an RCT of a small sample size had revealed improved survival, reduced ICU length of stay, a shorter duration of mechanical ventilation, and a lower incidence of ventilator-associated pneumonia (VAP) with an early tracheostomy [14]. Subsequently, an Italian RCT found no difference in the incidence of VAP; however, it suggested significantly more ventilator and ICU-free days, and a higher likelihood of weaning with early tracheostomy. In the largest RCT so far that evaluated the timing of tracheostomy, the TracMan trial provided robust evidence that performing a tracheostomy within 4 days of admission is unlikely to improve clinical outcomes, including mortality and the duration of stay in the ICU or hospital.

References

1. Colice GL. Chapter 1. Historical perspective on the development of mechanical ventilation. In: Tobin MJ, editor. Principles and practice of mechanical ventilation [Internet]. 3rd ed. New York: The McGraw-Hill Companies; 2013. [cited 2023 Jan 8]. Available from: accessmedicine.mhmedical.com/content.aspx?aid=57060501.
2. Jackson C. Tracheotomy. Laryngoscope. 1909;19(4):285–90.
3. Galloway TC. Tracheotomy in bulbar poliomyelitis. JAMA J Am Med Assoc. 1943;123(17):1096–7.
4. Trubuhovich RV. August 26th 1952 at Copenhagen: "Bjørn Ibsen's Day"; a significant event for Anaesthesia. Acta Anaesthesiol Scand. 2004;48(3):272–7.
5. Pollock RA. Percutaneous tracheostomy and percutaneous angiography: the diuturnity of Sven-Ivar Seldinger of Mora, Pasquale Ciaglia of Utica. Craniomaxillofac Trauma Reconstr. 2016;9(4):323–34.
6. Ciaglia P, Firsching R, Syniec C. Elective percutaneous dilatational tracheostomy. A new simple bedside procedure; preliminary report. Chest. 1985;87(6):715–9.
7. Combes A, Luyt CE, Nieszkowska A, Trouillet JL, Gibert C, Chastre J. Is tracheostomy associated with better outcomes for patients requiring long-term mechanical ventilation? Crit Care Med. 2007;35(3):802–7.

8. Freeman BD, Morris PE. Tracheostomy practice in adults with acute respiratory failure. Crit Care Med. 2012;40(10):2890–6.
9. Krishnan K, Elliot SC, Mallick A. The current practice of tracheostomy in the United Kingdom: a postal survey. Anaesthesia. 2005;60(4):360–4.
10. Veenith T, Ganeshamoorthy S, Standley T, Young P. Intensive care unit tracheostomy: a snapshot of UK practice. Int Arch Med. 2008;1(1):21.
11. Rumbak MJ, Newton M, Truncale T, Schwartz SW, Adams JW, Hazard PB. A prospective, randomized, study comparing early percutaneous dilational tracheotomy to prolonged translaryngeal intubation (delayed tracheotomy) in critically ill medical patients*. Crit Care Med. 2004;32(8):1689–94.
12. Griffiths J, Barber VS, Morgan L, Young JD. Systematic review and meta-analysis of studies of the timing of tracheostomy in adult patients undergoing artificial ventilation. BMJ. 2005;330(7502):1243.
13. Young D, Harrison DA, Cuthbertson BH, Rowan K, TracMan Collaborators. Effect of early vs late tracheostomy placement on survival in patients receiving mechanical ventilation: the TracMan randomized trial. JAMA. 2013;309(20):2121–9.
14. Rumbak MJ, Newton M, Truncale T, Schwartz SW, Adams JW, Hazard PB. A prospective, randomized, study comparing early percutaneous dilational tracheotomy to prolonged translaryngeal intubation (delayed tracheotomy) in critically ill medical patients. Crit Care Med. 2004;32(8):1689–94.

High-Frequency Oscillation in Acute Respiratory Distress Syndrome: The OSCILLATE Trial

5

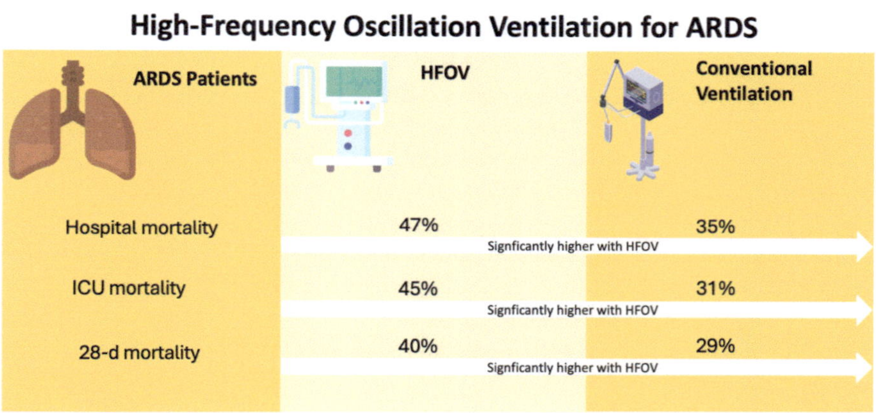

Ferguson et al. (NEJM, 2013)

Quick Take

Does high-frequency oscillatory ventilation (HFOV) improve survival in ARDS?

The OSCILLATE trial evaluated the efficacy of HFOV compared with conventional lung-protective ventilation in patients with moderate-to-severe acute respiratory distress syndrome (ARDS). This multicenter randomized controlled trial, conducted across 39 ICUs in five countries, planned to enrol 1200 patients but was stopped early after 548 patients were randomized due to safety concerns. The study found that HFOV increased in-hospital mortality. Besides, patients in the HFOV

Ferguson ND, Cook DJ, Guyatt GH, Mehta S, Hand L, Austin P, et al. High-frequency oscillation in early acute respiratory distress syndrome. N Engl J Med. 2013 Feb 28;368(9):795–805.

J. Chacko et al., *Landmark Studies in Critical Care*,
https://doi.org/10.1007/978-981-95-0673-6_5

group required higher doses of vasoactive drugs, suggesting hemodynamic compromise as a potential cause of harm. These findings indicate that early HFOV does not reduce and may increase mortality in ARDS, and should not be routinely used as a first-line ventilation strategy.

5.1 Introduction

Although mechanical ventilation is a life-saving intervention in acute respiratory distress syndrome (ARDS), injudicious modalities of support may perpetuate lung injury. Particularly, cyclical inflation and collapse of the alveoli may provoke an intense local and systemic inflammatory response that may trigger multiorgan failure and lead to adverse outcomes, including mortality [1]. The landmark ARDSNet trial had firmly established the safety of low tidal volume ventilation with increased levels of PEEP among patients with severe ARDS [2]. However, mortality continues to be high, necessitating alternate approaches to promote recruitment while protecting the lung [3].

High-frequency oscillation ventilation (HFOV) delivers minute tidal volumes of 1–2 ml/kg at a very high frequency, ranging between 3 and 15 breaths/second [4, 5]. Although earlier randomized controlled trials (RCTs) had demonstrated improved oxygenation and survival with HFOV, these studies employed outdated, possibly injurious ventilatory strategies in the control arm [6, 7].

Considering the largely unproven benefit of HFOV, the Canadian Critical Care Trials group designed an RCT to evaluate its efficacy compared with a lung-protective strategy of conventional ventilation, using low tidal volumes and high PEEP levels among patients with moderate-to-severe ARDS [4].

5.2 Population and Design

The OSCILLATE trial was conducted across 39 centers in Canada, the United States, Saudi Arabia, Chile, and India. Mechanically ventilated patients with symptom onset within the previous 2 weeks with bilateral air-space opacities on the chest radiograph and a PaO_2/FiO_2 ratio ≤200 mm Hg were eligible for inclusion.

5.2.1 Excluded

Patients who had met the eligibility criteria for >72 h were excluded from the study. Those with hypoxia secondary to raised left atrial pressure, neuromuscular disorders with the likely requirement for prolonged ventilator support, severe chronic respiratory disease, and raised intracranial pressure were also excluded.

5.3 Initial Ventilatory Management

Following enrolment, ventilator settings were standardized. Ventilation was in the pressure-controlled mode, aiming for a tidal volume of 6 ml/kg, a PEEP level of 10 cm H_2O or higher as appropriate, and an FiO_2 of 0.6. Patients in whom the PaO_2/FiO_2 ratio remained ≤200 mm Hg after 30 min at this setting were randomized. If the PaO_2/FiO_2 ratio was >200 mm Hg, they were reassessed for up to 72 h for possible randomization.

Those eligible were randomized to undergo HFOV or conventional ventilation. Randomization was in blocks of 2–4 and stratified by center.

5.3.1 HFOV Group

In the HFOV group, the first step was a recruitment maneuver with the application of a sustained airway pressure of 40 cm H_2O for 40 s aimed at opening closed lung units. Thereafter, HFOV was commenced at a mean airway pressure of 30 cm H_2O; the pressure was adjusted based on a protocol, aiming for a PaO_2 of 55–80 mm Hg. The tidal volume was maintained as low as feasible, with the highest oscillation frequency to maintain the arterial pH >7.25. The investigators used the Sensor Medics 3100B oscillator to deliver HFOV. Conventional ventilation was reinstated if the mean airway pressure could be maintained ≤24 cm H_2O for 12 h; the transition being mandatory when it dropped to 20 cm H_2O.

Mechanical ventilation was continued as in the control group after switching to conventional ventilation. HFOV could be recommenced if the FiO_2 was higher than 0.4 or the PEEP level exceeded 14 cm H_2O for >1 h to achieve target oxygenation.

5.3.2 Conventional Ventilation

A recruitment maneuver was carried out as in the HFOV group. Ventilation was in the pressure-controlled mode with a PEEP level of 20 cm H_2O and adjusted according to an FiO_2-based protocol. A tidal volume of 6 ml/kg was targeted, maintaining the plateau pressure at ≤35 cm H_2O. Alternatively, the volume-assist controlled mode or pressure-support could be employed with the set tidal volume and airway pressure limits. Weaning was carried out based on a protocol that included daily spontaneous breathing trials.

5.4 Common Management

In patients with persisting hypoxia despite an FiO_2 of ≥0.9, rescue therapies could be instituted, including prone ventilation and inhaled nitric oxide, while adhering to the assigned treatment protocol. Other therapies, including crossover from the conventional ventilation to the HFOV arm, were allowed in patients with refractory hypoxia, barotrauma, or refractory acidosis. The administration of intravenous fluids, sedatives, and muscle relaxants was at the clinician discretion.

5.5 Sample Size

The authors assumed a mortality of 45% in the control group. A sample size of 1200 patient provided the study with 80% power for a relative risk reduction of 20% with HFOV, even with a lower mortality of 37% in the control group, at a two-sided alpha level of 0.05.

5.6 Results

The trial was terminated after enrolment of 571 patients—275 in the HFOV group and 273 in the conventional ventilation group. At this stage of the trial, the hospital mortality was higher in the HFOV group.

5.7 Mortality

The hospital mortality was significantly higher in the HFOV group (47% vs. 35%, $P = 0.005$). The results were similar on multivariable analysis. The ICU mortality (45% vs. 31%) and the 28-day mortality (40% vs. 29%) were also higher in the HFOV group. On subgroup analysis, there was no interaction of mortality with the severity of hypoxia, the body mass index, vasopressor use, and experience of the study center.

5.8 Physiological Parameters

Although vasopressor use was similar at baseline, it increased significantly within 4 h of initiation of HFOV compared with the conventional ventilation group (73% vs. 62%, $P = 0.01$). The use of muscle relaxants was similar in both groups. The mean FiO_2 decreased similarly in the HFOV and conventional ventilation groups after 4 h of initiation and the following day.

5.9 Co-interventions

The use of vasoactive drugs was significantly higher in the HFOV group (91% vs. 84%, $P = 0.01$). Sedatives and opioids were administered for a similar duration in both groups during the study period. Prone positioning, renal replacement therapy, and glucocorticoid administration were similar in both groups.

Table 5.1 Main study outcomes

Outcome	HFOV	Conventional ventilation	Significance
Hospital mortality	47%	35%	$P = 0.005$
ICU mortality	45%	31%	$P = 0.001$
28-day mortality	40%	29%	$P = 0.004$
Median ICU stay	15 days	14 days	$P = 0.93$
Median hospital stay	30 days	25 days	$P = 0.74$

Abbreviation: *HFOV* high-frequency oscillation ventilation

5.10 Other Outcomes

Although refractory hypoxia occurred more commonly with conventional ventilation, mortality due to refractory hypoxia was similar. Life support was withdrawn at similar rates. Barotrauma occurred more commonly with HFOV, although the difference was not statistically significant. Among survivors, the duration of mechanical ventilation and ICU stay was not significantly different. The main study results are summarized in Table 5.1.

5.11 Strengths

The OSCILLATE trial addressed a key rescue intervention that was widely employed in ARDS with severe hypoxia. The multicentric, randomized controlled design enhanced the robustness of the trial and added external validity. Both arms of the study followed a protocolized line of care. The study focused on important clinical outcomes, including mortality.

5.12 Limitations

HFOV was employed as a rescue intervention in most clinical settings—however, the wide inclusion criteria of the study may not have focused on subgroups of patients who might have benefited from the intervention. The trial was ceased prematurely as increased mortality was noted in the HFOV group; however, the predefined threshold P value for stopping the trial was not met. The relatively small sample size may have led to a type II error. HFOV may have been associated with hemodynamic instability and barotrauma, but the trial lacked detailed subgroup analyses to explore these effects in detail. Although the study followed a strictly protocolized approach, it may not reflect pragmatic, real-world practice. Thirty-four patients (12%) crossed over from the conventional ventilation group to receive HFOV. While 31 of the 34 crossovers were per protocol, the remaining 3 occurred in violation of the protocol. Crossover may have led to an imbalance between groups and may have led to bias.

5.13 Study Conclusion

The authors concluded that early application of HFOV in moderate-to-severe ARDS, targeting lung recruitment, does not reduce mortality compared with a conventional mechanical ventilation strategy of low tidal volumes and high PEEP levels. On the contrary, the broad application of HFOV among these patients may increase mortality.

5.14 Summary

The OSCILLATE trial is considered a landmark study in the management of ARDS, which addressed the role of HFOV. Its relevance is underscored when considered alongside other pivotal trials that investigated the same question, including the OSCAR trial. Both trials demonstrated no benefit of HFOV in reducing mortality in ARDS, with OSCILLATE uniquely highlighting a possible association with increased mortality. This finding contrasts with earlier smaller studies and observational data suggesting potential benefits of HFOV in improving oxygenation and lung recruitment.

The methodology of the OSCILLATE trial, including its robust multicenter randomized design and rigorous adherence to protocol, provides high-quality evidence that challenged prior assumptions about HFOV. The trial also emphasized the possibility of hemodynamic instability induced by HFOV, which was less apparent in previous studies.

In the broader context, the OSCILLATE trial helped strengthen the shift away from HFOV as a routine strategy in ARDS management. It reinforced the efficacy of conventional mechanical ventilation strategies, such as low tidal volume ventilation with high PEEP, as validated by the earlier ARDSNet trial. Together, these findings have significantly influenced clinical guidelines, emphasizing the importance of evidence-based approaches to optimize ARDS outcomes.

References

1. Tremblay LN, Slutsky AS. Ventilator-induced lung injury: from the bench to the bedside. Intensive Care Med. 2006;32(1):24–33.
2. Acute Respiratory Distress Syndrome Network, Brower RG, Matthay MA, Morris A, Schoenfeld D, Thompson BT, et al. Ventilation with lower tidal volumes as compared with traditional tidal volumes for acute lung injury and the acute respiratory distress syndrome. N Engl J Med. 2000;342(18):1301–8.
3. Terragni PP, Rosboch G, Tealdi A, Corno E, Menaldo E, Davini O, et al. Tidal hyperinflation during low tidal volume ventilation in acute respiratory distress syndrome. Am J Respir Crit Care Med. 2007;175(2):160–6.

4. Ferguson ND, Cook DJ, Guyatt GH, Mehta S, Hand L, Austin P, et al. High-frequency oscillation in early acute respiratory distress syndrome. N Engl J Med. 2013;368(9):795–805.
5. Froese AB. High-frequency oscillatory ventilation for adult respiratory distress syndrome: let's get it right this time! Crit Care Med. 1997;25(6):906–8.
6. Derdak S, Mehta S, Stewart TE, Smith T, Rogers M, Buchman TG, et al. High-frequency oscillatory ventilation for acute respiratory distress syndrome in adults: a randomized, controlled trial. Am J Respir Crit Care Med. 2002;166(6):801–8.
7. Bollen CW, van Well GTJ, Sherry T, Beale RJ, Shah S, Findlay G, et al. High frequency oscillatory ventilation compared with conventional mechanical ventilation in adult respiratory distress syndrome: a randomized controlled trial [ISRCTN24242669]. Crit Care. 2005;9(4):R430–9.

High-Frequency Oscillation in Acute Respiratory Distress Syndrome: The OSCAR Trial

6

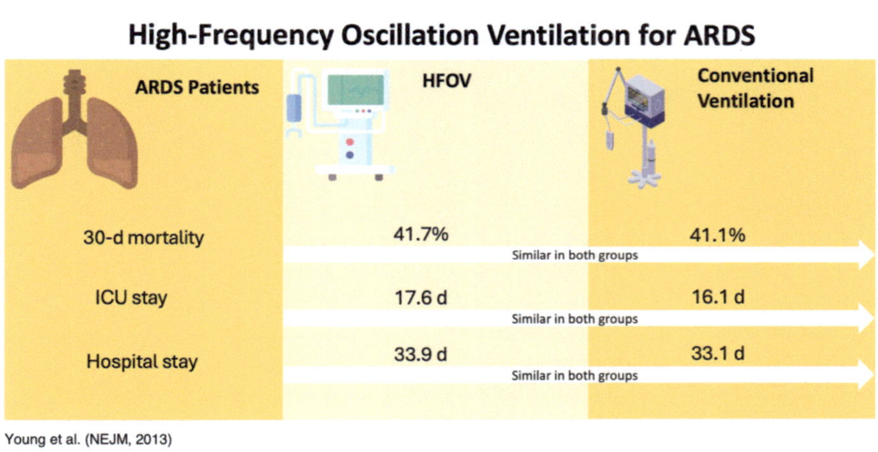

Quick Take

Does high-frequency oscillatory ventilation (HFOV) improve survival in ARDS?

The OSCAR trial evaluated the efficacy of HFOV compared to conventional ventilation in patients with acute respiratory distress syndrome (ARDS). This multicenter randomized controlled trial (RCT) enrolled over 800 patients with moderate-to-severe ARDS. The results showed no significant difference in 30-day mortality between the HFOV and the conventional ventilation groups. Additionally, HFOV was associated with a higher risk of adverse events, including hemodynamic

---

Young D, Lamb SE, Shah S, MacKenzie I, Tunnicliffe W, Lall R, et al. High-frequency oscillation for acute respiratory distress syndrome. N Engl J Med. 2013 Feb 28;368(9):806–13.

J. Chacko et al., *Landmark Studies in Critical Care*,
https://doi.org/10.1007/978-981-95-0673-6_6

instability. The findings suggest that HFOV does not confer a survival benefit in ARDS and should not be routinely used as a first-line ventilation strategy.

6.1 Introduction

The use of high-frequency oscillation ventilation (HFOV) dates to the early 1970s, following pioneering studies by Charles Bryan and Alan Laws in Toronto [1]. They used an oscillating loudspeaker diaphragm to deliver cyclical pressure to the airway at high frequency [1]. The technique in current use maintains lung inflation at a preset pressure, while carbon dioxide removal occurs through the back-and-forth movement of small volumes of gas at 3–15 Hz [2]. The tidal volumes generated are well below the dead space volume of the respiratory system, ranging between 1 and 2 ml/kg. The maintenance of constant inflation aims to obviate lung damage caused by the cyclical opening and closing of lung units during conventional mechanical ventilation [2]. Considering its potential to reduce volutrauma, HFOV has been in use as a rescue maneuver in patients who fail to improve with conventional mechanical ventilation [3]. However, evidence regarding efficacy was limited to small trials that used outdated ventilation strategies in the control group [4]. Against this background, the National Institute for Health Research in the United Kingdom designed an RCT to evaluate the utility of HFOV as a treatment modality among patients with ARDS [5].

6.2 Population and Design

The OSCAR trial was conducted between December 2007 and July 2012 across 27 ICUs in the United Kingdom. The study population included patients with acute respiratory distress syndrome (ARDS) with a PaO_2/FiO_2 ratio ≤200 mm Hg and a PEEP ≥5 cm H_2O. Bilateral pulmonary infiltrates on the chest radiograph, with no evidence of left atrial hypertension and the expectation of at least 2 more days of mechanical ventilation were required for study eligibility.

6.2.1 Exclusion

Patients <16 years old or with body weight <35 kg were excluded. Those who had undergone mechanical ventilation for ≥7 days, those with pre-existing lung disease and obstructive features or air trapping, or a history of recent lung surgery were also ineligible.

6.3 HFOV Group

HFOV was performed using a Novalung R100 ventilator (Metran) until the commencement of weaning. The initial settings were as follows.

- Frequency: 10 Hz
- Mean airway pressure: 5 cm H_2O above the plateau pressure on conventional ventilation
- Bias flow: 20 l/min
- Cycle volume: 100 ml (the actual tidal volume is only a fraction of the cycle volume)
- I:E ratio: 1:1
- FiO_2: 1.0

An algorithmic approach was followed to adjust HFOV settings based on the clinical situation. The pH level was maintained >7.25 by controlling the $PaCO_2$ level. As the first step, the cycle volume was increased to the maximum level for the set frequency. If the $PaCO_2$ levels continued to remain high, the frequency was reduced by 1 Hz at a time to a minimum frequency of 5 Hz. Additional measures were undertaken based on the recommendations of the study clinician.

The PaO_2 level was maintained between 60 and 75 mm Hg. If hypoxia occurred, the mean airway pressure was increased first, followed by an increase in the FiO_2. The modality of support was switched to pressure-controlled ventilation with the aim to wean once the FiO_2 had come down to 0.4, the mean airway pressure was maintained at 24 cm H_2O, and the PaO_2 was $\geq$60 mm Hg for $\geq$12 h. HFOV could be recommenced within 2 days if required.

6.4 Conventional Ventilation Group

In the conventional ventilation group, ventilator support was based on local practice. Pressure-controlled ventilation was encouraged, with a tidal volume of 6–8 ml/kg and FiO_2_PEEP combinations based on the ARDSNet protocol. All other modalities of treatment were based on clinician judgment.

6.5 Sample Size

The estimated mortality rate in the control group was 45%. HFOV was expected to reduce mortality by 9 percentage points. Enrolment of 503 patients in each group provided the study with 80% power to detect this difference at a two-sided *P*-value of 0.05.

6.6 Results

A total of 795 patients underwent randomization and were included in the primary analysis—397 received HFOV, while 398 underwent conventional ventilation. The median duration of HFOV use was 3 days; the longest duration was 24 days. The mean PaO_2/FiO_2 ratio was 113 mm Hg in both groups. The mean duration of ventilation before randomization was 2.2 days in the HFOV group and 2.1 days in the conventional ventilation group. Most patients (76.2%) had an underlying pulmonary cause for the ARDS. Over the first 3 days after randomization, the oxygenation improved, while the carbon dioxide levels rose in the HFOV group. Neuromuscular blockade was more commonly employed among patients who received HFOV.

6.7 The Primary Outcome: 30-Day Mortality

The 30-day all-cause mortality was not significantly different between the HFOV and conventional ventilation groups (41.7% vs. 41.1%, $P = 0.85$). Mortality rates remained similar between groups on adjusted analysis based on the study center, the baseline APACHE II score, and the PaO_2/FiO_2 ratio.

6.8 Secondary Outcomes

The all-cause mortality rates were also similar between the HFOV and conventional ventilation groups at first discharge from the ICU (44.1% vs. 42.1%, $P = 0.57$) and from the hospital (50.1% vs. 48.4%, $P = 0.62$). The duration of ICU stay (17.6 ± 16.6 vs. 16.1 ± 15.2 days, $P = 0.18$) and hospital stay (33.9 ± 41.6 vs. 33.1 ± 44.3 days $P = 0.79$) were not significantly different between groups. Among the other secondary outcomes, there was no significant difference in the duration of vasoactive drugs and receipt of antimicrobial agents. The main study outcomes are summarized in Table 6.1.

Table 6.1 Main study outcomes

Outcome	HFOV	Conventional ventilation	Significance
30-day mortality	166/398 (41.7%)	163/397 (41.1%)	$P = 0.85$
Duration of ICU stay	17.6 ± 16.6 days	16.1 ± 15.2 days	$P = 0.18$
Duration of hospital stay	33.9 ± 41.6 days	33.1 ± 44.3 days	$P = 0.79$
Vasoactive drug use	2.9 ± 4.5 days	2.8 ± 5.6 days	$P = 0.74$
Antimicrobial use	12.8 ± 12.0 days	12.4 ± 10.3 days	$P = 0.56$

Abbreviation: *HFOV* high-frequency oscillation ventilation

6.9 Study Conclusion

The authors concluded that the use of HFOV did not lead to any benefit or harm in patients with ARDS. They recommended that this technique not be routinely employed.

6.10 Strengths

The OSCAR trial was an adequately powered, multicentric trial that provided internal and external validity. The study included patients with severe ARDS who were mechanically ventilated for more than 48 h. Patients were severely ill at baseline, as evidenced by the high APACHE II scores. HFOV ventilation was continued until weaning from mechanical ventilation was considered feasible. Analysis was by intention to treat and there was no loss of follow-up, adding to the strengths of the study.

6.11 Limitations

Although they had intensive training, most participating centers were inexperienced with HFOV at the commencement of the study. A large number of patients were excluded; although 2769 patients were screened, only 795 patients were randomized. A new device, hitherto untested in clinical trials, was employed to deliver HFOV (the OSCAR study used the Novalung R100 ventilator, as opposed to the SensorMedics 3100B ventilators in common use during the study period). Ten patients assigned to conventional ventilation received HFOV, while 10 patients who were randomized to HFOV did not receive the assigned treatment. The study did not assess long-term outcomes, including quality of life among survivors.

6.12 Other Evidence

The results of the OSCILLATE trial were published in the same issue of the New England Journal of Medicine in January 2013 [6]. The trial was carried out across 39 ICUs in Canada, the United States, Saudi Arabia, Chile, and India. Adults with moderate to severe ARDS were randomized to HFOV or conventional mechanical ventilation. The study protocol was different from the OSCAR trial. The investigators performed a lung recruitment maneuver, applying an airway pressure of 40 cm H_2O for 40 s before initiating HFOV. HFOV was commenced at a mean airway pressure of 30 cm H_2O, with tidal volumes optimized by adjusting the frequency, aimed to maintain the blood pH above 7.25. In the control group, a tidal volume of 6 ml/kg was targeted, aiming to keep the plateau pressure <35 cm H_2O with high levels of PEEP.

The study was terminated early based on a strong signal of increased mortality with HFOV after enrolling 548 patients instead of the planned sample size of 1200 patients. At the time of cessation of the study, the in-hospital mortality was significantly higher in the HFOV group (47% vs. 35%, $P = 0.005$). The mortality difference was independent of baseline abnormalities in oxygenation and respiratory system compliance. The poor outcomes with HFOV may have been related to hemodynamic compromise that occurred more often compared with conventional mechanical ventilation, with a higher use of vasoactive drugs (91% vs. 84%, $P = 0.01$).

The higher use of sedatives and muscle relaxants in the HFOV group in both the OSCAR and OSCILLATE trials may have contributed to the poor outcomes.

Maitra et al. performed a meta-analysis of 1759 patients from seven RCTs that compared HFOV with lung-protective mechanical ventilation in adult patients with ARDS [7]. The in-hospital or 30-day mortality was similar with HFOV compared to conventional lung-protective ventilation (37.9% vs. 42.1%, $P = 0.70$). There was a trend toward a longer duration of mechanical ventilation among HFOV-treated patients (mean difference, 1.18 days; 95% CI, 0.00–2.35 days; $P = 0.05$). Refractory hypoxemia occurred less often with HFOV; moreover, HFOV use was not associated with a higher incidence of barotrauma or hemodynamic compromise.

6.13 Summary

HFOV was introduced in the 1970s, with sporadic use among clinicians as a rescue maneuver among patients with severe ARDS who do not improve with conventional mechanical ventilation. By maintaining a relatively constant inflation pressure and tidal volumes less than the anatomical dead space, HFOV was considered less likely to cause ventilator-induced lung injury. However, no adequately powered RCT had previously addressed its efficacy in real-world practice. Against this background, the National Institute of Health Research in the United Kingdom conducted an RCT that compared HFOV with usual ventilatory care in patients with ARDS. Patients with a PaO_2/FiO_2 of ≤ 200 mm Hg and expected to require mechanical ventilation for at least 2 days were included. The primary outcome of all-cause mortality at 30 days was similar in both groups. Furthermore, the duration of ICU and hospital stays was comparable. The findings of the OSCAR trial suggested that HFOV should not be routinely employed as a ventilatory strategy in ARDS.

References

1. Bohn D. The history of high-frequency ventilation. Respir Care Clin N Am. 2001;7(4):535–48.
2. Meyers M, Rodrigues N, Ari A. High-frequency oscillatory ventilation: a narrative review. Can J Respir Ther. 2019;55:40–6.
3. Chan KPW, Stewart TE, Mehta S. High-frequency oscillatory ventilation for adult patients with ARDS. Chest. 2007;131(6):1907–16.
4. Sud S, Sud M, Friedrich JO, Meade MO, Ferguson ND, Wunsch H, et al. High frequency oscillation in patients with acute lung injury and acute respiratory distress syndrome (ARDS): systematic review and meta-analysis. BMJ. 2010;340:c2327.
5. Young D, Lamb SE, Shah S, MacKenzie I, Tunnicliffe W, Lall R, et al. High-frequency oscillation for acute respiratory distress syndrome. N Engl J Med. 2013;368(9):806–13.
6. Ferguson ND, Cook DJ, Guyatt GH, Mehta S, Hand L, Austin P, et al. High-frequency oscillation in early acute respiratory distress syndrome. N Engl J Med. 2013;368(9):795–805.
7. Maitra S, Bhattacharjee S, Khanna P, Baidya DK. High-frequency ventilation does not provide mortality benefit in comparison with conventional lung-protective ventilation in acute respiratory distress syndrome: a meta-analysis of the randomized controlled trials. Anesthesiology. 2015;122(4):841–51.

7 Positive End-Expiratory Pressure Setting in Acute Respiratory Distress Syndrome: The ExPress Trial

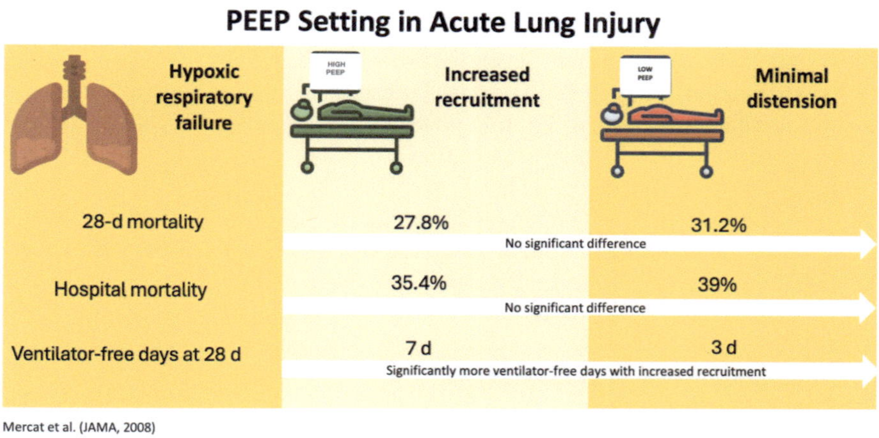

Quick Take

Do higher PEEP levels improve outcomes in acute lung injury (ALI) and acute respiratory distress syndrome (ARDS)?

The EXPRESS trial examined the optimal setting of positive end-expiratory pressure (PEEP) in patients with ALI and ARDS. This multicenter, randomized controlled trial (RCT) compared high versus low levels of PEEP in patients receiving mechanical ventilation. The study found that higher levels of PEEP improved

---

Mercat A, Richard JCM, Vielle B, Jaber S, Osman D, Diehl JL, et al. Positive end-expiratory pressure setting in adults with acute lung injury and acute respiratory distress syndrome: a randomized controlled trial. JAMA. 2008 Feb 13;299(6):646–55.

J. Chacko et al., *Landmark Studies in Critical Care*,
https://doi.org/10.1007/978-981-95-0673-6_7

oxygenation and reduced the need for additional interventions, including prone positioning, but it did not result in improved survival rates. The increased recruitment strategy reduced the time spent on mechanical ventilation; moreover, organ failures were also lower. Oxygenation and respiratory system compliance were also significantly better with the increased recruitment strategy. Suggesting that while it may benefit some aspects of respiratory function, it does not necessarily confer a survival advantage in this patient population.

7.1 Introduction

The application of an optimal level of positive end-expiratory pressure (PEEP) is the key component of a lung-protective ventilation strategy [1]. The beneficial effects of PEEP may be mediated by improved alveolar recruitment, greater homogeneity of ventilation, and protection of lung surfactant [2]. The use of low tidal volumes with high PEEP levels enables greater lung recruitment compared with the use of high tidal volumes, at any level of airway pressure [3].

The application of higher PEEP levels also carries the risk of hyperinflation. The use of low tidal volumes and limiting plateau pressures may mitigate this effect. Another approach may be the minimization of alveolar distension using low tidal volumes combined with moderate levels of PEEP. The ExPress trial aimed to compare the application of two different PEEP strategies – a low tidal volume with high PEEP aimed to increase recruitment compared with a low tidal volume and a moderate PEEP strategy to minimize distension.

7.2 Population and Design

The ExPress trial was conducted across 37 ICUs in France between September 2002 and December 2005 [4]. Adult patients with acute hypoxemic respiratory failure, receiving mechanical ventilation, were eligible. The inclusion criteria, present for not more than 48 h before enrollment, were a PaO_2:FiO_2 ratio $\leq$300 mm Hg, bilateral lung infiltrates, and no clinical features suggestive of left atrial hypertension (or a pulmonary capillary wedge pressure of <18 if available).

7.2.1 Excluded

Among those excluded were patients with raised intracranial pressure, chronic respiratory disease on home oxygen or ventilation, body weight >1 kg/cm, severe chronic liver disease, pneumothorax, and an expected duration of ventilation of less than 48 h.

7.3 Increased Recruitment Strategy (Intervention Group)

A maximal level of PEEP was applied while maintaining the inspiratory plateau pressure less than 28–30 cm H_2O. The PEEP level was titrated entirely based on the plateau pressure, regardless of the impact on oxygenation.

7.4 Minimal Distension Strategy (Control Group)

The PEEP and inspiratory plateau pressures were maintained at the lowest possible levels. The total PEEP (external + intrinsic PEEP) was maintained between 5 and 9 cm H_2O.

7.5 Both Groups

Patients in both groups were ventilated in the volume-assist controlled mode with a tidal volume of 6 ml/kg of predicted body weight. The PEEP level could be reduced to a minimum level of 5 cm of H_2O to ensure a plateau pressure of <30 cm H_2O. If the plateau pressure rose to >32 cm H_2O, the tidal volume was reduced in steps of 1–4 ml/kg body weight. If the plateau pressure remained higher than 32 cm H_2O with a pH of <7.15, the PEEP could be reduced to <5 cm H_2O in the minimal distension group.

The target oxygenation was a PaO_2 of 55 mm Hg and SpO_2 of 88–95%. If the oxygenation target was not met despite an FiO_2 of 1.0, the PEEP level could be increased to 12 cm H_2O in the minimal distension group; in the increased recruitment group, the PEEP level was increased up to a maximum plateau pressure of 32 cm H_2O. Recruitment maneuvers were not recommended; however, the decision was left to the clinician judgment.

Weaning from mechanical ventilation was protocolized. On day 4, if the PaO_2:FiO_2 ratio was >150 mm Hg, with an FiO_2 of ≤0.6, the PEEP level was weaned down. The patient was recommenced on the previous ventilator setting if there was a worsening of oxygenation during the weaning process. Pressure support or assist control ventilation was used as the weaning modality, based on clinician judgment. A spontaneous breathing trial was carried out once the PEEP level was weaned down to 5 cm H_2O, sedative agents and vasopressors were turned off, and the patient was responsive to verbal commands with an adequate cough response. T-piece breathing or pressure support ventilation with an inspiratory pressure of 7 cm H_2O was used during the spontaneous breathing trial, for up to 2 h. The decision to extubate was based on physician's judgment after the completion of the spontaneous breathing trial.

7.6 Sample Size

The authors assumed 40% mortality in the minimal distension group and a 10% absolute reduction in mortality with the increased recruitment strategy. A sample size of 400 patients provided the study with 80% power at a two-sided alpha level of 0.05.

7.7 Results

After 768 patients were enrolled, the study was terminated for futility of the primary endpoint, the 28-day mortality. The final analysis included 382 patients in the minimal distension group and 385 in the increased recruitment group. At baseline, 84% of patients had a PaO_2:FiO_2 ratio ≤200 mm Hg, suggestive of acute respiratory distress syndrome (ARDS); 95% were on a PEEP of ≥5 cm H_2O.

At each time point (days 1, 3, and 7) the PEEP level, plateau pressures, the respiratory system compliance, and the PaO_2/FiO_2 ratios were significantly higher in the increased recruitment group.

7.7.1 The Primary Outcome: 28-Day Mortality

The 28-day mortality was similar in the increased recruitment and the minimal distension groups (27.8% vs. 31.2%, $P = 0.31$).

7.7.2 Secondary Outcomes

Among the secondary outcomes, the hospital mortality (35.4% vs. 39.0%, $P = 0.30$) and the 60-day mortality (35.9% vs. 39.5%, $P = 0.31$) were not significantly different between the two groups. At 28 days, patients in the increased recruitment group experienced significantly higher ventilator-free days (median: 7 days vs. 3 days; $P = 0.04$) and organ failure-free days (median: 6 days vs. 2 days; $P = 0.04$) compared with the minimal distension group. Rescue therapies, including prone ventilation and inhaled nitric oxide, were used less often in the increased recruitment group (18.7% vs. 34.6%).

7.8 Adverse Events

The incidence of pneumothorax was similar in both groups (minimal distension: 5.8% vs increased recruitment: 6.8%, $P = 0.57$). The volume of resuscitation fluid infused was higher in the increased recruitment group; however, vasopressor use was similar in both groups. Extubation failure occurred at similar rates in both groups.

Table 7.1 The main study outcomes

Outcomes	Increased recruitment group ($n = 385$)	Minimal distension group ($n = 382$)	P-value
28-day mortality (n, %)	107 (27.8)	119 (31.2)	0.31
Hospital mortality (n, %)	136 (35.4)	149 (39.0)	0.30
60-day mortality (n, %)	138 (35.9)	151 (39.5)	0.31
Ventilation-free days at 28 day (median, IQR)	7 (0–19)	3 (0–17)	0.04
Organ-failure free days at 28 day (median, IQR)	6 (0–18)	2 (0–16)	0.04
Rescue therapies (n, %)	72 (18.7)	132 (34.6)	<0.001

Abbreviations: *IQR*, interquartile range

7.9 Cointerventions and Adjunctive Therapies

Fluid boluses to maintain hemodynamic stability were administered more often in the increased recruitment group during the first 72 h. Corticosteroids were administered at similar rates in both groups. The use of prone ventilation and inhaled nitric oxide as rescue therapy was higher in the minimal distension group. Patients who underwent rescue therapies experienced a similar high mortality (48.5% overall) in both groups. The main study outcomes are summarized in Table 7.1.

7.10 Strengths

The ExPress trial was a multicentric randomized controlled trial that evaluated a higher compared with a lower PEEP strategy. Mechanical ventilation was carried out based on a standard low tidal volume strategy. The weaning process was protocolized, reducing the risk of bias.

7.11 Limitations

The unblinded nature of the study may have biased the results. No formal evaluation of adherence to the study protocol was carried out; hence, the overall rate of compliance was unclear. Rescue interventions, including prone ventilation and nitric oxide, were employed based on clinician judgment alone. Most patients had ARDS related to pulmonary etiology; the extrapolation of the study findings to patients with extrapulmonary ARDS may be questionable. A higher PEEP level may be more beneficial in the most severely hypoxic patients. The ExPress trial included patients with a PaO_2/FiO_2 ratio of <300, and hence, does not address the impact of higher PEEP levels in patients with severe ARDS.

7.12 Study Conclusion

The authors concluded that a higher PEEP strategy in patients with ARDS led to improved lung recruitment, but did not significantly reduce the 28-day mortality compared to a lower PEEP strategy. There was improved oxygenation and a lower incidence of organ failure with the higher PEEP strategy, with no increase in barotrauma.

7.13 Subsequent Evidence

The PHARLAP study evaluated an open lung ventilation strategy, including recruitment maneuvers, and titrated PEEP with a conventional lung-protective ventilation strategy with PEEP levels based on the ARDSNet low PEEP table [5]. No significant difference was observed in the 28-day, ICU, and hospital mortality. The mortality at 90 days and 6 months, and the duration of ICU and hospital stay were also similar in both groups.

The multicenter ART trial compared a strategy of lung recruitment maneuvers combined with PEEP titrated to best compliance with a low PEEP strategy in patients with moderate to severe ARDS [6]. The recruitment and PEEP titration strategy was associated with a significantly higher 28-day mortality. Following three cardiac arrests, the original recruitment protocol had to be modified, with the application of lower airway pressures.

Kacmarek et al. evaluated an open-lung ventilation strategy, including a recruitment maneuver followed by downward titration of PEEP [7]. The control arm received the ARDSNet-low PEEP protocol-based strategy. The authors observed no significant difference in mortality or ventilation-free days between the two groups. However, improved oxygenation, lung mechanics, and lower driving pressures were observed with the open-lung ventilation strategy.

7.14 Summary

The ExPress trial compared two PEEP strategies in a multicentric RCT. A strategy of increased recruitment with titration of PEEP to a plateau pressure of 28–30 cm H_2O was compared with a minimal distension strategy aiming to maintain moderate PEEP levels between 5 and 9 cm H_2O. Mortality at 28 and 60 days did not differ significantly between the two groups. However, other important clinical outcomes were more favorable with the higher levels of PEEP employed in the increased recruitment strategy group. The increased recruitment strategy reduced the time spent on mechanical ventilation; moreover, organ failures were also lower. Oxygenation and respiratory system compliance were also significantly better with the increased recruitment strategy. Furthermore, rescue interventions, including prone ventilation and inhaled nitric oxide, were used less often in this group of patients.

The ExPress trial and subsequent trials suggest that empirically applied high levels of PEEP may not improve outcomes in a heterogenous group of ARDS patients. Subgroups of patients who are severely hypoxic and have the potential for recruitment may respond to higher levels of PEEP, calling for an individualized approach. Further studies are required to assess the potential for recruitment, to allow the individualized titration of PEEP to an optimal level.

References

1. Ashbaugh DG, Bigelow DB, Petty TL, Levine BE. Acute respiratory distress in adults. Lancet. 1967;2(7511):319–23.
2. Haitsma JJ, Lachmann RA, Lachmann B. Lung protective ventilation in ARDS: role of mediators, PEEP and surfactant. Monaldi Arch Chest Dis. 2003;59(2):108–18.
3. Richard JC, Maggiore SM, Jonson B, Mancebo J, Lemaire F, Brochard L. Influence of tidal volume on alveolar recruitment. Respective role of PEEP and a recruitment maneuver. Am J Respir Crit Care Med. 2001;163(7):1609–13.
4. Mercat A, Richard JCM, Vielle B, Jaber S, Osman D, Diehl JL, et al. Positive end-expiratory pressure setting in adults with acute lung injury and acute respiratory distress syndrome: a randomized controlled trial. JAMA. 2008;299(6):646–55.
5. Hodgson CL, Cooper DJ, Arabi Y, King V, Bersten A, Bihari S, et al. Maximal recruitment open lung ventilation in acute respiratory distress syndrome (PHARLAP). A Phase II, multicenter randomized controlled clinical trial. Am J Respir Crit Care Med. 2019;200(11):1363–72.
6. Cavalcanti AB, Suzumura ÉA, Laranjeira LN, Paisani D d M, Damiani LP, Guimarães HP, et al. Effect of lung recruitment and titrated positive end-expiratory pressure (PEEP) vs low PEEP on mortality in patients with acute respiratory distress syndrome. JAMA. 2017;318(14):1335–45.
7. Kacmarek RM, Villar J, Sulemanji D, Montiel R, Ferrando C, Blanco J, et al. Open lung approach for the acute respiratory distress syndrome: a pilot, randomized controlled trial. Crit Care Med. 2016;44(1):32–42.

Comparison of Different Methods of Weaning from Mechanical Ventilation

8

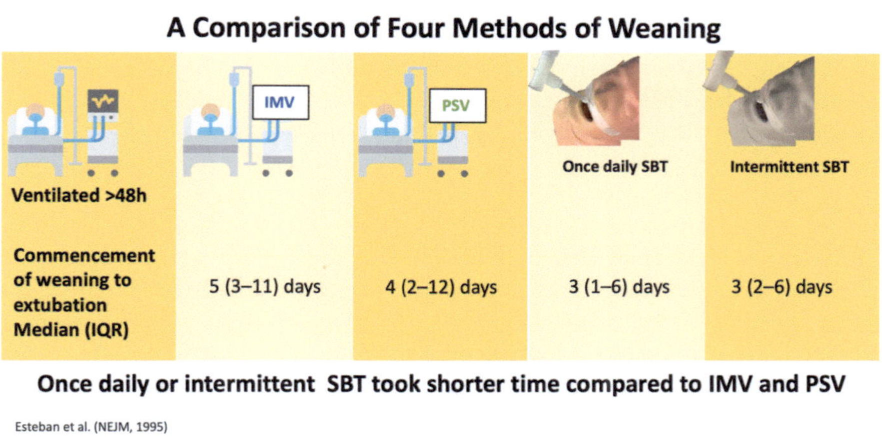

Quick Take

Which is the most efficient method of weaning from mechanical ventilation?

This multicenter, randomized trial compared four different methods for weaning patients off mechanical ventilation in the ICU. The methods compared were intermittent mandatory ventilation, pressure support ventilation, intermittent spontaneous breathing trials (SBT) carried out two or more times a day, or once daily SBT through a T-piece. The study found that there was no significant difference in

---

Esteban A, Frutos F, Tobin MJ, Alía I, Solsona JF, Valverdú I, et al. A comparison of four methods of weaning patients from mechanical ventilation. Spanish Lung Failure Collaborative Group. N Engl J Med. 1995 Feb 9;332(6):345–50.

J. Chacko et al., *Landmark Studies in Critical Care*,
https://doi.org/10.1007/978-981-95-0673-6_8

mortality, but patients weaned using a once daily SBT strategy were more likely to have a shorter duration of mechanical ventilation compared to other methods—extubation occurred thrice as quickly compared with intermittent mandatory ventilation and twice as quickly compared with pressure support ventilation.

8.1 Introduction

Although mechanical ventilation is lifesaving, it may be associated with complications, leading to poor outcomes [1]. Hence, it is imperative to expedite weaning and reduce the duration of ventilator support in critically ill patients. Approximately 40% of the time spent on mechanical ventilation is devoted to weaning [2]. However, a standardized approach to weaning was not in common practice, with several approaches available to the bedside clinician [2]. In a patient being ventilated in the synchronized intermittent mandatory ventilation mode, the ventilator rate may be gradually decreased. A spontaneous breathing trial (SBT) is another viable option and may be carried out using different approaches. The patient may be allowed to breathe through a T-piece with supplemental oxygen, without ventilatory assistance. An alternative strategy is switching over to the pressure support mode, with a titrated level of inspiratory pressure, usually between 5 and 8 cm H_2O [3]. Intermittent mandatory ventilation was considered superior to conventional approaches to weaning as it was believed to reduce the work of breathing by allowing the patient to breathe spontaneously between machine-delivered breaths [4].

In their 1995 trial, Esteban et al. designed a randomized controlled trial (RCT) comparing different weaning strategies in a subgroup of patients who were deemed difficult to wean [5]. They compared the efficacy of four different weaning techniques—intermittent mandatory ventilation, pressure support ventilation, spontaneous breathing trials (SBTs) performed several times a day, and once daily SBT.

8.2 Population and Design

Esteban et al. conducted their study over a 1-year period between October 1992 and October 1993 [5]. The study included patients admitted to 14 medical-surgical ICUs in Spain. Patients who had invasive mechanical ventilation for >24 h for acute respiratory failure were eligible. For study enrolment, patients should have improved or recovered sufficiently from the underlying cause of acute respiratory failure with a PaO_2/FiO_2 ratio >200 and a PEEP level of 5 cm H_2O. Other inclusion criteria were a core temperature <38 °C, hemoglobin level of >10 g/dl, and cessation of sedative and vasoactive agents. Besides, the patient was considered to be in a stable condition and ready for weaning according to clinician judgment. The study excluded patients on tracheostomy.

Eligible patients underwent a spontaneous breathing trial (SBT) with supplemental oxygen for 2 h through a T-tube circuit. According to pre-defined criteria, those who did not experience weaning failure were extubated. Assist control ventilation was recommenced in patients who experienced weaning failure and defined as “difficult to wean.”

Those designated as difficult to wean were randomly assigned to one of four methods of weaning.

8.3 Weaning Methods in the Difficult-to-Wean Patients

8.3.1 Intermittent Mandatory Ventilation

The ventilator rate was set at half of the rate used during assist control ventilation; mechanical breaths were synchronized with patient effort. The ventilator rate was reduced by 2–4 breaths/min at a time, at least twice a day; the rate was reduced more rapidly if tolerated. Patients who tolerated a set ventilator rate of 5 breaths/min for 2 h with no signs of distress were extubated.

8.3.2 Pressure Support Ventilation

The inspiratory pressure was titrated to maintain a respiratory rate of no more than 25/min. The pressure support level was reduced by 2–4 cm H_2O at least twice a day, based on patient tolerance, aiming to wean down to 5 cm of H_2O. Patients who were able to tolerate a support level of 5 cm H_2O for 2 h were extubated.

8.3.3 Intermittent SBTs

In this group, patients were disconnected from the ventilator and allowed to breathe spontaneously through a T-tube or a circuit that provided a continuous positive pressure level of 5 cm of H_2O. SBTs were attempted at least twice a day, and the duration gradually increased. Assist control ventilation, lasting at least 1 h, was reinstituted between trials of spontaneous breathing. Those who were able to sustain spontaneous breathing without assistance for at least 2 h were extubated.

8.3.4 Once-Daily SBT

In this group, patients breathed spontaneously through a T-tube circuit for up to two hours each day. Those who tolerated the 2-h trial of SBT were extubated; if there were signs of distress, they were recommenced on assist control ventilation, continued for the next 24 h, followed by another trial of SBT.

8.3.5 All Groups

Weaning was considered successful if extubation occurred within 14 days of commencement of weaning attempts, and reintubation was not carried out within 48 h.

8.4 Sample Size

The authors calculated a sample size of 31 patients in each group, providing the study with 80% power to identify a difference in the time for weaning between groups of 2 days, at a two-sided alpha level of 0.05.

8.5 Results

Among the 546 study patients, the initial spontaneous breathing trial was successful in 416 patients. The remaining 130 patients experienced poor tolerance to weaning and were designated as difficult to wean. These patients were randomized to undergo one of four weaning methods—intermittent mandatory ventilation (29 patients), pressure support ventilation (37 patients), intermittent SBTs (33 patients), or once-daily SBT (31 patients). Patient characteristics were similar in all four groups regarding the indication for mechanical ventilation and respiratory function.

8.5.1 Rate of Successful Weaning

Patient age, the duration of ventilator support before commencement of weaning, the weaning technique, and time to failure of the first SBT were predictors of successful weaning. After adjustment for covariates, the rate of successful weaning was significantly higher with once-daily SBT compared to intermittent mandatory ventilation or pressure support ventilation. However, successful weaning rates were similar between once-daily SBT and intermittent trials of spontaneous breathing. There was no significant difference in the adjusted rate of successful weaning between pressure support ventilation and intermittent mandatory ventilation.

8.5.2 Time to Extubation

The time to extubation was shortest with a once-daily trial of spontaneous breathing—it was about three times as rapid compared with intermittent mandatory ventilation and twice as quick compared with pressure-support ventilation. The duration between initiation of weaning and successful extubation was most rapid in the once-daily SBT group [median: 3 days, (IQR = 1–6 days)], followed by the intermittent SBT group [median: 3 days (IQR = 2–6 days)], and the pressure support ventilation

Table 8.1 Adjusted rate of successful weaning with different techniques

Comparison of techniques	Relative rate of successful weaning (95% CI)	*P* value
Once-daily SBT vs. IMV	2.83 (1.36–5.89)	<0.006
Once-daily SBT vs. PSV	2.05 (1.04–4.04)	<0.004
Once-daily SBT vs. intermittent SBT	1.24 (0.64–2.41)	0.54

Abbreviations: *CI* confidence interval, *SBT* spontaneous breathing trial, *IMV* intermittent mandatory ventilation, *PSV* pressure support ventilation

group [median: 4 days (IQR = 2–12 days)]; it was longest in the intermittent mandatory ventilation group [median: 5 days (IQR = 3–11 days)].

At 14 days, a significantly higher number of patients continued to require ventilator support in the intermittent mandatory ventilation group compared to patients who received once-daily SBT or intermittent SBTs. The extubation and reintubation rates were similar in all four groups. The main study outcomes are summarized in Table 8.1.

8.6 Strengths

The RCT that compared weaning techniques by Esteban et al. was one of the first to systematically evaluate different approaches to weaning among patients who are difficult to wean. Contrary to the conventional wisdom prevalent at the time, the study demonstrated that the use of synchronized intermittent mandatory ventilation with a gradual reduction in the respiratory rate may be an inferior weaning strategy compared with daily SBTs.

8.7 Limitations

The study revealed that the duration of weaning was shorter and extubation occurred earlier in the once-daily SBT group; however, the rates of successful extubation and reintubation were similar in all four groups. The study included a relatively small number of patients in each group, with the likelihood of outcomes being related to chance alone. Outliers who experienced difficult weaning and required extended periods of ventilation could have impacted the outcome of the whole group, particularly considering the limited number of patients in each group. As an example, patients with chronic obstructive pulmonary disease, likely to experience difficult weaning, varied from 27.6% in the intermittent mandatory ventilation group to 45.2% in the once-daily SBT group. The study did not evaluate the efficacy of a full ventilation mode interspersed with pressure support ventilation, a common weaning strategy in current practice. The weaning strategy may need to be flexible and individualized depending on the clinical status; this may be particularly relevant among patients on longer-term ventilatory support.

8.8 Study Conclusion

The authors concluded that a once-daily trial of spontaneous breathing led to successful extubation three times as rapidly compared with intermittent mandatory ventilation and twice as rapidly compared to pressure support ventilation. Multiple daily trials of spontaneous breathing were similarly successful.

8.9 Subsequent Evidence

Subirà et al. compared a less demanding, pressure support strategy with a potentially more demanding, T-piece technique of weaning among patients who were considered ready to wean following at least 24 h of mechanical ventilation [6]. Patients in the pressure support group underwent a 30-min SBT with an inspiratory pressure of 8 cm of H_2O and PEEP of zero, while the T-piece trial lasted 2 h. Among the 1018 patients who completed the trial, successful extubation was performed significantly more often in the pressure support group compared to the T-piece group (82.3% vs. 74.0%, $P = 0.001$). Besides, hospital and 90-day mortality were also lower in the pressure support group. The findings of this study suggested that a shorter, less demanding strategy using pressure support ventilation may be superior to T-piece weaning and result in more favorable outcomes.

In a more recent RCT, patients at high risk of extubation failure were randomly assigned to undergo SBT with pressure support ventilation (inspiratory pressure: 8 cm H_2O, PEEP: zero) or T-piece [7]. Among the 969 patients studied (pressure support: 484 vs. T-piece: 485 patients), the number of ventilation-free days at day 28 was similar in both groups. The time to extubation and reintubation rates were also similar in both groups.

Considering the lack of firm evidence, current international guidelines do not recommend a specific SBT strategy [8].

8.10 Summary

Historically, the strategy of weaning from mechanical ventilation had been variable with no systematic study comparing different approaches. Esteban et al. evaluated a total of 546 study patients; 130 were designated as difficult to wean following a 2-h spontaneous breathing trial and randomized to undergo one of four strategies of weaning—intermittent mandatory ventilation with gradual reduction of the ventilator rate, pressure support ventilation with periodic reduction in the inspiratory pressure, once-daily SBT or intermittent trials of spontaneous breathing through a T-tube. Weaning success, defined as extubation within 14 days of commencement of weaning attempts without the requirement for reintubation, was highest with once-daily SBT compared with intermittent mandatory ventilation and pressure support ventilation. Weaning success was similar between once-daily compared to multiple SBTs. The median duration of weaning was also shorter with spontaneous breathing trials compared with intermittent mandatory ventilation and pressure support ventilation.

References

1. Tobin MJ. Mechanical ventilation. N Engl J Med. 1994;330(15):1056–61.
2. Esteban A, Alía I, Ibañez J, Benito S, Tobin MJ. Modes of mechanical ventilation and weaning. A national survey of Spanish hospitals. The Spanish Lung Failure Collaborative Group. Chest. 1994;106(4):1188–93.
3. Brochard LJ, Lellouche F. Chapter 8. Pressure-support ventilation. In: Tobin MJ, editor. Principles and practice of mechanical ventilation [Internet]. 3rd ed. New York: The McGraw-Hill Companies; 2013. [cited 2024 Jun 7]. Available from: accessmedicine.mhmedical.com/content.aspx?aid=57062930.
4. Downs JB, Klein EF, Desautels D, Modell JH, Kirby RR. Intermittent mandatory ventilation: a new approach to weaning patients from mechanical ventilators. Chest. 1973;64(3):331–5.
5. Esteban A, Frutos F, Tobin MJ, Alía I, Solsona JF, Valverdú I, et al. A comparison of four methods of weaning patients from mechanical ventilation. Spanish Lung Failure Collaborative Group. N Engl J Med. 1995;332(6):345–50.
6. Subirà C, Hernández G, Vázquez A, Rodríguez-García R, González-Castro A, García C, et al. Effect of pressure support vs T-piece ventilation strategies during spontaneous breathing trials on successful extubation among patients receiving mechanical ventilation: a randomized clinical trial. JAMA. 2019;321(22):2175–82.
7. Thille AW, Gacouin A, Coudroy R, Ehrmann S, Quenot JP, Nay MA, et al. Spontaneous-breathing trials with pressure-support ventilation or a T-piece. N Engl J Med. 2022;387(20):1843–54.
8. Evans L, Rhodes A, Alhazzani W, Antonelli M, Coopersmith CM, French C, et al. Surviving sepsis campaign: international guidelines for management of sepsis and septic shock 2021. Intensive Care Med. 2021;47(11):1181–247.

9 Non-invasive Ventilation for Acute Exacerbation of Chronic Obstructive Pulmonary Disease: Brochard et al.

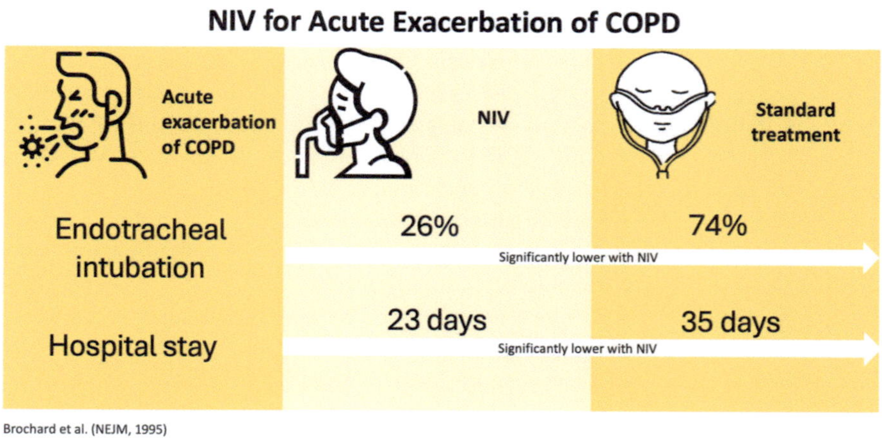

Quick Take

Can non-invasive ventilation improve outcomes in exacerbations of chronic obstructive pulmonary disease (COPD)?

This pivotal trial assessed the effectiveness of non-invasive ventilation in patients with acute exacerbations of COPD. In a multicenter, randomized trial, 136 patients with acute respiratory failure due to COPD exacerbation were assigned to receive either conventional treatment or NIV. The results

---

Brochard L, Mancebo J, Wysocki M, Lofaso F, Conti G, Rauss A, et al. Noninvasive ventilation for acute exacerbations of chronic obstructive pulmonary disease. N Engl J Med. 1995 Sep 28;333(13):817–22.

J. Chacko et al., *Landmark Studies in Critical Care*,
https://doi.org/10.1007/978-981-95-0673-6_9

demonstrated that NIV significantly reduced the need for endotracheal intubation and decreased in-hospital mortality compared to conventional therapy. The study provided strong evidence that NIV could be a life-saving intervention in managing acute exacerbations of COPD, transforming the management of this condition in critically ill patients.

9.1 Introduction

The application of non-invasive mechanical ventilation in acute respiratory failure, delivered through a mask interface, came into widespread use from the 1980s. The upsurge of interest in non-invasive ventilation was triggered by its efficacy when applied through a nasal mask in sleep apnea [1], and feasibility among patients who were unsuitable for endotracheal intubation. The potential benefits of avoiding invasive mechanical ventilation, with the complications associated with its use, were readily apparent. The mask interfaces also underwent refinement over the years, adding to patient comfort. Short-term respiratory support with non-invasive ventilation seemed rational in respiratory failure that may be rapidly reversible. It appeared to be the logical initial modality of support for acute exacerbations of chronic obstructive pulmonary disease (COPD) among patients with hypercapnic respiratory failure that typically resulted in rapid clinical improvement.

In an early study from 1989, Meduri et al. evaluated the use of non-invasive ventilation in ten patients with acute respiratory failure. Six patients had hypercapnic, and four, acute hypoxemic respiratory failure. The mask was tightly strapped to the face; the pressure support or pressure-controlled mode was employed for ventilatory support. Although three patients eventually required intubation, the authors observed that the physiological response was comparable to invasive mechanical ventilation. They suggested that non-invasive face mask ventilation may be an effective modality of support in acute respiratory failure [2]. A year later, Brochard et al. published a case-control study that evaluated the physiological effects of non-invasive pressure support delivered using a face mask in patients with acute exacerbation of COPD [3]. After 45 min of application of non-invasive ventilation, they observed a reduction in the PCO_2 level, an increase in the PO_2 level, and a rise in pH. This was accompanied by a marked improvement in tachypnea. There was just a lone patient in this cohort of 13 who required tracheal intubation, compared with 11 of 13 patients in a historical control group. Besides, the ICU length of stay was also shorter in patients who received non-invasive ventilation.

A randomized controlled trial (RCT) compared intermittent positive pressure ventilation (IPPV) applied through a nasal mask with conventional therapy in patients with acute exacerbation of COPD. Application of nasal IPPV resulted in lower $PaCO_2$ levels and a rise in pH. Furthermore, the 30-day mortality was lower in patients who received nasal IPPV after exclusion of patients who could not tolerate mask application [4].

Despite the putative physiological benefits of non-invasive ventilation in acute exacerbations of COPD, the impact on clinical outcomes, including mortality, had not been adequately established in a controlled trial. Brochard et al. designed an RCT to evaluate the clinical efficacy of non-invasive ventilation applied through a face mask in patients admitted to the ICU with acute exacerbation of COPD—specifically to assess whether it could reduce the requirement for invasive mechanical ventilation [5].

9.2 Population and Design

The trial was carried out between September 1990 and November 1991, in five hospitals—three from Paris in France, and one each from Italy and Spain. The enrolled patients had known COPD or had a high probability of the disease, based on clinical features and the chest radiograph, with hypercapnia and a high bicarbonate level. Other eligibility criteria included exacerbation of dyspnea of less than 2 weeks, with at least two of the following criteria: a respiratory rate >30/min, PaO_2 <45 mm Hg, and an arterial pH of <7.35 while breathing room air for 10 min. Patients were randomly assigned to receive standard treatment alone or standard treatment combined with non-invasive ventilation.

9.2.1 Exclusion

- Respiratory rate <12/min, or requirement for emergent intubation
- Administration of sedative agents within 12 h of randomization
- A neurological disorder leading to hypoxia, or hypercapnic encephalopathy
- Cardiac arrest
- Cardiogenic pulmonary edema
- Kyphoscoliosis leading to chronic respiratory failure
- Upper airway obstruction
- Bronchial asthma
- A precipitating cause leading to decompensation (e.g., sepsis, acute myocardial infarction)
- Facial deformity that precluded mask application

9.3 Standard Treatment

In this group, patients received supplemental oxygen through nasal prongs (maximum 5l/min) to achieve a target oxygen saturation of >90%. Subcutaneous heparin for prophylaxis against deep vein thrombosis, antibiotics, bronchodilators, aminophylline, and correction of dyselectrolytemias were part of standard care.

9.4 Non-invasive Ventilation

Patients in this group received standard care combined with non-invasive ventilation. The initial inspiratory pressure support level was set at 20 cm of H_2O applied through a face mask, specially designed for the study. Ventilatory support was flow-triggered and flow-cycled. No end-expiratory pressure was applied. Supplemental oxygen was titrated to maintain an oxygen saturation >90%. Patients received non-invasive ventilatory support for at least 6 h per day; the duration could be extended if tolerated. Each day, a 2-h period was allowed without non-invasive ventilatory support. The duration of non-invasive ventilatory support was based on clinical criteria and arterial blood gas analysis; the final decision to cease support was based on clinician judgment.

9.5 Both Groups

Endotracheal intubation was carried out based on pre-defined objective criteria. Those who required endotracheal intubation were ventilated in the assist-control mode; weaning was performed in the pressure-support mode.

9.6 Results

During the study period, 275 patients with acute exacerbation of COPD were admitted to the participating centers; 85 were randomized—42 were assigned to the standard care group and 43 to receive non-invasive ventilation combined with standard care. Patient characteristics were similar in both groups at baseline. A similar number of patients had undergone mechanical ventilation previously; the medications administered to both groups of patients were also similar.

9.7 The Primary Outcome: Requirement for Endotracheal Intubation

A significantly higher number of patients underwent endotracheal intubation in the standard care group compared with the non-invasive ventilation group (74% vs. 26%, $P < 0.001$). The rate of endotracheal intubation was consistent across the participating centers. In the standard treatment group, 17 patients required intubation within an hour of randomization; in the non-invasive ventilation group, only three patients underwent intubation within the first hour.

9.8 Other Outcomes

The duration of non-invasive ventilation was 4 ± 4 days.

The encephalopathy score, respiratory rate, PaO_2, and the pH level significantly improved within the first hour of commencement of treatment in the non-invasive ventilation group. In contrast, a worsening of the encephalopathy score, a rise in the $PaCO_2$ level, and a lower arterial pH were observed in the standard treatment group.

Among those who were successfully treated with non-invasive ventilation, the respiratory rate decreased progressively compared with baseline, while the encephalopathy score improved. The mean duration of invasive mechanical ventilation among the 31 patients who required intubation was 17 ± 21 days in the standard care group; it was 25, ±17 days among the 11 patients who underwent intubation and invasive ventilation in the non-invasive ventilation group.

The in-hospital mortality was significantly lower in the non-invasive ventilation group [4/43 (9%) vs. 12/42 (29%), $P = 0.02$]. On adjusted analysis, endotracheal intubation was the main factor leading to a difference in mortality between the two groups. Complications were more often encountered in patients who received standard care compared with those who underwent non-invasive ventilation (48% vs. 16%, $P = 0.001$).

The duration of hospital stay was significantly shorter in the non-invasive ventilation group (23 ± 17 vs. 35 ± 33 days, $P = 0.02$).

Pulmonary function tests within 3 months of randomization, including the forced expiratory volume in one second, the vital capacity, and the ratio of the two measures, were similar in both groups. The main study outcomes are summarized in Table 9.1.

Table 9.1 Main study outcomes

Outcome	NIV plus standard care	Standard care alone	P value
Requirement for intubation	31/42 (74%)	11/43 (26%)	<0.001
Duration of invasive ventilation among those intubated	17 ± 21 days	25 ± 17 days	
In-hospital mortality	4/43 (9%)	12/42 (29%)	0.02
Duration of hospital stay	23 ± 17 days	35 ± 33 days	0.02
Complications	16% of patients	48% of patients	0.001

Abbreviation: *NIV* non-invasive ventilation

9.9 Strengths

The Brochard et al. study was a pioneering, multicentric clinical trial that compared clinical outcomes with non-invasive ventilation applied through a face mask in patients with acute exacerbation of COPD. The authors evaluated robust endpoints, including the requirement for intubation. The study was designed to enrol patients with a high likelihood of requiring invasive ventilation. Intubation was carried out based on predefined criteria, thus reducing the possibility of bias. Based on the findings of this trial, non-invasive ventilation was widely accepted as the initial modality of support among patients with acute exacerbation of COPD, and has hence become the standard of care.

9.10 Limitations

The authors did not cite a baseline rate of intubation and the likely impact of non-invasive ventilation; no sample size was calculated. The intubation rate in the standard care group was higher than expected (74%), raising questions about the management in the control group. The fragility index for 30-day mortality was 1—just one additional death in the non-invasive ventilation group would have rendered the difference between groups non-significant. The population enrolled was highly selective—only 31% of patients admitted with COPD during the study period were included.

9.11 Study Conclusion

The authors concluded that in patients with acute exacerbation of COPD, the use of non-invasive ventilation leads to less requirement for endotracheal intubation, reduces hospital mortality, and reduces the duration of hospital stay.

9.12 Subsequent Evidence

A large retrospective study evaluated outcomes in 25,628 patients admitted with acute exacerbation of COPD who were treated with non-invasive ventilation compared to those who underwent invasive mechanical ventilation. On propensity-adjusted analysis, non-invasive ventilation was associated with a lower risk of mortality compared with invasive ventilation. Besides, the incidence of hospital-acquired pneumonia was lower and the duration of hospital stay shorter in patients who underwent non-invasive ventilation. The cost of care was also lower with non-invasive compared to invasive mechanical ventilation [6].

A Cochrane review evaluated the efficacy of non-invasive ventilation in hypercapnic respiratory failure due to acute exacerbation of COPD [7]. The authors performed a meta-analysis of 854 patients from 12 RCTs. Non-invasive ventilation was associated with a 46% reduction in the risk of mortality compared to usual care. Furthermore, a 65% reduction in intubation rates was observed among patients who underwent non-invasive ventilation. The efficacy appeared to be similar in patients with mild (pH 7.30–7.35) or more severe (pH < 7.30) acidosis.

9.13 Summary

The landmark trial by Brochard et al. was conducted during an era when non-invasive ventilation was being increasingly employed in acute respiratory failure. Earlier studies had suggested improvement in physiological parameters the plausibility of clinical benefit in acute exacerbation of COPD. The study randomly assigned patients with acute exacerbation of COPD to undergo non-invasive pressure support ventilation delivered through a face mask or to a control group that received standard treatment. The requirement for endotracheal intubation was lower among patients who received non-invasive ventilation. Besides, the duration of hospital stay was lower among patients who received non-invasive ventilation. The in-hospital mortality and the incidence of complications were also lower in the non-invasive ventilation group. This ground-breaking clinical trial firmly entrenched non-invasive ventilation as the initial modality of respiratory support in most patients with acute exacerbation of COPD.

References

1. Sullivan CE, Issa FG, Berthon-Jones M, Eves L. Reversal of obstructive sleep apnoea by continuous positive airway pressure applied through the nares. Lancet. 1981;1(8225):862–5.
2. Meduri GU, Conoscenti CC, Menashe P, Nair S. Noninvasive face mask ventilation in patients with acute respiratory failure. Chest. 1989;95(4):865–70.
3. Brochard L, Isabey D, Piquet J, Amaro P, Mancebo J, Messadi AA, et al. Reversal of acute exacerbations of chronic obstructive lung disease by inspiratory assistance with a face mask. N Engl J Med. 1990;323(22):1523–30.
4. Bott J, Carroll MP, Conway JH, Keilty SE, Ward EM, Brown AM, et al. Randomised controlled trial of nasal ventilation in acute ventilatory failure due to chronic obstructive airways disease. Lancet. 1993;341(8860):1555–7.
5. Brochard L, Mancebo J, Wysocki M, Lofaso F, Conti G, Rauss A, et al. Noninvasive ventilation for acute exacerbations of chronic obstructive pulmonary disease. N Engl J Med. 1995;333(13):817–22.
6. Lindenauer PK, Stefan MS, Shieh MS, Pekow PS, Rothberg MB, Hill NS. Outcomes associated with invasive and noninvasive ventilation among patients hospitalized with exacerbations of chronic obstructive pulmonary disease. JAMA Intern Med. 2014;174(12):1982–93.
7. Osadnik CR, Tee VS, Carson-Chahhoud KV, Picot J, Wedzicha JA, Smith BJ. Non-invasive ventilation for the management of acute hypercapnic respiratory failure due to exacerbation of chronic obstructive pulmonary disease. Cochrane Database Syst Rev. 2017;2017(7):CD004104.

Part II

Fluid Management

10 Albumin vs. Normal Saline for Resuscitation: The SAFE Trial

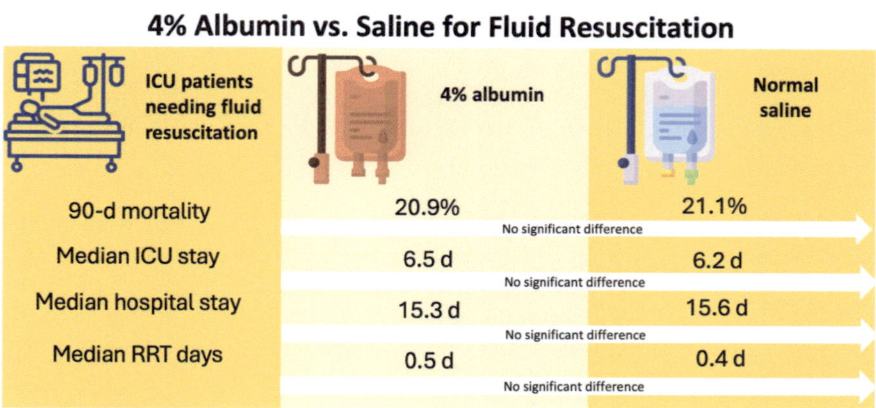

The SAFE Study Investigators (NEJM, 2004)

Quick Take

In critically ill patients requiring fluid resuscitation, does albumin improve outcomes compared to normal saline?

This landmark randomized controlled trial evaluated the safety and efficacy of albumin versus normal saline for fluid resuscitation in ICU patients. A total of 6997 patients from 16 ICUs in Australia and New Zealand were randomized to receive 4% albumin or normal saline for resuscitation. The study found no significant difference in 28-day mortality between the albumin and saline groups. Subgroup

---

Finfer S, Bellomo R, Boyce N, et al. A comparison of albumin and saline for fluid resuscitation in the intensive care unit. N Engl J Med. 2004;350(22):2247–2256.

J. Chacko et al., *Landmark Studies in Critical Care*,
https://doi.org/10.1007/978-981-95-0673-6_10

analyses showed no benefit of albumin in specific populations, including those with sepsis or trauma. Importantly, there was no significant difference in the incidence of new organ failure, length of ICU or hospital stay, or the need for renal replacement therapy between the groups.

The findings demonstrated that albumin is as safe as saline for fluid resuscitation in critically ill patients but does not confer a survival advantage. This trial remains a cornerstone in guiding fluid therapy choices in the ICU.

10.1 Introduction

The so-called "colloid vs. crystalloid debate" had gone on for over fifty years without resolution. There is a biological rationale for the infusion of colloidal solutions, particularly albumin, to maintain colloid osmotic pressure and to minimize the volume needed to be infused to achieve a specific resuscitation endpoint. There is very little clinical evidence to support this practice, however, and the strongest influence on the choice of fluid to use is geography, with marked variation around the world [1]. There are significant cost implications to the choice of fluid, with more than a hundred-fold difference between the cheapest and most expensive resuscitation fluid, and the global albumin market in 1996 was estimated to be worth US$1.5 billion.

In 1998, the Cochrane Collaboration published a systematic review and meta-analysis (SRMA) of all trials of albumin infusion in intensive care [2]. There was significant heterogeneity between patient groups, including burns and neonates, and many old and small studies were included, with a total of 1419 patients from 24 studies. A 6% excess mortality (95% CI 3–9%) was reported for patients who received albumin while in the ICU. This finding was widely publicized in the media, and the Director of the UK Cochrane Centre, Iain Chalmers, stated publicly, "What would I want if I or someone I cared for was critically ill? If I survived, I would attempt to sue anyone who had given me an infusion of albumin; I would not give my informed consent to take part in a randomized trial." A more restrained editorial comment in the *BMJ* recommended, "the administration of albumin should be halted until the results of a high quality large clinical trial are available" [3].

10.2 Background to the Study

Following the global furore caused by the 1998 Cochrane analysis, a further SRMA was performed examining 55 trials with 3504 patients and concluded there was no significant increase in the risk of death [4]. Pilot work conducted by the Australian and New Zealand Intensive Care Society (ANZICS) Clinical Trials Group found that almost exactly 50% of intensive care patients received albumin at some point during their intensive care stay. There was, therefore, a need to address the question of whether or not the use of albumin in the ICU was associated with excess mortality.

10.3 Population and Design

The SAFE trial was conducted over 18 months in 16 ICUs in Australia and New Zealand. A total of 6997 patients were randomized, making this one of the largest randomized controlled trials (RCTs) in intensive care medicine [5]. All adult patients in the ICU who were judged by the treating clinician to require fluid resuscitation to maintain or increase intravascular volume, supported by at least one objective criterion, were eligible for the trial. Patients admitted after cardiac surgery, liver transplantation, or treatment of burns were excluded. Patients who were able gave prospective consent, but the majority were recruited with a waiver of prior consent, with subsequent consent to use data and for follow-up, from patients or their surrogate decision makers. As SAFE was a process of care trial evaluating a readily available treatment already administered to a significant number of patients, this waiver of consent was approved in all jurisdictions under Australian and New Zealand law. Of the 6997 patients, 3497 were assigned to albumin, and 3500 were assigned 0.9% saline. Of these, 94.7% were recruited using an initial waiver of consent.

A total of 7000 patients were initially randomized, of whom 3499 were allocated to albumin and 3501 were allocated to saline. There were 26 and 41 patients, respectively, lost to follow-up, including three double randomizations. The primary endpoint was available for 3473 (99.25%) vs. 3460 (98.25%), which were analyzed.

10.4 Intervention

The intervention was specially manufactured 500 ml glass bottles of 4% human albumin solution (Albumex, CSL), used for all fluid resuscitation episodes (boluses of fluid) for the duration of stay up to 28 days.

10.5 Control

The control fluid was 0.9% saline, manufactured in the same 500 ml glass bottle and presented in the same masking carton and administered with the same masked infusion set. A formal evaluation of the effectiveness of the masking (blinding) confirmed that clinicians were less than 50% accurate when asked to guess which fluid they were administering.

10.6 Statistical Analysis

The sample size was derived from the results of the 1996 Cochrane SRMA, which suggested a 6% excess mortality from albumin. The lower 95% confidence interval (3%) was considered still a clinically significant difference, so SAFE was designed to have a 90% power to detect a 3% absolute mortality difference based on a predicted 15% baseline mortality. This would require a total of 7000 patients.

Proportions were compared with the chi-square or Fisher's exact test, and continuous variables were compared using unpaired t-tests. Survival times were compared by means of the log-rank test and presented as Kaplan–Meier curves, and heterogeneity of treatment effect was assessed with the test for a common relative risk. All analyses were intention-to-treat.

The primary outcome was all-cause mortality 28 days after randomization. This was also determined in six predefined subgroups (trauma, sepsis, or the acute respiratory distress syndrome at baseline). This became important when considering heterogeneity of results. Secondary outcomes included survival time during the first 28 days, the proportion of patients who developed new organ failures while in the trial, and the duration of mechanical ventilation, renal replacement therapy and ICU and hospital stay.

10.7 Results

The study fluid was administered to all but 197 (2.8%) of patients.

Examining the physiological effects of fluid resuscitation, clinical endpoints were achieved over the first four days with a smaller volume of albumin compared with saline, in a ratio of 1:1.4 overall. Patients in the saline group had a higher central venous pressure and patients in the albumin group had a higher measured serum albumin.

Overall, there was no difference in outcome between groups, with 28-day mortality 20.9% vs. 21.1% and relative risk of death 0.99 (95% CI 0.91–1.09). There was no difference in survival time between groups, with identical Kaplan-Meier estimates of the probability of survival. There was no difference in the number of patients with new organ failures, nor ICU and hospital length of stay and duration of mechanical (MV) and renal replacement therapy (RRT).

There may have been heterogeneity between pre-specified subgroups. The relative risk of death for trauma patients administered albumin was 1.36 compared to the corresponding risk of death for patients without trauma (0.96) ($p = 0.04$ by the test for a common relative risk). This difference was restricted to those with traumatic brain injury—there was no difference in outcome in patients with trauma without a brain injury.

In severe sepsis, the relative risk of death in those administered albumin was 0.87, compared to 1.05 in those without severe sepsis ($p = 0.06$ by the test for a common relative risk). The main study outcomes are summarized in Table 10.1.

Table 10.1 Main study outcomes

Outcome	Albumin group n = 3473	Saline group n = 3460	Relative risk (95% CI)	Absolute difference (95% CI)	P value
Status at 28 days—no (%)					
Dead	726 (20.9)	729 (21.1)	0.99 (0.91–1.09)		0.87
Alive in ICU	111 (3.2)	87 (2.5)	1.27 (0.96–1.68)		0.09
Alive in hospital	793 (22.8)	848 (24.5)	0.93 (0.86–1.01)		0.10
Length of stay in ICU - days	6.5 ± 6.6	6.2 ± 6.2		0.24 (−0.06–0.54)	0.44
Length of stay in hospital—days	15.3 ± 9.6	15.6 ± 9.6		−0.24 (−0.70–0.21)	0.30
Duration of MV—days	4.5 ± 6.1	4.3 ± 5.7		0.19 (−0.08–0.47)	0.74
Duration of RRT - days	0.48 ± 2.28	0.39 ± 2.0		0.09 (0.0–0.19)	0.41
Subgroups—death within 28 days					
Trauma	81/596 (13.6)	59/590 (10.0)	1.36 (0.99–1.86)		0.06
Severe sepsis	185/603 (30.7)	217/615 (35.3)	0.87 (0.74–1.02)		0.09
ARDS	24/61 (39.3)	28/66 (42.4)	0.93 (0.61–1.41)		0.72

10.8 Strengths

This was a well-conducted, large, pragmatic, double-blinded RCT of two resuscitation fluids in the ICU, with broad and rapid recruitment and minimal loss to follow-up. Resuscitation was to pre-specified hemodynamic endpoints, and more saline was required to achieve the same clinical endpoint, though the consistent ratio of 1:1.4; in contrast to the 1:3 ratio quoted in textbooks derived from animal studies in the 1950s. The physiological importance of this finding from SAFE has been under-recognized and probably represents the effect of endothelial damage in critical illness compared to the normal endothelium of healthy experimental animals.

10.9 Limitations

Despite its size, the trial did not have the power to detect small but important differences between subgroups. There appears to be heterogeneity between pre-specified groups, with significantly worse outcomes in trauma patients resuscitated with albumin and non-significantly better outcomes in severe sepsis. The albumin group received more blood transfusions, and the reasons for this are speculative.

The primary criticism that has been leveled against SAFE, and other clinical trials of similar design, is that it does not reflect the "real world," where a variety of fluids are administered to patients, but rather that participating patients always received the "study fluid" whenever a fluid bolus was required while in the ICU. This can also be considered a strength as it removes a lot of the irrational variations in day-to-day clinical practice. Fluid administration before and after the intensive care stay could not be controlled.

10.10 Subsequent Evidence

The SAFE Study investigators conducted several post-hoc evaluations to explore the meaning of their findings. The most important of these was SAFE-TBI, where the traumatic brain injury cohort was followed to a 24-month endpoint [6]. Of the trauma cohort, 460 patients were identified as having trauma with an abnormal cerebral CT scan and a Glasgow Coma Score (GCS) of 13 or lower, and these were further divided into severe TBI with initial GCS of 3–8 and moderate TBI with initial GCS of 9–13. At 24 months, 71/214 (33.2%) of the albumin group had died compared with 42/206 (29.4%) of the saline group [relative risk 1.63, 95% CI 1.17–2.26, $p = 0.003$]. These findings provided convincing evidence of harm using albumin to fluid resuscitate traumatic brain injury patients.

Another sub-study (SAFE-BSA) evaluated patients with various baseline serum albumin levels in a post-hoc analysis but could not detect any threshold at which there was a benefit of the administration of albumin to correct hypoalbuminemia [7].

The findings in the severe sepsis group are tantalizing and have led to several subsequent international trials examining the place of albumin specifically in the fluid resuscitation of severe sepsis.

Overall, the findings of the SAFE trial have generally been used to confirm the pre-existing biases of the readers. The trial was designed in response to an SRMA suggesting a 6% excess mortality when albumin was administered to intensive care patients. It was not possible to duplicate that finding in a large, well-conducted RCT; hence, on the one hand, the administration of albumin (with the exception of traumatic brain injury) is indeed "safe." However, albumin is a scarce and expensive blood product (in some parts of the world) and may be hard to justify on economic grounds in these countries.

The SAFE study investigators have followed this up with a series of short prevalence studies looking at changes in fluid resuscitation practice over time [1, 8]. A similar methodology has been used in other major fluid resuscitation trials comparing hydroxyethyl starch with saline, and balanced salt solution with saline, and these will be separately discussed in this book [9, 10].

10.11 Summary

SAFE was one of the first large, pragmatic, investigator-initiated clinical trials in intensive care medicine. It was conducted rigorously and proved the feasibility of a blinded fluid resuscitation trial. It recruited quickly with a simple and pragmatic design, and at the time was one of the largest trials conducted in intensive care medicine. Like all good trials, it answered questions but also raised new ones, which led to further research.

References

1. Finfer S, Liu B, Taylor C, Bellomo R, Billot L, Cook D, Du B, McArthur C, Myburgh J for the SAFE TRIPS Investigators. Resuscitation fluid use in critically ill adults: an international cross-sectional study in 391 intensive care units. Crit Care. 2010;14:R185.
2. Cochrane Injuries Group Albumin Reviewers. Human albumin administration in critically ill patients: systematic review of randomized controlled trials. BMJ. 1998;317:235–40.
3. Offriga M. Excess mortality after human albumin administration in critically ill patients. Clinical and pathophysiological evidence suggests albumin is harmful. BMJ. 1998;317:223–4.
4. Choi PT, Yip G, Quinonez LG, Cook DJ. Crystalloids vs colloids in fluid resuscitation: a systematic review. Crit Care Med. 1999;27:200–10.
5. Finfer S, Bellomo R, Boyce N, et al. A comparison of albumin and saline for fluid resuscitation in the intensive care unit. N Engl J Med. 2004;350(22):2247–56. https://doi.org/10.1056/NEJMoa040232.
6. The SAFE Study Investigators. Saline or albumin for fluid resuscitation in patients with traumatic brain injury. N Engl J Med. 2007;357:874–84.
7. Saline versus Albumin Fluid Evaluation Investigators. Effect of baseline serum albumin concentration on outcome of resuscitation with albumin or saline in patients in intensive care units: analysis of data from the SAFE study. Br Med J. 2006;333:1044–9.
8. Hammond NE, Taylor C, Saxena M, Liu B, Finfer S, Glass P, Seppelt I, Willenberg L, Myburgh J for the George Institute for Global Health and the Australian and New Zealand Intensive Care Society Clinical Trials Group. Resuscitation fluid use in Australian and New Zealand intensive care units between 2007 and 2013. Intensive Care Med. 2015;41(9):1611–9.
9. Myburgh JA, Finfer S, Bellomo R, Billot L, Cass A, Gattas D, Glass P, Lipman J, Liu B, McArthur C, McGuinness S, Rajbhandari D, Taylor CB, Webb SA, CHEST Investigators; Australian and New Zealand Intensive Care Society Clinical Trials Group. Hydroxyethyl starch or saline for fluid resuscitation in intensive care. N Engl J Med. 2012;367(20):1901–11.
10. Finfer S, Micxallef S, Hammond N, Navarra L, Bellomo R, Billot L, Delaney A, Gallagher M, Gattas D, Li Q, Mackle D, Mysore J, Saxena M, Raylor C, Young P, Myburgh J, PLUS Study Investigators and the Australian and New Zealand Intensive Care Society Clinical Trials Group. Balanced multielectrolyte solution versus saline in critically ill adults. N Engl J Med. 2022;386(9):815–26.

Albumin Replacement in Severe Sepsis and Septic Shock: The ALBIOS Trial

11

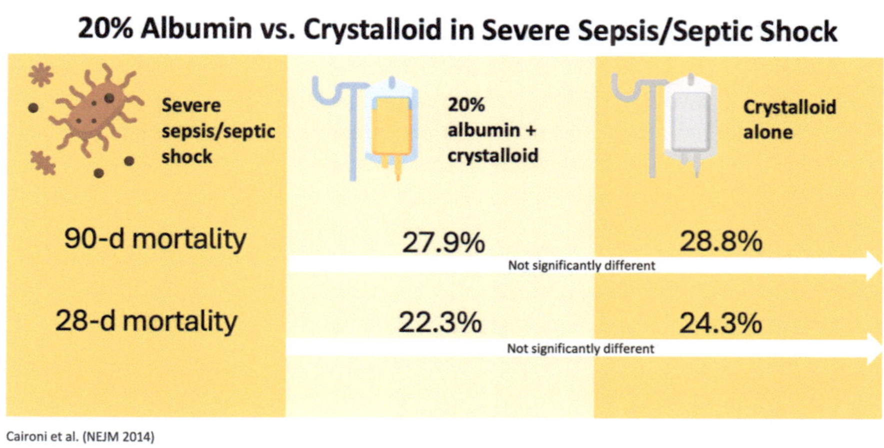

Quick Take

Does albumin infusion play a role in sepsis management?

The ALBIOS trial investigated the role of albumin in patients with severe sepsis or septic shock. This large, multicenter, randomized controlled trial (RCT) included 1800 patients who were randomized to receive either albumin (along with crystalloids) or crystalloids alone for fluid resuscitation. The study found no significant difference in 28-day mortality between the albumin group and the control group. However, patients who received albumin required less vasopressor support and

---

Caironi P, Tognoni G, Masson S, Fumagalli R, Pesenti A, Romero M, et al. Albumin Replacement in Patients with Severe Sepsis or Septic Shock. N Engl J Med. 2014 Apr 10;370(15):1412–21

J. Chacko et al., *Landmark Studies in Critical Care*,
https://doi.org/10.1007/978-981-95-0673-6_11

experienced a shorter duration of ICU stay. A post hoc subgroup analysis also suggested improved survival in patients with septic shock with the use of albumin. This trial provided important insights into fluid resuscitation in sepsis, suggesting that while albumin did not improve survival, it may be useful in reducing vasopressor dependency.

11.1 Introduction

There is a strong physiological rationale behind albumin administration in septic patients—one of the main purported benefits is the maintenance of the colloidal osmotic pressure. In 1979, Weil et al. observed that the iatrogenic dilution of plasma proteins due to what they referred to as "overzealous administration of crystalloids" may be detrimental [1].

Oxidative stress constitutes one of the hallmarks of sepsis. The thiol groups, abundant in albumin solution, are electron acceptors and act as powerful antioxidants. Albumin administration to septic patients was shown to produce a sustained increase in thiol levels, suggesting an important mechanism of clinical benefit [2]. Furthermore, albumin solutions may exert anti-inflammatory and immunomodulating effects that may impart beneficial effects in sepsis. Albumin may also attenuate sepsis-induced vascular dysfunction through its nitric oxide scavenging properties [3].

The SAFE trial had previously compared 4% albumin with normal saline as resuscitation fluid in critically ill patients. Overall, there was no difference in the 28-day mortality, duration of mechanical ventilation, ICU stay, or the duration of renal replacement therapy between the two groups. However, a pre-defined subgroup analysis of patients with severe sepsis revealed a lower risk of death with albumin administration [4]. Another RCT in a medical-surgical ICU compared albumin administration among patients with hypoalbuminemia (serum albumin ≤30 g/L) with a control group that received no albumin. Improved organ function, based on the Sequential Organ Failure Assessment (SOFA) score, was observed in the albumin group, mainly related to improved respiratory, cardiovascular, and central nervous system function [5].

In a later meta-analysis, Delaney et al. included RCTs that employed albumin-containing solutions compared with other types of fluid for fluid resuscitation among patients with sepsis. They included 1977 patients from 17 studies. Eight studies evaluated patients with sepsis, while in nine studies, septic patients represented a subgroup of the study population. Albumin use for resuscitation of septic patients was associated with lower mortality in the pooled estimate [6].

Against this background, the ALBIOS study investigators conducted an RCT to evaluate the efficacy of albumin in septic patients. They compared clinical outcomes using a combination of 20% albumin and crystalloids with a control group that received crystalloids alone among patients with severe sepsis and septic shock [7].

11.2 Population and Design

The ALBIOS (Albumin Italian Outcome Sepsis) study was conducted between August 2008 to February 2012 across 100 ICUs in Italy. Adult patients ≥18 years of age with severe sepsis by clinical criteria at any time during their ICU stay, within 24 h of meeting the inclusion criteria, were eligible.

11.2.1 Excluded

Patients who were terminally ill, those with traumatic brain injury, and congestive cardiac failure (New York Heart Association class of 3 or 4) were excluded. Patients in whom albumin was clinically indicated (cirrhosis with ascites, nephrotic syndrome, burns, etc.) were also excluded. Eligible patients were randomly allocated to receive a combination of 20% albumin with crystalloids (albumin group) or crystalloid solutions alone (crystalloid group) for 28 days after randomization or until ICU discharge.

11.3 The Albumin Group

Following randomization, 300 ml of 20% albumin was administered. On subsequent days until day 28 or ICU discharge, 20% albumin was administered every day, aiming to maintain the serum albumin level ≥30 g/L. Crystalloids were administered as clinically indicated, based on clinician judgment.

11.4 The Crystalloid Group

In this group, patients received crystalloids alone based as considered appropriate by the treating clinician. Emergency use of albumin was allowed in this group, although it was considered a violation of the study protocol.

11.5 Management in Both Groups

During the initial phase of resuscitation, both groups received intravenous fluids based on the early goal-directed therapy (EGDT) protocol proposed by Rivers et al. [8]. Synthetic colloids were not allowed; crystalloid administration was at the clinician discretion. All other aspects of care were left to the clinician judgment.

11.6 Sample Size

The sample size was calculated based on the 28-day mortality, the primary outcome. The authors assumed a baseline mortality of 45% with a 7.5% difference between groups. A sample size of 1350 patients provided the study with 80% power with a two-sided P value of <0.05. The sample size was increased to 1800 patients following an interim analysis.

11.7 Results

The study randomized a total of 1818 patients, including 910 in the albumin group and 908 in the crystalloid group. After the exclusion of eight patients, 1810 were included in the final analysis. Patients were well-matched at baseline, except for a marginal difference between groups in the central venous oxygen saturation and the number of patients with organ dysfunction. The indication for ICU admission was mostly medical; the common foci of infection were the lung and abdomen, followed by the urinary tract. The total volume of fluids administered was similar in both groups over the first 7 days. The serum albumin level was higher in the albumin group until day 28. The mean arterial pressure was higher, and the heart rate was slower in the albumin group over the first 7 days.

11.7.1 The Primary Outcome: Mortality at 28 Days

The 28-day mortality was similar in both groups—285 of 895 (31.8%) of patients had died compared to 288 of 900 (32%) of patients in the crystalloid group. The relative risk in the albumin group was 1.00, with a 95% confidence interval (CI) of 0.87–1.14 ($P = 0.94$).

11.7.2 Secondary Outcomes

The 90-day all-cause mortality, the main secondary outcome, was also similar in both groups. By 90 days, 365 of 888 (41.1%) patients had died in the albumin group compared to 389 of 893 (43.6%) patients in the crystalloid group (relative risk, 0.94; 95% CI, 0.85–1.05, $P = 0.29$). The overall SOFA score did not differ significantly between the two groups; however, the cardiovascular component of the SOFA score was lower in the albumin group, while the coagulation and liver dysfunction scores were higher. The higher coagulation sub-score was attributable to the lower platelet count, and the liver sub-score to a higher bilirubin level in the albumin group.

11.7.3 Tertiary Outcomes

The development of new organ dysfunction was similar in both groups. The incidence of acute kidney injury, the use of renal replacement therapy, and the duration of mechanical ventilation were also similar in both groups. Vasopressors were ceased earlier in the albumin compared to the crystalloid group. On subgroup analysis, no difference in outcomes was observed when patients were stratified based on the interval between meeting clinical criteria for severe sepsis and randomization.

11.7.4 Post Hoc Analysis

On post hoc univariate and multivariate analysis, outcomes were analyzed among 1121 patients with septic shock. The 90-day mortality was significantly lower in the albumin group among patients with septic shock (relative risk, 0.87; 95% CI, 0.77–0.99). In contrast, among patients with severe sepsis without shock, the mortality was higher in the albumin group, although the difference was not statistically significant. The main study outcomes are summarized in Table 11.1.

Table 11.1 Main study outcomes

Outcome	Albumin group (903 patients)	Crystalloid group (907 patients)	Significance
28-day mortality	285/895 (31.8%)	288/900 (32.0%)	RR: 1.00 (0.87–1.14) Not significant
90-day mortality	365/888 (41.1%)	389/893 (43.6%)	RR: 0.94 (0.85–1.05) Not significant
SOFA score (median, IQR)	6.00 (4.00–8.50)	5.62 (3.92–8.28)	Not significant
New-onset organ failure	464/836 (55.5%)	458/841 (54.5%)	Not significant
AKI	183/834 (21.9%)	190/837 (22.7%)	Not significant
Days to vasopressor cessation (median, IQR)	3 (1–6)	4 (2–7)	$P = 0.007$, significant
Septic shock, 90-day mortality	243/557 (43.6%)	281/563 (49.9%)	RR: 0.87 (0.77–0.99) $P = 0.03$, significant

Abbreviations: *SOFA* sequential organ failure assessment, *RR* relative risk, *IQR* interquartile range, *AKI* acute kidney injury

11.8 Study Conclusion

In patients with severe sepsis, the administration of albumin in addition to crystalloids, targeting a serum albumin level of ≥30 g/L, did not lead to improved survival compared to crystalloids alone.

Patients in the albumin group appeared to maintain better hemodynamic stability, with relatively higher mean arterial pressures, slower heart rates, and more rapid weaning of vasoactive drugs. These findings may support a physiological benefit of albumin use with greater fluid distribution within the intravascular compartment.

11.9 Strengths

The ALBIOS trial was an adequately powered, multicentric RCT that compared albumin with crystalloids among patients with severe sepsis. It was a pragmatic study that addressed an important clinical question regarding the appropriate type of fluid therapy in severe sepsis. There was minimal loss to follow-up.

11.10 Limitations

The study was unblinded and may have led to bias. The power calculation was based on a 28-day mortality of 45%, well below the observed mortality of 32%, and could have resulted in an underpowered study with a false negative result. The improved survival noted with albumin among patients with septic shock was based on post-hoc analysis, with a high likelihood of bias. In contrast to the SAFE trial that used a 4% albumin solution, the ALBIOS trial used 20% albumin, aiming for a serum albumin level of ≥30 g/L. Thus, albumin was not primarily administered as resuscitation fluid. Furthermore, most patients were enrolled in the later phase of severe sepsis. In the crystalloid group, 37% of patients received albumin, which may have affected outcomes.

11.11 Subsequent Analyses

A secondary analysis of the ALBIOS trial among immunocompromised patients did not reveal any advantage with the use of albumin in this subgroup of patients [9]. Another retrospective analysis of the ALBIOS trial compared the 90-day mortality among patients defined by Shock-2 and Shock-3 criteria. The patient cohort as defined by the Shock-3 criteria, based on the Sepsis-3 guidelines, was smaller, but carried higher mortality. The mortality benefit from albumin was no longer significant when septic shock was defined by the Shock-3 criteria [10].

11.12 Summary

The use of albumin in sepsis carries several putative physiological benefits. It maintains colloidal osmotic pressure besides exerting potential anti-inflammatory, immunomodulating, and nitric oxide scavenging effects. However, improved clinical outcomes with albumin administration in severe sepsis remained contentious. The SAFE trial had suggested improved survival with the use of 4% albumin as resuscitation fluid compared with normal saline among critically ill patients. Against this background, the ALBIOS investigators evaluated the efficacy of combining 20% albumin with crystalloids among patients with severe sepsis, targeting an albumin level of 30 g/L. The control group received crystalloids alone. This adequately powered RCT failed to reveal improved 28- or 90-day survival with the use of albumin, although the hemodynamic indices were more favorable in the albumin group, with earlier cessation of vasopressor support. A post hoc subgroup analysis suggested improved survival in patients with septic shock with the use of albumin; however, this finding requires validation in adequately powered RCTs.

References

1. Weil MH, Henning RJ, Puri VK. Colloid oncotic pressure: clinical significance. Crit Care Med. 1979;7(3):113–6.
2. Quinlan GJ, Margarson MP, Mumby S, Evans TW, Gutteridge JM. Administration of albumin to patients with sepsis syndrome: a possible beneficial role in plasma thiol repletion. Clin Sci Lond Engl 1979. 1998;95(4):459–65.
3. Stamler JS, Jaraki O, Osborne J, Simon DI, Keaney J, Vita J, et al. Nitric oxide circulates in mammalian plasma primarily as an S-nitroso adduct of serum albumin. Proc Natl Acad Sci USA. 1992;89(16):7674–7.
4. SAFE Study Investigators, Finfer S, McEvoy S, Bellomo R, McArthur C, Myburgh J, et al. Impact of albumin compared to saline on organ function and mortality of patients with severe sepsis. Intensive Care Med. 2011;37(1):86–96.
5. Dubois MJ, Orellana-Jimenez C, Melot C, De Backer D, Berre J, Leeman M, et al. Albumin administration improves organ function in critically ill hypoalbuminemic patients: A prospective, randomized, controlled, pilot study. Crit Care Med. 2006;34(10):2536–40.
6. Delaney AP, Dan A, McCaffrey J, Finfer S. The role of albumin as a resuscitation fluid for patients with sepsis: a systematic review and meta-analysis. Crit Care Med. 2011;39(2):386–91.
7. Caironi P, Tognoni G, Masson S, Fumagalli R, Pesenti A, Romero M, et al. Albumin replacement in patients with severe sepsis or septic shock. N Engl J Med. 2014;370(15):1412–21.
8. Rivers E, Nguyen B, Havstad S, Ressler J, Muzzin A, Knoblich B, et al. Early goal-directed therapy in the treatment of severe sepsis and septic shock. N Engl J Med. 2001;345(19):1368–77.
9. Cortegiani A, Grasselli G, Meessen J, Moscarelli A, Ippolito M, Turvani F, et al. Albumin replacement therapy in immunocompromised patients with sepsis – secondary analysis of the ALBIOS trial. J Crit Care. 2021;63:83–91.
10. Vasques F, Duscio E, Romitti F, Pasticci I, Caironi P, Meessen J, et al. Septic shock-3 vs 2: an analysis of the ALBIOS study. Crit Care. 2018;22:237.

Hydroxyethyl Starch vs. Normal Saline for Fluid Resuscitation: The CHEST Trial

12

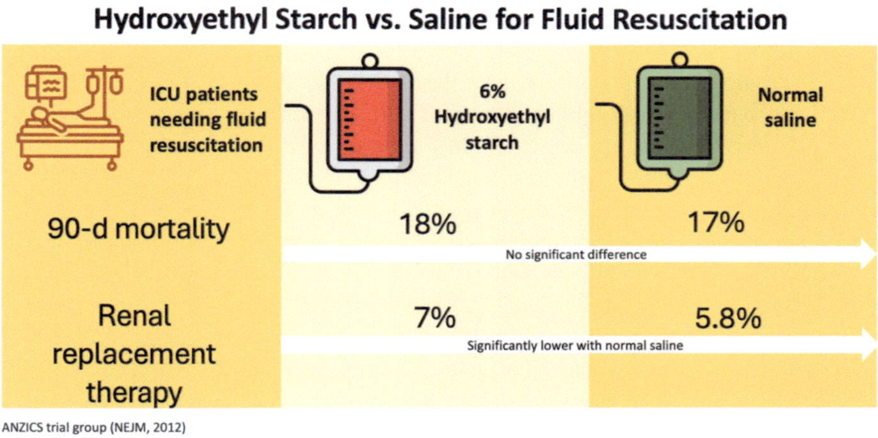

Quick Take

Does resuscitation with the synthetic colloid, hydroxyethyl starch (HES) impact outcomes in ICU patients?

This large, multicenter, randomized trial compared the use of HES with normal saline for fluid resuscitation in critically ill patients. The study involved 7000 patients and aimed to assess whether HES, a synthetic colloid, offered any advantage over the commonly used crystalloid, normal saline, in terms of mortality or kidney function. The results showed no significant difference in 90-day mortality

---

Myburgh JA, Finfer S, Bellomo R, Billot L, Cass A, Gattas D, et al. Hydroxyethyl Starch or Saline for Fluid Resuscitation in Intensive Care. N Engl J Med. 2012 Nov 15;367(20):1901–11.

J. Chacko et al., *Landmark Studies in Critical Care*,
https://doi.org/10.1007/978-981-95-0673-6_12

between the two groups. However, significantly more patients in the HES group required renal replacement therapy. The trial raised important concerns about the safety of HES in intensive care, leading to changes in fluid resuscitation practices in critical care settings worldwide.

12.1 Introduction

In the late nineteenth century, physiologists were fascinated by the movement of fluid between the intravascular and interstitial compartments and its effect on the circulating volume. Ernest Starling, working from his laboratory at Guy's Hospital in London, proposed that the net transudation of fluid depends on two forces. The capillary pressure tends to drive fluid out, while the colloid osmotic pressure, driven by proteins, enables reabsorption of fluid into the intravascular compartment. The pursuit of synthetic colloids with the potential to remain in circulation for a longer duration compared with crystalloids became the focus of interest in the early twentieth century.

The commercial starch solution, available from the early 1960s, was manufactured from potatoes or sorghum, a type of corn. Starch solutions, composed primarily of amylopectin, are unstable and undergo enzymatic degradation in the blood. They are treated with ethylene oxide to prevent enzymatic hydrolysis, resulting in the creation of the hydroxyethyl compound. Hydroxyethyl starch was considered superior to crystalloid solutions. It was reasonably priced and with a molecular weight of around 400,000, it persisted in circulation for a longer duration—sometimes for several weeks [1]. Even in the early days of clinical use, questions were raised regarding assimilation into tissues, with possible adverse outcomes. Initial studies revealed efficacy in animal models of hemorrhagic shock [2]. A later clinical trial suggested that plasma volume expansion may be almost twice as much with hydroxyethyl starch solutions compared with plasma, gelatin solutions, or dextran 70 [3].

Shortly after its introduction to clinical practice, concerns were raised regarding the safety profile of hydroxyethyl starch. Excessive bleeding was reported, possibly related to the depletion of clotting factors, including factor VIII, fibrinogen, and Von Willebrand factor [4]. Microcirculatory abnormalities and platelet dysfunction were also implicated. Renal dysfunction related to hydroxyethyl starch use was reported in patients with pre-existing nephropathy who underwent hemodilution [5]. Besides, histological lesions in transplanted kidneys were also observed [6]. Adding fuel to the fire were accusations of fraud and falsification of data in numerous trials of hydroxyethyl starch by Joachim Boldt, a German anesthesiologist. Subsequently, more than 90 studies authored by Boldt that favored the use of hydroxyethyl starch were withdrawn by international medical journals [7]. A subsequent meta-analysis of clinical trials that excluded studies by Boldt revealed significantly higher mortality and acute kidney injury with hydroxyethyl starch compared to other resuscitation fluids [8].

12.2 Background to the Trial

Subsequent clinical trials underscored the risk of acute kidney injury with the use of hydroxyethyl starch, particularly with the 10% solutions [9, 10]. A large randomized controlled trial (RCT) from Scandinavia also reported increased mortality with the use of 6% hydroxyethyl starch for the resuscitation of septic patients [11]. The Australian and New Zealand Intensive Care Society (ANZICS) Clinical Trials Group conducted the CHEST (Crystalloid versus Hydroxyethyl Starch Trial) RCT to evaluate the efficacy and safety of fluid resuscitation with a 6% hydroxyethyl starch solution in saline with a molecular weight of 130 kD (HES) in a heterogeneous group of ICU patients. The study fluid was compared with a control group who underwent resuscitation with normal saline [12].

12.3 Population and Design

The CHEST trial was a multicentric RCT conducted across 32 medical-surgical ICUs in Australia and New Zealand between December 2009 and January 2012. Patients admitted to the ICU who required fluid resuscitation according to the treating clinician were eligible. Fluid resuscitation was defined as any bolus administration in addition to maintenance or replacement fluids. The requirement for bolus fluid was based on clinician judgment, supported by objective criteria. The volume of fluid administered was titrated based on clinical findings. The study excluded patients who received ≥1000 ml of HES before ICU admission and those in whom renal replacement therapy was ongoing or imminent. Patients with intracranial hemorrhage, burns, and those who underwent cardiac surgery or liver transplant were also excluded. HES was ceased if renal replacement therapy was required. Among these patients, normal saline was recommended; however, any alternative, appropriate fluid could be used. The administration of resuscitation fluids in locations outside the ICU (e.g., intraoperative fluid administration) was not controlled.

12.4 Intervention

Patients were randomized to receive HES for resuscitation. HES was administered up to a maximum limit of 50 ml/kg/day; if any extra fluid was required, open-label normal saline was administered.

12.5 Control

Normal saline was administered in identical 500 ml bags.

12.6 Common Management

The use of maintenance fluids, nutrition, type of hemodynamic monitoring, vasoactive medication, respiratory, and renal support was based on clinician discretion. The pre-assigned fluid type was administered until discharge from the ICU, death, or 90 days post-randomization.

12.7 Sample Size

The authors estimated a baseline mortality of 26%. The study was powered to detect a 3.5% absolute difference in the 90-day mortality. A sample size of 7000 patients was calculated to provide 90% power at an alpha level of 0.05, assuming a 5% loss to follow-up. Furthermore, the study had 90% power at an alpha level of 0.05 to identify an absolute increase in the incidence of acute kidney injury (AKI) of 1.5%, assuming a baseline of 6%. Analysis was by intention-to-treat.

12.8 Results

A total of 7000 patients, with 3500 in each group, were randomized. After excluding patients who withdrew consent and were lost to follow-up, 3315 patients in the HES group and 3336 patients in the saline group were included in the 90-day analysis. The median APACHE II score was 17.0 in both groups. The incidence of AKI by the Risk, Injury, Failure, Loss, and End-stage renal failure (RIFLE) criteria was 36% in both groups. In the HES group, 29.2% of patients had sepsis compared with 28.4% in the normal saline group. Patients in the HES group received less fluid compared with the normal saline group in the first 4 days of ICU admission (526 ml vs. 616 ml); however, HES-treated patients received more blood products compared with normal saline.

12.8.1 The Primary Outcome: 90-Day Mortality

The 90-day mortality was not significantly different between the HES and the normal saline groups (18% vs. 17%; RR: 1.06, 95% CI: 0.96–1.18). On predefined subgroup analysis, the 90-day survival was similar in subgroups of patients with acute kidney injury, sepsis, trauma, traumatic brain injury, an APACHE II score of >25, and those who received HES before randomization.

12.8.2 Secondary Outcomes

Among the secondary outcomes, acute kidney injury requiring renal replacement therapy was significantly higher among HES-treated patients (7% vs. 5.8%; relative risk 1.21, 95% CI: 1.00–1.45; $p = 0.04$). Besides, based on RIFLE criteria, significantly more patients in the HES group sustained RIFLE-F type of dysfunction, while RIFLE-R and RIFLE-I were more common with normal saline.

No difference was observed between the two groups in the mortality in the ICU, hospital, or at 28 days. The duration of mechanical ventilation, renal replacement therapy, and hospital stay was also similar between the two groups. The incidence of new-onset hepatic failure was more common in the HES group, while new-onset cardiovascular failure was more common in the saline group.

On post hoc analysis, the urine output was significantly lower, and the serum creatinine levels were significantly higher in the HES group during the first week of treatment.

12.9 Adverse Events

The incidence of adverse events was significantly higher with HES compared with saline (4.6% vs. 3.3%); however, these were generally mild, with pruritus and rash being the most common. The main study outcomes are summarized in Table 12.1.

Table 12.1 Main study outcomes

Outcome	HES	NS	Significance
90-day mortality	18%	17%	$P = 0.26$
RRT	7%	5.8%	$P = 0.04$
New-onset cardiovascular failure	36.5%	39.9%	$P = 0.03$
ICU mortality	11%	10.8%	$P = 0.81$
Hospital mortality	14.6%	13.7%	$P = 0.3$

Abbreviations: *HES* hydroxyethyl starch, *NS* normal saline, *RRT* renal replacement therapy

12.10 Strengths

The CHEST trial was an adequately powered, multicentric RCT that evaluated the safety and efficacy of HES compared with normal saline as the resuscitation fluid. The study was double-blinded, thus minimizing bias. It was a pragmatic trial, with the requirement for fluid resuscitation based mainly on clinician judgment, and the volume of fluid administered was based on clinical assessment. The statistical analysis was planned a priori, and the analysis was by intention to treat.

12.11 Weaknesses

In the saline group, 15% of patients received HES before randomization, which may have affected the results. There was a 5% loss to follow-up; however, this was accounted for in the calculation of the sample size. The sample size calculation was wbased on a mortality rate of 26%; however, the actual mortality was much lower in both groups—this may have resulted in a false negative conclusion. The main secondary outcome was the requirement for renal replacement therapy. However, the decision to perform renal replacement therapy was not based on predefined criteria. The possibility of bias was considered low as the treating clinicians were blinded to the fluid assignment. The administration of resuscitation fluids in locations outside the ICU was not according to assignment and was not considered in the analysis.

The CHEST trial led to the restriction of HES use based on the recommendation by regulatory authorities. Following this, manufacturers of HES appealed against these recommendations, citing inaccuracies and misinterpretations of the trial. The trial sponsor, the George Institute for Global Health, initiated an independent re-analysis of the trial. Although minor differences were observed in some of the secondary and tertiary outcomes, these did not affect the conclusions drawn from the trial. The analysis of the primary and patient-centered outcomes revealed findings that were almost identical to the original trial, thus confirming the integrity of the trial and its conclusions [13].

12.12 Study Conclusion

In critically ill patients, the use of 6% HES compared with normal saline for resuscitation does not offer any clinical benefit. The requirement for renal replacement therapy may be higher with the use of HES.

12.13 Summary

The CHEST trial, along with the Scandinavian 6S trial that preceded it, settled the seemingly never-ending controversy over the use of HES, a synthetic colloid, as resuscitation fluid in critically ill patients. The use of HES as the resuscitation fluid led to a 21% relative increase in the requirement for renal replacement therapy, thus, convincingly establishing its adverse impact on renal function. The 90-day mortality was not significantly different between the HES and saline groups. The trial results indicated a mortality effect ranging between a relative decrease of 4% to a relative increase of 18% with the use of HES. The serum creatinine levels were consistently higher in HES-treated patients, further reinforcing the adverse impact on renal function. Furthermore, new-onset hepatic dysfunction was also more common with HES resuscitation. Globally, the pendulum has swung away from the use of HES, with many regulatory bodies placing stringent restrictions on its use.

References

1. Maguire LC, Strauss RG, Koepke JA, Bowman RJ, Zelenski KR, Lambert RM, et al. The elimination of hydroxyethyl starch from the blood donors experiencing single of multiple intermittent-flow centrifugation leukapheresis. Transfusion (Paris). 1981;21(3):347–53.
2. Ballinger WF, Solanke TF, Thompson WL. The effect of hydroxyethyl starch upon survival of dogs subjected to hemorrhagic shock. Surg Gynecol Obstet. 1966;122(1):33–6.
3. Solanke TF, Khwaja MS, Madojemu EI. Plasma volume studies with four different plasma volume expanders. J Surg Res. 1971;11(3):140–3.
4. Alexander B, Odake K, Lawlor D, Swanger M. Coagulation, hemostasis, and plasma expanders:a quarter century enigma. Fed Proc. 1975;34(6):1429–40.
5. Waldhausen P, Kiesewetter H, Leipnitz G, Scielny J, Jung F, Bambauer R, et al. Hydroxyethyl starch-induced transient renal failure in preexisting glomerular damage. Acta Med Austriaca. 1991;18(Suppl 1):52–5.
6. Legendre C, Thervet E, Page B, Percheron A, Noël LH, Kreis H. Hydroxyethylstarch and osmotic-nephrosis-like lesions in kidney transplantation. Lancet Lond Engl. 1993;342(8865):248–9.
7. Tramèr MR. The Boldt debacle. Eur J Anaesthesiol. 2011;28(6):393–5.
8. Antonelli M, Sandroni C. Hydroxyethyl starch for intravenous volume replacement: more harm than benefit. JAMA. 2013;309(7):723–4.
9. Schortgen F, Lacherade JC, Bruneel F, Cattaneo I, Hemery F, Lemaire F, et al. Effects of hydroxyethylstarch and gelatin on renal function in severe sepsis: a multicentre randomised study. Lancet Lond Engl. 2001;357(9260):911–6.
10. Dart AB, Mutter TC, Ruth CA, Taback SP. Hydroxyethyl starch (HES) versus other fluid therapies: effects on kidney function. Cochrane Database Syst Rev. 2010;2013(1):CD007594.
11. Perner A, Haase N, Guttormsen AB, Tenhunen J, Klemenzson G, Åneman A, et al. Hydroxyethyl Starch 130/0.42 versus Ringer's Acetate in Severe Sepsis. N Engl J Med. 2012;367(2):124–34.
12. Myburgh JA, Finfer S, Bellomo R, Billot L, Cass A, Gattas D, et al. Hydroxyethyl starch or saline for fluid resuscitation in intensive care. N Engl J Med. 2012;367(20):1901–11.
13. Patel A, Pieper K, Myburgh JA, Perkovic V, Finfer S, Yang Q, et al. Reanalysis of the crystalloid versus hydroxyethyl starch trial (CHEST). N Engl J Med. 2017;377(3):298–300.

Balanced Crystalloid vs. Normal Saline for Resuscitation: The SMART Trial

13

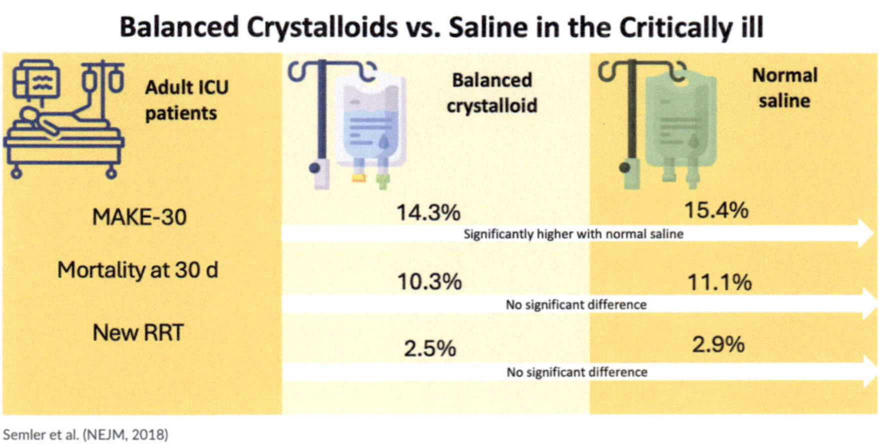

Quick Take

In critically ill adults, does the use of balanced crystalloids improve clinical outcomes compared to normal saline for fluid resuscitation?

This cluster-randomized, multiple-crossover trial enrolled 15,802 ICU patients across five US medical centers to evaluate the impact of balanced crystalloids (Lactated Ringer's or Plasma-Lyte A) versus saline. The study demonstrated that balanced crystalloids significantly reduced the incidence of the composite outcome compared to saline, particularly in minimizing kidney injury and improving

Semler MW, Self WH, Wanderer JP, Ehrenfeld JM, Wang L, Byrne DW, et al. Balanced crystalloids versus saline in critically ill adults. N Engl J Med. 2018 Mar 1;378(9):829–839.

J. Chacko et al., *Landmark Studies in Critical Care*,
https://doi.org/10.1007/978-981-95-0673-6_13

metabolic outcomes. There was no increase in adverse events in the balanced crystalloids group, highlighting their safety.

These findings established balanced crystalloids as a preferred option over saline for fluid resuscitation in critically ill patients, influencing clinical guidelines and practice globally.

13.1 Introduction

For decades, 0.9% sodium chloride (normal saline) has been the most commonly used intravenous fluid for resuscitation in critically ill patients. While inexpensive and universally available, saline contains a relatively high chloride concentration (154 mmol/L). Besides, it lacks buffer compounds and may induce hyperchloremic metabolic acidosis, with possible impairment of renal function [1]. Balanced crystalloids such as lactated Ringer's solution and Plasma-Lyte A more closely resemble plasma in composition and include buffers like lactate or acetate.

Several observational studies and randomized controlled trials (RCTs) have suggested that balanced crystalloids may reduce the risk of acute kidney injury (AKI), the need for renal replacement therapy (RRT), and even mortality when compared to saline [2–4]. However, two pilot trials—SPLIT and the SALT—found no significant difference in outcomes between saline and balanced fluids [5, 6]. The SMART trial was designed to definitively determine whether the composition of intravenous fluid impacts clinical outcomes in critically ill adults [7].

13.2 Population and Design

The SMART (Isotonic Solutions and Major Adverse Renal Events Trial) was a pragmatic, unblinded, cluster-randomized, multiple-crossover study conducted in five ICUs at Vanderbilt University Medical Center from June 2015 to April 2017 [8]. The participating ICUs included medical, surgical, trauma, neurological, and cardiac ICUs.

Each ICU was randomized monthly to use either balanced crystalloids or saline. During each calendar month, all patients admitted to a particular ICU received the fluid assigned for that month. The alternating crossover design mitigated selection bias and allowed early initiation of the assigned therapy.

All adults (≥18 years) admitted to one of the ICUs during the study period were included. Patients could be re-enrolled if they were readmitted to an ICU during the trial.

13.2.1 Exclusion

There were no patient-level exclusions; however, clinicians could override the fluid assignment if they considered it to be unsafe. Relative contraindications to balanced crystalloids included hyperkalemia and traumatic brain injury.

Patients already on RRT before ICU admission were excluded from specific renal outcome analyses, although they were still included in the composite primary outcome if they died during hospitalization.

13.3 Intervention

Patients in ICUs assigned to the intervention arm received balanced crystalloids—either lactated Ringer's or Plasma-Lyte A—for all isotonic crystalloid administration during ICU and hospital stay. The specific fluid chosen was left to the preference of the treating clinician.

13.4 Control

Patients in control ICUs received 0.9% sodium chloride (saline) exclusively for isotonic fluid therapy throughout their ICU and hospital stay.

13.5 Common Management

All other management strategies, including hemodynamic monitoring, vasopressor use, ventilation, nutrition, and medication, were left to the clinician discretion. The use of non-isotonic fluids, blood products, and medications was not protocolized. Coordination with the emergency department and operating rooms ensured that the assigned fluid was administered across care settings when feasible.

13.6 Sample Size Calculation

The initial plan was to enrol 8000 patients over 60 unit-months, assuming a 22% event rate in the saline group, aiming to detect a 12% relative risk reduction in the primary outcome with 90% power. Observational data later suggested a lower baseline event rate (approximately 15%), prompting extension of the trial to 82 unit-months and increasing the sample size to 14,000 participants. The final enrolment was 15,802 patients (7942 in the balanced crystalloids group and 7860 in the saline group).

13.7 Results

13.7.1 Primary Outcome

The primary outcome was a major adverse kidney event within 30 days (MAKE30), a composite of:

- Death from any cause
- New initiation of RRT
- Persistent renal dysfunction (final creatinine ≥200% of baseline)

This was censored at hospital discharge or 30 days after ICU admission, whichever came first.

The primary outcome occurred in 14.3% of the balanced crystalloids group vs. 15.4% in the saline group (adjusted OR 0.90, 95% CI 0.82–0.99; $P = 0.04$).

13.7.2 Secondary Outcomes

The secondary outcomes included the three components of the primary outcome.

- 30-day in-hospital mortality: 10.3% in the balanced group vs. 11.1% in the saline group ($P = 0.06$).
- New RRT: 2.5% vs. 2.9% ($P = 0.08$).
- Persistent renal dysfunction: 6.4% vs. 6.6% ($P = 0.60$).

The number of ICU-free, ventilator-free, and vasopressor-free days were similar in both groups. However, the mean RRT-free days was marginally higher (although not clinically significant) in the balanced crystalloid group (25.0 vs. 24.8 days; $P = 0.01$).

13.8 Subgroup Analyses

In prespecified subgroups, the benefit of balanced crystalloids was most pronounced among septic patients—MAKE30 was 25.2% with balanced fluids vs. 29.4% with saline (adjusted OR 0.80, 95% CI 0.67–0.97; $P = 0.02$). Besides, the beneficial effect of balanced crystalloids compared with saline appeared to be more pronounced among those who received larger volumes.

The main study outcomes are summarized in Table 13.1.

Table 13.1 Main study outcomes

Outcome	Balanced crystalloids	Saline	Significance
Major adverse kidney event (MAKE30)	14.3%	15.4%	$P = 0.04$
In-hospital mortality (30 days)	10.3%	11.1%	$P = 0.06$
New renal replacement therapy	2.5%	2.9%	$P = 0.08$
Persistent renal dysfunction	6.4%	6.6%	$P = 0.60$
ICU-free days (median)	25.3 days	25.3 days	$P = 0.94$
Ventilator-free days (median)	28.0 days	28.0 days	$P = 0.22$
Vasopressor-free days (median)	28.0 days	28.0 days	$P = 0.26$
RRT-free days (mean ± SD)	25.0 ± 8.6 days	24.8 ± 8.9 days	$P = 0.01$

13.9 Study Conclusion

In critically ill adults, the use of balanced crystalloids for intravenous fluid therapy resulted in a modest but statistically significant reduction in the composite outcome of death, new RRT, or persistent renal dysfunction at 30 days compared with saline. These benefits were more pronounced in septic patients and those receiving larger fluid volumes.

13.10 Strengths

The large sample size with >15,000 patients allowed the detection of small differences in outcome. The design was pragmatic, including all ICU admissions, enhancing real-world validity. The study interventions occurred early on during ICU admission. There was a low potential for selection bias; most patients who were admitted to the ICU during the study period were included in the study. Data collection was comprehensive from electronic health records. The authors conducted sensitivity analyses that enhanced the robustness of findings.

13.11 Weaknesses

The SMART trial was a single-center study and may limit generalizability. The unblinded design allowed knowledge of fluid type, which may have influenced RRT decisions. Patients staying across calendar months could receive both fluids. The follow-up was relatively short-term, with data censored at 30 days or discharge and may have missed later events. The trial was not designed to differentiate between lactated Ringer's and Plasma-Lyte A—as they were used interchangeably based on clinician preference.

13.12 Other Evidence

SMART results were corroborated by the SALT-ED [9] trial conducted simultaneously in non-critically ill patients in the emergency department. The two trials jointly shifted clinical guidelines towards the preferential use of balanced crystalloids in both ICU and ED settings.

13.13 Summary

The SMART trial convincingly demonstrated that, compared to saline, balanced crystalloids are associated with a lower incidence of major adverse kidney events in critically ill adults. While the absolute difference was modest, the implications are substantial given the widespread use of IV fluids in ICUs. With strong internal validity and practical applicability, SMART has helped clinicians reconsider the fluid resuscitation strategy, favoring balanced crystalloids in most critically ill patients.

References

1. Yunos NM, Kim IB, Bellomo R, et al. The biochemical effects of restricting chloride-rich fluids in intensive care. Crit Care Med. 2011;39(11):2419–24.
2. Shaw AD, Raghunathan K, Peyerl FW, et al. Association between IV chloride load during resuscitation and in-hospital mortality among patients with SIRS. Intensive Care Med. 2014;40(12):1897–905.
3. Rochwerg B, Alhazzani W, Sindi A, et al. Fluid resuscitation in sepsis: a systematic review and network meta-analysis. Ann Intern Med. 2014;161(5):347–55.
4. Raghunathan K, Shaw A, Nathanson B, et al. Association between the choice of IV crystalloid and in-hospital mortality among critically ill adults with sepsis. Crit Care Med. 2014;42(7):1585–91.
5. Young P, Bailey M, Beasley R, et al. Effect of a buffered crystalloid solution vs saline on acute kidney injury in the ICU: the SPLIT randomized trial. JAMA. 2015;314(16):1701–10.
6. Semler MW, Wanderer JP, Ehrenfeld JM, et al. Balanced crystalloids versus saline in the intensive care unit: the SALT randomized trial. Am J Respir Crit Care Med. 2017;195(10):1362–70.
7. Semler MW, Self WH, Wang L, et al. Balanced crystalloids vs saline in the ICU: study protocol for a cluster-randomized, multiple-crossover trial. Trials. 2017;18:129.
8. Semler MW, Self WH, Wanderer JP, et al. SMART Investigators and the Pragmatic Critical Care Research Group. Balanced crystalloids versus saline in critically ill adults. N Engl J Med. 2018;378(9):829–39.
9. Self WH, Semler MW, Wanderer JP, et al. Balanced crystalloids vs saline in noncritically ill adults. N Engl J Med. 2018;378(9):819–28.

Balanced Crystalloid vs. Normal Saline for Resuscitation: The BaSICS Trial

14

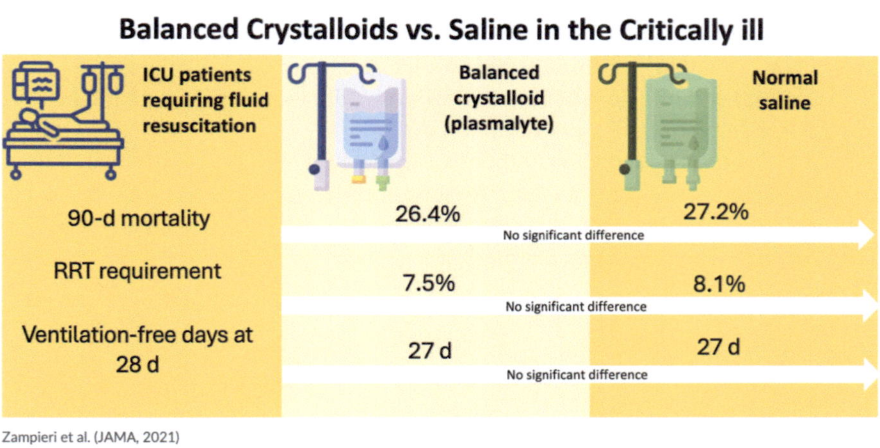

14.1 Introduction

The administration of intravenous fluids represents a key area of practice in the management of critically ill patients. Saline (0.9% sodium chloride) often constitutes the traditional choice of fluid; however, it may be associated with hyperchloremia and acidosis due to its high chloride content (154 mmol/L). Balanced

Zampieri FG, Machado FR, Biondi RS, et al. Effect of intravenous fluid treatment with a balanced solution vs 0.9% saline solution on mortality in critically ill patients: the BaSICS randomized clinical trial. JAMA. 2021;326(9):818–829.

J. Chacko et al., *Landmark Studies in Critical Care*,
https://doi.org/10.1007/978-981-95-0673-6_14

crystalloids such as Plasma-Lyte 148 are formulated to approximate plasma electrolyte composition more closely and contain buffer compounds like acetate and gluconate instead of chloride.

Evidence from observational studies and single-center trials, including the SMART and SALT-ED trials, has suggested improved outcomes with balanced crystalloids, with reduced renal complications and possibly lower mortality [1–3]. However, these trials were unblinded single-center studies. The BaSICS trial was designed to address this evidence gap through a large, multicenter, double-blind randomized controlled design, evaluating the effect of a balanced crystalloid compared to saline on 90-day mortality in critically ill patients [4].

14.2 Population and Design

The BaSICS trial was a multicenter, double-blind, 2 × 2 factorial randomized controlled trial conducted in 75 ICUs across Brazil, conducted between May 29, 2017, and March 2, 2020 [4]. The trial tested two interventions: fluid type (balanced solution vs saline) and infusion speed (rapid vs slow); the present report focused on the comparison between the types of fluid.

Eligible patients were adults admitted to the ICU with an anticipated stay of >24 h who required at least one fluid expansion and met at least one high-risk criterion (e.g., age >65, hypotension or vasopressor use, sepsis, mechanical ventilation ≥12 h, kidney dysfunction, or liver failure).

14.3 Exclusion

Patients were excluded if they had any of the following:

- Imminent death within 24 h.
- Brain death or receiving palliative care alone.
- Severe electrolyte disturbances (Na ≤120 or ≥160 mmol/L).
- Those who were already receiving or imminently required RRT (within 6 h).
- Prior enrolment in the study.

Hyperkalemia (>5.5 mEq/L) was an initial exclusion criterion initially but was removed following an interim analysis.

14.4 Intervention

Patients randomized to the intervention group received Plasma-Lyte 148 as the intravenous fluid during the ICU stay, including bolus therapy, maintenance fluids, and drug infusions >100 mL. The fluid was administered in coded, identical bags, ensuring blinding of clinicians and study personnel.

14.5 Control

The control group received 0.9% sodium chloride (normal saline), also in coded, indistinguishable bags. As with the intervention group, saline was used for all fluid requirements in the ICU, including bolus administration and infusions exceeding 100 mL.

14.6 Common Management

All other aspects of ICU management were determined by treating physicians. The study fluid administration was mandated for all eligible indications during the ICU stay. Drug infusions ≤100 mL and fluids outside the ICU (e.g., in the operating rooms or the emergency department) were not protocolized. Clinicians remained blinded to fluid assignment; adherence was regularly monitored on days 1, 2, 3, and 7 after randomization.

14.7 Sample Size Calculation

The authors assumed a 90-day mortality rate of 35% in the control group and targeted detection of a 10% relative reduction (HR 0.90) with 89% power and $\alpha = 0.05$. The study aimed to enrol 11,000 patients. A total of 11,052 were randomized according to plan; 10,520 were included in the final analysis after accounting for post-randomization exclusions due to withdrawal of consent or duplication.

14.8 Results

14.8.1 Primary Outcome

The primary outcome was 90-day survival. Mortality occurred in 26.4% of patients in the balanced solution group vs 27.2% in the saline group [adjusted hazard ratio (HR) 0.97; 95% CI, 0.90–1.05; $P = 0.47$]; the difference was not statistically significant.

14.8.2 Secondary Outcomes

Secondary outcomes included the need for RRT, acute kidney injury (AKI) incidence, organ dysfunction scores, and ventilator-free days; none of these were significantly different between the two groups.

- RRT within 90 days: 7.5% (balanced) vs 8.1% (saline); RR 0.95 (95% CI, 0.83–1.08).

- AKI by KDIGO stage ≥2 at day 3: 27.2% (balanced) vs 27.8% (saline); OR 0.99 (95% CI, 0.88–1.11).
- SOFA score at day 7: Median 4 in both groups; difference was driven by worse neurological scores in the balanced group.
- Neurological SOFA >2 at day 7: 32.1% (balanced) vs 26.0% (saline); OR 1.40 (95% CI, 1.18–1.66).
- Days alive and free of mechanical ventilation at 28 days: Similar (median 27 days in both groups).

14.8.3 Tertiary Outcomes

- ICU mortality: 17.4% (both groups).
- Hospital mortality: 22.6% (balanced) vs 23.0% (saline); OR 0.98 (95% CI, 0.88–1.09).
- Median ICU and hospital LOS: 3 and 8–9 days, respectively, for both groups.

The main study outcomes are summarized in Table 14.1.

Table 14.1 Main study outcomes

Outcome	Balanced solution	Saline	Significance
90-day mortality	26.4%	27.2%	$P = 0.47$
Use of RRT within 90 days	7.5%	8.1%	*RR* = 0.95 (95% CI 0.83–1.08)
KDIGO stage ≥2 at day 3	27.2%	27.8%	*OR* = 0.99 (95% CI 0.88–1.11)
Neurological SOFA >2 at day 7	32.1%	26.0%	*OR* = 1.40 (95% CI 1.18–1.66)
Median ICU length of stay	3 days	3 days	*P* = NS
Median hospital length of stay	8 days	9 days	*P* = NS
Median ventilator-free days (28 day)	27 days	27 days	*P* = NS
ICU mortality	17.4%	17.4%	*P* = NS
Hospital mortality	22.6%	23.0%	*OR* = 0.98 (95% CI 0.88–1.09)

14.9 Study Conclusion

In this large, double-blind, multicenter trial, the use of a balanced solution (Plasma-Lyte 148) did not significantly reduce 90-day mortality compared with saline among critically ill adults requiring bolus fluid therapy. These results contrasted with previous single-center trials such as SMART and SALT-ED and did not support a mortality benefit of Plasma-Lyte over saline.

14.10 Strengths

The large sample size and high event rate ensured sufficient power for detecting modest treatment effects. The double-blind design with indistinguishable fluid bags minimized ascertainment bias. The multicentric design across 75 ICUs enhances external validity and generalizability. The study followed a standardized protocol for fluid use during ICU stay with good adherence rates (80%+). Data collection was rigorous, including SOFA scores, chloride levels, and longitudinal outcomes.

14.11 Weaknesses

The non-protocolized administration of fluid before ICU admission may have diluted the treatment effect. The mortality was lower than expected and may have reduced the statistical power to detect differences. The study population was heterogeneous, including nearly 50% elective surgical patients with relatively low severity of illness. The findings with the use of a single balanced solution tested (Plasma-Lyte 148) may not be generalizable to other balanced fluids like lactated Ringer's. Neurological outcomes were worse with balanced fluids among patients with traumatic brain injury; the clinical significance of this finding remains unclear.

14.12 Other Evidence

The BaSICS trial contrasts with the SMART trial, which demonstrated a statistically significant reduction in the composite outcome with balanced crystalloids compared with normal saline [1]. However, while SMART was an unblinded, single-center study, BaSICS represents more rigorous, multicenter, blinded data. The conflicting findings of these trials have led to a continued debate about the optimal fluid for resuscitation, particularly in patients without large-volume needs and those who undergo elective surgery. The PLUS trial, published subsequently, also showed no mortality benefit of balanced fluids over saline in a broad ICU population [5].

Current guidelines now take a more nuanced approach, recommending balanced fluids for patients at high risk for kidney injury or receiving large volumes, while acknowledging that evidence does not clearly favor one fluid for all ICU patients [6].

14.13 Summary

The BaSICS trial showed that the use of a balanced crystalloid (Plasma-Lyte 148) compared to saline in critically ill patients did not reduce 90-day mortality or major secondary outcomes, including the need for RRT or the hospital length of stay. This high-quality, double-blind multicenter trial contrasts with prior observational and single-center studies, and calls into question the assumption that balanced fluids are universally superior. Subgroup signals of harm in traumatic brain injury also raise caution and need further investigation. The findings of the BaSICS trial reinforce the need for individualized fluid choice, guided by clinical context, patient characteristics, and volume requirements.

References

1. Semler MW, Self WH, Wanderer JP, et al. Balanced crystalloids versus saline in critically ill adults. N Engl J Med. 2018;378(9):829–39.
2. Self WH, Semler MW, Wanderer JP, et al. Balanced crystalloids vs saline in noncritically ill adults. N Engl J Med. 2018;378(9):819–28.
3. Yunos NM, Bellomo R, Hegarty C, et al. Association between a chloride-liberal vs chloride-restrictive fluid strategy and kidney injury in critically ill adults. JAMA. 2012;308(15):1566–72.
4. Zampieri FG, Machado FR, Biondi RS, et al. Effect of intravenous fluid treatment with a balanced solution vs 0.9% saline solution on mortality in critically ill patients: the BaSICS randomized clinical trial. JAMA. 2021;326(9):818–29.
5. Finfer S, Mouncey PR, Hammond NE, et al. Balanced multielectrolyte solution versus saline in critically ill adults. N Engl J Med. 2022;386(9):815–26.
6. National Institute for Health and Care Excellence (NICE). Intravenous fluid therapy in adults in hospital. Clinical guideline [CG174]. Published 2013. Updated 2021.

Balanced Multielectrolyte Solution vs. Normal Saline for Resuscitation: The PLUS Trial

15

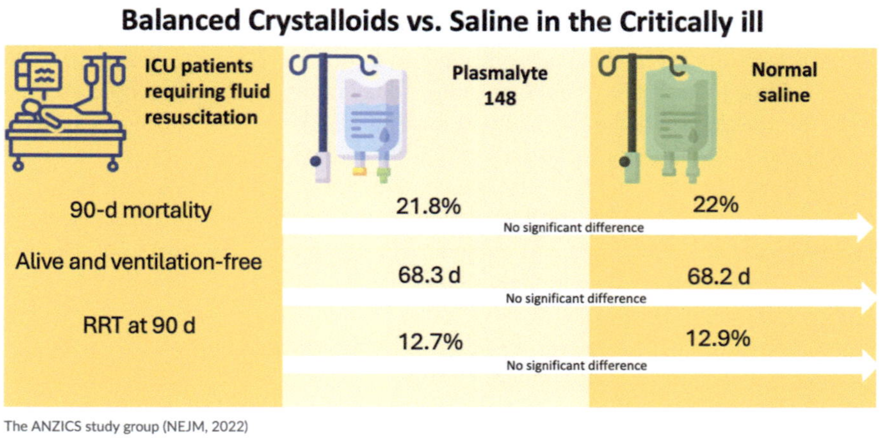

Quick Take

In critically ill adults, does a balanced multielectrolyte solution improve outcomes compared to saline for fluid resuscitation?

This key randomized controlled trial enrolled 5037 ICU patients across multiple centers in Australia and New Zealand to compare the effects of Plasma-Lyte 148 (a balanced multielectrolyte solution) versus 0.9% saline. The study found no

---

Zampieri FG, Machado FR, Biondi RS, et al. Effect of intravenous fluid treatment with a balanced solution vs 0.9% saline solution on mortality in critically ill patients: the BaSICS randomized clinical trial. JAMA. 2021;326(9):818–829.

J. Chacko et al., *Landmark Studies in Critical Care*,
https://doi.org/10.1007/978-981-95-0673-6_15

significant difference in 90-day mortality between the balanced solution and saline groups. Additionally, there were no substantial differences in secondary outcomes, including renal complications or other adverse events. The trial demonstrated the safety of both fluids while highlighting that neither offered a clear advantage in overall mortality or key clinical outcomes.

These results provide critical insights into fluid management in the ICU, affirming that balanced multielectrolyte solutions and saline are both acceptable options for fluid resuscitation, with decisions likely best guided by individual patient needs and clinician preference.

15.1 Introduction

Intravenous fluid therapy is one of the most widely used interventions in intensive care. Historically, 0.9% sodium chloride (saline) has been the default choice due to its isotonicity and broad compatibility. However, the high chloride content and absence of buffering agents can contribute to hyperchloremic metabolic acidosis; adverse clinical outcomes, including acute kidney injury (AKI) and increased mortality, have been reported in critically ill patients [1, 2].

Balanced crystalloids—Plasma-Lyte 148 and lactated Ringer's—resemble plasma more closely in their electrolyte content and contain buffers including acetate and gluconate. These fluids have a more favorable impact on the acid-base status and have been associated with a lower risk of AKI and improved outcomes in previous observational and interventional studies [3, 4].

The Plasma-Lyte 148 versus Saline (PLUS) trial was designed to definitively assess whether use of a balanced multielectrolyte solution compared with saline improves survival in a broad population of ICU patients [5].

15.2 Population and Design

The PLUS trial was a double-blind, multicenter, randomized controlled trial conducted across 53 ICUs in Australia and New Zealand between September 2017 and December 2020 [5]. Adult patients ($\geq$18 years) were eligible if they had been admitted to an ICU in the preceding 24 h and were expected to stay in the ICU and receive intravenous fluids for at least 3 days.

Randomization was stratified by site; patients were assigned in a 1:1 ratio to receive either Plasma-Lyte 148 or saline (0.9% sodium chloride) for fluid therapy during their ICU stay.

15.3 Exclusion

Patients with a specific indication for or contraindication to either study fluid (e.g., cerebral edema, hyponatremia, hyperkalemia), and those who received >500 mL of the non-assigned fluid during ICU stay were not included in the study. Those with traumatic brain injury, advanced directives for limiting care, or expected to die were also excluded.

15.4 Intervention

Patients in the intervention arm received Plasma-Lyte 148, a buffered, balanced multielectrolyte solution containing sodium 140 mmol/L, chloride 98 mmol/L, and acetate and gluconate buffers. It was used for all compatible intravenous therapies, including boluses, infusions, and maintenance fluids, for up to 90 days in the ICU.

15.5 Control

The control group received 0.9% sodium chloride (saline) in an identical packaging and followed the same protocol for administration.

15.6 Common Management

Other aspects of ICU care were left to the discretion of treating teams. Fluids could be withheld or changed only if deemed clinically necessary. Use of open-label fluids outside the ICU was permitted and not restricted by the protocol.

15.7 Sample Size Calculation

The trial originally planned to enrol 8800 patients, assuming a baseline 90-day mortality of 23% and targeting a 2.9% absolute reduction in mortality, providing the study with 90% power. Due to recruitment delays during the COVID-19 pandemic, the sample size was reduced to 5037 patients—the revised sample was powered to detect an absolute reduction in mortality by 3.8% at a two-sided α level of 0.05.

15.8 Results

15.8.1 Primary Outcome

The 90-day mortality was similar in both groups—21.8% in the BMES group vs 22.0% in the saline group. The adjusted risk difference was −0.15 percentage points (95% CI, −3.60 to 3.30), $P = 0.90$; adjusted odds ratio: 0.99 (95% CI, 0.86–1.14).

15.8.2 Secondary Outcomes

Among the secondary outcomes, the requirement for renal replacement therapy was similar in both groups (Plasma-Lyte 148: 12.7% vs. saline: 12.9%(saline). The maximum creatinine rise was 0.41 mg/dL in both groups. The ICU mortality (16.2% vs 15.4%), hospital mortality (20.7% vs 21.2%), and the 28-day mortality (18.5% vs 18.4%) were not significantly different. The number of ventilator-free days also did not differ significantly in both groups (~68.3 days). The chloride levels were lower and the arterial pH higher in the Plasma-Lyte 148 group. The main study findings are summarized in Table 15.1.

Table 15.1 Main study findings

Outcome	Balanced solution	Saline	Significance
90-day mortality	21.8%	22.0%	$P = 0.90$
New renal replacement therapy	12.7%	12.9%	Not significant
Maximum creatinine rise in ICU	0.41 mg/dL	0.41 mg/dL	Not significant
ICU mortality	16.2%	15.4%	Not significant
Hospital mortality	20.7%	21.2%	Not significant
28-day mortality	18.5%	18.4%	Not significant
Ventilator-free days (90 days)	68.3 days	68.3 days	Not significant
Chloride level (day 1–7)	Lower	Higher	Biochemical difference
pH (day 1–7)	Higher	Lower	Biochemical difference

15.9 Study Conclusion

The use of Plasma-Lyte 148 in critically ill adults did not reduce 90-day mortality compared to saline. There were no significant differences in renal outcomes or other secondary endpoints, despite the modest biochemical differences observed.

15.10 Strengths

The PLUS study followed a robust, double-blind, placebo-controlled design. The multicentric study, including 53 ICUs, offers external validity. There was strict adherence to the study protocol with detailed follow-up. The authors carried out a comprehensive evaluation of hard-core clinical outcomes.

15.11 Weaknesses

Open-label use of fluid was allowed outside the ICU. Besides, the non-study fluid was administered to some patients in both groups, which could have impacted the results. A reduction in the sample size, inevitable as it may have been due to the COVID-19 pandemic, could also have limited the power of the study to detect differences between groups. The volume of fluid administered may have been modest. Longer-term outcomes that may have been relevant were not reported.

15.12 Subsequent Evidence

The findings of the PLUS trial are consistent with the BaSICS trial [6], which also found no significant benefit of balanced fluids over saline. However, they contrast with the SMART trial [4], which showed reduced kidney injury and mortality with balanced crystalloids. Meta-analyses suggest any benefit may be confined to high-risk subgroups or those receiving large volumes of fluid [7].

15.13 Summary

The PLUS trial demonstrated that use of a balanced multielectrolyte solution did not reduce 90-day mortality or renal complications in critically ill adults compared to saline. While balanced fluids may result in a more favorable biochemical profile, they do not seem to impact clinical outcomes, particularly in the volumes commonly employed. These studies underline the need for individualized fluid strategies.

References

1. Yunos NM, Bellomo R, Hegarty C, Story D, Ho L, Bailey M. Association between a chloride-liberal vs chloride-restrictive intravenous fluid administration strategy and kidney injury in critically ill adults. JAMA. 2012;308(15):1566–72.
2. Shaw AD, Raghunathan K, Peyerl FW, et al. Association between intravenous chloride load during resuscitation and in-hospital mortality among patients with systemic inflammatory response syndrome. Intensive Care Med. 2014;40(12):1897–905.
3. Raghunathan K, Shaw A, Nathanson B, et al. Association between the choice of intravenous crystalloid and in-hospital mortality among critically ill adults with sepsis. Crit Care Med. 2014;42(7):1585–91.
4. Semler MW, Self WH, Wanderer JP, et al. Balanced crystalloids versus saline in critically ill adults. N Engl J Med. 2018;378(9):829–39.
5. Finfer S, Micallef S, Hammond N, et al. Balanced multielectrolyte solution versus saline in critically ill adults. N Engl J Med. 2022;386(9):815–26.
6. Zampieri FG, Machado FR, Biondi RS, et al. Effect of intravenous fluid treatment with a balanced solution vs 0.9% saline solution on mortality in critically ill patients: the BaSICS randomized clinical trial. JAMA. 2021;326(9):818–29.
7. Hammond NE, Bellomo R, Gallagher M, et al. Balanced crystalloids versus saline in critically ill adults: a systematic review and meta-analysis. Crit Care Med. 2022;50(3):432–41.

16 Conservative vs. Liberal Fluid Management in ARDS: The FACTT Trial

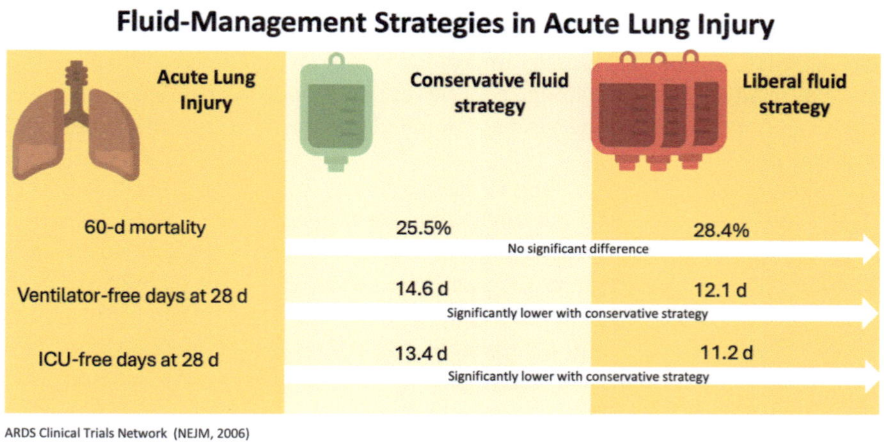

Quick Take

Can less fluid be more in acute lung injury (ALI) and acute respiratory distress syndrome (ARDS)?

This FACTT randomized controlled trial compared two fluid-management strategies in patients with acute lung injury (ALI) or acute respiratory distress syndrome (ARDS): a conservative versus a liberal fluid strategy. The conservative approach

---

National Heart, Lung, and Blood Institute Acute Respiratory Distress Syndrome (ARDS) Clinical Trials Network, Wiedemann HP, Wheeler AP, Bernard GR, Thompson BT, Hayden D, et al. Comparison of two fluid-management strategies in acute lung injury. N Engl J Med. 2006 Jun 15;354(24):2564–75.

J. Chacko et al., *Landmark Studies in Critical Care*,
https://doi.org/10.1007/978-981-95-0673-6_16

aimed to minimize fluid overload by using lower volumes of intravenous fluids, while the liberal approach allowed for more fluid resuscitation. The 60-day mortality, the primary outcome, was not different between the two groups. However, a conservative strategy resulted in improved lung function, with better lung injury scores and oxygenation indexes, and, importantly, a shorter duration of mechanical ventilation and ICU stay.

16.1 Introduction

Fluid accumulation in the lung provoked by increased capillary permeability is the hallmark of the adult respiratory distress syndrome (ARDS). Lung edema is perpetuated by an increase in the capillary hydrostatic pressure and a reduction in the oncotic pressure. The optimal fluid management strategy in ARDS had remained contentious. The adoption of a conservative approach with limitation of intravenous fluid administration and augmentation of urine output using diuretics may alleviate lung edema, thereby improving ventilatory parameters. Such a strategy may enable earlier weaning from ventilator support and improve survival. Conversely, a fluid-restrictive strategy might also reduce cardiac output and lead to organ dysfunction.

Evaluation of a restrictive fluid strategy among patients with ARDS had been largely confined to observational studies, and the results remained inconclusive.

In a retrospective study, ARDS patients with a low cumulative fluid balance and a weight loss of >3 kg had improved survival compared to their counterparts with a higher cumulative balance and net weight gain [1]. Another retrospective analysis suggested that a reduction in the pulmonary capillary wedge pressure by ≥25% resulted in improved survival in ARDS patients [2]. Martin et al. conducted an RCT of 37 mechanically ventilated patients with acute lung injury and a serum total protein level ≤5.0/dl [3]. In the intervention arm, they administered 25 g of human albumin/8 h with a continuous infusion of furosemide for 5 days. The control arm received a dual placebo. They observed improved PaO_2/FiO_2 ratios in the treatment group, although the respiratory mechanics and hospital mortality were similar.

Considering the lack of robust evidence to support a conservative fluid strategy, the National Heart, Lung, and Blood Institute Acute Respiratory Distress Syndrome (ARDS) Clinical Trials Network designed an RCT that compared a fluid-conservative with a liberal strategy among patients with acute lung injury (ALI) and its impact on clinical outcomes [4]. The study also aimed to compare central venous pressure with pulmonary artery occlusion pressure monitoring to assess the filling status.

16.2 Population and Design

The Fluid and Catheter Therapy Trial (FACTT) enrolled patients with ALI from 20 North American centers between June 2000 and October 2005. For eligibility, patients had to be on mechanical ventilation with a PaO_2/FiO_2 ratio of <300 and bilateral lung infiltrates on chest radiography consistent with pulmonary edema, with no features suggestive of left atrial hypertension. Eligible patients were randomized to undergo a conservative or a liberal fluid management strategy for 7 days. In a two-by-two design, they were also randomized to receive a central venous or pulmonary artery catheter to assess volume status within 4 h post-randomization.

16.2.1 Exclusion

Patients with ALI of >48 h duration and those with a pulmonary artery catheter after the onset of ALI were excluded. Those with chronic comorbidities that could impact survival, affect weaning from ventilator support, or influence compliance with the trial protocol (e.g., severe lung disease, neuromuscular disorders, dialysis dependence) were not eligible. Terminally ill patients with an estimated 6-month mortality of >50% (e.g., advanced malignancy) were also excluded.

A predefined protocol was followed in the conservative and liberal fluid management groups. The protocol was determined every 4 h based on 20 predefined cells, based on the following parameters:

- Central venous pressure (CVP) or pulmonary artery occlusion pressure (PAOP), based on group assignment.
- The presence of shock—defined as a mean arterial pressure (MAP) of <60 mm Hg or the requirement for any dose of vasopressor, except dopamine 5 mcg/kg/min.
- Oliguria—defined as urine output of <0.5 ml/kg/h.
- Effectiveness of circulation—ineffective circulation was defined as a cardiac index of <2.5 l/min/m^2 in the pulmonary artery catheter group. In the central venous catheter group, cold, mottled skin and a capillary refill time of >2 s represented ineffective circulation.

16.3 The Fluid-Conservative Strategy

In the conservative arm, normotensive patients with "effective" circulation without oliguria received furosemide, aiming for a CVP of <4 mm Hg or a PAOP of <8 mm Hg. The furosemide dose was guided by the urine output in the preceding hours; it was withheld if the patient was in shock within the previous 12 h.

16.4 The Fluid-Liberal Strategy

In the liberal arm, they received intravenous fluids aiming for higher filling pressures—a CVP of 10–14 mm Hg or a PAOP of 14–18 mm Hg.

16.5 Both Groups

The choice of intravenous fluid was left to the clinician discretion; however, the volume of fluid to be administered was defined in the protocol. Among patients in shock, the management was left to the clinician judgment; once the blood pressure was stable, weaning of vasopressor support was protocol-based.

Mechanical ventilation was carried out based on the ARDS-Network low tidal volume protocol. Weaning from ventilation was also protocolized. The assigned strategy was commenced within 2 h of catheter insertion (central venous or pulmonary artery catheter) and continued for 7 days or after 12 h of unassisted breathing. The pulmonary artery catheter could be replaced with a central venous catheter after 3 days if hemodynamic stability was achieved.

16.6 Sample Size

The primary outcome was in-hospital mortality at 60 days post-randomization. The authors assumed a mortality reduction of 10 percentage points (from 31% to 21%). A sample size of 1000 patients provided the study with 90% power to assess in-hospital mortality.

16.7 Results

Among the 1000 patients randomized, 503 were included in the conservative group and 497 in the liberal group. The study population included mostly medical patients (66%). Baseline characteristics, including age, gender, cause of ALI, severity of illness, organ dysfunction, fluid balance before study commencement, presence of shock, and vasopressor use, were similar in both groups. The underlying etiology of ALI included pneumonia (47%), followed by sepsis (25%), and pulmonary aspiration (14%).

There was a substantial difference in the 7-day cumulative fluid balance between the liberal and conservative groups (6992 ± 502 ml vs. 136 ± 491 ml, $P < 0.001$). The difference was even more profound among patients with shock at baseline—10,138 ± 922 vs. 2904 ± 1008 ml ($P < 0.001$). The liberal group received more fluid compared to the conservative group on every study day between days 1—4. The cardiac index and MAP were marginally lower in the conservative strategy group.

16.8 The Primary Outcome: Death at 60 Days

The 60-day in-hospital mortality was similar in both groups (conservative vs. liberal: 25.5% vs. 28.4%, $P = 0.30$).

16.9 Other Outcomes

At 28 days post-randomization, patients in the conservative strategy group experienced significantly higher ventilator-free days (14.6 ± 0.5 vs. 12.1 ± 0.5 days, $P < 0.001$). Patients in the conservative strategy group also spent less time in the ICU. The number of ICU-free days was longer between days 1–7 (0.9 ± 0.1 vs. 0.6 ± 0.1 days) and between days 1–28 (13.4 ± 0.4 vs. 11.2 ± 0.4 days) in the conservative group. The number of organ failure-free days (cardiovascular, renal, and hepatic) was similar in both groups at 28 days. The requirement for renal replacement therapy (RRT) was similar in both groups at 60 days. The number of days of renal support among those who required RRT was also similar.

16.10 Safety Outcomes

Electrolyte abnormalities were reported more often in the conservative strategy group, although there were no associated arrhythmias. Hypokalemia and metabolic alkalosis were observed more commonly in the conservative strategy group. The main study outcomes are summarized in Table 16.1.

Table 16.1 Main study outcomes

Outcome	Conservative	Liberal	P-value
7-day cumulative fluid balance	136 ± 491 ml	6992 ± 502 ml	<0.001
In-hospital mortality at 60 days	25.5%	28.4%	0.30
Ventilator-free days at day 28	14.6 ± 0.5	12.1 ± 0.5	<0.001
ICU-free days at 1–7 days	0.9 ± 0.1	0.6 ± 0.1	<0.001
ICU-free days at 1–28 days	13.4 ± 0.4	11.2 ± 0.4	<0.001

16.11 Comparison between Pulmonary Artery Catheter vs. Central Venous Catheter

The main clinical outcomes were uninfluenced by the type of monitoring—CVP vs PAOP. However, catheter-related complications were twice as high with pulmonary artery catheters compared to central venous catheters, primarily related to arrhythmias. Patients who underwent pulmonary artery catheterization received more blood transfusions compared to those who underwent central venous catheterization (38% vs. 30%).

16.12 Strengths

The FACTT trial was a multicentric RCT powered to evaluate clinical outcomes. The study followed a strictly protocolized approach with a clear-cut decision-making tree based on hemodynamic parameters. The study personnel underwent extensive training to familiarize themselves with the study protocol. Compliance with the study protocol was monitored twice daily; the adherence rate was high (approximately 90%) and similar in both groups. Follow-up was nearly complete, except for the sole patient who withdrew consent. Analysis was performed on an intention-to-treat basis. There was a clear separation in the cumulative fluid balance between the study arms at the end of the study week, rendering the comparison meaningful.

16.13 Limitations

A large number of patients (91%) were excluded, raising the possibility of selection bias. The main reasons for exclusion were chronic lung disease, end-stage renal disease on dialysis, chronic liver disease, and acute myocardial infarction. The study findings may not be applicable to these subgroups of patients. Lack of blinding may also have led to bias; however, a rigid protocol was followed and reviewed periodically, and could have mitigated the impact of bias on clinical outcomes. The majority of patients (66%) were medical; hence, extrapolation of the study findings to surgical patients may be limited. The trial used a meticulous, labor-intensive protocol that may be difficult to reproduce in the real world. Besides, after decades of controversy surrounding its use, currently, the pulmonary artery catheter is rarely used by clinicians among the general critically ill population.

There was a 24-hour gap between the diagnosis of ALI and the study intervention. Would the results be different with earlier intervention? The FACTT trial also revealed no improvement in survival or organ function with pulmonary artery catheter compared with central venous catheter-guided therapy. The lower duration of mechanical ventilation and ICU stay observed in the conservative group were secondary outcomes, for which the study was not powered.

16.14 Study Conclusions

A fluid-conservative compared to a fluid-restrictive strategy did not significantly impact the 60-day mortality among patients with ALI or ARDS. However, a conservative strategy led to improved lung function, with more favorable lung injury scores and oxygenation indexes. The duration of mechanical ventilation and ICU stay was shorter with a fluid-conservative approach.

16.15 Subsequent Evidence

Stewart et al. performed a subgroup analysis of 244 surgical patients enrolled in the FACTT trial [5]. A conservative fluid strategy and CVP-guided therapy resulted in a shorter duration of mechanical ventilation and ICU stay. Furthermore, a conservative strategy did not result in a higher incidence of acute kidney injury. The 60-day mortality did not differ between the two groups, regardless of catheter type or fluid strategy.

Later studies from the Acute Respiratory Distress Syndrome Network used a simpler conservative protocol called "FACTT Lite." This protocol applied to patients who were off vasopressors for >12 h and had a MAP of >60 mm Hg. Fluid boluses or furosemide were administered based on the central venous pressure and the urine output. Grissom et al. performed a retrospective comparison of the liberal and conservative strategies of the FACTT trial and the FACTT lite protocol [6]. The cumulative fluid balance over 7 days was 918 ± 323 ml, 6992 ± 502 ml, and −136 ± 491 ml in the FACTT Lite, liberal, and conservative groups, respectively. The number of ventilator-free days was similar in the FACTT lite and conservative arms and significantly higher compared to the liberal arm. The incidence of acute kidney injury was also similar in the FACTT Lite and conservative groups. FACTT lite may be simpler and easier to perform at the bedside, with clinical outcomes similar to the FACTT-conservative strategy.

16.16 Summary

The optimal fluid management among patients with acute lung injury was unclear, with no robust evidence to support a conservative compared with a liberal strategy. The National Heart, Lung, and Blood Institute Acute Respiratory Distress Syndrome (ARDS) Clinical Trials Network group conducted an RCT that compared a fluid-restrictive with a liberal strategy. Patients were also randomized to undergo pulmonary artery or central venous catheterization in a two-by-two factorial design.

A conservative fluid strategy resulted in improved lung function, with better lung injury scores and oxygenation indexes, and, importantly, a shorter duration of mechanical ventilation and ICU stay. The volume of fluid administered was considerably lower in the conservative group; however, it did not lead to a higher incidence of organ failures or shock. The findings of the FACTT trial drove home the importance of titrated fluid resuscitation during the "ebb" phase of shock, and scaling it down once the "flow" phase has reached—with normalization of cardiac output and reversal of shock. Taking it one step further would be the strategy of "de-resuscitation" during the flow phase, including the use of diuretics that may have salutary effects on lung function. However, the switch from the "ebb" to the "flow" phase may represent a grey zone; hence, appropriate timing of the de-resuscitation strategy is crucial. Overall, the FACTT trial supported a conservative compared with a liberal fluid strategy among patients with acute lung injury. The choice of catheter—central venous or pulmonary artery catheter—did not impact outcomes.

References

1. Simmons RS, Berdine GG, Seidenfeld JJ, Prihoda TJ, Harris GD, Smith JD, et al. Fluid balance and the adult respiratory distress syndrome. Am Rev Respir Dis. 1987;135(4):924–9.
2. Humphrey H, Hall J, Sznajder I, Silverstein M, Wood L. Improved survival in ARDS patients associated with a reduction in pulmonary capillary wedge pressure. Chest. 1990;97(5):1176–80.
3. Martin GS, Mangialardi RJ, Wheeler AP, Dupont WD, Morris JA, Bernard GR. Albumin and furosemide therapy in hypoproteinemic patients with acute lung injury. Crit Care Med. 2002;30(10):2175–82.
4. National Heart, Lung, and Blood Institute Acute Respiratory Distress Syndrome (ARDS) Clinical Trials Network, Wiedemann HP, Wheeler AP, Bernard GR, Thompson BT, Hayden D, et al. Comparison of two fluid-management strategies in acute lung injury. N Engl J Med. 2006;354(24):2564–75.
5. Stewart RM, Park PK, Hunt JP, McIntyre RC, McCarthy J, Zarzabal LA, et al. Less is more: improved outcomes in surgical patients with conservative fluid administration and central venous catheter monitoring. J Am Coll Surg. 2009;208(5):725–35. discussion 735-737
6. Grissom CK, Hirshberg EL, Dickerson JB, Brown SM, Lanspa MJ, Liu KD, et al. Fluid management with a simplified conservative protocol for the acute respiratory distress syndrome*. Crit Care Med. 2015;43(2):288–95.

Part III

Cardiopulmonary Resuscitation

17 Compression-Only Cardiopulmonary Resuscitation in Out-of-Hospital Cardiac Arrest: The DART Trial

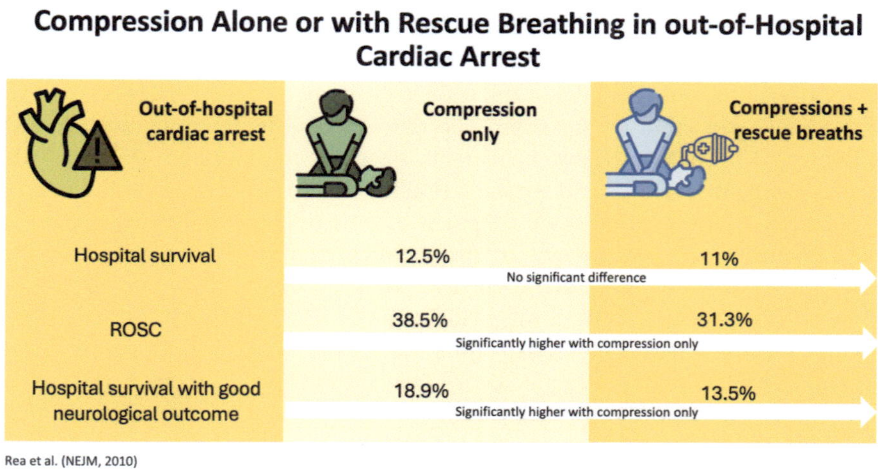

Quick Take

Bystander-initiated cardiopulmonary resuscitation (CPR) with chest compressions alone or with rescue breathing: which saves more lives?

This study evaluated the outcomes of bystander-initiated CPR using either chest compressions alone or conventional CPR with rescue breathing in out-of-hospital cardiac arrest cases. Including 1941 patients, the findings revealed that compression-only CPR was at least as effective as conventional CPR in improving survival

---

Rea TD, Fahrenbruch C, Culley L, Donohoe RT, Hambly C, Innes J, et al. CPR with chest compression alone or with rescue breathing. N Engl J Med. 2010 Jul 29; 363(5):423–33.

J. Chacko et al., *Landmark Studies in Critical Care*,
https://doi.org/10.1007/978-981-95-0673-6_17

rates and favorable neurological outcomes. Its simplicity may increase bystander willingness to perform CPR, potentially saving more lives. However, the study acknowledged that conventional CPR might still be preferred in specific circumstances, such as in pediatric cases or arrests of respiratory origin.

17.1 Introduction

Internal cardiac massage was employed to resuscitate the arrested heart from the late nineteenth century. This technique was largely confined to intraoperative cardiac arrest in anesthetized patients. If the abdomen was open, the surgeon would attempt subdiaphragmatic compression, a technique later found to be largely ineffective. Hence, if spontaneous cardiac activity did not occur, the diaphragm was incised, and direct compression of the heart was carried out. In their treatise of 1952, Bost et al. described a success rate of one-third with this technique [1].

The adequacy of external chest compression had been evaluated in animals much earlier, followed by several reports in humans. However, by the early twentieth century, external compressions had been all but given up in favor of direct massage through an open chest or abdomen. The efficacy of external compressions was rediscovered by William Kouwenhoven, an electrical engineer, during his experiments with defibrillation techniques at the Johns Hopkins University in Baltimore. He had placed heavy paddles on the chest of a dog while investigating external defibrillation. The sheer weight of the paddles increased the blood pressure. Furthermore, rhythmic pressure applied to the sternum seemed to maintain adequate circulation to the brain. It was evident that compression of the chest resulted in forward flow from the heart, while relaxation enabled refilling. William Kouwenhoven, with his colleagues James Jude and Guy Knickerbocker, reported a series of five patients who suffered cardiac arrest followed by successful resuscitation with external cardiac compressions [2]. They affirmed, "Anyone, anywhere, can now initiate cardiac resuscitative procedures. All that is needed are two hands." This report marked the rebirth of the era of external cardiac compressions as we know it today.

The importance of early initiation of cardiopulmonary resuscitation (CPR) was clearly the need of the hour. By the 1980s, telephonic instructions to provide CPR were provided to bystanders who sought assistance for out-of-hospital cardiac arrest, while emergency personnel were on the way. By the turn of the new millennium, dispatcher-assisted CPR was established in many emergency medical systems across the world.

17.2 Background to the Study

Historically, recommendations for out-of-hospital CPR by lay public included chest compressions combined with rescue breathing. A compression-only strategy avoided interruptions and had the potential to offer enhanced circulatory support

[3]; besides, it may be more acceptable among the lay public [4]. Attempts at rescue breathing during CPR may also lead to a rise in the intrathoracic pressure, reduction in the venous return, cardiac output, and impaired coronary flow. While a compression-only strategy may be advantageous if the underlying etiology is of cardiac origin, a primary respiratory cause clearly requires expeditious respiratory support. Animal studies suggested the efficacy of a tailored strategy based on the etiology of cardiac arrest [5]. Observational studies comparing a compression-only strategy with conventional CPR had revealed similar survival rates, although the findings were limited by confounders [6, 7]. A randomized controlled trial (RCT) that compared chest compression-only CPR with compressions interspersed with mouth-to-mouth respiration revealed improved survival to hospital discharge. Bystanders performed CPR based on instructions provided telephonically by dispatchers. Survival to hospital discharge was higher among those who received compression-only CPR, although the difference was not statistically significant (14.6% vs. 10.4%) [8].

The Dispatcher-Assisted Resuscitation Trial (DART) RCT compared two CPR approaches—chest compression-only vs. compressions combined with rescue breathing, carried out based on dispatcher instructions [9].

17.3 Population and Design

Three emergency services—two in the US (Washington state) and one in the UK (the London Ambulance Service) participated in the trial, conducted between 2004–2008. The trial considered emergency calls from bystanders for adult patients (>18 years) who had sustained out-of-hospital cardiac arrest. Patients who were deemed to be unconscious and not breathing normally by the dispatcher were eligible if CPR had not already been initiated. Randomization was carried out to one of two groups—compression-only CPR, or standard CPR with chest compression combined with rescue breathing. Randomization was stratified according to the dispatch center and carried out in blocks of 10.

17.4 Exclusion

Cardiac arrest due to trauma, drowning, asphyxiation, and those with a do-not-resuscitate order were excluded upon evaluation by the dispatcher. Patients could be excluded post-randomization; final eligibility required basic and advanced care from the emergency medical services (EMS). Patients who were judged to be not in cardiac arrest by the dispatcher, and those who were considered irreversible by the EMS, were also excluded.

17.5 Compression-Only Group

The dispatcher provided instructions to perform 50 consecutive compressions (one cycle). After completion of one cycle, the dispatcher enquired about signs of life; instructions were provided to continue compressions as appropriate.

17.6 Compressions with Rescue Breathing (Standard CPR Group)

Fifteen chest compressions were followed by two rescue breaths, with subsequent cycles in the same ratio. The dispatcher assessed the situation telephonically and provided instructions to continue CPR as appropriate.

17.7 Sample Size

The investigators designed the trial to identify a difference in survival by 3.5% points between the two groups, at a two-sided alpha level of 0.05 with 80% power.

17.8 Results

A total of 5525 patients were presumed to be in cardiac arrest and randomization envelopes were opened. Among these patients, 1941 fulfilled the inclusion criteria—981 in the compression-only group and 960 in the conventional group. An underlying cardiac cause was present in 70%; less than half were witnessed arrests, and about one-third presented with a shockable rhythm. The average time from dispatch to arrival of EMS personnel was 6.5 min. Baseline characteristics were similar in both groups. The location of the arrest—whether residential, nursing home, or at a public location was also similar.

17.9 The Primary Outcome: Survival to Hospital Discharge

Survival to hospital discharge could not be established in seven patients—three in the compression-only group and four in the conventional group. In the compression-only group, 122/978 (12.5%) patients survived to hospital discharge compared with 105/956 (11.0%) in the conventional group. The difference was not statistically significant ($p = 0.31$).

17.9.1 Subgroup Analysis

On predefined subgroup analysis, there was a trend toward improved survival to hospital discharge with compression-only CPR among patients with an underlying cardiac cause for the arrest (15.5% vs. 12.3%, $P = 0.09$). A similar trend favoring compression-only CPR was also observed among patients who had a shockable rhythm (31.9% vs. 25.7%, $p = 0.09$).

17.10 Secondary Outcomes

Return of spontaneous circulation at the end of EMS care was significantly higher in the compression-only group compared to the standard group (38.5% vs. 31.3%, $p = 0.005$). Survival to hospital discharge with a favorable neurological outcome, defined as a Cerebral Performance Category (CPC) score of 1 or 2, was similar between the two groups. However, among patients with an underlying cardiac cause for the arrest, survival to hospital discharge with a good neurological outcome was significantly higher in the compression-only group (18.9% vs. 13.5%, $p = 0.03$). The main study outcomes are summarized in Table 17.1.

Table 17.1 Main study outcomes

Outcome	Compression-only CPR	Compression + rescue breathing	Significance
Survival to hospital discharge	12.5%	11%	$P = 0.31$
Survival to hospital discharge in patients with shockable rhythm	31.9%	25.7%	$P = 0.09$
Survival to hospital discharge with favorable neurological outcome	14.4%	11.5%	$P = 0.13$
Survival to hospital discharge in patients with cardiac causes	15.5%	12.3%	$P = 0.09$
ROSC at end of EMS care	38.5%	31.3%	$P = 0.005$

Abbreviations: *CPR* cardiopulmonary resuscitation, *ROSC*, return of spontaneous circulation, *EMS* Emergency Medical Services

17.11 Strengths

The outcomes from out-of-hospital cardiac arrest have remained abysmal. CPR by the lay public may be of crucial importance in improving outcomes. The DART RCT addressed a simplified, compression-only approach to out-of-hospital CPR by the untrained. This large RCT involved three EMS providers and addressed clinically meaningful outcomes. The study offered sound evidence that compression-only CPR is at least equally effective compared with the standard approach of rescue breathing interspersed with compressions. Furthermore, a simplified approach may curtail fears of transmission of infection during rescue breathing. The study design and its systematic conduct, including validation of randomization by audio review, enabled tenability across a wider community.

17.12 Limitations

Although a large RCT, the study may still have lacked the requisite power to evaluate survival with favorable neurological outcomes. The neurological status was evaluated in only two of the three centers that participated in the study. The efficacy of interventions—including the depth of chest compression—was not objectively assessed. The study excluded patients with asphyxia, drowning, and trauma. Hence, the results cannot be generalized to heterogeneous causes of cardiac arrest. The compression to ventilation ratio followed was 15:2, although the American Heart Association (AHA) currently recommends a 30:2 ratio. Needless to emphasize, the efficacy of compression-only CPR in out-of-hospital cardiac arrest does not apply to trained rescuers.

17.13 Study Conclusions

The DART trial compared CPR instructions to the lay public in patients who suffered out-of-hospital cardiac arrest. Instructions were provided to perform chest compressions alone compared with compressions and rescue breathing. The overall survival to hospital discharge, the primary outcome, did not differ significantly between these strategies. However, subgroup analysis revealed that a compression-only strategy may improve survival in patients with an underlying cardiac cause and those with a shockable rhythm. Furthermore, survival to hospital discharge with a favorable neurological outcome was also higher in patients who received compression-only CPR.

17.14 Evidence from Other Studies

Yet another RCT comparing compression-only with standard CPR was published in the same issue of the New England Journal of Medicine. This study was conducted by the Swedish Emergency Medical Services, and included 1276 patients—620 patients were assigned to receive compression-only CPR and 656 to a standard strategy of two ventilations alternating with 15 compressions [10]. There was no significant difference in the 30-day survival between the two groups (compression-only vs. standard CPR: 8.7% vs. 7.0%, $p = 0.29$). Subgroup analysis revealed similar 30-day survival regardless of the location of the arrest, the time to EMS response, and the presenting cardiac rhythm.

A meta-analysis by Cabrini et al. included three RCTs that compared compression-only with standard CPR among patients with witnessed or unwitnessed cardiac arrest [11]. The meta-analysis included 3737 patients—1895 received compression-only CPR, while 1842 received standard CPR. Survival to hospital discharge was higher with compression-only CPR (11.5% vs. 9.4%, $p = 0.04$). These findings were echoed in the meta-analysis by Hüpfl et al. The primary meta-analysis of RCTs revealed that dispatcher-assisted compression-only CPR by lay public resulted in a 22% improvement in survival compared with standard CPR [12].

17.15 Summary

Standard CPR—with compressions interspersed with rescue breathing may have limitations when performed by the lay public. The efficacy of mouth-to-mouth respiration is questionable; besides, attempts at rescue breathing lead to undesirable interruption to compressions, likely to adversely impact the quality of CPR. Rescue breaths may also be detrimental during the early phase of CPR due to increased intrathoracic pressures, leading to reduced venous return. The lay public may also be reluctant to perform mouth-to-mouth rescue breathing on an unidentified victim, thereby exposing themselves to the possibility of transmission of infections. The concept of compression-only CPR had already been in vogue at the time of publication of the DART trial. This large RCT cemented the feasibility and efficacy of compression-only CPR, with the likelihood of improved outcomes, particularly among patients with an underlying cardiac cause for arrest. The authors suggested that attempts at rescue breathing by the lay public would likely have a deleterious impact emanating from the interruption of compressions. The American Heart Association recommends compression-only CPR by the lay public in patients with out-of-hospital cardiac arrest [3]. However, trained EMS personnel must continue to practice standard CPR in out-of-hospital cardiac arrest. Ventilation may be crucial with an underlying non-cardiac cause, especially related to primary respiratory failure.

References

1. Bost TC. Cardiac arrest during anesthesia and surgical operations. Am J Surg. 1952;83(2):135–42.
2. Kouwenhoven WB, Jude JR, Knickerbocker GG. Closed-chest cardiac massage. JAMA. 1960;173:1064–7.
3. Sayre MR, Berg RA, Cave DM, Page RL, Potts J, White RD, et al. Hands-only (compression-only) cardiopulmonary resuscitation: a call to action for bystander response to adults who experience out-of-hospital sudden cardiac arrest: a science advisory for the public from the American Heart Association emergency cardiovascular care committee. Circulation. 2008;117(16):2162–7.
4. Locke CJ, Berg RA, Sanders AB, Davis MF, Milander MM, Kern KB, et al. Bystander cardiopulmonary resuscitation. Concerns about mouth-to-mouth contact. Arch Intern Med. 1995;155(9):938–43.
5. Berg RA. Role of mouth-to-mouth rescue breathing in bystander cardiopulmonary resuscitation for asphyxial cardiac arrest. Crit Care Med. 2000;28(11 Suppl):N193–5.
6. Paredes VL, Rea TD, Eisenberg MS, Cobb LA, Copass MK, Cagle A, et al. Out-of-hospital care of critical drug overdoses involving cardiac arrest. Acad Emerg Med Off J Soc Acad Emerg Med. 2004;11(1):71–4.
7. Bohm K, Rosenqvist M, Herlitz J, Hollenberg J, Svensson L. Survival is similar after standard treatment and chest compression only in out-of-hospital bystander cardiopulmonary resuscitation. Circulation. 2007;116(25):2908–12.
8. Hallstrom A, Cobb L, Johnson E, Copass M. Cardiopulmonary resuscitation by chest compression alone or with mouth-to-mouth ventilation. N Engl J Med. 2000;342(21):1546–53.
9. Rea TD, Fahrenbruch C, Culley L, Donohoe RT, Hambly C, Innes J, et al. CPR with chest compression alone or with rescue breathing. N Engl J Med. 2010;363(5):423–33.
10. Svensson L, Bohm K, Castrèn M, Pettersson H, Engerström L, Herlitz J, et al. Compression-only CPR or standard CPR in out-of-hospital cardiac arrest. N Engl J Med. 2010;363(5):434–42.
11. Cabrini L, Biondi-Zoccai G, Landoni G, Greco M, Vinciguerra F, Greco T, et al. Bystander-initiated chest compression-only CPR is better than standard CPR in out-of-hospital cardiac arrest. HSR Proc Intensive Care Cardiovasc Anesth. 2010;2(4):279–85.
12. Hüpfl M, Selig HF, Nagele P. Chest-compression-only versus standard cardiopulmonary resuscitation: a meta-analysis. Lancet. 2010;376(9752):1552–7.

Part IV

Neurosciences

18 Intracranial Pressure Monitoring and Outcomes in Traumatic Brain Injury: The BEST-TRIP Trial

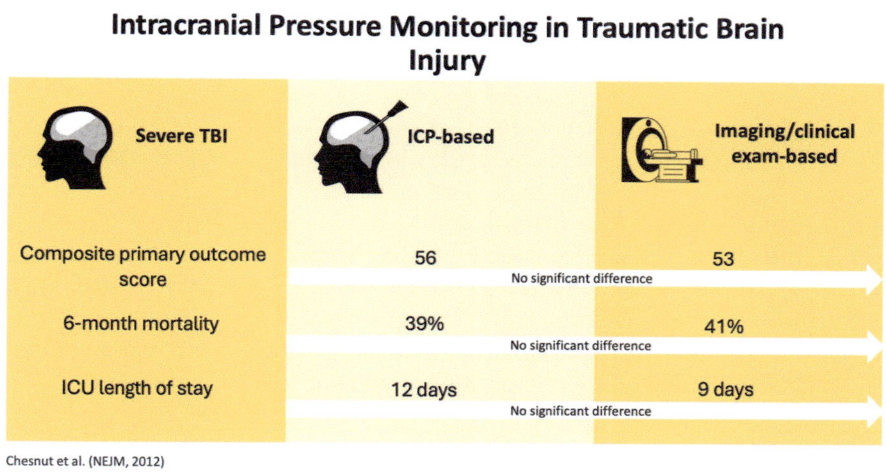

Quick Take

Does monitoring intracranial pressure improve survival in traumatic brain injury (TBI)?

The BEST-TRIP landmark trial explored the effectiveness of intracranial pressure (ICP) monitoring in improving outcomes among patients with severe TBI. A total of 324 patients with severe TBI were randomized to either receive ICP monitoring or standard clinical management without ICP monitoring. The study found

---

Chesnut RM, Temkin N, Carney N, Dikmen S, Rondina C, Videtta W, et al. A Trial of Intracranial-Pressure Monitoring in Traumatic Brain Injury. N Engl J Med. 2012 Dec 27;367(26):2471–81.

J. Chacko et al., *Landmark Studies in Critical Care*,
https://doi.org/10.1007/978-981-95-0673-6_18

no significant difference in mortality or functional outcomes between the two groups, suggesting that ICP monitoring did not confer a clear survival advantage. Despite its widespread use, the results of this trial raised questions about the utility of routine ICP monitoring in TBI management, challenging long-held practices in neurocritical care.

18.1 Introduction

In 1960, Nils Lundberg, a Swedish neurosurgeon, measured the intraventricular pressure (ICP) in 64 patients [1]. He inserted a plastic catheter into the frontal horn of the lateral ventricle and connected it to a strain gauge pressure transducer. Recording was carried out with an ink-writing potentiometer. Although archaic by modern standards, he used this equipment to identify three types of intracranial pressure waves. The large plateau-type "A" waves suggested a very high ICP of >50 mm Hg and imminent deterioration. This phase strongly correlated with symptoms of raised intracranial pressure (ICP), including headache, vomiting, irregular respirations, and hypertension. The rhythmically oscillating "B" waves at a frequency of 1–2/min suggested a lower ICP between 30 and 50 mm Hg, and the higher frequency "C" waves denoted an ICP of <30 mm Hg. Initially, neurosurgeons of that era were understandably reluctant to resort to invasive monitoring. By the 1970s and 80 s, Lundberg's technique gained more acceptance and was being increasingly employed in subarachnoid hemorrhage and traumatic brain injury. However, a 1978 survey of neurosurgical training programs in the USA revealed that ICP monitoring was rarely employed by neurosurgeons [2]. With increasing experience, more widespread use followed; between 1995 and 2005, ICP monitoring in traumatic brain injury had more than doubled in the USA.

Sahjpaul et al. conducted a survey of Canadian neurosurgeons regarding the utilization of ICP monitoring in traumatic brain injury more than two decades ago [3]. There appeared to be universal acceptance of ICP monitoring; however, only 20.4% of respondents expressed a high level of confidence in the efficacy of ICP monitoring to improve clinical outcomes. The majority of respondents believed that a prospective trial to evaluate the efficacy of ICP monitoring is warranted, considering the uncertainty regarding its clinical utility. A year later, Stocchetti et al. performed a questionnaire-based study on severe traumatic brain injury and ICP monitoring practices in Europe [4]. There was a wide variability in ICP and cerebral perfusion pressure monitoring among centers. Monitoring of ICP was a reliable tool in identifying intracranial hypertension when clinical signs alone were inconclusive. The incidence of complications related to ICP monitoring was low.

In the days before ICP monitoring became commonplace, surgical intervention for mass lesions was the only specific treatment modality available for traumatic brain injury. Identification of mass lesions was based on the limited diagnostic tools of the pre-CT era. With the advent of ICP monitoring, other therapeutic measures, including mechanical ventilation, sedation, and fluid management, could be instituted and titrated to the desired effect. In the meantime, CT imaging became widely available in the 1970s, allowing regular, rigorous evaluation of the injured brain, thus facilitating aggressive therapeutic interventions. The advent of CT technology led to a dramatic improvement in clinical outcomes following traumatic brain injury from the mid-1970s to the 1990s. However, from the 1990s onwards, clinical outcomes largely remained static. A 1995 survey involving trauma centers in the USA revealed that only 28% of centers routinely performed ICP monitoring in traumatic brain injury [5].

18.2 Background to the Trial

The evolution of ICP-based management has been intertwined with advances in other facets of care in the management of patients with severe traumatic brain injury. These advancements involved pre-hospital and emergency department care, besides groundbreaking improvements in neurointensive care and neurorehabilitation. It remained unclear if the improved clinical outcomes could be attributed to ICP measurement and monitoring or confounded by advancements in overall care. Observational studies revealed worse outcomes with an ICP-guided approach to managing severe traumatic brain injury, with a longer duration of mechanical ventilation, worse functional status, a higher risk of pneumonia, renal dysfunction, and mortality [6, 7]. Clinical guidelines also cite inadequate evidence to support the efficacy of ICP monitoring [8]. Although a randomized controlled trial (RCT) was called for, ethical considerations arose from having a control group without ICP monitoring, especially in settings where it was routine practice in severe traumatic brain injury.

In Latin America, intensivists routinely managed severe traumatic brain injury without recourse to ICP monitoring. There was a sufficient level of equipoise among them that allowed the conduct of an RCT to evaluate the efficacy of ICP monitoring without facing an ethical dilemma. The BEST-TRIP trial was conceptualized to include patients with severe traumatic brain injury from two Latin American countries—Bolivia and Ecuador, where ICP monitoring was not routinely carried out.

18.3 Study Hypothesis

The BEST-TRIP investigators compared a management protocol based on ICP monitoring with management guided by clinical examination and serial CT imaging. They hypothesized that ICP-guided management would lead to lower mortality, improved neuropsychological, and functional outcomes at 6 months.

18.4 Population and Design

The BEST-TRIP trial was a multicenter RCT conducted across six sites—four in Bolivia and two in Ecuador—among patients with severe traumatic brain injury [9]. The study was conducted between September 2008 and May 2012. Patients were randomized to undergo management based on ICP monitoring (the ICP group) or imaging and clinical examination (the I-CE group). Randomization was stratified by age, severity of injury, and study site. The study sites were staffed by intensivists and had round-the-clock neurosurgical cover and access to CT scan.

18.5 Inclusion Criteria

The study patients were ≥13 years with traumatic brain injury and a score on the Glasgow Coma Scale (GCS) between 3 and 8 on presentation, or within 48 h of injury. Among patients who were intubated and mechanically ventilated, the motor component of the GCS had to be between 1–5 for study inclusion.

18.6 Excluded

Patients with a GCS score of 3 and bilateral fixed, dilated pupils were excluded. Patients who were considered unlikely to survive were also excluded.

18.7 The ICP Group

Patients allocated to the ICP group underwent insertion of an intraparenchymal catheter as soon as feasible. Treatment measures were aimed at maintaining the ICP below 20 mm of Hg according to standard guidelines. Ventriculostomy was performed if cerebrospinal fluid drainage was necessary.

18.8 The I-CE (Control) Group

In this group, management was based on clinical examination and CT imaging as appropriate. Therapeutic modalities included a protocol-based administration of hyperosmolar therapy, mild hyperventilation to $PaCO_2$ levels of 30–35 mm Hg, and ventricular drainage if appropriate. If cerebral edema persisted, high-dose barbiturates and decompressive craniectomy were considered.

18.9 Common Management in both Groups

A CT scan of the brain was performed at baseline, 48 h, and 5–7 days after admission, or otherwise as considered necessary. Analgesia, sedation, and muscle relaxants were administered as required to both groups. Surgical evacuation of mass lesions and decompressive craniectomy were performed as appropriate. A protocolized approach was followed if neurological worsening occurred.

18.10 Sample Size

The authors calculated a sample size of 324 patients to provide 80% power to identify an increase by 10% points in the number of patients with a good outcome or moderate disability based on the Glasgow Outcome Score-Extended (GOS-E).

18.11 Results

The study enrolled 324 patients as planned—157 in the ICP group and 167 in the I-CE group. The median motor component of the GCS was 5 (3–5) and 4 (3–5), respectively. In the ICP group, the catheter was maintained for a median duration of 3.6 days. There were signs of raised ICP on the initial CT scan in 90% of patients in the ICP group compared with 89% in the control group. Midline shift by more than 5 mm was evident in 34% and 39% respectively. A mass lesion was evacuated in 31% of patients in the ICP group and 35% in the control group. Osmotherapy and hyperventilation were more often resorted to in the I-CE compared to the ICP group.

18.11.1 The Primary Outcome

The primary outcome was a composite of 21 parameters. The individual components of the composite outcome included survival time, impairment of the conscious level, the functional status at 3 and 6 months, and the neuropsychological status at 6 months. The outcome was expressed as a percentile between 0 and 100, with a higher percentile indicating better outcomes. Evaluation was carried out at 3 and 6 months by trained assessors, who were blinded to group assignment. There was no significant difference in the composite primary outcome between the ICP and the I-CE groups. The median percentile in the ICP group was 56 (22–27) compared with 53 (21–26) in the control group (OR: 0.49; 95% CI; 0.74–1.58).

The composite primary outcome was similar between the two groups when the analysis was restricted to survivors alone. Besides, on pre-defined subgroup analysis, there was no difference in the primary outcome based on age, gender, study site, and CT findings.

18.11.2 Secondary Outcomes

Among the secondary outcomes, the 14-day mortality was similar in both groups. The cumulative mortality at 6 months was also similar—39% in the ICP and 41% in the I-CE groups (OR: 1.10; 95% CI, 0.77–1.5). The GOS-E, ranging from 1 (death) to 8 (most favorable recovery), was evaluated at 6 months. A score of 2–4 was considered an unfavorable outcome and 5–8 a favorable outcome. The number of patients who died or experienced favorable and unfavorable outcomes were similar in both groups.

18.11.3 Other Outcomes

The hospital length of stay was marginally lower in the I-CE group. No significant differences were observed in the ICU length of stay, the duration of ventilator support, and the incidence of non-neurological complications. A greater number of patients were treated with high-dose barbiturates, hypertonic saline, and hyperventilation in the I-CE group. The duration of treatment with mannitol or hypertonic saline was also longer in the I-CE group. No significant difference was observed in the number of patients who underwent decompressive craniectomy between the two groups. The main outcomes are summarized in Table 18.1.

Table 18.1 Main study outcomes

Outcome	ICP group ($N = 157$)	Control group ($N = 167$)	Significance
Primary composite outcome, expressed as a percentile (0–100). Higher = better outcome	56	53	$P = 0.49$
Mortality at 6 months	39%	41%	$P = 0.6$
GOS-E at 6 months: favorable outcome (score 5–8)	44%	39%	
GOS-E at 6 months: unfavorable outcome (score 2–4)	17%	17%	
ICU length of stay	12 days	9 days	$P = 0.25$

Abbreviations: *ICP* intracranial pressure, *GOS-E* Extended Glasgow Outcome Scale

18.12 Adverse Events

There were ten adverse events related to the ICP catheter; these included catheter malfunction (3%), accidental removal (3%), and hemorrhage [1]. Serious adverse events occurred in 45% of patients in the ICP group and 46% of patients in the control group.

18.13 Study Conclusions

Among patients with severe traumatic brain injury, management based on maintenance of ICP ≤20 mm Hg was not superior to imaging and clinical examination-based management.

18.14 Strengths

The BEST-TRIP trial was the first large RCT that evaluated clinical outcomes using an ICP-guided approach compared with a clinical examination and CT-guided approach to managing patients with severe traumatic brain injury. The multi-centric study had robust internal validity. The investigators meticulously evaluated a broad array of relevant endpoints based on in-hospital morbidity, mortality, and quality of life. The assessors were blinded to the assignment arm, thus reducing the risk of bias. Although conducted in two low-income countries, the care provided was of a high standard and complied with the trial design.

18.15 Limitations

The composite primary outcome, including 21 parameters, may not be ideal. Although the 14- and 30-day mortality rates were similar in both groups, the study was not powered for these endpoints.

Although the treatment in both groups was protocolized, there were some key differences in the therapeutic strategy. In the ICP group, CSF drainage was one of the modalities employed to reduce ICP, while it was not part of the treatment strategy in the IC-E group. In the IC-E group, more patients underwent osmotherapy and hyperventilation, while the ICP group received barbiturates more often. The difference in treatment intensity between groups is difficult to explain. The study did not provide information regarding the number of CT scans performed in each group, which contributes to the cost of care and exposure to radiation.

Clinical outcomes following traumatic injury may depend on the specific area of compression, especially the brain stem, thalamus, and the reticular activating system. Injury to these areas occurs due to local mechanical displacement of brain tissue. Therapeutic interventions aimed to reduce ICP—the average pressure within the cranial cavity—may not always alleviate injury mediated by mechanical displacement.

The commonly followed ICP threshold of 20 mm Hg based on arbitrary guidelines may be considered too low. Indeed, the window of opportunity for interventions based on intracranial hypertension may be narrow. Patients at either end of the spectrum may be unaffected by ICP-based therapeutic interventions. Those with a relatively low ICP may have favorable outcomes without specific interventions, while those with catastrophic intracranial hypertension have poor outcomes regardless of the monitoring modality employed.

The trial was conducted in countries where clinicians were well-versed in management based on clinical signs and CT findings. A deviation from the usual approach, although based on a standard protocol, may result in unfamiliarity with a novel strategy that may have impacted outcomes. On the contrary, the results of the trial may not be applicable in healthcare settings that routinely measure ICP as an important facet of care in patients with severe traumatic brain injury. Furthermore, the pre-hospital care and transfer of patients may vary considerably in other parts of the world, where the results of the trial may not be valid. Post-discharge care, including rehabilitation, holds the key to outcomes in traumatic brain injury. The details of this vital aspect of care were unclear.

The authors emphasized that the study does not challenge the use of ICP monitoring in the management of severe traumatic brain injury—they only sought to test the monitoring-based treatment algorithm. It is also plausible that a one-size-fits-all approach with the use of a universal ICP threshold may not be the most efficacious strategy. The ICP trend over time may be more relevant than individual, instantaneous values. Furthermore, a rigid management strategy based on a fixed level of ICP may not be the optimal approach in different subtypes of injury.

18.16 Summary

Measurement of ICP was introduced in the 1960s as a monitoring tool to evaluate the well-being of the brain at the bedside. Over the next several decades, it evolved into a standard monitoring tool and was engrained into protocols for the management of traumatic brain injury. In the meantime, questions arose regarding the utility of ICP monitoring—particularly with observational trials suggesting adverse outcomes. However, observational studies always carry a risk of bias; ICP monitoring may often be employed in the sickest of patients who are prone to poor outcomes. Clinical guidelines cited inadequate evidence to support the efficacy of

ICP monitoring in traumatic brain injury. An adequately powered RCT was called for, considering the uncertainty regarding the efficacy of ICP monitoring. The BEST-TRIP trial took up the challenge of questioning what was considered to be "standard of care." The trial findings did not support the superiority of ICP monitoring-based management compared with a clinical examination and CT-guided approach. However, as the authors themselves aver, the study may not apply to healthcare settings that use ICP monitoring as a standard monitoring tool. Continuous monitoring may be particularly necessary in patients with severe intracranial hypertension; the trial did not specifically evaluate this subgroup of patients. The study provided evidence that a clinical examination and CT scan-based management may be appropriate in resource-poor settings where ICP monitoring is not routinely performed.

References

1. Lundberg N. Continuous recording and control of ventricular fluid pressure in neurosurgical practice. Acta Psychiatr Scand Suppl. 1960;36(149):1–193.
2. Saunders RL. Intracranial pressure monitoring survey. Neurosurgery. 1978;3(1):130.
3. Sahjpaul R, Girotti M. Intracranial pressure monitoring in severe traumatic brain injury—results of a Canadian survey. Can J Neurol Sci. 2000;27(2):143–7.
4. Stocchetti N, Longhi L, Magnoni S, Roncati Zanier E, Canavesi K. Head injury, subarachnoid hemorrhage and intracranial pressure monitoring in Italy. Acta Neurochir. 2003;145(9):761–5. discussion 765
5. Ghajar J, Hariri RJ, Narayan RK, Iacono LA, Firlik K, Patterson RH. Survey of critical care management of comatose, head-injured patients in the United States. Crit Care Med. 1995;23(3):560–7.
6. Griesdale DEG, McEwen J, Kurth T, Chittock DR. External ventricular drains and mortality in patients with severe traumatic brain injury. Can J Neurol Sci. 2010;37(1):43–8.
7. Shafi S, Diaz-Arrastia R, Madden C, Gentilello L. Intracranial pressure monitoring in brain-injured patients is associated with worsening of survival. J Trauma. 2008;64(2):335–40.
8. Brain Trauma Foundation, American Association of Neurological Surgeons, Congress of Neurological Surgeons, Joint Section on Neurotrauma and Critical Care, AANS/CNS, Carney NA, Ghajar J. Guidelines for the management of severe traumatic brain injury. Introduction. J Neurotrauma. 2007;24(Suppl 1):S1–2.
9. Chesnut RM, Temkin N, Carney N, Dikmen S, Rondina C, Videtta W, et al. A trial of intracranial-pressure monitoring in traumatic brain injury. N Engl J Med. 2012;367(26):2471–81.

19 Methylprednisolone in Severe Traumatic Brain Injury: The CRASH Trial

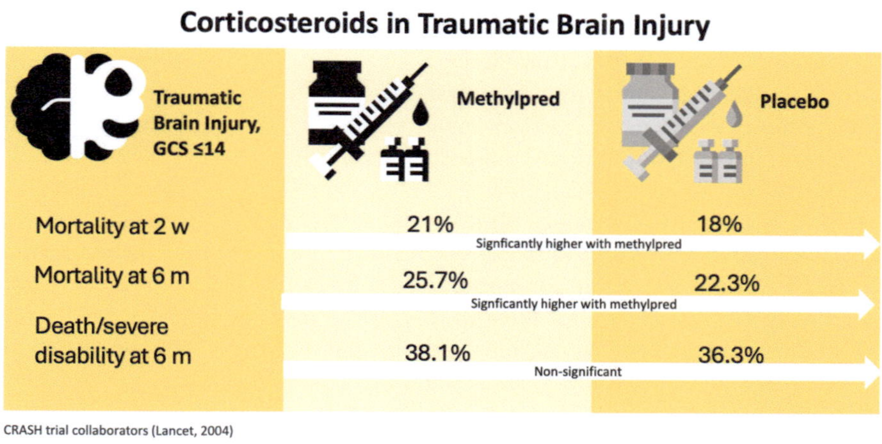

Quick Take

Could corticosteroids impact outcomes in traumatic brain injury?

This large, multicenter, randomized, placebo-controlled trial investigated the effect of intravenous corticosteroids on mortality in patients with clinically significant head injuries. A total of 10,008 adults were enrolled, with the intervention group receiving corticosteroids and the control group receiving placebo. The study

Roberts I, Yates D, Sandercock P, Farrell B, Wasserberg J, Lomas G, et al. Effect of intravenous corticosteroids on death within 14 days in 10008 adults with clinically significant head injury (MRC CRASH trial): randomised placebo-controlled trial. Lancet Lond Engl. 2004 Oct 9;364(9442):1321–8.

J. Chacko et al., *Landmark Studies in Critical Care*,
https://doi.org/10.1007/978-981-95-0673-6_19

revealed that methylprednisolone administration within 8 h of traumatic brain injury could lead to possible harm with higher mortality at 2 weeks and 6 months and more severe disability among survivors. These findings led to a change in practice, with corticosteroid therapy being largely abandoned for the management of severe head trauma. The trial emphasized the importance of evidence-based interventions in trauma care, revealing that corticosteroids were not beneficial and could be harmful in this context.

19.1 Introduction

Several million people around the globe suffer accidental injury every year. Severe traumatic brain injury leads to substantial mortality and severe disability among survivors. Raised intracranial pressure leading to fatal brain herniation is a leading cause of mortality. Most of the damage occurs at the time of injury; however, a later inflammatory reaction may contribute to secondary neuronal degeneration and lead to adverse clinical outcomes. Considering their powerful anti-inflammatory effect, corticosteroids have been in use for several decades in traumatic brain injury.

A 1996 survey evaluated practices among patients with traumatic brain injury in 39 ICUs in the United Kingdom. Corticosteroids were used to treat raised intracranial pressure in 19 units [1]. The practice in the United States was similar—a survey revealed that 64% of study centers used corticosteroids in traumatic brain injury [2]. Alderson et al. performed a systematic review of randomized controlled trials (RCTs) on the use of corticosteroids in traumatic brain injury [3]. They included 2073 patients enrolled in 14 RCTs from 1966 until December 1995. This study pointed to an absolute risk reduction of death by 1–2% with corticosteroid use; however, the confidence interval suggested reduced mortality by 6% to an increase in mortality by 2%. Hence, the findings of this review suggested the likelihood of modest benefit or possible harm with corticosteroid use in traumatic brain injury. Inflammation is considered to be a key driver behind the pathophysiology of traumatic brain injury, with the release of immune mediators within minutes of the primary injury [4]. However, the overall impact of the inflammatory response on brain tissue is unknown—is it beneficial, or does it contribute to secondary brain damage? Specifically, the question of whether the anti-inflammatory effect of corticosteroids could be potentially beneficial in traumatic brain injury remained unresolved.

The 1990s witnessed increasing enthusiasm for corticosteroid use in traumatic spinal cord injury. The NASCIS-2 trial revealed a salutary effect with a 24-hour dose of methylprednisolone administered within 8 h of injury. At 6 months, the methylprednisolone-treated patients revealed improved motor function, sensation to pinprick and touch compared to placebo [5]. The NASCIS-3 trial, published 7 years later, compared methylprednisolone administration for 24 vs. 48 h after spinal cord injury [6]. When methylprednisolone was administered within 3–8 h after injury, the 48-hour dose appeared to be more efficacious, with improved motor recovery at 6 weeks and 6 months. The modest benefits of corticosteroids observed in spinal cord injury spurred interest regarding potential benefits among patients with traumatic brain injury.

The CRASH (corticosteroid randomization after significant head injury) trial sought to evaluate the impact of methylprednisolone on clinical outcomes following traumatic brain injury, in light of the beneficial effects observed in spinal cord injury. Considering the massive global burden of traumatic brain injury, even a modest benefit could potentially impact mortality and favorably impact the lives of survivors.

19.2 Population and Design

The CRASH trial enrolled patients from 239 hospitals across 49 countries between April 1999 and May 2004 [7]. The study population included adult patients (16 years and older) who were within 8 h of traumatic brain injury, with a Glasgow coma score of ≤14. Patients were screened for eligibility based on the "uncertainty" principle—the clinician was substantially uncertain whether to use corticosteroids or not. Patients who had a clear indication for corticosteroids (e.g., spinal cord injury), and those with a clear contraindication were excluded. Eligible patients were randomly allocated to the methylprednisolone or placebo group.

19.2.1 Methylprednisolone Group

Patients received a loading dose of methylprednisolone 2 g in 100 ml normal saline as an intravenous infusion over 1 h. This was followed by 0.4 mg/h for 48 h as an intravenous infusion at 20 ml/h.

19.2.2 Placebo Group

In the control group, an identical placebo was infused using the same volumes as in the methylprednisolone group.

19.3 Sample Size

The investigators estimated a mortality risk of 15% in the placebo group. They contended that even a 2% improvement in survival may be clinically important given the global burden of traumatic brain injury. A sample size of 20,000 patients provided 90% power to demonstrate a 2% difference in survival to achieve $p < 0{\cdot}01$. All analyses were based on intention-to-treat.

19.4 Results

In May 2004, 5 years after the commencement of recruitment, the data monitoring and ethics committee disclosed the unmasked results of the study; by this time, a total of 10,008 patients had been randomized. The study was terminated at this stage as mortality at 2 weeks was higher in the corticosteroid group.

The mean age of the study population was 37 years, and the median time from injury to randomization was 3 h. Patient characteristics, including the cause of injury, presence of extracranial injuries, and CT findings, were similar in both groups.

19.5 The 2-Week Mortality

The 2-week mortality data were available for 9964 patients. At this point, mortality was signficantly higher in the methylprednisolone group; 1052 of 4985 patients in the methylprednisolone group (21%) and 893 of 4979 patients in the placebo group (18%) had died (relative risk of death with methylprednisolone: 1.18 (95% CI 1·09–1·27; p = 0·0001). The relative risk of death remained similar regardless of injury severity or the time since injury. The mortality at 2 weeks was also analyzed based on the CT findings. The relative risk of death at 2 weeks was not significantly different between the two groups in subgroups of patients with a normal CT, petechial hemorrhages, obliteration of the third ventricle or basal cisterns, subarachnoid hemorrhage, midline shift >5 mm, contusions, or non-evacuated hematoma.

19.6 Complications

There was no increase in the incidence of complications associated with methylprednisolone. The incidence of seizures, hematemesis, or melaena requiring transfusion, wound infections, pneumonias, other nosocomial infections, and the requirement for neurosurgical intervention was similar in both groups.

19.7 Follow-Up Study

In a later report, the authors published follow-up data at 6 months on 9673 patients [8]. Mortality at 6 months was significantly higher among patients who received methylprednisolone (1248 of 4854 patients, 25·7%) compared with placebo (1075 of 4819 patients, 22·3%). The relative risk of mortality in the methylprednisolone group for mortality at 6 months was 1·15 (95% CI 1·07–1·24; p = 0·0001). Death or severe disability on the Glasgow outcome scale was also higher in the methylprednisolone group [relative risk: 1·05 (95% CI 0·99–1·10; p = 0·079)]. The relative risk for death or severe disability remained higher in the methylprednisolone group when patients were stratified by the severity of injury or time since injury. Main outcomes are represented in Table 19.1.

Table 19.1 Main outcomes

Outcome	Methylprednisolone	Placebo	Relative risk
Mortality at 2 weeks	1052/4985 (21%)	893/4979 (18%)	1.18 (95% CI 1·09–1·27; $p = 0{\cdot}0001$)
Mortality at 6 months	1248/4854 (25·7%)	1075/4819 (22·3%)	1·15 (95% CI 1·07–1·24; $p = 0{\cdot}0001$)
Death or severe disability at 6 months	1828 (38·1%)	1728 (36·3%)	1·05 (95% CI 0·99–1·10; $p = 0{\cdot}079$

19.8 Study Conclusion

Methylprednisolone administration among patients with traumatic brain injury resulted in an increase in the all-cause mortality at 2 weeks and 6 months compared to placebo. The composite of death or severe disability at 6 months was also higher with methylprednisolone. The findings remained the same regardless of the severity of injury or time to administration of methylprednisolone. The authors concluded that corticosteroids are not indicated in traumatic brain injury, irrespective of the severity.

19.9 Strengths

The CRASH trial was randomized and double-blinded, adding to its robustness. The multinational design, including more than 200 centers from 49 countries, offered external validity and applicability in real-world practice. Baseline characteristics and prognostic factors were well-balanced between the two groups. The 2-week mortality data were available for >99% of patients, with analysis performed on an intention-to-treat basis.

19.10 Limitations

The study was terminated before the sample size was attained. Concurrent management of traumatic brain injury and other injuries was based on local practices; no data were provided. However, a similar number of patients were allocated to either arm in all hospitals, and hence the likelihood of bias may be low. Details on the cause of death were unavailable; it is plausible that mortality may have been due to concomitant injuries, unrelated to traumatic brain injury. The authors were unable to explain the reason for higher mortality with methylprednisolone—especially considering similar complication rates in both groups. The higher incidence of hyperglycemia may have unblinded clinicians to patients in the methylprednisolone group, leading to bias.

19.11 Summary

Corticosteroid use in severe traumatic brain injury was commonplace before the CRASH trial. The findings of the CRASH trial contrasted with the physiological plausibility of improved outcomes related to the anti-inflammatory effect of corticosteroids. The study revealed that methylprednisolone administration within 8 h of traumatic brain injury could lead to possible harm with higher mortality at 2 weeks and 6 months and more severe disability among survivors. The CRASH trial, including 10,008 patients, was among the largest clinical trials in patients with traumatic brain injury and provided a robust answer to an intriguing clinical question. The incidence of complications—infective or otherwise— was no higher with methylprednisolone; hence, the mechanism behind adverse outcomes with corticosteroids remained unexplained. The landmark CRASH trial provided the key message that injudicious use of unproven therapy could potentially lead to harm in large numbers of patients.

References

1. Jeevaratnam DR, Menon DK. Survey of intensive care of severely head injured patients in the United Kingdom. BMJ. 1996;312(7036):944–7.
2. Ghajar J, Hariri RJ, Narayan RK, Iacono LA, Firlik K, Patterson RH. Survey of critical care management of comatose, head-injured patients in the United States. Crit Care Med. 1995;23(3):560–7.
3. Alderson P, Roberts I. Corticosteroids in acute traumatic brain injury: systematic review of randomised controlled trials. BMJ. 1997;314(7098):1855–9.
4. Morganti-Kossmann MC, Rancan M, Stahel PF, Kossmann T. Inflammatory response in acute traumatic brain injury: a double-edged sword. Curr Opin Crit Care. 2002;8(2):101–5.
5. Bracken MB, Shepard MJ, Collins WF, Holford TR, Young W, Baskin DS, et al. A randomized, controlled trial of methylprednisolone or naloxone in the treatment of acute spinal-cord injury. Results of the second national acute spinal cord injury study. N Engl J Med. 1990;322(20):1405–11.
6. Bracken MB, Shepard MJ, Holford TR, Leo-Summers L, Aldrich EF, Fazl M, et al. Administration of methylprednisolone for 24 or 48 hours or tirilazad mesylate for 48 hours in the treatment of acute spinal cord injury. Results of the third National Acute Spinal Cord Injury Randomized Controlled Trial. National Acute Spinal Cord Injury Study. JAMA. 1997;277(20):1597–604.
7. Roberts I, Yates D, Sandercock P, Farrell B, Wasserberg J, Lomas G, et al. Effect of intravenous corticosteroids on death within 14 days in 10008 adults with clinically significant head injury (MRC CRASH trial): randomised placebo-controlled trial. Lancet. 2004;364(9442):1321–8.
8. Edwards P, Arango M, Balica L, Cottingham R, El-Sayed H, Farrell B, et al. Final results of MRC CRASH, a randomised placebo-controlled trial of intravenous corticosteroid in adults with head injury-outcomes at 6 months. Lancet. 2005;365(9475):1957–9.

20 Thrombectomy at 6 to 24 Hours Following Stroke with Mismatch between Deficit and Infarct Size: The DAWN Trial

Mechanical Thrombectomy vs. Standard Care Alone in Acute Stroke

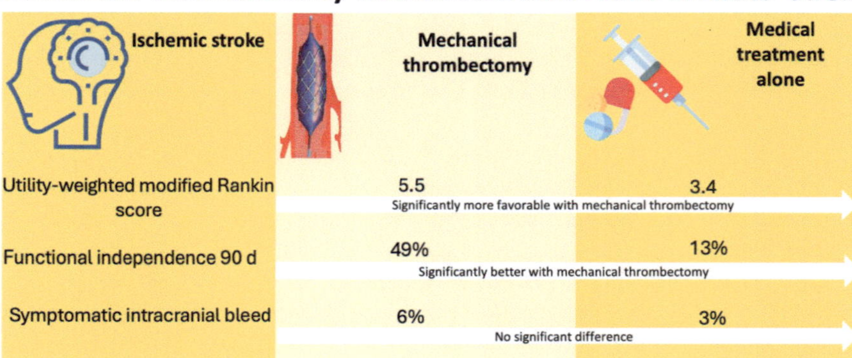

Nogueira et al. (NEJM, 2018)

Quick Take

Can the clock be stretched for stroke treatment? Would endovascular thrombectomy beyond 6 h improve outcomes in patients with clinical deficits out of proportion to the volume of infarct on imaging?

The DAWN trial investigated the benefits of endovascular thrombectomy in patients with acute ischemic stroke treated between 6 and 24 h after symptom onset. The trial enrolled patients with a mismatch between clinical deficit severity and

---

Nogueira RG, Jadhav AP, Haussen DC, Bonafe A, Budzik RF, Bhuva P, et al. Thrombectomy 6 to 24 Hours after Stroke with a Mismatch between Deficit and Infarct. N Engl J Med. 2018 Jan 4;378(1):11–21.

J. Chacko et al., *Landmark Studies in Critical Care*,
https://doi.org/10.1007/978-981-95-0673-6_20

infarct size (clinical deficits out of proportion to the volume of infarct on imaging). The results demonstrated that endovascular thrombectomy significantly improved functional outcomes compared to standard medical therapy alone, with a higher proportion of patients achieving independence at 90 days. The trial established that selected patients, even with delayed presentation, could benefit from mechanical thrombectomy, challenging the conventional treatment window for stroke intervention.

20.1 Introduction

Endovascular therapy for acute ischemic stroke was investigated more than two decades ago, especially among patients with large or more proximal occlusion. Conventional intravenous thrombolysis among patients with large, proximal occlusions may not be efficacious and carries the risk of fatal intracranial hemorrhage. The PROACT trials of the late 1990s evaluated the use of intra-arterial thrombolysis with pro-urokinase in acute ischemic stroke and revealed a trend towards improved neurological outcomes [1]. Subsequently, early trials of mechanical thrombectomy using retriever devices suggested effective recanalization in large-vessel occlusive disease [2, 3].

The identification of penumbral tissue in the brain—areas that are ischemic, but not infarcted—has been previously investigated. Such areas carry the potential for early reperfusion and salvage, thereby improving functional outcomes [1, 4]. Goyal et al. performed a meta-analysis of five randomized controlled trials (RCTs) between 2010 and 2014 that evaluated the efficacy of endovascular thrombectomy compared with standard care alone among patients with acute ischemic stroke [5]. These trials included patients with occlusion of the proximal anterior artery circulation who underwent thrombectomy within 12 h of the onset of symptoms. Among 1287 patients included in the meta-analysis, 634 were assigned to thrombectomy, while 653 were in the control group. Disability at 90 days, assessed using the modified Rankin Scale, was significantly lower in the thrombectomy group. On subgroup analysis, favorable outcomes were also observed among patients who presented more than 5 h after the onset of symptoms and those who were ineligible for intravenous thrombolysis. Another meta-analysis of the same RCTs revealed that the favorable outcomes with thrombectomy were directly related to the duration between the onset of symptoms and arterial puncture. A gradual decline of favorable effects was observed with every hour of delay to reperfusion.

The efficacy of thrombectomy performed >6 h after the time that the patient was last known to be well remained unclear. Would thrombectomy improve outcomes in patients presenting with ischemic brain tissue that had not yet undergone infarction, and hence, may be potentially salvageable? The presence of clinical deficits out of proportion to the volume of infarct on imaging may help identify patients who may have ischemic brain tissue that may be amenable to reperfusion with mechanical thrombectomy. A retrospective analysis suggested that endovascular therapy may be safely carried out beyond 8 h from the time last seen well, when patients were selected based on MRI or CT perfusion imaging [6]. Another observational study also suggested that improved outcomes following endovascular reperfusion may not be time-dependent in the presence of salvageable brain tissue, as evident on MRI [7].

The DAWN (DWI or CTP Assessment with Clinical Mismatch in the Triage of Wake-Up and Late Presenting Strokes Undergoing Neurointervention with Trevo) investigators evaluated neurological outcomes with endovascular thrombectomy compared to standard care alone among patients with acute ischemic stroke who were last known to be well 6–24 h earlier, and had a mismatch between infarct size and clinical deficit [8].

20.2 Population and Design

The DAWN trial was a multicenter, prospective, randomized, open-label trial conducted between September 2014 through February 2017 across 26 centers in the United States, Canada, Europe, and Australia. Patients with ischemic stroke were eligible if they had occlusion of the intracranial internal carotid artery, the proximal segment of the middle cerebral artery, or both, as evident on CT angiography or magnetic resonance angiography. A disproportionately severe neurological deficit compared to the infarct volume was required for eligibility. Patients were divided into three groups based on the infarct volume—clinical deficit mismatch.

Group A: ≥80 years, infarct volume <21 ml, a score of ≥10 on the National Institutes of Health Stroke Scale (NIHSS, ranging from 0 to 42).
Group B: <80 years, infarct volume <31 ml, a score of ≥10 or higher on the NIHSS.
Group C: <80 years, infarct volume of 31–50 ml, a score of ≥20 or higher on the NIHSS.

The other inclusion criteria were a duration of 6–24 h between the time the patient was last known to be well and randomization, a score of 0 or 1 on the modified Rankin scale at baseline, absence of intracranial hemorrhage, and involvement of less than one-third of the middle cerebral artery territory. Those who were ineligible for thrombolysis due to late presentation or had persistent vessel occlusion despite thrombolytic treatment were also eligible.

20.2.1 Thrombectomy Group

Mechanical thrombectomy was performed in addition to standard medical therapy. The investigators employed a retrievable, self-expanding stent to remove occlusive thrombi and restore flow. Rescue interventions with reperfusion therapy or other devices were not allowed. Concurrent stenting of the cervical internal carotid artery was not permitted; however, carotid angioplasty could be performed if considered necessary to deploy the retriever device.

20.2.2 Control Group

The control group received standard medical treatment alone, based on local guidelines.

20.2.3 Common Management

Patients enrolled in the trial were admitted to ICUs or stroke units. Those who did not undergo thrombolysis with intravenous alteplase could be treated with antiplatelet agents within 24 h of randomization. Aspirin was administered in a dose of 81 mg; prophylaxis against deep vein thrombosis was according to local guidelines. Patients also underwent a comprehensive post-stroke rehabilitation program.

20.3 Statistical Methodology

The DAWN trial was based on the hypothesis that patients with small-sized infarcts and disproportionately higher clinical deficits would most likely benefit from thrombectomy. However, the maximum core infarct size that may offer the most benefit was unclear. Hence, patients were divided into subgroups based on the infarct volume. At interim analyses, the adaptive trial design enabled reducing the largest infarct volume eligible for the trial based on the results already observed. The first primary analysis evaluated the probability that thrombectomy combined with standard care may result in less clinical disability at 90 days compared with standard care alone using a Bayesian model based on the baseline infarct volume. The adaptive design offered a flexible sample size ranging from 150 to 500 patients.

The trial was terminated at the first pre-specified interim analysis following the enrollment of 206 patients, as thrombectomy revealed a predictive probability of superiority of at least 95%.

20.4 Results

20.4.1 Baseline Characteristics

A total of 206 patients were enrolled—107 were assigned to thrombectomy, while 99 received standard medical treatment alone. Stroke severity was similar, with a median NIHSS score of 17 in both groups. The median infarct volume was 7.6 ml in the thrombectomy group and 8.9 ml in the standard care group. The median duration between when the patient was last known to be well and randomization was similar between groups (12.2 vs. 13.3 h). There were more patients in the thrombectomy group with atrial fibrillation and wake-up stroke; alteplase was more commonly used in the control group. Sixty-seven of 107 patients (63%) in the thrombectomy group and 47 of 99 (47%) in the control group were wake-up strokes with an unknown time of symptom onset.

20.5 Primary Endpoint

The study evaluated two co-primary endpoints. The utility-weighted modified Rankin scale ranges from 0 (death) to 10 (no disability), with higher scores indicating more favorable outcomes. The mean score on the utility-weighted modified Rankin scale was significantly higher with thrombectomy compared with standard care, suggesting improved outcomes (5.5 ± 3.8 vs. 3.4 ± 3.1, posterior probability of superiority >0.999).

The other co-primary endpoint was the level of functional independence, assessed using the modified Rankin scale, ranging from 0 (no disability) to 6 (death). A score of 0, 1, or 2 indicates functional independence. Functional independence at 90 days was significantly greater in the thrombectomy group (49% vs. 13%, posterior probability of superiority >0.999).

Sensitivity analysis was carried out, adjusting for between-group differences at baseline. The superiority of thrombectomy persisted for both co-primary endpoints.

20.6 Secondary Endpoints

Early neurological response, assessed using the NIHSS score, was greater in the thrombectomy group (48% vs. 19%). The rate of recanalization and change in the infarct volume from baseline to 24 h was also more favorable with thrombectomy compared with standard care. In the thrombectomy group, 84% of patients achieved a mTICI score (modified Thrombolysis in Cerebral Infarction) of 2b or 3, indicating reperfusion of >50% of the affected infarct territory. The size of the core infarct reduced significantly in the thrombectomy group compared with the control group (8 versus 22 mL; $P \leq 0.001$).

20.7 Safety Endpoints

The safety endpoints evaluated included stroke-related mortality at 90 days, all-cause mortality at 90 days, and symptomatic intracerebral hemorrhage. These endpoints were similar in both groups. Neurological deterioration occurred more often in the control group. The main study results are summarized in Table 20.1.

Table 20.1 Main study outcomes

Outcome	Thrombectomy	Control	Significance
Utility-weighted modified Rankin score at 90 days (0–10; higher score = better outcome)	5.5 ± 3.8	3.4 ± 3.1	Higher with thrombectomy
Functional independence at 90 days	49%	13%	Higher with thrombectomy
Early neurological response	48%	19%	$P < 0.001$
Recanalization at 24 h	77%	39%	$P < 0.001$
Infarct volume at 24 h	8 ml	22 ml	$P < 0.001$

20.8 Study Conclusions

Among patients with stroke due to occlusion of the intracranial internal carotid or proximal middle cerebral artery, who were last known to be well 6–24 h earlier, with a disproportionately severe deficit compared to stroke volume, functional outcomes were more favorable with thrombectomy compared with standard medical care alone. The favorable outcomes associated with thrombectomy were consistent across subgroups of patients based on age, severity of stroke, site of occlusion, and the time to treatment.

20.9 Strengths

The DAWN trial was a multicentric RCT that addressed the efficacy of a thrombectomy, a key intervention among patients who present late, up to 24 h after stroke onset. Assessors of the primary endpoint were blinded to the allocation arm. The scores on the modified Rankin scale, one of the co-primary outcomes, were dichotomized, allowing comparison with other trials. A good clinical outcome ranged from 0 to 2 on the modified Rankin scale, indicating functional independence with only slight disability.

20.10 Limitations

Functionally independent outcomes in the control group were worse than expected compared with previous studies. This could have been related to the less frequent use of thrombolysis due to later presentation. Besides, patients were older and experienced more severe strokes based on the NIHSS scale. Although randomization was stratified based on prognostic parameters that the authors considered relevant, there were baseline imbalances between groups—with more patients with atrial fibrillation and wake-up stroke in the thrombectomy group, while alteplase was more often used in the control group. However, on post-hoc sensitivity analysis adjusting for these differences, the benefit of thrombectomy persisted. The use of co-primary endpoints is unconventional; besides, the utility-weighted modification of the usual Rankin scale, one of the endpoints, may not capture individual variation in utility values and thereby reduce statistical power [9]. In 21% of patients, outcome assessment was carried out through a telephonic interview with the patient or caregivers—less than ideal compared with physical evaluation.

20.11 Summary

Patients in the DAWN trial presumably had large penumbral areas, considering the disproportionately severe neurological deficits in relation to the volume of the infarct. The findings of the trial reinforced the likelihood of improved outcomes with thrombectomy for up to 24 h after symptom onset among patients who had proximal vessel occlusion with a mismatch between infarct size and neurological deficits. The most crucial facet of this strategy is the identification of penumbral zones in the brain through appropriate imaging. The DAWN trial employed CT angiography or MRI scans to establish the presence of large penumbral tissue that held the potential for reperfusion.

Overall, patients who underwent thrombectomy were twice as likely to experience an improvement in neurological status and more likely to be functionally independent at 90 days compared with the control group. Participants randomized to the active arm were two-fold more likely to have an improvement in their neurological status (odds ratio, 2.1; 95% confidence interval, 1.20–3.12). The number needed to treat was just 2 for any lower disability at the pre-specified time. The DAWN trial heralded a new paradigm with clinical deficit to core mismatch emerging as the key criterion in the likelihood of successful thrombectomy, independent of the time of onset of symptoms.

References

1. Furlan A, Higashida R, Wechsler L, Gent M, Rowley H, Kase C, et al. Intra-arterial prourokinase for acute ischemic stroke. The PROACT II study: a randomized controlled trial. Prolyse in Acute Cerebral Thromboembolism. JAMA. 1999;282(21):2003–11.
2. Smith WS, Sung G, Saver J, Budzik R, Duckwiler G, Liebeskind DS, et al. Mechanical thrombectomy for acute ischemic stroke: final results of the multi MERCI trial. Stroke. 2008;39(4):1205–12.
3. Penumbra Pivotal Stroke Trial Investigators. The penumbra pivotal stroke trial: safety and effectiveness of a new generation of mechanical devices for clot removal in intracranial large vessel occlusive disease. Stroke. 2009;40(8):2761–8.
4. del Zoppo GJ, Higashida RT, Furlan AJ, Pessin MS, Rowley HA, Gent M. PROACT: a phase II randomized trial of recombinant pro-urokinase by direct arterial delivery in acute middle cerebral artery stroke. PROACT Investigators. Prolyse in Acute Cerebral Thromboembolism. Stroke. 1998;29(1):4–11.

5. Goyal M, Menon BK, van Zwam WH, Dippel DWJ, Mitchell PJ, Demchuk AM, et al. Endovascular thrombectomy after large-vessel ischaemic stroke: a meta-analysis of individual patient data from five randomised trials. Lancet. 2016;387(10029):1723–31.
6. Jovin TG, Liebeskind DS, Gupta R, Rymer M, Rai A, Zaidat OO, et al. Imaging-based endovascular therapy for acute ischemic stroke due to proximal intracranial anterior circulation occlusion treated beyond 8 hours from time last seen well: retrospective multicenter analysis of 237 consecutive patients. Stroke. 2011;42(8):2206–11.
7. Lansberg MG, Cereda CW, Mlynash M, Mishra NK, Inoue M, Kemp S, et al. Response to endovascular reperfusion is not time-dependent in patients with salvageable tissue. Neurology. 2015;85(8):708–14.
8. Nogueira RG, Jadhav AP, Haussen DC, Bonafe A, Budzik RF, Bhuva P, et al. Thrombectomy 6 to 24 hours after stroke with a mismatch between deficit and infarct. N Engl J Med. 2018;378(1):11–21.
9. Dijkland SA, Voormolen DC, Venema E, Roozenbeek B, Polinder S, Haagsma JA, et al. Utility-weighted modified Rankin scale as primary outcome in stroke trials. Stroke. 2018;49(4):965–71.

Decompressive Craniectomy in Severe Diffuse Traumatic Brain Injury: The DECRA Trial

21

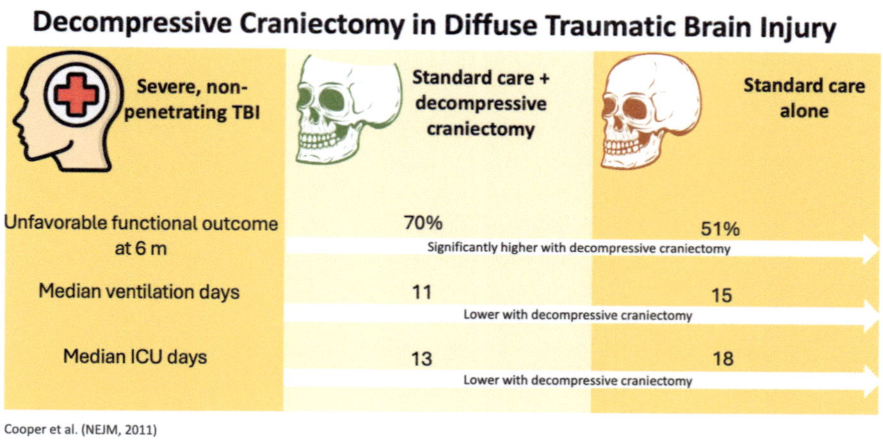

Quick Take

Does decompressive craniectomy improve functional outcomes in severe traumatic brain injury (TBI) and refractory intracranial hypertension?

The DECRA trial explored the role of early decompressive craniectomy in patients with severe diffuse TBI and refractory intracranial hypertension. The study compared outcomes between patients receiving decompressive craniectomy versus standard care. Despite effectively lowering intracranial pressure, the trial found that decompressive craniectomy was associated with worse functional

Cooper DJ, Rosenfeld JV, Murray L, Arabi YM, Davies AR, D'Urso P, et al. Decompressive craniectomy in diffuse traumatic brain injury. N Engl J Med. 2011 Apr 21;364(16):1493–502.

J. Chacko et al., *Landmark Studies in Critical Care*,
https://doi.org/10.1007/978-981-95-0673-6_21

outcomes at 6 months, as measured by the Extended Glasgow Outcome Scale. These findings suggested that while the procedure reduces intracranial pressure, it may not improve—and could even worsen—long-term recovery in this patient population.

21.1 Introduction

Historically, surgical decompression was employed as a desperate measure to reduce pressure within the skull in life-threatening brain injury. At the turn of the twentieth century, Theodor Kocher first proposed the potential of decompressive craniotomy to reduce intracranial pressure (ICP) in patients with traumatic brain injury (TBI). In 1901, he wrote that favorable clinical outcomes might ensue with "decompression of the brain by wide opening of the skull to decrease the intracranial pressure." The current concept of decompressive craniectomy was proposed by Harvey Cushing, involving the removal of a segment of the skull, enabling a reduction in pressure by opening the intracranial compartment [1].

In the *Proceedings of the Society of British Neurological Surgeons* in 1971, Ranashoff and Benjamin presented their experience with decompressive craniectomy as a life-saving intervention in patients with acute subdural hematoma within the first 24 h of injury [2]. In the pre-CT era, diagnosis was by expeditious angiography soon after securing the airway by endotracheal intubation, administration of osmotic agents, and continued resuscitative measures as appropriate. They removed a large fronto-temporo-occipital flap, with the removal of the squamous temporal bone to the base of the skull. Eight of 20 patients who underwent decompressive craniectomy were able to return to their previous level of employment, while two others made a partial recovery.

Seven years later, Britt and Hamilton reported a series of 42 patients with acute subdural hematoma. Evaluation was based on plain radiography or angiography. A CT scan, in the early days of its introduction to widespread practice, was performed in five patients. The authors performed a large decompressive craniotomy with evacuation of the hematoma, attainment of hemostasis, and patch-grafting of the dura. Although 14 patients were discharged home, many were left severely disabled with cognitive deficits, motor weakness, and aphasia [3].

By the late 1970s, decompressive craniectomy was considered a reasonable option to reduce the ICP rise associated with severe TBI. A reduction in the ICP resulted in improved cerebral perfusion, thus preventing ischemic injury. If cerebral edema worsened, brain herniation would occur through the craniectomy, thus preventing tentorial herniation and fatal brain stem compression. However, anecdotally, massive cerebral edema was occasionally observed at the craniectomy site. Cooper et al. noted in 1979 that the edema in patients who underwent craniectomy might even be more severe compared to those who were not subjected to decompression, although the ICP decreased dramatically [4]. The findings of an experimental model suggested that the removal of a bone segment may lead to a drastic reduction in the interstitial pressure in the brain tissue; the intravascular pressure, acting largely unopposed, may drive excessive edema formation [4].

The 1980s witnessed a resurgence of interest in decompressive craniectomy following TBI. Gaab et al. conducted a prospective observational study of 37 patients aged 40 years or less with TBI. The ICP could not be controlled despite optimizing conservative measures; rapid clinical deterioration followed. Decompressive craniectomy was performed within 5 h to 10 days of trauma. Among these patients, 32 (86%) survived with a mild or moderate level of disability. The authors observed that an initial GCS of ≥7 was the best predictor of a favorable outcome [5].

21.2 Background to the DECRA Trial

In more than a decade preceding the DECRA trial, decompressive craniectomies were being carried out extensively in TBI. Between 2009 and 2010, 143 papers were published on the topic, for different types of neurological disorders [6]. However, only a single randomized controlled trial (RCT) including 27 children had been carried out. This small RCT showed that very early decompressive craniectomy combined with medical therapy leads to a better functional outcome and improved quality of life compared to medical therapy alone [7]. The DECRA trial was designed to answer the question of whether decompressive craniectomy would improve neurological outcomes in patients with TBI, in whom conventional measures had failed to control ICP.

21.3 Study Population and Design

The DECRA trial was conducted by the Australian and New Zealand Intensive Care Society Clinical Trials Group between 2002 and 2010 across 15 ICUs in Australia, New Zealand, and Saudi Arabia. The study included patients aged 15–59 years with severe, non-penetrating TBI [8]. Severe TBI was defined as a score of 3–8 on the Glasgow Coma Scale or Marshall class III injury on CT imaging, representing moderate diffuse involvement. Patients in whom continued aggressive treatment was considered unlikely to benefit were excluded. Patients with bilateral dilated, non-reactive pupils, mass lesions, spinal cord injury, and those who suffered cardiac arrest at the scene were also excluded.

21.4 Standard Care

The ICP was monitored through an external ventricular drain or a parenchymal catheter. A rise in the ICP above 20 mm Hg triggered first-tier therapeutic interventions, including optimization of sedation, use of neuromuscular blocking agents, maintenance of normocapnia, osmotherapy including mannitol or hypertonic saline, and external ventricular drainage as appropriate. A spontaneous, persistent rise in the ICP for more than 15 min over a 1-h period despite these measures, either continuously or intermittently, was considered refractory intracranial hypertension.

21.5 Randomization

Patients were randomly assigned to undergo continued standard care alone or combined with decompressive craniectomy within the first 72 h if first-tier therapies failed to control ICP. Randomization was stratified according to center and the ICP monitoring technique, in blocks of two or four patients. In patients randomized to decompressive craniectomy, a standard surgical technique was followed. A large, bifrontotemporoparietal craniectomy with opening of the dura was performed to maximize the impact on ICP reduction. The excised bone segment was preserved at −70 °C or placed subcutaneously on the abdominal wall according to the preference of the surgeon. The bone flap was replaced after 2–3 months, after local swelling and infection had subsided.

21.6 Interventions for Refractory Intracranial Hypertension

Second-tier interventions were resorted to in both groups if the ICP remained persistently high. Such measures included mild induced hypothermia to 35 °C and barbiturate infusions. Among patients receiving standard care, decompressive craniectomy could be performed as a life-saving measure after 72 h of admission.

21.7 Sample Size

The initial sample size of 210 patients was calculated based on a 20% increase in favorable neurological outcomes with decompressive craniectomy, defined as a score of 5–8 on the extended Glasgow Outcome Scale. On interim analysis, the sample size was revised to 150 patients (75 in each group) to detect a difference in the median score of 1.5 between groups by ordinal logistic regression. The reduced sample size was aimed at completing the study within a reasonable time frame. If loss to follow-up occurred, an additional 15 patients could be recruited.

21.8 Results

Among the 3478 patients who were eligible, 155 were enrolled; the majority of patients were from Australia and New Zealand (88%). Early decompressive craniectomy was performed in 73 patients, while 82 received standard care. Patients were relatively young, with a median age of 23.7 years in the decompressive craniectomy group and 24.6 years in the standard care group. There were more patients with unreactive pupils in the decompressive craniectomy group. Patients were transferred to the hospital with minimum delay; the median duration from the time of injury to hospitalization was 1 h in the decompressive craniectomy group and 1.2 h in the standard care group. Decompressive craniectomy was performed as a life-saving intervention in 15 patients (18%) who were assigned to the standard care group.

21.8.1 Intracranial Pressure

Decompressive craniectomy resulted in a dramatic fall in the ICP. The mean ICP was 14.4 mm Hg post-decompressive craniectomy compared to 19.1 mm in the standard care arm. However, did the reduction in ICP improve functional outcomes?

21.8.2 Primary Outcome

The primary outcome was the functional status assessed by the Extended Glasgow Outcome Scale. Despite lower ICPs and fewer interventions for ICP control, patients who underwent decompressive craniectomy experienced worse functional outcomes. Unfavorable outcomes, defined as death, vegetative state, or severe disability, representing a score of 1–4 on the Extended Glasgow Outcome scale, occurred more frequently with decompressive craniectomy [51/73 (70%) vs. 42/82 (51%)]; odds ratio, 2.21; 95% CI, 1.14 to 4.26; $P = 0.02$. The risk of an unfavorable functional outcome with decompressive craniectomy remained high after adjustment for predefined covariates.

21.8.3 Secondary Outcomes

Mortality at 6 months was similar between the two groups. The duration of mechanical ventilation and ICU stay was significantly shorter in the decompressive craniectomy group. The duration of hospital stay was similar between the two groups. The main study outcomes are summarized in Table 21.1.

Table 21.1 Main study outcomes

Outcome	Standard care + decompressive craniectomy	Standard care alone	Significance
Death, vegetative state, or severe disability	70%	51%	$P = 0.02$
Ventilation days	11	15	$P < 0.001$
ICU days	13	18	$P < 0.001$
Hospital days	28	37	$P = 0.82$

21.9 Study Conclusions

Among patients with severe diffuse TBI and refractory intracranial hypertension, decompressive craniectomy decreased the intracranial pressure, the duration of ventilator support, and ICU stay. However, clinical outcomes assessed using the Extended Glasgow Outcome Scale were significantly worse at 6 months compared with standard care alone.

21.10 Comments

The DECRA trial demonstrated that in patients with severe TBI and refractory intracranial hypertension, early decompressive craniectomy resulted in worse functional outcomes at 6 months. The ICP levels were markedly lower following decompressive craniectomy; however, neurological outcomes remained poor compared to the standard care group. Although the duration of mechanical ventilation and ICU stay were shorter among patients who underwent decompressive craniectomy, the duration of hospital stay was similar in both groups.

Why did the functional outcomes remain poor despite a reduction in the ICP as expected? The authors hypothesized that extension of brain swelling outside the skull, with the resultant axonal stretch, may have triggered poor clinical outcomes, as suggested by Cooper et al. [4] several decades ago. The surgical technique employed may also have influenced outcomes. The bilateral approach followed in the DECRA trial has been associated with complications compared with a unilateral procedure [9]. The sagittal sinus and the falx cerebri were left intact in contrast to the procedure originally described by Polin et al. [10], although there is a likelihood of complications with both techniques. Thus, the findings of the study may apply to the specific surgical technique employed.

21.11 Limitations

The investigators were aware of the study groups as blinding was not possible; this may have resulted in bias. Although the trial was multicentric, the majority of patients were recruited from Australia and New Zealand; in fact, one-third of all study patients were from a single center. There were more patients with unreactive pupils in the decompressive craniectomy group at baseline, which may have contributed to poor outcomes; however, adjusted analysis after taking this difference into account did not impact the overall effect size. The sample size was scaled down after the first interim analysis with a view to the completion of the study within a reasonable time frame, which may constitute a suboptimal design. The study took 8 years to complete; changes may have occurred in the overall care of patients over this period that may have impacted outcomes. The performance of decompressive surgery after only 15 min of ICP rise above 20 mm Hg over a 1-h period may have been too early. As allowed by the study protocol, 18% of patients in the standard care group crossed over to undergo decompressive craniectomy after 72 h, which may have affected outcomes on intention-to-treat analysis.

21.12 The Post-DECRA Era

The RESCUEicp trial (2016) randomized 408 patients in 52 centres across 20 countries [11]. The patients were initially treated with stage 1 measures, including head end elevation, sedation, analgesia, and neuromuscular blockade. If the ICP remained high, stage 2 measures were applied, including ventriculostomy, osmotherapy, moderate hypocapnia, and therapeutic hypothermia. If the ICP remained >25 mm Hg for 1–12 h despite these measures, patients were randomized to undergo decompressive craniectomy or continued medical therapy. The primary outcome was the Extended Glasgow Outcome Score at 6 months. Mortality at 6 months was lower in the decompressive craniectomy group; however, there was a significantly higher incidence of vegetative state and severe disability compared to standard medical care alone. In contrast to the DECRA trial, the RESCUEicp trial employed decompressive craniectomy as a last-tier treatment.

21.13 Summary

Although decompressive surgery had been in widespread use at the time, the DECRA trial was the first large RCT to evaluate its efficacy in severe TBI with refractory intracranial hypertension compared with standard care alone. Although decompressive craniectomy resulted in lower ICP levels as expected, the reduction in intracranial pressure did not translate to improved functional outcomes. Indeed, early decompressive craniectomy, performed after 15 min of ICP rise above 20 mm Hg over a 1-h period, led to worse functional outcomes at 6 months. The subsequent RESUCEicp trial resorted to a more delayed approach to decompressive craniectomy after the failure of stage 1 and 2 measures to control the ICP. Although mortality was lower at 6 months, neurological disability was more severe among survivors. Both these trials point towards a judicious approach to decision-making in severe TBI with refractory intracranial hypertension, with due consideration of adverse functional outcomes among survivors.

References

1. Cushing HI. Subtemporal decompressive operations for the intracranial complications associated with bursting fractures of the skull. Ann Surg. 1908;47(5):641–644.1.
2. Ransohoff J, Benjamin V. Hemicraniectomy in the treatment of acute subdural haematoma. J Neurol Neurosurg Psychiatry. 1971;34(1):106.
3. Britt RH, Hamilton RD. Large decompressive craniotomy in the treatment of acute subdural hematoma. Neurosurgery. 1978;2(3):195–200.

4. Cooper PR, Hagler H, Clark WK, Barnett P. Enhancement of experimental cerebral edema after decompressive craniectomy: implications for the management of severe head injuries. Neurosurgery. 1979;4(4):296–300.
5. Gaab MR, Rittierodt M, Lorenz M, Heissler HE. Traumatic brain swelling and operative decompression: a prospective investigation. Acta Neurochir Suppl (Wien). 1990;51:326–8.
6. Servadei F. Clinical value of decompressive Craniectomy. N Engl J Med. 2011;364(16):1558–9.
7. Taylor A, Butt W, Rosenfeld J, Shann F, Ditchfield M, Lewis E, et al. A randomized trial of very early decompressive craniectomy in children with traumatic brain injury and sustained intracranial hypertension. Childs Nerv Syst. 2001;17(3):154–62.
8. Cooper DJ, Rosenfeld JV, Murray L, Arabi YM, Davies AR, D'Urso P, et al. Decompressive craniectomy in diffuse traumatic brain injury. N Engl J Med. 2011;364(16):1493–502.
9. Gooch MR, Gin GE, Kenning TJ, German JW. Complications of cranioplasty following decompressive craniectomy: analysis of 62 cases. Neurosurg Focus. 2009;26(6):E9.
10. Polin RS, Shaffrey ME, Bogaev CA, Tisdale N, Germanson T, Bocchicchio B, et al. Decompressive bifrontal craniectomy in the treatment of severe refractory posttraumatic cerebral edema. Neurosurgery. 1997;41(1):84–92; discussion 92–94.
11. Hutchinson PJ, Kolias AG, Timofeev IS, Corteen EA, Czosnyka M, Timothy J, et al. Trial of decompressive Craniectomy for traumatic intracranial hypertension. N Engl J Med. 2016;375(12):1119–30.

22 Decompressive Craniectomy for Intracranial Hypertension Following Traumatic Brain Injury: The RESCUEicp Trial

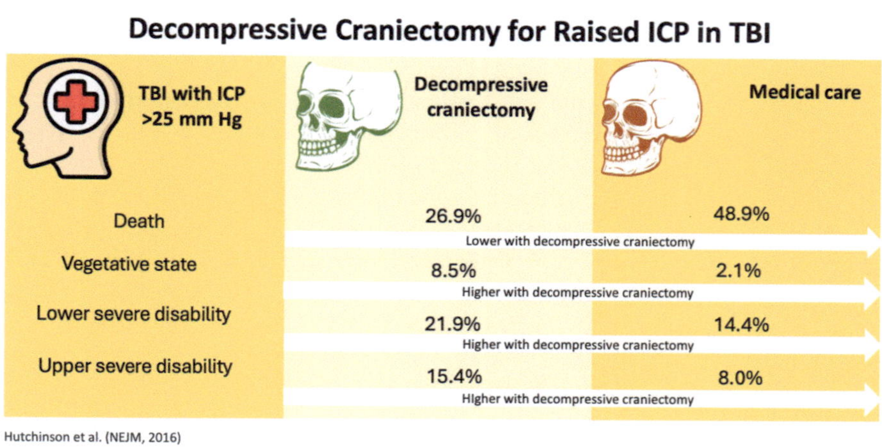

Quick Take

In patients with traumatic brain injury (TBI) and refractory intracranial hypertension, does decompressive craniectomy improve outcomes compared to medical management alone?

The RESCUEicp trial, a multicenter randomized controlled study, investigated this question in patients with refractory intracranial hypertension above 25 mm Hg despite optimal medical therapy. Patients were randomized to undergo

---

Hutchinson PJ, Kolias AG, Timofeev IS, Corteen EA, Czosnyka M, Timothy J, et al. Trial of Decompressive Craniectomy for Traumatic Intracranial Hypertension. N Engl J Med. 2016 Sep 22;375(12):1119–30.

J. Chacko et al., *Landmark Studies in Critical Care*,
https://doi.org/10.1007/978-981-95-0673-6_22

decompressive craniectomy or continued medical management. The trial found that decompressive craniectomy significantly reduced mortality; however, survivors in the surgical group had higher rates of severe disability, vegetative state, or dependence compared to the medical group. These findings highlight the dilemma of balancing improved survival with the risk of significant neurological disability. The study underscores the need for careful patient selection and individualized decision-making when considering decompressive craniectomy for TBI with refractory intracranial hypertension.

22.1 Introduction

The intracranial pressure (ICP) is often raised following severe traumatic brain injury (TBI) [1]. Uncontrolled intracranial hypertension leads to a reduction in the cerebral perfusion pressure [2] and carries an increased risk of death [3]. In intractable cases, decompressive craniectomy may be performed to reduce the ICP [4]. This procedure involves the removal of a large section of the skull and opening the dura mater that lies underneath [5]. A primary decompressive craniectomy is carried out following the evacuation of an intracranial hematoma in the early phase of TBI [5]. Among patients with refractory intracranial hypertension, a stepwise protocol is often followed, including the performance of a secondary decompressive craniectomy to maintain cerebral perfusion pressure. The earlier DECRA trial had evaluated the efficacy of decompressive craniectomy in patients who experienced an ICP of >20 mm Hg for >15 min during a 1-h period [6]. Decompressive craniectomy may also be resorted to as a last-tier intervention when all other measures fail.

The RESCUEicp Trial Collaborators aimed to evaluate the efficacy of decompressive craniectomy as a last-tier intervention among patients with refractory intracranial hypertension following TBI [7].

22.2 Population and Design

The multicentric trial was conducted between January 2004 and March 2014 across 52 centers in 20 countries [7]. The study population included patients with TBI with an abnormal CT scan and a raised ICP of >25 mm Hg for 1–12 h despite stage 1 and 2 therapies. Patients who had bilateral fixed dilated pupils, a bleeding tendency, and those considered unlikely to survive were excluded.

Patients were randomly assigned to undergo a last-tier secondary decompressive craniectomy or continued medical management for uncontrolled intracranial hypertension following TBI.

22.3 Initial Common Management

A stepwise, tiered protocol was followed to maintain the ICP below 25 mm Hg. The first stage of interventions included the administration of sedatives, analgesics, and neuromuscular blockade as appropriate. The cerebral perfusion pressure was targeted to >60 mm Hg. Normothermia and normoglycemia were maintained. The $PaCO_2$ was maintained between 34 and 38 mm Hg, and the oxygen saturation was >97%. If the ICP remained high, the second-stage measures were employed, including ventriculostomy, osmotherapy, moderate reduction of the $PaCO_2$ levels to 30–34 mm Hg, maintenance of adequate blood pressure, and therapeutic hypothermia (not <34 °C).

Despite these measures, if the ICP remained >25 mm Hg for 1–12 h, patients were randomized to undergo decompressive craniectomy or continued medical management.

22.3.1 Decompressive Craniectomy

The study recommended unilateral frontotemporoparietal craniectomy for patients with unilateral hemispheric swelling. Among patients with diffuse cerebral edema, a bifrontal craniectomy was recommended. The exact type of surgical intervention was left to the discretion of the surgeon. Decompressive craniectomy had to be performed within 4–6 h of randomization.

22.3.2 Continued Medical Therapy

Patients in this group were continued on conservative measures; intravenous barbiturate infusions could be added to the treatment regimen to control intracranial hypertension.

22.4 Sample Size

The authors calculated a sample size of 400 patients to identify a difference of 15 percentage points in favorable outcomes. A favorable outcome was defined as upper severe disability or better on the 8-point Extended Glasgow Outcome Scale (GOS-E) (Table 22.1). The sample size provided the study with 80% power at 5% significance level, allowing a 15% loss to follow-up.

Table 22.1 The Extended Glasgow Outcome Scale (GOS-E)

Extended Glasgow Outcome Scale (GOS-E) category	Description
Upper good recovery	Full recovery or minor symptoms that do not impact daily life
Lower good recovery	Able to return to previous roles in life; some symptoms are impacting daily life
Upper moderate disability	Independent at home and outside; able to return to previous life roles. Some physical or mental disability
Lower moderate disability	Independent, but cannot return to previous life roles
Upper severe disability	Independent at home; needs help with activities outside home
Lower severe disability	Dependent, with requirement for frequent assistance with activities of daily living
Vegetative	Lack of awareness of self or surroundings
Dead	

22.5 Results

At the 6-month follow-up, there were 201 patients in the decompressive craniectomy group and 188 patients who underwent medical therapy. The baseline characteristics were similar at baseline. Among those allocated to surgery, 92.6% underwent decompressive craniectomy, with a median time from randomization to surgery of 2.2 h. Decompressive craniectomy was also performed in 37.2% of patients randomized to the medical group.

22.5.1 The Primary Outcome: Extended Glasgow Outcome Scale (GOS-E) at 6 Months After Randomization

The primary outcome in each category of GOS-E at 6 months is summarized in Table 22.2.

On prespecified sensitivity analysis, a larger number of patients experienced upper severe disability or better, defined as a favorable outcome, in the surgical decompressive craniectomy group, although the difference was not statistically significant (42.8% vs. 34.6%, $P = 0.12$).

22.5.2 Secondary Outcomes

The secondary outcomes included GOS-E at 12 months, summarized in Table 22.3.

Table 22.2 Primary outcomes in each category of the Extended Glasgow Outcome Scale (GOS-E) at 6 months

Outcome	Decompressive craniectomy	Continued medical therapy
Death	26.9%	48.9%
Vegetative state	8.5%	2.1%
Lower severe disability	21.9%	14.4%
Upper severe disability	15.4%	8%
Moderate disability	23.4%	19.7%
Good recovery	4.0%	6.9%

Table 22.3 Primary outcomes in each category of the Extended Glasgow Outcome Scale (GOS-E) at 12 months

Outcome	Decompressive craniectomy	Continued medical therapy
Death	30.4%	52%
Vegetative state	6.2%	1.7%
Lower severe disability	18%	14%
Upper severe disability	13.4%	3.9%
Moderate disability	22.2%	20.1%
Good recovery	9.8%	8.4%

On prespecified sensitivity analysis, a significantly larger number of patients in the decompressive craniectomy group experienced a favorable outcome, defined as upper severe disability or better at 12 months (45.4% vs. 32.4%, $P = 0.01$). Among every 100 patients who underwent decompressive craniectomy, there were 22 more who survived. Among these 22 survivors, 9 (41%) were in a vegetative state or experienced lower severe disability—considered an unfavorable outcome. Thirteen patients (59%) experienced upper severe disability or better function, which was considered a favorable outcome.

As expected, ICP control was better achieved in the decompressive craniectomy group. Among survivors, the median time to discharge from ICU was shorter in the decompressive craniectomy group (15 vs. 20.8 days, $P = 0.01$). Adverse events occurred significantly more often in the decompressive craniectomy group (16.3% vs. 9.2%, $P = 0.03$). Common adverse events encountered included pneumonia, postoperative hematoma, and wound infection.

22.6 Study Conclusion

Among patients who underwent decompressive craniectomy for severe, refractory intracranial hypertension following TBI, the mortality was significantly lower compared to those who underwent continued medical therapy. Decompressive craniectomy also resulted in higher rates of vegetative state, lower severe disability, and higher severe disability according to the GOS-E outcomes. The rates of good recovery and moderate disability were similar in both groups.

22.7 Strengths

The randomized controlled design reduced the likelihood of bias. The large sample size across multiple centers with the availability of neurosurgical services around the clock provided external validity. Standardized protocols were followed in both arms of the study. The outcome assessment, using the extended Glasgow Outcome Scale at 6 and 12 months, was robust.

22.8 Weaknesses

The study included patients with varied severity of TBI, which could limit the generalizability of the results. Recruitment was slow, taking over 10 years to complete. Although therapeutic hypothermia was employed in the study, subsequent evidence from the EUROTHERM trial did not support its use [8]. Clinicians were aware of the assignment arm as blinding was not feasible. A substantial proportion of patients (37%) in the medical therapy group underwent decompressive craniectomy, which may have impacted the results. Some patients were excluded from the final analysis due to withdrawal of consent or loss to follow-up, which may have affected the results.

22.9 Subsequent Study—Follow-Up at 24 Months

In their secondary analysis, Kolias et al. evaluated 24-month outcomes for patients included in the RESCUEicp randomized controlled trial [9]. The authors observed lower mortality in the decompressive craniectomy group at 24 months (33.5% vs. 54%). More patients remained vegetative in the surgical group at this point. The rates of lower or upper moderate disability and lower or upper severe disability were higher among those who underwent decompressive craniectomy, indicating more favorable outcomes. However, the rates of good recovery—upper and lower—were similar in both groups. The authors concluded that a sustained reduction in mortality with higher rates of vegetative state, severe and moderate disability persisted at 24 months. More patients who underwent decompressive craniectomy improved with time compared to those who underwent medical management.

22.10 Summary

The RESCUEicp investigators evaluated the efficacy of decompressive craniectomy as a last-tier intervention against the background of the adverse outcomes observed in the DECRA trial with earlier intervention. The study included adults with severe TBI and refractory intracranial hypertension, despite maximal medical therapy. In the surgical group, patients underwent a unilateral frontotemporoparietal or a bifrontal craniectomy, based on the extent of hemispheric involvement and the judgment of the surgeon. In the medical therapy group, conservative measures were continued with intravenous barbiturate infusions if appropriate. Mortality at 6 months was lower in the surgical group, although more patients remained in a vegetative state. The rates of lower severe and upper severe disability were also higher. Moderate disability and good recovery occurred at similar rates in both groups.

The RESCUE-ICP trial provided compelling evidence that decompressive craniectomy saves lives in patients with refractory intracranial hypertension; however, it also raised important ethical and quality-of-life considerations. Decision-making should be individualized and weigh the life-saving potential of decompressive craniectomy against functional outcomes.

References

1. Stocchetti N, Maas AIR. Traumatic intracranial hypertension. N Engl J Med. 2014;371(10):972.
2. Hutchinson PJ, Kolias AG, Czosnyka M, Kirkpatrick PJ, Pickard JD, Menon DK. Intracranial pressure monitoring in severe traumatic brain injury. BMJ. 2013;346:f1000.
3. Balestreri M, Czosnyka M, Hutchinson P, Steiner LA, Hiler M, Smielewski P, et al. Impact of intracranial pressure and cerebral perfusion pressure on severe disability and mortality after head injury. Neurocrit Care. 2006;4(1):8–13.
4. Sahuquillo J, Arikan F. Decompressive craniectomy for the treatment of refractory high intracranial pressure in traumatic brain injury. Cochrane Database Syst Rev. 2006;(1):CD003983.
5. Kolias AG, Kirkpatrick PJ, Hutchinson PJ. Decompressive craniectomy: past, present and future. Nat Rev Neurol. 2013;9(7):405–15.
6. Cooper DJ, Rosenfeld JV, Murray L, Arabi YM, Davies AR, D'Urso P, et al. Decompressive craniectomy in diffuse traumatic brain injury. N Engl J Med. 2011;364(16):1493–502.
7. Hutchinson PJ, Kolias AG, Timofeev IS, Corteen EA, Czosnyka M, Timothy J, et al. Trial of decompressive craniectomy for traumatic intracranial hypertension. N Engl J Med. 2016;375(12):1119–30.
8. Andrews PJD, Sinclair HL, Rodriguez A, Harris BA, Battison CG, Rhodes JKJ, et al. Hypothermia for intracranial hypertension after traumatic brain injury. N Engl J Med. 2015;373(25):2403–12.
9. Kolias AG, Adams H, Timofeev IS, Corteen EA, Hossain I, Czosnyka M, et al. Evaluation of outcomes among patients with traumatic intracranial hypertension treated with decompressive craniectomy vs standard medical care at 24 months: a secondary analysis of the RESCUEicp randomized clinical trial. JAMA Neurol. 2022;79(7):664–71.

23 Decompressive Craniectomy in Older Patients with Extensive Middle-Cerebral-Artery Stroke: The DESTINY II Trial

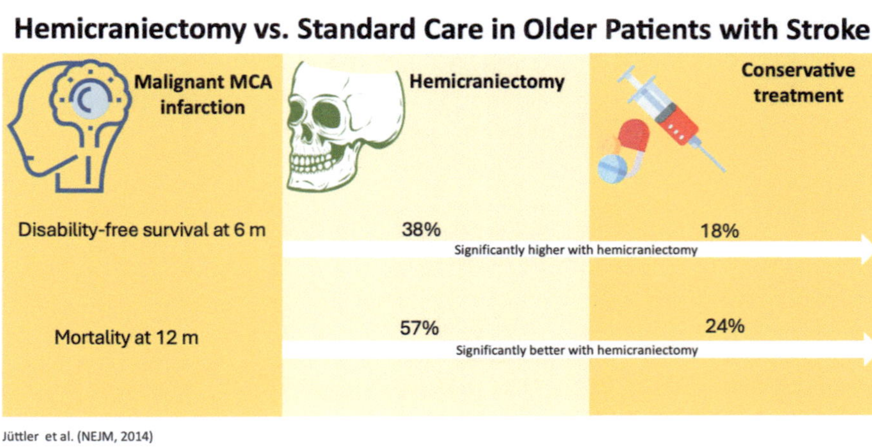

Quick Take

Does decompressive hemicraniectomy improve survival without severe disability in patients aged >60 years with malignant middle cerebral artery (MCA) infarction?

Patients were randomized to undergo hemicraniectomy within 48 h of symptom onset or receive conservative medical treatment. The primary outcome was survival with a modified Rankin Scale (mRS) score of 4 or lower at 6 months. The trial demonstrated that hemicraniectomy significantly improved survival compared to

---

Jüttler E, Unterberg A, Woitzik J, Bösel J, Amiri H, Sakowitz OW, et al. Hemicraniectomy in Older Patients with Extensive Middle-Cerebral-Artery Stroke. N Engl J Med. 2014 Mar 20;370(12):1091–100.

J. Chacko et al., *Landmark Studies in Critical Care*,
https://doi.org/10.1007/978-981-95-0673-6_23

conservative treatment but resulted in higher rates of survivors with mRS scores of 4 or 5, indicating severe disability. While some survivors reported acceptable quality of life, the clinical benefit must be weighed against the likelihood of significant disability. DESTINY II emphasized the importance of patient and caregiver preferences when deciding on hemicraniectomy in older patients with malignant MCA infarction.

23.1 Introduction

Massive hemispheric involvement occurs in up to 10% of patients with supratentorial infarcts [1]. Life-threatening cerebral edema often follows, referred to as malignant middle-cerebral-artery syndrome [2], with a mortality of 70–80% [3]. The onset of clinical deterioration usually occurs between 3 and 5 days of stroke onset, characterized by increasing drowsiness, leading to coma. Therapeutic modalities commonly employed include sedation, mechanical ventilation with maintenance of hypocapnia, corticosteroids, and osmotherapy. However, there is no evidence to support the efficacy of these measures [4, 5]; some reports suggest that they may indeed be harmful [6]. Beginning from the 1950s, surgical decompression with hemicraniectomy and duraplasty was proposed as a rescue measure in this situation [7].

Nearly five decades ago, Ivamoto et al. published a detailed case report of a 49-year-old housewife who presented with flaccid hemiplegia, homonymous hemianopia, and Babinsky's sign following extensive infarction involving the right middle-cerebral-artery territory [8]. Her condition deteriorated gradually; by the third day of her illness, she lay in a stuporous state, with irregular respirations and progressive bradycardia. Her right pupil was blown and was hardly reacting to light, suggesting impending herniation. A bolus dose of 20% mannitol led to transient improvement; however, death appeared imminent. Her surgeon decided to perform decompressive surgery as a last resort to save her life. She underwent a large craniotomy and subtemporal craniectomy with an anterior dural incision. Her intracranial pressure, measured using a fiberoptic device, reduced dramatically following the procedure; by early next morning, she was alert and orientated, with normal pupils and respiration. She was discharged home 3 weeks later; her left hemiparesis had marginally improved by that time. The authors reviewed an additional 17 cases of decompressive craniectomy performed for ischemic stroke reported in the literature. They concluded that large cerebral infarcts may lead to significant edema and cause a life-threatening rise in intracranial pressure. These effects may be alleviated by a life-saving decompressive craniectomy; however, they proposed controlled trials to evaluate the true clinical efficacy of this procedure.

Hemicraniectomy enables the creation of space to accommodate the swollen brain and ameliorate raised intracranial pressure, thereby preventing fatal brain herniation. The turn of the millennium witnessed the commencement of three randomized controlled trials (RCT)—DESTINY, DECIMAL, and HAMLET—to evaluate the efficacy of decompressive craniectomy compared with conservative management among patients with malignant middle-cerebral-artery syndrome [9–11]. A pooled analysis of these trials revealed improved 1-year survival with early hemicraniectomy compared with conservative management (78% vs. 29%) [12]. Furthermore, functional outcomes were superior following hemicraniectomy, with 43% experiencing relatively good outcomes with mild or moderate disability compared to 21% in the control group.

Enrolment was limited to patients who were 60 years old or less in all three RCTs. Hence, the possible efficacy of hemicraniectomy among older patients with ischemic stroke was unclear. A systematic review of 19 studies found higher mortality with decompressive craniectomy following malignant middle-cerebral-artery stroke among those >60 years old compared to younger patients. Besides, clinical outcomes among survivors were less favorable in this age group [13]. A database analysis evaluated outcomes following decompressive craniectomy among patients with infarction involving the middle-cerebral-artery. On multivariate analysis, age >50 years was a predictor of unfavorable outcomes [14]. Death or significant disability was also found to be more common among patients >50 years of age who underwent decompressive craniectomy following large hemispheric infarcts [15]. Considering the lack of robust evidence and conflicting results from observational trials, a compelling need arose for an RCT to evaluate the possible benefit of decompressive craniectomy in extensive middle-cerebral-artery stroke among older patients.

The DESTINY II investigators sought to evaluate outcomes following early hemicraniectomy compared with conservative management among patients >60 years old with malignant middle-cerebral-artery infarction [16].

23.2 Population and Design

The DESTINY II trial recruited patients between August 2009 and May 2013 across 13 centers in Germany. Patients ≥61 years old, with malignant middle-cerebral artery infarction, were randomized in a 1:1 ratio to conservative treatment or hemicraniectomy. The eligibility criteria included an NIHSS (National Institutes of Health Stroke Scale) score >14 in a nondominant hemisphere and >19 in a dominant hemisphere stroke, with impaired consciousness. Besides, the infarct had to involve at least two-thirds of the middle-cerebral-artery territory, including the basal ganglia.

23.2.1 Excluded

Patients with a premorbid score of >1 on the modified Rankin scale were excluded (patients included in the trial had no significant disability and were able to carry out all usual activities at baseline). Patients with a pre-existing score of <95 on the Barthel index were also excluded (patients included in the trial were almost totally independent with activities of daily living at baseline). Also excluded were patients with absent pupillary reflexes, a score of <6 on the Glasgow Coma Scale (GCS), intracranial hemorrhage, contraindications for surgery, and a life expectancy of <3 years. Randomization was carried out within 48 h of symptom onset. Treatment was commenced in both groups within 48 h of symptom onset and not later than 6 h after randomization.

23.3 The Conservative Treatment Group

In the conservative arm, treatment was based on a consensus protocol. Osmotherapy included mannitol, hypertonic hydroxyethyl starch, or glycerol; invasive mechanical ventilation with hypocapnia to 28–32 mm Hg was resorted to as appropriate.

23.4 The Hemicraniectomy Group

A large hemicraniectomy with duraplasty was performed with a bone flap of at least 12 cm, including the frontal, parietal, temporal, and part of the occipital squamae. Among survivors, cranioplasty was carried out at 6 weeks to 8 months using the stored bone flap or an artificial flap. In the postoperative period, the systolic blood pressure was maintained between 140 and 160 mm Hg for the first 8 h to prevent intracranial bleeding.

23.5 Common Management

The appropriate use of sedatives and measurement of intracranial pressure were left to the clinician's judgment. Normothermia was aimed for, and the blood glucose level was maintained between 80 and 110 mg/dl, with an upper level not to exceed 140 mg/dl. The hemoglobin level was maintained above 10 g/dl; low molecular weight heparin was recommended as prophylaxis against deep vein thrombosis.

23.6 Sample Size

The primary endpoint was a score of 0–4 on the modified Rankin scale at 6 months (Table 23.1). The authors used a sequential methodology with pre-planned stoppage of the trial at any stage when efficacy, harm, or futility was evident on interim analysis. They calculated the sample size assuming a success rate of 31% for the primary endpoint in the hemicraniectomy group and 8.6% in the control group, thus providing the study with 90% power.

Table 23.1 The modified Rankin Scale

Score	Description
0	No symptoms
1	Some symptoms, but able to perform all routine activities
2	Mild disability, unable to perform *all* previous activities; able to look after own affairs unassisted
3	Moderate disability, requires some help. *Able to walk without assistance*
4	Moderately severe disability. *Unable to walk without assistance; unable to attend to bodily needs without assistance*
5	Severe disability; bedridden, incontinent, and requires nursing care
6	Death

23.7 Results

Based on pre-specified stopping rules, the study was terminated after the recruitment of 112 patients—49 in the hemicraniectomy group and 63 in the control group. The median age was 70 years, and the modified Rankin score was similar at baseline in both groups. The median NIHSS score was 20 in the hemicraniectomy group and 21 in the control group among those who were assessable. The median GCS was 12 in the hemicraniectomy group and 10 in the control group.

23.8 The Primary Endpoint

At 6 months, a score of 0–4 on the modified Rankin scale (from no symptoms to moderately severe disability—inability to walk and attend to bodily needs without assistance), considered a favorable outcome, was significantly higher in the hemicraniectomy group (20/49 vs. 10/63). The bias-corrected estimate of survival without severe disability was significantly greater with hemicraniectomy (38% vs. 18%, odds ratio, 2.91; 95% CI, 1.06–7.49, $p = 0.04$). Analysis based on a sequential proportional-odds model confirmed the beneficial impact of hemicraniectomy. However, hemicraniectomy did not reveal a significant benefit when scores were dichotomized to 0–3 (able to walk unassisted) vs. 4–6 (unable to walk unassisted, moderate to severe disability, or death).

There were no patients in either group with a score of 0–2 (ability to take care of their own affairs without support). In the hemicraniectomy group, 7% of patients had a score of 3 compared with 3% in the control group; a score of 4 occurred in 32% of the hemicraniectomy group compared with 15% in the control group.

23.9 Secondary Endpoints

The 12-month survival was significantly higher in the hemicraniectomy group (57% vs. 24%). Other secondary endpoints included the score on the modified Rankin scale, the NIHSS score, the Barthel index score (the level of activities of daily living), the HDRS score (level of depression), the SF-36 score (quality of life), and the EQ-5D score (self-report) at 12 months. All the above endpoints were more favorable in the hemicraniectomy group.

23.10 Safety Outcomes

The incidence of adverse events was similar between groups. Infective complications were more common in the hemicraniectomy group. Twenty-three complications were directly related to either the initial hemicraniectomy or reimplantation of the bone flap. In the control group, the most common adverse events were cerebral edema and herniation. The main study outcomes are summarized in Table 23.2.

Table 23.2 Main study outcomes

Outcome	Hemicraniectomy	Conservative	Significance
Favorable neurological outcome (0–4 on mRS)	38%	18%	Significantly better with hemicraniectomy
mRS 0–3 vs. 4–6 (able to walk unassisted)			Not significantly different
12-month survival	57%	24%	Significantly higher with hemicraniectomy

Abbreviation: mRS modified Rankin score

23.11 Study Conclusions

Hemicraniectomy significantly reduced mortality in patients aged ≥60 years with malignant middle cerebral artery (MCA) infarction compared to standard medical treatment. However, survivors were more likely to have severe disability, highlighting the need for judicious patient selection and shared decision-making regarding functional outcomes.

23.12 Strengths

Strokes are generally more common among the elderly and carry worse outcomes than in younger subjects. Hence, the DESTINY II investigators addressed an important clinical question regarding the efficacy of hemicraniectomy for malignant middle-cerebral-artery infarction among patients older than 60 years of age. The multicentric design adds to the external validity of the trial. The conclusions were robust and revealed significantly improved survival following hemicraniectomy among older patients with extensive hemispheric stroke, although most survivors required continued assistance with bodily needs.

23.13 Weakness

The outcome benefit was largely due to improved survival among patients who underwent hemicraniectomy. However, the level of disability among survivors was similar in both groups. At 1-year follow-up, nearly 50% of survivors in both groups were unable to walk or attend to bodily needs without assistance; one-third of patients in both groups were bedridden, incontinent, or required constant bedside care. Hence, although surgical intervention saved lives, the level of disability remained comparable. The trial was ceased early based on pre-defined stoppage rules, as the efficacy of hemicraniectomy appeared evident. However, early stoppage resulted in a reduced sample size that could have affected the results. A score of 3 on the modified Rankin scale, with the ability to walk unsupported, may be considered a preferred endpoint compared with a score of 2, with the inability to attend to bodily needs and walk unsupported. The study was not powered to evaluate the efficacy of hemicraniectomy for this more favorable endpoint.

23.14 Summary

Internal carotid or middle-cerebral-artery occlusion leads to massive hemispheric infarction in approximately 10% of ischemic strokes. Three RCTs were published between 2007 and 2009 that evaluated the efficacy of hemicraniectomy in malignant ischemic stroke within 48 h of symptom onset. The results from these studies revealed improved survival with favorable neurological outcomes among patients aged 18–60 years. However, ischemic strokes become more common with advancing age, leading to poorer clinical outcomes. The DESTINY II trial addressed the question of whether the favorable effects of hemicraniectomy in massive ischemic stroke may be applicable among older patients aged 61 years and above. The median age of patients included was 70 years. The study was stopped early as improved outcomes became evident in the hemicraniectomy group. A score of 0–4 on the modified Rankin scale, considered a favorable outcome, occurred in significantly more patients in the hemicraniectomy group. The outcome benefit was driven mainly by improved survival among patients who underwent hemicraniectomy; the level of disability among survivors remained similar in both groups. Indeed, there were no patients in either group who survived to a level of minor or no disability. Nearly all post-operative survivors were severely disabled. The study established improved survival with hemicraniectomy in patients >60 years old with malignant middle-cerebral-artery infarction. However, most survivors continued to require assistance with bodily needs.

Outcomes from malignant middle-cerebral-artery infarction remain poor, with a high mortality of close to 80% among the older population. The DESTINY II trial established improved survival with hemicraniectomy in this population. Most survivors experienced a high level of disability, being unable to walk unsupported and requiring assistance for bodily needs. It is important to understand the perspective of patients and families regarding what they may consider to be a reasonable outcome. When faced with the prospect of imminent death, many may consider life-saving measures as appropriate while remaining hopeful of reasonable long-term outcomes.

References

1. Heinsius T, Bogousslavsky J, Van Melle G. Large infarcts in the middle cerebral artery territory. Etiology and outcome patterns. Neurology. 1998;50(2):341–50.
2. Hacke W, Schwab S, Horn M, Spranger M, De Georgia M, von Kummer R. "Malignant" middle cerebral artery territory infarction: clinical course and prognostic signs. Arch Neurol. 1996;53(4):309–15.
3. Berrouschot J, Sterker M, Bettin S, Köster J, Schneider D. Mortality of space-occupying ('malignant') middle cerebral artery infarction under conservative intensive care. Intensive Care Med. 1998;24(6):620–3.
4. Bereczki D, Liu M, do Prado GF, Fekete I. Mannitol for acute stroke. Cochrane Database Syst Rev. 2001;(1):CD001153.
5. Hofmeijer J, van der Worp HB, Kappelle LJ. Treatment of space-occupying cerebral infarction. Crit Care Med. 2003;31(2):617–25.

6. Schwarz S, Schwab S, Bertram M, Aschoff A, Hacke W. Effects of hypertonic saline hydroxyethyl starch solution and mannitol in patients with increased intracranial pressure after stroke. Stroke. 1998;29(8):1550–5.
7. King AB. Massive cerebral infarction producing ventriculographic changes suggesting a brain tumor. J Neurosurg. 1951;8(5):536–9.
8. Ivamoto HS, Numoto M, Donaghy RM. Surgical decompression for cerebral and cerebellar infarcts. Stroke. 1974;5(3):365–70.
9. Jüttler E, Schwab S, Schmiedek P, Unterberg A, Hennerici M, Woitzik J, et al. Decompressive surgery for the treatment of malignant infarction of the middle cerebral artery (DESTINY): a randomized, controlled trial. Stroke. 2007;38(9):2518–25.
10. Vahedi K, Vicaut E, Mateo J, Kurtz A, Orabi M, Guichard JP, et al. Sequential-design, multicenter, randomized, controlled trial of early decompressive craniectomy in malignant middle cerebral artery infarction (DECIMAL trial). Stroke. 2007;38(9):2506–17.
11. Hofmeijer J, Kappelle LJ, Algra A, Amelink GJ, van Gijn J, van der Worp HB, et al. Surgical decompression for space-occupying cerebral infarction (the Hemicraniectomy After Middle Cerebral Artery infarction with Life-threatening Edema Trial [HAMLET]): a multicentre, open, randomised trial. Lancet Neurol. 2009;8(4):326–33.
12. Vahedi K, Hofmeijer J, Juettler E, Vicaut E, George B, Algra A, et al. Early decompressive surgery in malignant infarction of the middle cerebral artery: a pooled analysis of three randomised controlled trials. Lancet Neurol. 2007;6(3):215–22.
13. Arac A, Blanchard V, Lee M, Steinberg GK. Assessment of outcome following decompressive craniectomy for malignant middle cerebral artery infarction in patients older than 60 years of age. Neurosurg Focus. 2009;26(6):E3.
14. Uhl E, Kreth FW, Elias B, Goldammer A, Hempelmann RG, Liefner M, et al. Outcome and prognostic factors of hemicraniectomy for space occupying cerebral infarction. J Neurol Neurosurg Psychiatry. 2004;75(2):270–4.
15. Gupta R, Connolly ES, Mayer S, Elkind MSV. Hemicraniectomy for massive middle cerebral artery territory infarction: a systematic review. Stroke. 2004;35(2):539–43.
16. Jüttler E, Unterberg A, Woitzik J, Bösel J, Amiri H, Sakowitz OW, et al. Hemicraniectomy in older patients with extensive middle-cerebral-artery stroke. N Engl J Med. 2014;370(12):1091–100.

24 Intravenous Thrombolysis Between 3 and 4.5 h After Ischemic Stroke: The ECASS III Trial

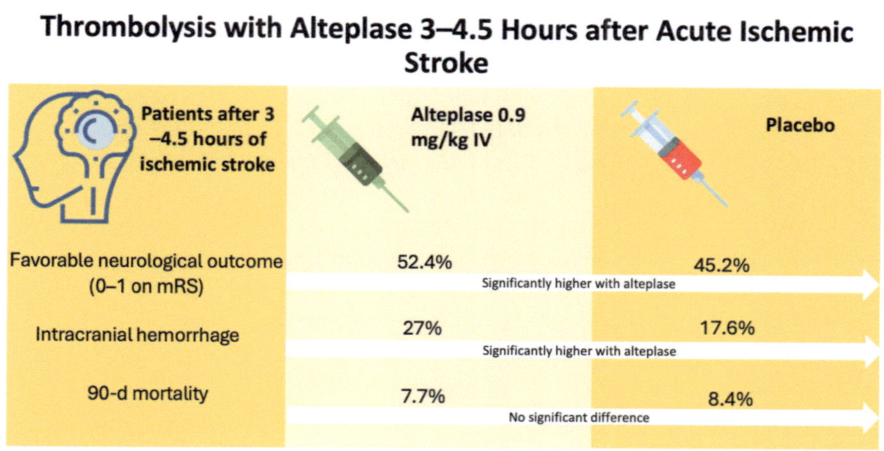

Hacke et al. (NEJM, 2008)

Quick Take

Could the time window be extended for thrombolytic treatment in acute ischemic stroke?

The ECASS III trial evaluated the safety and efficacy of intravenous alteplase (tPA) administered between 3 and 4.5 h after symptom onset in patients with acute ischemic stroke. This randomized, double-blind study found that patients receiving alteplase had significantly better functional outcomes at 90 days compared to those

---

Hacke W, Kaste M, Bluhmki E, Brozman M, Dávalos A, Guidetti D, et al. Thrombolysis with Alteplase 3 to 4.5 Hours after Acute Ischemic Stroke. N Engl J Med. 2008 Sep 25;359(13):1317–29.

J. Chacko et al., *Landmark Studies in Critical Care*,
https://doi.org/10.1007/978-981-95-0673-6_24

receiving a placebo. However, the treatment group also experienced a higher rate of symptomatic intracranial hemorrhage. These results extended the therapeutic window for thrombolytic therapy in selected patients, offering a critical opportunity to improve stroke outcomes.

24.1 Introduction

Acute ischemic stroke remains one of the few neurological disorders in which expeditious diagnosis and treatment could potentially lead to complete recovery. In 1995, the National Institute of Neurological Disorders and Stroke (NINDS) study group published their landmark randomized controlled trial (RCT) of intravenous thrombolysis with alteplase compared to placebo in acute ischemic stroke [1]. Patients treated with intravenous alteplase within 3 h of symptom onset were more likely to have minimal or no disability at 3 months compared with placebo, despite a higher incidence of symptomatic intracerebral hemorrhage. Two further RCTs followed; the ECASS trial included patients within 6 h of symptom onset. Functional outcomes were more favorable with alteplase in patients with moderate to severe neurological deficits without extended signs of infarct on initial CT imaging [2]. The ECASS II trial, published 3 years later, stratified patients according to the time since onset of symptoms, between 0 and 3 h or 3 and 6 h. No significant difference was observed in favorable neurological outcomes between the two groups, regardless of the duration of symptoms; however, most patients received treatment between 3 and 6 h [3].

Subsequently, a pooled analysis evaluated outcomes from 6 RCTs, including 2775 patients who used intravenous recombinant tissue plasminogen activator (rt-PA) in acute ischemic stroke [4]. Compared with placebo, the authors reported favorable clinical outcomes when thrombolytic treatment was administered between 3 and 4.5 h after symptom onset. Furthermore, the extended time window did not result in an increased incidence of intracranial hemorrhage or death.

The ECASS III trial was designed to evaluate the efficacy of intravenous thrombolysis with alteplase among patients who present between 3 and 4.5 h after the onset of stroke symptoms [5].

24.2 Population and Design

The ECASS III RCT was a double-blind, parallel-group trial conducted across multiple centers in Europe. The study was conducted from July 2003 to November 2007 across 130 sites in 19 countries. Patients between 18 and 80 years old with a clinical diagnosis of stroke were eligible if the study drug could be administered within 3–4 h of symptom onset. The time interval was extended to 4.5 h after the enrollment of 228 patients, considering newly available evidence and slower than expected recruitment rate. Stroke symptoms had to persist for $\geq$30 min with no sign of improvement in between for eligibility.

24.2.1 Exclusion

Patients with intracranial hemorrhage and those in whom the time of symptom onset was unknown, those with severe stroke, and intracranial hemorrhage were excluded. Those with seizures, previous stroke or severe traumatic brain injury in the preceding 3 months, thrombocytopenia (platelet count <100,000), hypertension (systolic BP >185 or diastolic BP >110 mm Hg), extremes of blood glucose levels (<50 or >400 mg/dl), major surgery or severe trauma within the previous 3 months, and major disorders with an increased risk of bleeding were also excluded. Randomization was carried out at study centers in a 1:1 ratio, in blocks of four, to allow a balanced distribution of assignment to groups.

24.2.2 Alteplase Group

Patients received alteplase, 0.9 mg/kg, intravenously, to a maximum dose of 90 mg. Ten percent of the dose was administered as a bolus, followed by the remaining dose over 60 min.

24.2.3 Placebo Group

A matching placebo consisting of an identical lyophilized powder reconstituted in water was administered over the same duration.

24.2.4 Common Management

During the first 24 h after the administration of the study drug, intravenous heparin, oral anticoagulants, aspirin, and volume expanders, including hetastarch or dextrans, were not allowed. Subcutaneous unfractionated or low molecular weight heparin was allowed as prophylaxis against deep vein thrombosis. CT or MRI scans were performed before the commencement of treatment and at 22–36 h later. Patients were evaluated on days 30 and 90 using the modified Rankin scale (Table 24.1).

Table 24.1 The modified Rankin scale

Score on the modified Rankin scale	Description
0	No symptoms
1	No significant disability. Able to carry out all usual activities, despite some symptoms
2	Slight disability. Able to look after own affairs without assistance, but unable to carry out all previous activities
3	Moderate disability. Requires some help, but able to walk unassisted
4	Moderately severe disability. Unable to attend to own bodily needs without assistance, or unable to walk unassisted
5	Severe disability. Requires constant nursing care and attention, bedridden, incontinent
6	Dead

24.3 Sample Size

The investigators calculated the sample size based on the primary efficacy end-point—disability on day 90. Disability was assessed using the modified Rankin scale and dichotomized to favorable (0 or 1) or unfavorable (2–6) scores. They assumed an odds ratio of 1.4 favoring alteplase based on data from the previous pooled analysis [4] that compared patients who received thrombolysis with placebo at 3–4.5 h after stroke onset. A sample size of 800 patients provided the study with 90% power to detect a favorable effect with thrombolysis.

24.4 Results

A total of 821 patients were randomized—418 patients were assigned to the alteplase group and 403 to the placebo group. Alteplase was administered at a median duration of 3 h and 59 min after the onset of symptoms. Most patients were randomized between 3.5–4 h (46.8%), followed by between 4–4.5 h (39.2%), and 3–3.5 h (10%). Stroke severity was higher in the placebo group (mean NIHSS score: 11.6 ± 5.9 vs. 10.7 ± 5.6). The incidence of previous stroke was also higher in the placebo group (14.1% vs. 7.7%). Apart from these characteristics, patients were well-matched at baseline.

24.4.1 The Primary Endpoint: Disability at Day 90

A favorable outcome, defined as a score of 0–1 on the modified Rankin scale (no symptoms or mild symptoms, but able to carry out all usual activities), was significantly greater with alteplase compared to placebo [52.4% vs. 45.2%, odds ratio:

1.34 (1.02–1.76), $p = 0.04$]. On post-hoc intention-to-treat analysis, after adjustment for confounding baseline characteristics, the favorable outcomes persisted with alteplase compared with placebo [odds ratio: 1.42 (1.02–1.98) $P = 0.04$).

24.4.2 The Secondary Endpoint: Global Outcome

The secondary endpoint was a global outcome measure that used a combination of outcomes at 90 days. The individual components of the global outcome included a score of 0 or 1 on the modified Rankin scale, a score of ≥95 on the Barthel Index, a score of 0 or 1 on the NIHSS, and a score of 1 on the Glasgow Outcome Scale. The Global outcome measure was more favorable in the alteplase group [odds ratio: 1.28 (1.0–1.65), $p = 0.05$]. The authors calculated the likelihood of a favorable outcome, with an independent lifestyle, to be 28% higher with alteplase compared with placebo.

The individual components of the global outcome measure were assessed at 30 and 90 days. A modified Rankin score of 0–2 and a Barthel Index score (ranging from a score of 0 for total dependence to 100 for independent living) of ≥95 were similar in both groups. An NIHSS score (0 to 42, with higher values reflecting more severe neurologic impairment) of 0 or 1, or >8-point improvement from baseline, was more favorable at 30 days in the alteplase group.

24.4.3 Safety Outcomes

A total of 66 patients died; mortality was not significantly different between the alteplase and placebo groups (7.7% vs. 8.4%, $p = 0.68$). The overall incidence of intracranial hemorrhage was higher with alteplase compared to placebo (27.0% vs. 17.6%, $p = 0.001$). Symptomatic intracranial hemorrhage, although uncommon, was significantly higher with alteplase (2.4% vs. 0.3%, $p = 0.008$). All cases of symptomatic intracranial hemorrhage occurred within 22–36 h of commencement of treatment. The incidence of symptomatic cerebral edema did not differ significantly between the two groups. Adverse events involving other organ systems were few and were similar in both groups. The main outcomes are summarized in Table 24.2.

Table 24.2 Summary of main outcomes

Outcome	Alteplase (418 patients)	Placebo (403 patients)	Odds ratio	*p*-value
mRS score of 0 or 1	219 (52.4%)	182 (45.2%)	1.34 (1.02–1.76)	0.04
Global outcome			1.28 (1.00–1.65)	0.05
90-d mortality	32 (7.7%)	34 (8.4%)	0.90 (0.54–1.49)	0.68
Symptomatic ICH	10 (2.4%)	1 (0.2%)	9.85 (1.26–77.32)	0.008

Abbreviations: *mRS* modified Rankin Scale, *ICH* intracranial hemorrhage

24.5 Study Conclusions

Intravenous alteplase administered between 3 and 4.5 h after acute ischemic stroke significantly improved functional outcomes at 90 days compared to placebo, with a higher likelihood of achieving independent recovery. However, delayed thrombolysis was associated with an increased risk of symptomatic intracranial hemorrhage, though it did not significantly affect overall mortality.

24.6 Strengths

The NINDS trial had previously reported significantly favorable outcomes among stroke patients who received thrombolytic treatment within 3 h of symptom onset. The ECASS III trial evaluated the efficacy of thrombolysis beyond this time window for up to 4.5 h. This landmark trial represented an important milestone in stroke therapy, establishing the efficacy of thrombolysis in patients who may present beyond the previously studied time window of 3 h after the onset of symptoms. The study had a robust design and was well-conducted. The authors applied multiple, pre-specified analytical approaches to overcome potential confounders. The outcomes studied were pre-specified and clinically relevant. The study raised optimism of improved neurological outcomes among patients who may present beyond the conventionally accepted window of 3 h after the onset of symptoms following ischemic stroke.

24.7 Limitations

The investigators excluded patients with severe stroke. A subgroup analysis of the NINDS trial had in fact, revealed improved outcomes with thrombolytic treatment in severe stroke among older patients. There were imbalances between groups at baseline; patients in the placebo group had more severe strokes by the NIHSS criteria and a higher incidence of previous stroke. Besides, in the placebo group, the incidence of large vessel occlusion was higher, smokers were more common, and fewer patients were on aspirin. The fragility index of the study was just 1—which meant that the difference between groups would have been statistically non-significant if one additional patient in the placebo group had a favorable primary outcome. The study protocol was revised midway through the trial, with the time window for thrombolysis being extended from 4 to 4.5 h. The number of patients with diabetes was relatively low compared to previous stroke trials. Would the results be generalizable to diabetic patients?

24.8 Re-analysis of ECASS III

In 2020, Alper et al. performed a re-analysis of the ECASS III data, adjusting for differences in baseline characteristics between the alteplase and placebo groups [6]. They carried out multivariable and stratified analyses; sensitivity analysis was performed for missing data. Baseline imbalances were identified between groups in regard to the NIHSS score and previous history of stroke. The ECASS III paper had reported that their methodology of assessment of stroke severity was based on a range of 0–42 based on 15 parameters. However, the analysis was actually carried out on a score ranging from 0 to 46 that included two additional components of distal motor function. On re-analysis based on the standard NIHSS scale of 0–42, a favorable primary outcome of 0 or 1 on the modified Rankin scale at 90 days was not significantly greater in the alteplase group.

Further re-analysis after adjusting for baseline imbalances revealed that none of the secondary outcomes were significantly more favorable in the alteplase group; however, the significantly higher incidence of intracerebral hemorrhage persisted. This re-analysis of the ECASS III trial raises concerns regarding bias arising from baseline imbalances that could have confounded the results. However, as the authors of the re-analysis themselves state, although their findings may alter the certainty behind the unadjusted analysis of the original study, they can only be considered hypothesis-generating.

24.9 Summary

Thrombolysis, administered in a timely manner, was established as the definitive therapy for acute ischemic stroke within the first 3 h of onset of symptoms following the NINDS study. The benefit of later administration of thrombolysis remained contentious despite RCTs and pooled analyses that followed. The ECASS III investigators conducted a multicentric, adequately powered RCT to evaluate the efficacy of alteplase compared with placebo among stroke patients between 3 and 4.5 h after symptom onset. Compared with placebo, intravenous thrombolysis with alteplase resulted in improved neurological outcomes, resulting in more patients with either no disability or minimal deficit that did not restrict their usual activities. The incidence of intracranial hemorrhage was higher with alteplase; mortality was similar in both groups. Although the study was limited by imbalances between groups at baseline, it remains a landmark in the history of thrombolytic therapy for acute ischemic stroke and led to an extension of the time window for treatment.

References

1. National Institute of Neurological Disorders and Stroke rt-PA Stroke Study Group. Tissue plasminogen activator for acute ischemic stroke. N Engl J Med. 1995;333(24):1581–7.
2. Hacke W, Kaste M, Fieschi C, Toni D, Lesaffre E, von Kummer R, et al. Intravenous thrombolysis with recombinant tissue plasminogen activator for acute hemispheric stroke. The European Cooperative Acute Stroke Study (ECASS). JAMA. 1995;274(13):1017–25.
3. Hacke W, Kaste M, Fieschi C, von Kummer R, Davalos A, Meier D, et al. Randomised double-blind placebo-controlled trial of thrombolytic therapy with intravenous alteplase in acute ischaemic stroke (ECASS II). Second European-Australasian Acute Stroke Study Investigators. Lancet Lond Engl. 1998;352(9136):1245–51.
4. Hacke W, Donnan G, Fieschi C, Kaste M, von Kummer R, Broderick JP, et al. Association of outcome with early stroke treatment: pooled analysis of ATLANTIS, ECASS, and NINDS rt-PA stroke trials. Lancet Lond Engl. 2004;363(9411):768–74.
5. Hacke W, Kaste M, Bluhmki E, Brozman M, Dávalos A, Guidetti D, et al. Thrombolysis with alteplase 3 to 4.5 hours after acute ischemic stroke. N Engl J Med. 2008;359(13):1317–29.
6. Alper BS, Foster G, Thabane L, Rae-Grant A, Malone-Moses M, Manheimer E. Thrombolysis with alteplase 3–4.5 hours after acute ischaemic stroke: trial reanalysis adjusted for baseline imbalances. BMJ Evid-Based Med. 2020;25(5):168–71.

A Comparison of Four Treatments for Generalized Convulsive Status Epilepticus: Treiman et al.

25

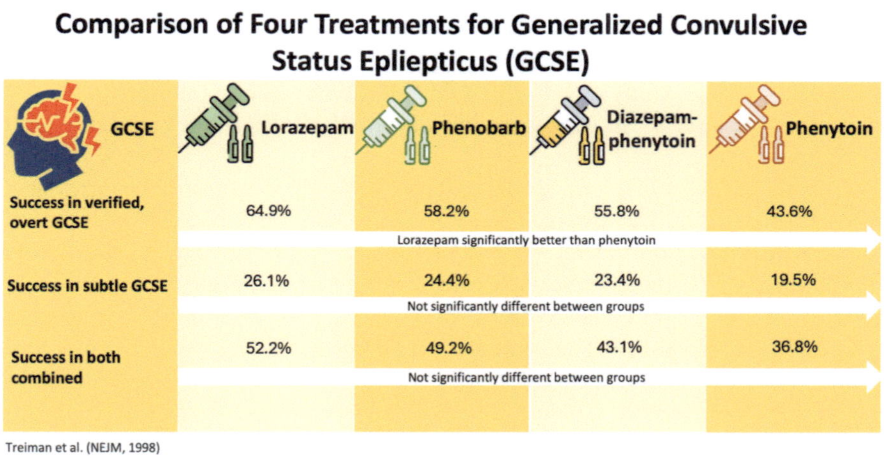

Quick Take

Which treatment is most effective for generalized convulsive status epilepticus (GCSE)?

The study by Treiman et al. compared the efficacy of different treatments for GCSE in a multicenter randomized controlled trial (RCT). The trial enrolled patients with GCSE and compared the outcomes with four treatments—diazepam followed by phenytoin, lorazepam, phenobarbital, and phenytoin. The results showed that

---

Treiman DM, Meyers PD, Walton NY, Collins JF, Colling C, Rowan AJ, et al. A comparison of four treatments for generalized convulsive status epilepticus. Veterans Affairs Status Epilepticus Cooperative Study Group. N Engl J Med. 1998 Sep 17;339(12):792–8.

J. Chacko et al., *Landmark Studies in Critical Care*,
https://doi.org/10.1007/978-981-95-0673-6_25

lorazepam was significantly more effective in controlling seizures compared to the other treatments, with fewer side effects. The study concluded that lorazepam should be the first-line treatment for GCSE, setting a new standard for managing this life-threatening condition in emergency settings.

25.1 Introduction and Background

Status epilepticus represents a neurological emergency that requires expeditious evaluation and treatment. Uncontrolled seizures often result in adverse neurological sequelae [1] and mortality [2]. The key to prompt seizure control centers around the administration of an anti-seizure agent with a rapid onset of action and sustained effect. At the time of the conduct of the Veterans Affairs Status Epilepticus Cooperative Study Group trial, clinicians commonly employed four treatment regimens for seizure control in status epilepticus—phenobarbital, phenytoin, a combination of phenytoin and diazepam, and lorazepam [3]. However, no large randomized controlled trial (RCT) had been performed to compare the relative efficacy of these drugs. The Veterans study was designed to compare the efficacy of standard dosing with these regimens in the management of generalized convulsive status epilepticus.

In an RCT from 1983, lorazepam was compared with diazepam in the treatment of status epilepticus. The trial included 78 patients who experienced 81 episodes of status epilepticus. Lorazepam, 4 mg, was compared with diazepam 10 mg, both administered intravenously. Seizure control with a single dose of the drug was higher with lorazepam compared with diazepam, although the difference was not statistically significant. Overall, seizure control with one or two doses was also higher with lorazepam (89% vs. 76%). The time to seizure control did not differ between the two drugs; the incidence of adverse effects was also similar [4]. Seizures were controlled in 89% of the episodes treated with lorazepam and in 76% of episodes treated with diazepam. The onset of action did not differ significantly between the two agents. Adverse effects occurred in 13% of the lorazepam-treated patients and in 12% of the diazepam-treated patients. Respiratory depression and arrest, the most frequent adverse effects, were treated symptomatically; no adverse sequelae ensued.

Considering the relative paucity of data regarding the efficacy of commonly used treatment regimens in status epilepticus, the Veterans Affairs Status Epilepticus Cooperative Study Group conducted an RCT to compare commonly used treatment modalities in the control of status epilepticus [5].

25.2 Population and Design

The double-blind study was conducted at 16 Veterans Affairs medical centers and 6 affiliated university hospitals in the USA during a 5-year period between 1990 and 1995. Patients with generalized convulsive status epilepticus were enrolled, regardless of prior treatment.

Generalized convulsive status epilepticus was defined as *overt* or *subtle*. *Overt* generalized convulsive status was defined as the occurrence of two or more generalized convulsions without full recovery of consciousness in between, or when seizure activity persisted for more than 10 min. Continuous coma with subtle motor convulsions was defined as generalized *subtle* generalized convulsive status epilepticus. A comatose state with seizure activity on the electroencephalogram, with or without subtle convulsions, was also considered subtle status epilepticus. The requirement for an electroencephalogram to diagnose generalized convulsive status was considered to indicate subtle generalized convulsive status epilepticus.

25.2.1 Excluded

Patients less than 18 years old and those with non-generalized status epilepticus were excluded. Other exclusion criteria were presentation with a neurological emergency requiring immediate surgical intervention, contraindication to hydantoin, benzodiazepine, or barbiturates, and pregnancy. If repeated episodes of generalized convulsive status epilepticus occurred, the first episode alone was included in the evaluation.

25.3 Treatment Groups

Patients were randomly assigned to one of four intravenous treatment regimens. The drug regimen kits were identical to ensure blinding.

25.3.1 Diazepam

In this group, diazepam was administered in a dose of 0.15 mg/kg, followed by phenytoin, 18 mg/kg, intravenously.

25.3.2 Lorazepam

In this group, lorazepam was administered in a dose of 0.1 mg/kg intravenously.

25.3.3 Phenobarbital

Patients received phenobarbital, 15 mg/kg, intravenously.

25.3.4 Phenytoin

A dose of phenytoin, 18 mg/kg intravenously, was administered to patients in this group.

25.3.5 Common Management

Intravenous access was secured, followed by infusion of normal saline. Electroencephalogram recording was commenced as early as feasible, without delaying treatment. The study period was 12 h, during which seizure activity was recorded every 5 min in the first 20 min, and every 10 min for the next 40 min. This was followed by hourly recording of the seizure activity and conscious level. Patients who did not respond to the first line of treatment received a second, and if necessary, a third treatment regimen. The alternate treatment options in non-responders were not randomized. Treatment success entailed cessation of all clinical and electrical evidence of seizures within 20 min of commencement of therapy; besides, no recurrence of seizures should occur between 20 and 60 min of treatment.

25.4 Statistical Analysis

Analysis was performed separately for patients with overt and subtle generalized convulsive status epilepticus. Analysis was carried out on an intention-to-treat basis, including patients mistakenly assigned to the wrong group (overt vs. subtle), those who presented with other types of status epilepticus, or did not actually experience status epilepticus. A separate analysis was performed exclusively for patients with a verified diagnosis of generalized convulsive status epilepticus.

25.5 Results

During the study period, 1705 patients were screened, of whom 570 were enrolled—of these, 395 had overt, and 175, subtle status epilepticus. Among 518 patients with a verified diagnosis of status epilepticus—384 experienced overt and 184 subtle status epilepticus. Among these patients with a verified diagnosis, lorazepam was administered in 136, phenobarbital in 124, diazepam-phenytoin combination in 131, and phenytoin alone in 127 patients. Baseline characteristics were similar in all four groups of patients. Lorazepam infusion was completed most rapidly among all treatments; regimens that included phenytoin took the longest to complete.

25.5.1 Successful Initial Treatment

Treatment success was defined as cessation of all clinical and electrical evidence of seizures within 20 min of commencement of therapy, with no recurrence of seizures occurring between 20 and 60 min of treatment. Overall, among 518 patients with a verified diagnosis of generalized convulsive status epilepticus, the initial treatment was successful in significantly more patients with overt compared to subtle status epilepticus (55.5% vs. 14.9%, $P = 0.02$).

Among patients with verified overt status epilepticus, lorazepam was the most successful (64.9%), followed by phenobarbital (58.2%), and the diazepam–phenytoin combination (55.8%); phenytoin was the least successful (43.6%). Lorazepam was significantly more successful compared with phenytoin (64.9% vs. 43.6%, $P = 0.002$). Pairwise comparisons between other treatments did not reveal a significant difference. The results were similar on intention-to-treat analysis, including all enrolled patients (as opposed to patients with a "verified" diagnosis).

In subtle status epilepticus, the success rate was much lower and did not differ between the four treatment regimens ($P = 0.18$).

When patients with overt and subtle status epilepticus were combined in a post hoc analysis, lorazepam remained the most effective (52.2%), followed by phenobarbital (49.2%), diazepam-phenytoin combination (43.1%), and phenytoin alone (36.8%). On paired analysis, lorazepam and phenobarbital were significantly more effective compared with phenytoin. Approximately 50% of patients with overt status epilepticus required a second antiseizure medication; however, when the initial treatment was unsuccessful, response to a second medication was poor (7%).

On intention-to-treat analysis, the trends in treatment efficacy were similar; however, no significant differences were observed between treatment groups in either overt or subtle status epilepticus.

The incidence of recurrent seizures was similar in all four groups of patients. At the end of the 12-h study period, none of the patients in the subtle status epilepticus group regained consciousness, compared with 17% who regained consciousness in the overt group.

25.5.2 30-Day Outcomes

At 30 days, patients with subtle status epilepticus experienced worse outcomes compared to those with overt status epilepticus; only 8.8% of patients with subtle status epilepticus were discharged from the hospital, compared with 50.1% in the overt group. The 30-day mortality was also higher with subtle compared to overt status epilepticus (64.7% vs. 27%). No differences in the 30-day outcomes were observed between the four treatment regimens in either group.

Table 25.1 Main outcomes

Outcome	Lorazepam	Phenobarbital	Diazepam-phenytoin	Phenytoin	Significance
Treatment success is verified, overt GCSE	64.9%	58.2%	55.8%	43.6%	Lorazepam superior to phenytoin ($P = 0.002$)
Treatment success in subtle GCSE	26.1%	24.4%	23.4%	19.5%	Not significant
Treatment success in overt and subtle combined	52.2%	49.2%	43.1%	36.8%	Not significant

Abbreviation: *GCSE* Generalized convulsive status epilepticus

Overall, patients who were successfully treated with the first study drug experienced more favorable outcomes. Mortality was twice as high in both overt and subtle status epilepticus when seizures were not controlled with the first dose of the drug. The main outcomes are summarized in Table 25.1.

25.6 Adverse Events

Hypotension, hypoventilation, and cardiac arrhythmias were the commonly reported adverse events; there was no significant difference in the incidence of adverse events among the four groups of patients. Hypotension was more often observed with subtle compared with overt status epilepticus.

25.7 Study Conclusions

The authors concluded that lorazepam is significantly more effective than phenytoin in the initial control of overt generalized convulsive status epilepticus. Lorazepam was the most effective drug in paired comparisons between different treatment regimens. Furthermore, it was the most convenient to use and took the least time to complete the administration. Recurrence of status during the 12-h study period was not significantly different between treatment regimens. The risk of drug-related adverse events was also similar among all four groups. The authors also observed that subtle status epilepticus was harder to control and associated with worse clinical outcomes, including mortality. Success with initial treatment was associated with more favorable clinical outcomes in both overt and subtle status epilepticus. The authors recommended lorazepam in the initial treatment of generalized convulsive status epilepticus until newer therapies were established.

25.8 Strengths

The Veterans trial evaluated the relative efficacy of commonly used anti-seizure medications in the control of status epilepticus, in a randomized four-armed design. The study suggested that lorazepam may be the most efficacious, while phenytoin appeared to be the least effective. The study included a broad subgroup of patients, although there was a relative preponderancy of male patients. The authors performed intention-to-treat analysis, including all patients; besides, patients with "verified" generalized convulsive status epilepticus were analyzed separately, adding to the robustness of the trial. The trial provided reasonably clear guidance regarding the optimal in-hospital management of status epilepticus.

25.9 Limitations

The definition of status epilepticus has changed over the years. The Veterans study defined status epilepticus as continuous seizure activity that lasted for 10 min. Currently, the Neurocritical Care Society guidelines (2012) define status epilepticus as clinical or electrographic seizure activity that continues for ≥5 min, with no recovery in between [6]. The term "subtle" status epilepticus used in the study probably represents non-convulsive status epilepticus according to the current definition. Continuous electroencephalographic monitoring was not in vogue during the study period. Cessation of seizures may have been difficult to interpret based on clinical signs alone. The current practice is to perform continuous electroencephalographic monitoring in patients with status epilepticus.

Several new anti-seizure drugs have been introduced since the publication of the trial, including fosphenytoin [7], which may be infused more rapidly (5–7 min) compared with phenytoin. Furthermore, it has fewer adverse effects compared with phenytoin. Levetiracetam is another newer agent that has been shown to be equally efficacious compared with lorazepam, with fewer adverse effects [8]. In patients with refractory and super-refractory status epilepticus, propofol and ketamine infusions are commonly used among patients who are intubated and mechanically ventilated [9]. The study included adult patients with generalized convulsive status epilepticus; the findings may not be extrapolatable to other types of seizures or among patients who undergo surgical procedures, including traumatic brain injury, and the treatment of children with generalized convulsive status epilepticus.

25.10 Subsequent Evidence

Although lorazepam continues to remain the initial drug of choice, intramuscular midazolam has emerged as a viable alternative for the pre-hospital treatment of status epilepticus following the RAMPART trial [10]. This double-blind RCT enrolled adults and children; intramuscular midazolam in a dose of 5 or 10 mg was compared with intravenous lorazepam, 2 or 4 mg, depending on the body weight. Seizures were absent on arrival to the emergency department in a similar proportion of patients in both groups. The requirement for endotracheal intubation and mechanical ventilation and the incidence of recurrent seizures were also similar. The authors concluded that intramuscular midazolam is at least as safe and effective as intravenous lorazepam in the pre-hospital control of seizures.

Since the publication of the Veterans trial, sodium valproate and levetiracetam have emerged as second-line drugs in the management of status epilepticus. Although the practice is variable, many clinicians choose alternative drugs in status epilepticus that do not respond to lorazepam, before employing anesthetic drugs as a last resort.

25.11 Summary

The most optimal initial management of generalized convulsive status epilepticus, a life-threatening emergency, was unclear in the era preceding the Veterans study. The authors embarked upon a comparative study of four intravenous treatment regimens commonly employed by clinicians in that period—diazepam followed by phenytoin, lorazepam, phenobarbital, and phenytoin alone. Among 384 patients with a verified diagnosis of overt generalized convulsive status epilepticus, lorazepam was most efficacious and significantly superior to phenytoin. In subtle generalized status epilepticus, the difference between the four treatment regimens was not statistically significant. The incidence of recurrent status epilepticus during the 12-h study period, the 30-day clinical outcomes, and adverse events were similar in all four groups of patients.

The authors concluded that in the control of overt generalized convulsive status epilepticus, lorazepam is superior to phenytoin. Besides, it was the easiest to administer, prompting the authors to recommend it as the preferred agent for the treatment of generalized convulsive status epilepticus.

References

1. DeLorenzo RJ, Hauser WA, Towne AR, Boggs JG, Pellock JM, Penberthy L, et al. A prospective, population-based epidemiologic study of status epilepticus in Richmond, Virginia. Neurology. 1996;46(4):1029–35.
2. Logroscino G, Hesdorffer DC, Cascino G, Annegers JF, Hauser WA. Short-term mortality after a first episode of status epilepticus. Epilepsia. 1997;38(12):1344–9.
3. Delgado-Escueta AV, Wasterlain C, Treiman DM, Porter RJ. Current concepts in neurology: management of status epilepticus. N Engl J Med. 1982;306(22):1337–40.
4. Leppik IE, Derivan AT, Homan RW, Walker J, Ramsay RE, Patrick B. Double-blind study of lorazepam and diazepam in status epilepticus. JAMA. 1983;249(11):1452–4.

5. Treiman DM, Meyers PD, Walton NY, Collins JF, Colling C, Rowan AJ, et al. A comparison of four treatments for generalized convulsive status epilepticus. Veterans Affairs Status Epilepticus Cooperative Study Group. N Engl J Med. 1998;339(12):792–8.
6. Brophy GM, Bell R, Claassen J, Alldredge B, Bleck TP, Glauser T, et al. Guidelines for the evaluation and management of status epilepticus. Neurocrit Care. 2012;17(1):3–23.
7. Luer MS. Fosphenytoin. Neurol Res. 1998;20(2):178–82.
8. Misra UK, Kalita J, Maurya PK. Levetiracetam versus lorazepam in status epilepticus: a randomized, open labeled pilot study. J Neurol. 2012;259(4):645–8.
9. Rai S, Drislane FW. Treatment of refractory and super-refractory status epilepticus. Neurother J Am Soc Exp Neurother. 2018;15(3):697–712.
10. Silbergleit R, Durkalski V, Lowenstein D, Conwit R, Pancioli A, Palesch Y, et al. Intramuscular versus intravenous therapy for prehospital status epilepticus. N Engl J Med. 2012;366(7):591–600.

Neurosurgical Clipping Versus Endovascular Coiling in Ruptured Intracranial Aneurysms: The ISAT Trial

26

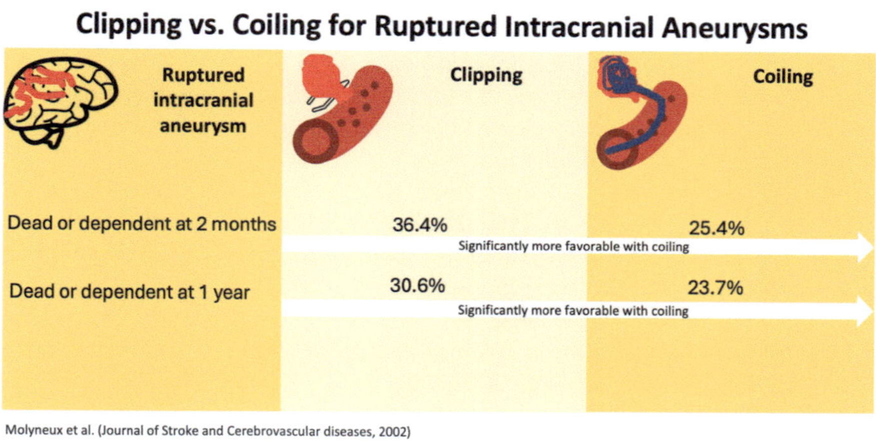

Quick Take

Which is more effective for ruptured intracranial aneurysms suitable for either modality: surgical clipping or endovascular coiling?

The ISAT trial was a landmark randomized controlled trial comparing neurosurgical clipping with endovascular coiling for the treatment of ruptured intracranial aneurysms. The study enrolled 2143 patients and demonstrated that patients treated

---

Molyneux A, Kerr R. and the International Subarachnoid Aneurysm Trial (ISAT) Collaborative Group. International Subarachnoid Aneurysm Trial (ISAT) of neurosurgical clipping versus *endovascular coiling in 2143 patients with ruptured intracranial aneurysms: A randomized trial. J Stroke Cerebrovasc Dis. 2002 Nov;11(6):304–14.*

J. Chacko et al., *Landmark Studies in Critical Care*,
https://doi.org/10.1007/978-981-95-0673-6_26

with endovascular coiling had a significantly lower rate of death or dependence at 1 year compared to those treated with surgical clipping. The findings indicated that endovascular coiling was associated with better outcomes in terms of functional recovery and reduced complications, leading to a shift in clinical practice towards preferring coiling over clipping for most patients with ruptured intracranial aneurysms.

26.1 Introduction

Intracranial aneurysms occur in about 5–8% of the population [1]. Aneurysmal rupture often leads to catastrophic outcomes, including substantial mortality [2]. Treatment modalities aim to achieve complete occlusion of the aneurysm while ensuring continued blood flow to the parent vessel, its branches, and perforating vessels.

In his 1933 report, Norman Dott described a 53-year-old man who presented with recurrent episodes of subarachnoid hemorrhage [3]. Through a left frontal approach, the culprit aneurysm was identified close to the bifurcation of the internal carotid artery. The vessel was cleared of clots all around and the aneurysm was wrapped with thin strips of muscle obtained from the patient's leg. In 1938, the legendary Walter Dandy, one of the founding fathers of neurosurgery, performed the first obliterative clipping of an intracranial aneurysm on a 43-year-old man who presented with a ruptured aneurysm of the internal carotid artery [4]. He described how the narrow aneurysmal neck offered an easy "surgical attack". A flat silver clip was placed on the neck of the aneurysm and tightly compressed, leading to complete obliteration. The aneurysm softened and ceased to pulsate almost instantaneously, heralding the era of surgical clipping.

The inherent complexity of surgical procedures paved the way for the genesis of endovascular techniques of aneurysm treatment. The quest for less invasive techniques led to the introduction of the detachable platinum coil device [5]. The aneurysm is densely packed with multiple coils, leading to thrombus and granulation tissue formation, thereby limiting blood flow to the lumen. The endovascular coiling technique gained wide acceptance, considering its relative simplicity and applicability in patients too sick to undergo major surgery.

Hand in hand, surgical interventions too were performed with increasing finesse, with the advent of the operating microscope, improved microsurgical techniques, and the development of vascular neurosurgery as a stand-alone specialty. However, by 1995, endovascular coiling was being increasingly employed as the preferred treatment modality for intracranial aneurysms. Robust evidence on the ideal modality of treatment remained elusive, with only a small randomized controlled trial (RCT) that compared neurosurgical clipping with endovascular coiling. This RCT included 109 patients who presented with subarachnoid hemorrhage following a ruptured aneurysm [6]. Patients were randomized to undergo surgical ligation or coil embolization. This study revealed more favorable angiographic results with surgical intervention in patients with anterior cerebral artery aneurysms, while endovascular treatment appeared more optimal among those with aneurysms in the posterior circulation. The need for an adequately powered RCT that compared endovascular coiling with neurosurgical clipping was sorely felt, leading to the study by the International Subarachnoid Aneurysm Trial (ISAT) Collaborative Group.

26.2 Population and Design

The ISAT multicentric RCT was conducted between Sept 12, 1994, and May 1, 2002, across 43 centers in Europe and North America [7]. Patients with ruptured intracranial aneurysms were randomized to conventional neurosurgical or endovascular treatment if they were considered suitable for both therapies. All participating sites were major neurosurgical centers, treating between 60 and 100 cases per year, with expertise in both treatment modalities.

26.2.1 Inclusion Criteria

Subarachnoid hemorrhage was proven by CT or lumbar puncture within 28 days preceding randomization. A causative intracranial aneurysm had to be demonstrated by conventional or CT angiography. Patients were deemed to require treatment by neurosurgical intervention or endovascular technique; either treatment modality was considered appropriate based on angiographic anatomy.

26.2.2 Excluded

Patients were excluded if >28 days had elapsed since the occurrence of subarachnoid hemorrhage or were considered ineligible for one or both treatment modalities.

26.3 Randomization and Procedure

Patients were randomized to craniotomy and micro-neurosurgical clipping or endovascular treatment using detachable platinum coils. A minimization algorithm was employed, aiming to balance both groups based on age, gender, clinical grade, location of the culprit aneurysm, and the extent of hemorrhage on the CT scan. Post-procedure angiography was mandated for endovascular procedures unless specifically contraindicated. Angiography was also recommended for patients who underwent clipping, but not mandated if it meant a change in practice for the center where the procedure was performed. Following the initial procedure, further interventions could be performed on the target lesion or other lesions as appropriate.

26.4 Sample Size

The authors assumed a reduction in the number of patients dead or dependent at 1 year from 24% in the surgical clipping group to 19% in the endovascular treatment arm. This represented a 25% relative reduction in unfavorable outcomes at 1 year. The trial aimed to recruit 2500 patients, providing the study with 90% power at a level of significance of 0.01.

26.5 Results

Recruitment was ceased following a planned interim analysis in May 2002. During the study period, 9559 patients were admitted with proven subarachnoid hemorrhage; following exclusion of 7416 patients, 2143 were randomized. Nearly all aneurysms (97.3%) involved the anterior circulation—most common locations were anterior cerebral, internal carotid, and middle cerebral arteries. The assigned modality of treatment was performed in 95.3% of patients. Nine patients who were randomized to the endovascular treatment group crossed over to surgical clipping, while 38 allocated to the surgical arm received endovascular treatment. Among patients randomized to the endovascular arm, the mean duration between randomization and performance of the procedure was 1.1 days; it was significantly longer in the neurosurgical group (1.7 days). The WFNS grade, size of the target aneurysm, and the number of aneurysms identified were similar in both groups. The endovascular procedure was successful in 92.5% of patients; the neurosurgical procedure was completed in 97.8% patients.

26.5.1 Clinical Outcomes at 2 Months

Among 1918 patients who were eligible for analysis at 2 months, data were available on 1906 patients. Clinical outcomes were evaluated based on the modified Rankin scale. The primary objective was to evaluate the proportion of patients who were dead or dependent, defined as a score of 3–6. At 2 months, there were significantly more patients who were dead or dependent in the neurosurgical group compared to the endovascular treatment group. In the endovascular treatment group, 254/959 (25.4%) patients were dead or dependent compared with 345/947 (36.4%) in the neurosurgery group (relative risk, 0.698; [95% CI: 0.609–0.801], $p = 0.0001$).

26.5.2 Clinical Outcomes at 1 Year

At 1 year, data were available on 1594 of 1624 patients who were eligible for analysis. Similar to outcomes at 2 months, patients who underwent endovascular treatment fared better compared with those who underwent neurosurgical procedures. Among 801 patients assigned to endovascular treatment, 190 (23.7%) were dead or dependent at 1 year, compared with 243/793 (30.6%) patients who were allocated to undergo neurosurgery (relative risk, 0.774; [95% CI: 0.658–0.911], $p = 0.0019$). This represented a relative risk reduction of 22.6% and an absolute risk reduction of 6.9% for patients who underwent endovascular procedures. The case fatality rate at 1 year did not differ significantly between the two groups (endovascular treatment: 8.1% vs. neurosurgery: 10.1%).

26.5.3 Rebleeding

Rebleeding before the assigned procedure occurred in 14 (7%) patients in the endovascular treatment group and 23 (16%) patients in the neurosurgical group. Rebleeding in the first 30 days after the procedure was more common in the endovascular treatment group (20 [10%] vs. 6 [3%] patients).

Among the 20 patients who rebled in the endovascular group, the aneurysm could not be occluded in five patients, while occlusion was incomplete in seven. In three patients, the aneurysm was considered fully occluded. The remaining five patients developed a thromboembolic complication following the endovascular procedure. They went on to receive thrombolytic therapy; however, there were no survivors.

Among the six patients in the neurosurgery group who rebled, occlusion of the aneurysm was incomplete in three patients, while the other three had undergone complete neurosurgical clipping.

The total incidence of rebleeding from initial rupture up to 1 year was similar in both groups. The risk of rebleeding after 1 year was low—two per 1276 patient-years in the endovascular treatment group and 0 per 1081 patient-years in the neurosurgical group. The main study outcomes are summarized in Table 26.1.

Table 26.1 Main study outcomes

Outcomes	Endovascular treatment	Surgical treatment	Significance
Dead or dependent at 2 months	25.4%	36.4%	$p = 0.0001$
Dead or dependent at 1 year	23.7%	30.6%	$p = 0.0019$
Risk of rebleeding at 1 year	2/1276 patients	0/1081 patients	

26.6 Study Conclusions

The ISAT trial demonstrated that in patients with ruptured intracranial aneurysms, disability-free survival is significantly greater with endovascular treatment using detachable platinum coils compared with neurosurgical intervention to clip the neck of the aneurysm. Early rebleeding was more common with endovascular coiling; however, the long-term risk of rebleeding was low with both therapies. The results of the trial apply to patients who are deemed to be appropriate for either intervention by the treating team. The case fatality rate at 1 year did not differ between the two groups.

26.7 Strengths

The ISAT trial addressed an important, but largely unanswered clinical question regarding the optimal modality of therapy in ruptured intracranial aneurysms. It was a multicentric trial with central randomization, providing external validity. Short and long-term follow-up was rigorous and unbiased.

26.8 Limitations

Although multicentric by design, most patients (77%) were recruited from the UK. A large number of patients were excluded, casting doubts on the generalizability of the study. Although 9559 patients were assessed for eligibility, only 2143 (22.4%) patients were randomized. The trial was ceased prematurely as an interim analysis revealed the likelihood of more favorable outcomes with endovascular coiling compared with neurosurgical intervention. Follow-up data were collected by a postal questionnaire, which may have been liable to subjective bias and misinterpretation. The outcomes from neurosurgical intervention were less favorable than those observed in previous studies. Although endovascular operators were required to meet pre-set experience criteria, no such eligibility rules were applied to neurosurgeons. Questions were raised as to whether a lack of experience with the surgical procedure may have resulted in suboptimal outcomes. Most centers were proficient with endovascular treatment; however, centers with adequate neurosurgical expertise were fewer. The study reported 92.5% of endovascular procedures as "completed"; however, the authors failed to provide angiographic data to substantiate this result. There was no report of procedure-related complications.

26.9 Comments

Rebleeding frequently occurred among patients who were awaiting neurosurgical intervention following the failure of endovascular treatment, suggesting that follow-up interventions must be carried out expeditiously unless contraindicated. The study did not suggest that neurosurgical intervention should be totally dispensed with; there are many patients who may not be amenable to endovascular treatment due to anatomical features or the clinical setting. Thrombolytic therapy was clearly shown to cause rebleeding and death; hence, antiplatelet agents are preferred for ischemic complications.

26.10 Follow-Up Studies

26.10.1 Complete 1-Year Follow-Up (2005)

The first ISAT study had complete 1-year follow-up data only for 1594 of 2143 patients who were randomized. In a later study, the ISAT authors reported on 1-year outcomes of 2118/2143 patients who were enrolled [8]. This included 1063 of 1073 patients originally allocated to endovascular treatment, and 1055 of 1070 patients assigned to neurosurgical treatment. Clinical outcomes were significantly more favorable in the endovascular treatment group at 1-year follow-up. In the endovascular treatment group, 250/1063 (23.5%) were dead or dependent at 1 year compared with 326/1055 (30.9%) in the neurosurgical treatment group. This represented an absolute risk reduction of 7.5% (95% CI, 3.6–11.2; $p = 0.0001$). The survival advantage following endovascular treatment was sustained for up to 7 years. Furthermore, the risk of epileptic seizures was lower among patients who underwent endovascular treatment.

26.10.2 Aneurysm Recurrence and Retreatment (2007)

Although long-term clinical outcomes were more favorable with endovascular treatment, concerns were raised regarding aneurysm recurrence due to inadequate initial occlusion or late reopening after coiling. In a follow-up report, retreatment was more often required with endovascular treatment compared with neurosurgical intervention (17.4% vs. 3.8%) [9]. Late retreatment was 6.9 times more frequent after endovascular intervention. Risk factors for late retreatment included younger age, larger lumen, and incomplete initial occlusion. Short-term follow-up imaging was insufficient to identify aneurysm recurrence.

26.10.3 The 6–14 Year Follow-Up (2009)

This follow-up report of the ISAT trial evaluated the risk of recurrent subarachnoid hemorrhage, death, and dependence based on data available from 2004 patients [10]. Rebleeding occurred in 24 patients more than 1 year after treatment—13 were from the originally treated aneurysm. Among these 13 rebleeds from the originally treated aneurysm, 10 occurred in the endovascular treatment group and 3 in the neurosurgical group. At 5 years of follow-up, mortality was higher in the neurosurgical compared to the endovascular group (14% vs. 11%, p = 0.03). Disability-free survival at 5 years was similar—83% in the endovascular and 82% in the neurosurgical group.

26.10.4 The 18-Year Follow-Up (2014)

In a later study, the ISAT investigators reported on the follow-up of 1644 patients enrolled in 22 UK neurosurgical centers for clinical outcomes between 10.0 and 18.5 years [11]. At 10 years of follow-up, 674/809 (83%) of patients in the endovascular coiling group and 657/835 (79%) patients in the neurosurgical group were alive; the difference was not statistically significant (odds ratio 1.35; 95% CI 1.06–1.73). Among 1003 subjects who answered the questionnaire at 10 years, 82% of patients in the endovascular coiling group and 78% of patients in the neurosurgical group were independent; the difference was not significant. Patients who underwent endovascular treatment were more likely to be alive and independent at 10 years (odds ratio 1.34; 95% CI 1.07–1.67). Although the overall incidence was low, rebleeding from the originally targeted aneurysm occurred more frequently in the endovascular treatment group (13 vs. 4 cases).

26.11 Summary

The ISAT RCT aimed to compare the safety and efficacy of endovascular coiling with neurosurgical clipping for aneurysms considered suitable for both modalities of treatment. The investigators enrolled 2143 patients—1073 were assigned to endovascular treatment and 1073 to neurosurgical clipping. Trial recruitment was ceased following a planned interim analysis that showed a likely benefit with endovascular treatment. Significantly more patients were dead or dependent at 1-year follow-up in the neurosurgical compared with the endovascular treatment group. The risk of rebleeding after 1 year was low; however, it was marginally higher with endovascular treatment. The study established that disability-free survival was higher with endovascular treatment compared with neurosurgical intervention among patients who were considered appropriate for either modality of treatment.

It is important to point out that both neurosurgical clipping and endovascular coiling remain effective treatment modalities for intracranial aneurysms. Refinements in technique have shifted the preference to endovascular treatment in recent years, especially considering the reduced procedural time and tolerability in sicker patients. However, not all aneurysms are amenable to intervention by the endovascular route; neurosurgical treatment using bypass techniques to direct the flow away from the aneurysm is still required in complex clinical situations.

References

1. Lee KS, Zhang JJY, Alalade AF, Vine R, Lanzino G, Park N, et al. Radiological surveillance of small unruptured intracranial aneurysms: a systematic review, meta-analysis, and meta-regression of 8428 aneurysms. Neurosurg Rev. 2021;44(4):2013–23.
2. van Gijn J, Kerr RS, Rinkel GJE. Subarachnoid haemorrhage. Lancet Lond Engl. 2007;369(9558):306–18.
3. Dott NM. Intracranial aneurysms: cerebral arterio-radiography: surgical treatment. Edinb Med J. 1933;40(12):T219–40.
4. Dandy WE. Intracranial aneurysm of the internal carotid artery: cured by operation. Ann Surg. 1938;107(5):654–9.
5. Guglielmi G. History of the genesis of detachable coils: a review. J Neurosurg. 2009;111(1):1–8.
6. Vanninen R, Koivisto T, Saari T, Hernesniemi J, Vapalahti M. Ruptured intracranial aneurysms: acute endovascular treatment with electrolytically detachable coils – a prospective randomized study. Radiology. 1999;211(2):325–36.
7. Molyneux A, Kerr R. and the International Subarachnoid Aneurysm Trial (ISAT) Collaborative Group. International Subarachnoid Aneurysm Trial (ISAT) of neurosurgical clipping versus endovascular coiling in 2143 patients with ruptured intracranial aneurysms: a randomized trial. J Stroke Cerebrovasc Dis. 2002;11(6):304–14.
8. Molyneux AJ, Kerr RSC, Yu LM, Clarke M, Sneade M, Yarnold JA, et al. International subarachnoid aneurysm trial (ISAT) of neurosurgical clipping versus endovascular coiling in 2143 patients with ruptured intracranial aneurysms: a randomised comparison of effects on survival, dependency, seizures, rebleeding, subgroups, and aneurysm occlusion. Lancet. 2005;366:809.
9. Campi A, Ramzi N, Molyneux AJ, Summers PE, Kerr RSC, Sneade M, et al. Retreatment of ruptured cerebral aneurysms in patients randomized by coiling or clipping in the International Subarachnoid Aneurysm Trial (ISAT). Stroke. 2007;38(5):1538–44.
10. Molyneux AJ, Kerr RS, Birks J, Ramzi N, Yarnold J, Sneade M, et al. Risk of recurrent subarachnoid haemorrhage, death, or dependence and standardised mortality ratios after clipping or coiling of an intracranial aneurysm in the International Subarachnoid Aneurysm Trial (ISAT): long-term follow-up. Lancet Neurol. 2009;8(5):427–33.
11. Molyneux AJ, Birks J, Clarke A, Sneade M, Kerr RSC. The durability of endovascular coiling versus neurosurgical clipping of ruptured cerebral aneurysms: 18 year follow-up of the UK cohort of the International Subarachnoid Aneurysm Trial (ISAT). Lancet. 2015;385(9969):691–7.

27 Tissue Plasminogen Activator for Acute Ischemic Stroke: The NINDS Trial

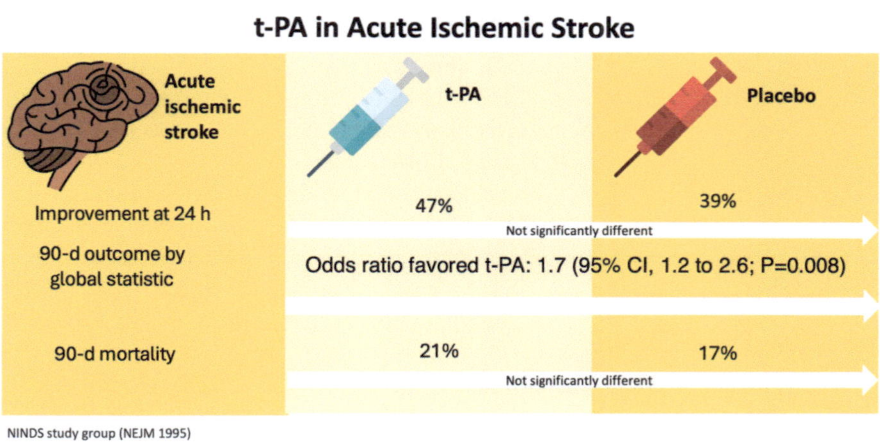

Quick Take

In patients with acute ischemic stroke, does intravenous t-PA administered within 3 h of symptom onset improve clinical outcomes?

The landmark NINDS randomized controlled trial assessed the efficacy and safety of intravenous tissue plasminogen activator (t-PA) administered within 3 h of symptom onset in patients with acute ischemic stroke. The trial was conducted in two parts. Part 1 focused on early neurological improvement at 24 h, while Part 2 evaluated long-term functional outcomes at 90 days. Patients receiving t-PA

National Institute of Neurological Disorders and Stroke rt-PA Stroke Study Group. Tissue plasminogen activator for acute ischemic stroke. N Engl J Med. 1995 Dec 14;333(24):1581–7.

J. Chacko et al., *Landmark Studies in Critical Care*,
https://doi.org/10.1007/978-981-95-0673-6_27

achieved significantly greater functional independence at 3 months, compared to those receiving a placebo. Notably, improvements were observed across four validated scales and a global test statistic. The incidence of symptomatic intracerebral hemorrhage was higher in the t-PA group. However, there was no difference in the 90-day mortality between the two groups. The study provided compelling evidence that early administration of tPA improves long-term outcomes in acute ischemic stroke within a 3-h therapeutic window. These findings represented a paradigm shift in the management of acute stroke, highlighting the critical importance of early recognition and treatment to optimize neurological recovery.

27.1 Introduction and Background

Thrombolytic therapy dates back to 1933 when Tillet and Garner serendipitously observed that some strains of streptococci could dissolve fibrin clots [1]. Early studies of thrombolysis in acute ischemic stroke were carried out with streptokinase and urokinase, with no discernible benefit; indeed, intracerebral bleed was the leading cause of treatment-related death [2]. By the mid-1970s, computerized tomography (CT) became available, enabling direct visualization of the brain, especially intracerebral hemorrhages. The 1980s witnessed investigations on thrombolysis in stroke with renewed vigor; the urokinase-dextran combination was shown to be safe and effective [3]. In the meantime, tissue plasminogen activator (t-PA) was being increasingly used to open blocked coronary arteries in acute myocardial infarction. Large-scale use followed the GUSTO trial of 1993, which clearly demonstrated improved survival in acute myocardial infarction treated with t-PA and intravenous heparin [4].

The first trial of t-PA in acute ischemic stroke, published in 1990, included 364 patients. In this study, outcomes were not significantly different compared with urokinase [5]. Two pilot studies followed, sponsored by the National Institute of Neurological Disorders and Stroke (NINDS) [6, 7]. They used escalating doses of 0.35–1.08 mg/kg t-PA in 94 patients overall within a time window of 3 h of stroke onset. These studies suggested that patients with acute ischemic stroke could be evaluated and t-PA administered within a 90-min window. Early neurological improvement was observed, albeit with an inherent risk of hemorrhage. The findings of these pilot studies justified a placebo-controlled randomized clinical trial. Against this background, the NINDS investigators designed a randomized controlled trial (RCT) to evaluate the safety and efficacy of intravenous t-PA in acute ischemic stroke [8].

27.2 Population and Design

The NINDS t-PA trial was conducted between January 1991 and October 1994, across eight major academic centers in the USA—all tertiary hospitals with expertise in acute stroke care. The study population included patients with acute ischemic stroke in whom the time of symptom onset was known, and the extent of deficit was measurable on the National Institutes of Health Stroke Scale, with no evidence of hemorrhage on the CT scan.

27.2.1 Exclusion

- Previous stroke or traumatic brain injury in the preceding 3 months
- Previous intracranial hemorrhage or symptoms suggestive of subarachnoid hemorrhage
- Major surgery within 14 days
- Systolic BP >185 mm Hg or diastolic BP >110 mm Hg
- Minor or rapidly improving deficits
- Gastrointestinal or urinary tract hemorrhage in the preceding 7 days
- Seizure at stroke onset
- Anticoagulant use
- Presence of coagulopathy (prothrombin time >15 s) or thrombocytopenia (platelet count <100,000/ cu mm)
- Blood glucose <50 mg/dL or >400 mg/dL

The study was conducted as two consecutive RCTs—part 1 and part 2. Part 1, conducted between January 1991 and October 1993, enrolled 291 patients; part 2 followed soon after, and continued until October 1994, including 333 patients. Patients in both parts of the study were randomized to receive intravenous tissue plasminogen activator (t-PA) or placebo. Patients were stratified by study center and time of onset of stroke to commencement of treatment—0 to 90 min or 91 to 180 min. The study was double-blinded. In part 1 of the study, the primary outcome was early neurological improvement at 24 h; however, these patients were followed up for the 90-day outcome (as a secondary endpoint). In part 2, the primary outcome was the 90-day functional outcome; early improvement (24 h) was secondary.

27.3 Primary Outcome: Part 1

The primary outcome evaluated in part 1 of the study was neurological improvement, defined as ≥4-point improvement in the NIH Stroke Scale (NIHSS) or complete resolution of neurological deficits within 24 h of stroke onset.

27.4 Primary Outcome: Part 2

A favorable outcome was defined according to four global disability/neurological scales at 90 days, as specified below.

- Modified Rankin scale (mRS of 0 or 1). The modified Rankin scale ranges from 0 (absence of symptoms) to 5 (severe disability)
- Barthel index (≥95). The Barthel index measures activities of daily living on a scale of 0–100 (100 denotes the ability to perform all activities of daily living independently)
- NIH Stroke Scale (NIHSS of 0 or 1). The NIHSS ranges from 0 to 42, with 0 indicating absence of neurological deficit, and higher scores indicating more severe deficit
- Glasgow Outcome Scale (Score = 1). The Glasgow outcome scale is a global assessment of function, with scores ranging from 1 (good recovery) to 5 (death)

Besides, the authors evaluated outcomes based on a global statistic derived from all four parameters.

27.5 Sample Size Calculation

In part 1 of the study, the authors calculated the sample size for an absolute difference of 24% in the primary outcome (early neurological improvement at 24 h), assuming a rate of 16% in the control group. Seventy patients in each stratum of the study (administration within 0–90 min and 91–180 min) for each group (total of 280 patients) provided the study with 90% power.

In part 2, the authors assumed a difference of 20 percentage points in the primary outcome (functional status at 90 days). The inclusion of 80 patients in each time stratum (320 patients overall) provided the study with 95% power.

Analyses were conducted separately for each phase (Part 1 and Part 2); additionally, pooled data from both phases were also analyzed.

27.6 t-PA Group

In this group, patients received intravenous recombinant t-PA in a dose of 0.9 mg/kg to a maximum dose of 90 mg within 180 min of acute ischemic stroke. Ten percent of the dose was administered as a bolus; the remaining 90% was infused over 1 h.

27.7 Control Group

A matching placebo infusion was administered using the same dosing scheme. Randomization was stratified according to center, and the time between stroke onset and commencement of treatment (0–90 min vs. 91–180 min).

27.8 Results

Overall, 624 patients were randomized over the nearly 4-year duration of the study. Patients were generally well-matched at baseline.

27.8.1 Part 1: The 24-h Outcome

There was no significant difference in the primary outcome—defined as ≥4-point improvement in the NIHSS between the t-PA and control groups. However, the median NIHSS score favored t-PA at most time strata, suggesting a trend toward early improvement.

27.8.2 Part 2: The 90-Day Outcome

The 90-day outcome was significantly more favorable in the t-PA group for each of the four measures of the primary outcome. According to the global statistic used, the odds ratio for a favorable outcome was 1.7 with t-PA (95% confidence interval, 1.2–2.6, $P = 0.008$). The number needed to treat for a favorable outcome was seven patients. This meant that for every seven patients treated with rt-PA, one additional patient would have a better outcome compared to those receiving a placebo. The outcome benefit was observed with t-PA in subgroups of patients based on age, stroke classification, severity, and use of aspirin before the stroke. Patients who received t-PA were 30% more likely to experience minimal or no disability at 90 days compared to the control group.

The favorable outcomes extended across subtypes of strokes—small vessel occlusive, large vessel occlusive, and embolic.

27.9 Combined Analysis Including Part 1 and Part 2

On pooled analysis of patients including those randomized to part 1 (the 24-h outcome) and part 2 (the 90-day outcome), the neurological outcomes at 90 days were significantly more favorable based on all five criteria of assessment. The favorable outcomes were observed among patients who received t-PA within 0–90 min or 91–180 min of stroke onset.

27.10 Intracerebral Hemorrhage

Symptomatic intracerebral hemorrhage at 36 h was more common in patients treated with t-PA (6.4% vs. 0.6%, $P < 0.001$). At 3 months, among the 28 patients with intracerebral hemorrhage, 17 had died (61%).

Table 27.1 Main study outcomes

Time Point	Outcome measure	Placebo group	t-PA group	Statistical significance
24 h	Early neurological improvement	39%	47%	$P = 0.21$
90 days	Modified Rankin Score 0–1	26%	39%	$P = 0.008$
	Barthel Index ≥95	39%	59%	$P < 0.001$
	NIHSS score 0 or 1	20%	38%	$P < 0.001$
	Glasgow Outcome Score = 1	32%	50%	$P < 0.001$
90 days	Mortality	21%	17%	$P = 0.30$
Within 36 h	Symptomatic intracerebral hemorrhage (ICH)	0.6%	6.4%	$P < 0.001$

27.11 Mortality at 90 Days

At 90 days after stroke onset, the mortality was not significantly different between the t-PA and the control groups (17% vs. 21%, $P = 0.30$). The main study outcomes are summarized in Table 27.1.

27.12 Follow-Up Study

In a subsequent follow-up of patients included in the NINDS trial, Kwiatkowski et al. analyzed outcomes at 6 and 12 months after stroke occurrence [9]. The primary outcome was evaluated based on a global statistic including the Barthel index, the modified Rankin Scale, and the Glasgow Outcome Scale. A favorable outcome was defined as minimal or no disability based on the global statistic.

A favorable outcome was significantly higher in the t-PA group at both 6 months (OR, 1.7; 95% confidence interval, 1.3–2.3) and 12 months (OR, 1.7; 95% confidence interval, 1.2–2.3). Mortality at 12 months did not differ significantly between the treatment and control groups (24% vs. 28%, $P = 0.29$). The outcomes were similar across the different types of strokes studied. The incidence of recurrent stroke was similar in both groups at 12 months.

27.13 Strengths

The NINDS trial followed a robust, double-blind, placebo-controlled design. It was the first major clinical trial to rigorously evaluate the impact of thrombolysis in stroke within a clinically relevant time window. The investigators used rigorous endpoints, including a global statistic to evaluate functional neurological outcomes. The benefits were observed across diverse subgroups of patients—based on age, severity of stroke, and prior use of aspirin. The study conclusively showed that patients receiving t-PA were more likely to experience functionally independent outcomes at 90 days—a hardcore clinical endpoint in stroke.

27.14 Limitations

The study was of a relatively small sample size—with 312 patients in each group, it had limited power for subgroup and safety analysis. Strict inclusion and exclusion criteria were followed, perhaps limiting generalizability in real-world practice at the time the study was conducted. The trial was conducted mostly in academic centers, all in the US, again raising questions about validity in other, especially resource-limited settings. Access to advanced imaging modalities commonly employed today, including detailed MRI imaging to identify the extent of damage and salvageable tissue, were not commonly in use at the time of the study.

Reviewers have also raised concerns about baseline imbalances in stroke severity—specifically, a higher severity of stroke in the placebo group [10]. However, subsequent adjusted analyses have allayed these concerns and confirmed the efficacy of t-PA [11].

27.15 Summary

The NINDS trial, conducted between 1991 and 1994, was a pivotal study that revolutionized the treatment of acute ischemic stroke. The trial investigated the efficacy of intravenous tissue plasminogen activator (t-PA) administered within 3 h of stroke onset.

The trial was divided into two parts: part 1 assessed early neurological improvement within 24 h, while part 2 evaluated sustained clinical benefits at 90 days. Patients were randomized to receive either t-PA or a placebo based on strict inclusion criteria.

The trial results revealed that t-PA significantly improved neurological outcomes at 90 days. However, there was no difference in mortality between groups; symptomatic intracranial hemorrhage occurred significantly more often with t-PA. Despite these risks, the findings of the trial led to FDA approval of t-PA in 1996, establishing it as an effective therapy for acute ischemic stroke.

The rigorous design and groundbreaking results of the NINDS trial set the foundation for modern stroke management. It emphasized the importance of timely intervention and reshaped the management of acute stroke.

References

1. Tillett WS, Garner RL. The fibrinolytic activity of hemolytic streptococci. J Exp Med. 1933;58(4):485–502.
2. Fletcher AP, Alkjaersig N, Lewis M, Tulevski V, Davies A, Brooks J, et al. A pilot study of urokinase therapy in cerebral infarction. Stroke. 1976;7(2):135–42.
3. Fujishima M, Omae T, Tanaka K, Iino K, Matsuo O, Mihara H. Controlled trial of combined urokinase and dextran sulfate therapy in patients with acute cerebral infarction. Angiology. 1986;37(7):487–98.

4. Gusto Investigators. An international randomized trial comparing four thrombolytic strategies for acute myocardial infarction. N Engl J Med. 1993;329(10):673–82.
5. Terashi A, Kobayashi Y, Katayama Y, Inamura K, Kazama M, Abe T. Clinical effects and basic studies of thrombolytic therapy on cerebral thrombosis. Semin Thromb Hemost. 1990;16(3):236–41.
6. Brott TG, Haley EC, Levy DE, Barsan W, Broderick J, Sheppard GL, et al. Urgent therapy for stroke. Part I. Pilot study of tissue plasminogen activator administered within 90 minutes. Stroke. 1992;23(5):632–40.
7. Haley EC, Levy DE, Brott TG, Sheppard GL, Wong MC, Kongable GL, et al. Urgent therapy for stroke. Part II. Pilot study of tissue plasminogen activator administered 91-180 minutes from onset. Stroke. 1992;23(5):641–5.
8. National Institute of Neurological Disorders and Stroke rt-PA Stroke Study Group. Tissue plasminogen activator for acute ischemic stroke. N Engl J Med. 1995;333(24):1581–7.
9. Kwiatkowski TG, Libman RB, Frankel M, Tilley BC, Morgenstern LB, Lu M, et al. Effects of tissue plasminogen activator for acute ischemic stroke at one year. National Institute of Neurological Disorders and Stroke Recombinant Tissue Plasminogen Activator Stroke Study Group. N Engl J Med. 1999;340(23):1781–7.
10. Mann J. The Efficacy Analysis of the NINDS Trial is Flawed. 2025 Apr 20 [Cited 2025 Apr 20]; Available From: https://www.Bmj.Com/Rapid-Response/2011/10/28/Efficacy-Analysis-Ninds-Trial-Flawed.
11. Mann J. The NINDS Reanalysis Committee Analysed The NINDS Trial From the Wrong Perspective. 2025 Apr 20 [Cited 2025 Apr 20]; Available From: https://www.Bmj.Com/Rapid-Response/2011/10/30/Ninds-Reanalysis-Committee-Analysed-Ninds-Trial-Wrong-Perspective.

28 Tranexamic Acid in Traumatic Brain Injury: The CRASH-3 Trial

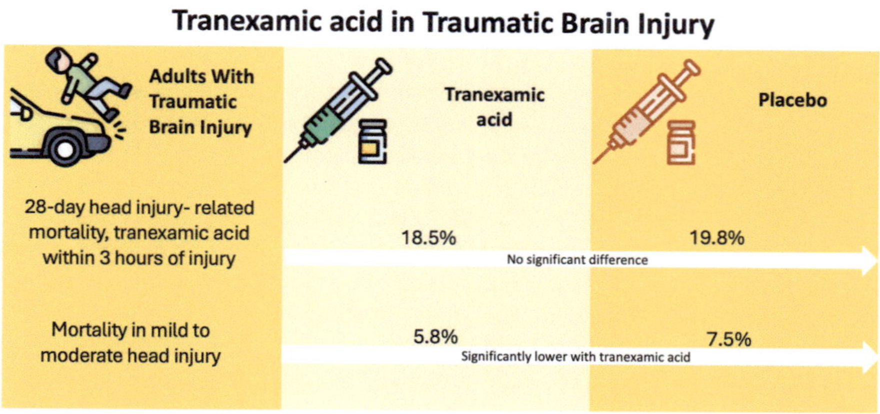

Quick Take
Can tranexamic acid improve outcomes in traumatic brain injury (TBI)?

The CRASH-3 trial evaluated the effects of tranexamic acid on patients with acute TBI. A total of 12,737 patients were randomized to receive either tranexamic acid or placebo within 3 h of injury. Improved survival with tranexamic acid was confined to patients who suffered mild and moderate head injury; no beneficial

---

CRASH-3 trial collaborators. Effects of tranexamic acid on death, disability, vascular occlusive events and other morbidities in patients with acute traumatic brain injury (CRASH-3): a randomised, placebo-controlled trial. Lancet Lond Engl. 2019 Nov 9;394(10210):1713–23.

J. Chacko et al., *Landmark Studies in Critical Care*,
https://doi.org/10.1007/978-981-95-0673-6_28

impact was observed among patients with severe injury. Disability among survivors was also similar. The treatment did not lead to a higher incidence of vascular occlusive events. The trial contributed to a more nuanced understanding of the role of tranexamic acid in the management of TBI, particularly focusing on early administration for hemorrhage control.

28.1 Introduction

Intracranial hemorrhage often leads to death or severe disability in TBI. Bleeding occurs at the moment of impact and may continue for several hours afterwards [1], leading to intracranial hypertension, coning, and death. Abnormalities of coagulation function have been established to be major contributors to the progression of hemorrhagic lesions and adverse outcomes in TBI; hyperactivity of the fibrinolytic pathway may provoke the progression of intracranial hematomas. The elevated levels of fibrinogen degradation products, often seen in TBI, suggest activation of the fibrinolytic pathway and predict expansion of intracranial hematomas [2].

Therapeutic strategies that seemed physiologically plausible have often met with failure in traumatic brain injury (TBI), including corticosteroids [3], and induced hypothermia [4]. Tranexamic acid, a potent anti-fibrinolytic agent, has been shown to improve outcomes in bleeding patients—including polytrauma [5] and postpartum hemorrhage [6]. The CRASH 2 trial had previously evaluated the effect of tranexamic acid in trauma patients with active bleeding or those at risk of significant bleeding. In this large randomized controlled trial (RCT), more than 20,000 patients were included. The study provided strong evidence that early treatment with tranexamic acid within the first hour of injury had the greatest impact in reducing the risk of death from bleeding; treatment between 1 and 3 h also significantly reduced the risk of death due to bleeding [5]. Considering the evidence of beneficial impact among bleeding patients from these studies, there was a strong physiological rationale that tranexamic acid may reduce expansion of intracranial hematomas, and thereby, prevent brain herniation and death among patients with TBI.

A meta-analysis of two small trials had shown a reduction in mortality with tranexamic acid in TBI; however, no data were available on the level of disability among survivors or adverse events [7]. The CRASH 3 investigators aimed to evaluate the impact of tranexamic acid on clinical outcomes among patients with TBI, including head injury-related death, disability, and adverse events [8].

28.2 Population and Design

The CRASH 3 randomized controlled trial (RCT) was conducted between July 2012 and January 2019 to evaluate the effect of tranexamic acid on death and disability among patients with traumatic brain injury (TBI). Adult patients within 3 h of TBI, and a Glasgow Coma Scale (GCS) score of ≤12, or any evidence of intracranial hemorrhage on the CT scan, were eligible. The appropriateness of tranexamic use had to be "substantially uncertain" to the treating clinician for study enrollment. The original time window for eligibility was within 8 h of TBI; however, the protocol was amended midway through the study, considering fresh evidence that suggested the lack of effectiveness of tranexamic acid if administration is delayed beyond 3 h. Patients with major extracranial bleed were excluded.

Patients were randomly assigned to receive tranexamic acid or a matching placebo as an intravenous infusion. Participants and staff were blinded to the assigned treatment.

28.2.1 Intervention

In the intervention group, patients received a loading dose of tranexamic acid, 1 g intravenously, administered over 10 min. This was followed by an infusion of 1 g over the next 8 h.

28.2.2 Control

In the control group, 0.9% saline was administered from identical packs.

28.3 Common Management

Considering the substantially variable modalities of treatments available depending on the clinical situation, participating centers followed local guidelines in the management of TBI. Tranexamic acid or a placebo was administered as an additional intervention.

28.4 Sample Size

The authors calculated a sample size of 10,000 patients within 3 h of TBI to detect a 15% relative reduction in the all-cause mortality from 20% in the placebo group to 17% in the tranexamic group. The time window for eligibility was originally 8 h; later, the protocol was revised to within 3 h post-injury. At the time of revision, about 3000 patients presenting >3 h after TBI had already been recruited. Hence, the sample size was increased to approximately 13,000 patients—this was expected to provide the study with 90% power at a two-sided alpha level of 1%.

28.5 Results

A total of 12,737 patients were enrolled; 12,561 received the initial bolus dose of the assigned treatment. Of these, 6314 patients were in the tranexamic acid group while 6247 received a placebo. Among patients who were randomized within 3 h of TBI, outcome data were available in 4613 patients who received tranexamic acid and 4514 who received a placebo. Baseline characteristics, including age, gender, time since injury, the systolic blood pressure, the GCS score, and the pupillary reaction, were similar in both groups.

28.6 The Primary Outcome: Head Injury-Related Death Within 28 Days of Injury

The in-hospital, head injury-related death within 28 days of injury was lower among patients who received tranexamic acid within 3 h of injury. In the tranexamic acid group, 855/4613 patients (18.5%) had died at 28 days, compared with 892/4514 in the placebo group. The relative risk of death with tranexamic acid use was 0.94 (95% CI, 0.86–1.02).

The relative risk of head injury-related death with tranexamic acid among patients randomized within 1 h of injury was 0.96 (95% CI, 0.79–1.17); it was 0.93 (95% CI, 0.85–1.02) between 1–3 h, and 0.94 (95% CI, 0.81–1.09) among those randomly assigned after 3 h of injury.

28.7 Head Injury-Related Death After Exclusion of Patients with GCS of 3 and Bilateral Unreactive Pupils

Considering the uniformly poor outcome of patients with GCS of 3 and bilateral unreactive pupils, the investigators performed a prespecified sensitivity analysis by excluding these patients. The head injury-related mortality appeared to favor tranexamic acid use in sensitivity analysis after excluding these patients. In the tranexamic acid group, the mortality was 485/3888 (12.5%) compared with 525/3757 (14.0%) in the placebo group (relative risk: 0.89; 95% confidence interval, 0.80–1.00).

28.8 Mortality Related to Baseline GCS

The severity of head injury was classified into mild (GCS: 14 or 15), moderate (GCS: 9–13), or severe (GCS: 3–8) after adjusting for the GCS score, age, and the systolic blood pressure. On this model, patients with mild to moderate head injury had a lower risk of mortality with tranexamic acid compared with placebo; however, there was no significant difference between groups among patients with severe head injury. On regression analysis, tranexamic acid improved survival among patients with less severe injury. Furthermore, mortality was lower with tranexamic acid among patients with reactive pupils.

28.9 Secondary Outcomes

Death within 24 h of injury was significantly lower in the tranexamic acid group (RR, 0.81; 95% CI [0.56–0.92]). Non-head injury-related mortality and all-cause mortality were not significantly different between groups. Disability among survivors was evaluated using the Disability Rating Scale; the mean disability scores were similar in both groups regardless of whether tranexamic acid was administered within 3 h or later. The functional status was also assessed based on being in an extreme category in six areas of function (walking, washing, pain and discomfort, anxiety or depression, agitation or aggressive behavior, and fatigue); there was no difference in the level of disability between groups.

The incidence of vascular occlusive events and seizures—potential risks with tranexamic acid use—was similar in both groups of patients.

Specifically, tranexamic acid was not associated with an increased risk of stroke. Other adverse events were also similar. The main trial outcomes are summarized in Table 28.1.

Table 28.1 Main study outcomes

Outcome	Tranexamic acid	Placebo	RR (95% CI)
Head injury-related death at 28 days	18.5%	19.8%	0.94 (0.86–1.02)
Head injury-related death at 24 h			0.81 (0.69–0.95)
Head injury-related death after exclusion of GCS 3 or bilateral non-reactive pupils	12.5%	14%	0.89 (0.80–1.00)
Mortality with mild to moderate TBI	5.8%	7.5%	0.78 (0.62–0.95)
Mortality with severe TBI	39.6%	40.1%	0.99 (0.91–1.07)

Abbreviations: RR relative risk, *CI* confidence interval, *TBI* traumatic brain injury, *GCS* Glasgow Coma Scale

28.10 Study Conclusions

The CRASH 3 trial suggested that tranexamic acid administration within 3 h of TBI was associated with a lower incidence of head injury-related mortality. Improved survival with tranexamic acid was confined to patients who suffered mild and moderate head injury; no beneficial impact was observed among patients with severe injury. Disability among survivors was also similar.

28.11 Strengths

The CRASH 2 trial was a large, adequately powered RCT that aimed to evaluate the impact of tranexamic acid among patients with TBI. It represents the first clinical trial that showed benefit with a pharmacological agent in TBI. It was a multicentric, pragmatic study that provided robust external validity. The patient groups were well-matched at baseline. There was minimal loss to follow-up, reducing the likelihood of attrition bias. The pre-specified subgroup analyses were relevant and important after exclusion of patients who were unlikely to survive and evaluation of mortality according to baseline GCS.

28.12 Limitations

Head injury-related mortality at 28 days, the primary outcome, may be subject to bias depending on the clinician interpretation of the cause of death. Besides, a substantial number of deaths may occur after 28 days in traumatic brain injury—this needs evaluation in a subsequent analysis. Would the neurological status have been a more meaningful primary outcome than mortality? The overall management was based on local practice—no data were available regarding pre-hospital care, and interventions carried out in the hospital. In absolute statistical terms, a significant difference in the head injury-related mortality, the primary outcome, was confined to the subgroup of patients with mild to moderate TBI. However, this was a clinically important finding in a predefined subgroup that included a large number (5615) of patients.

28.13 Summary

Activation of the fibrinolytic pathway may be a trigger for continued bleeding and adverse outcomes in trauma. Previous evidence had shown that tranexamic acid, an anti-fibrinolytic agent, improves clinical outcomes in trauma-related bleeding and postpartum hemorrhage. A meta-analysis of two previous trials had shown a reduction in mortality with tranexamic acid in patients with TBI. The CRASH 3 investigators embarked upon a large RCT to confirm these findings. This randomized, placebo-controlled trial was conducted across 175 hospitals in 29 countries. Patients with TBI received tranexamic acid, 1 g over 10 min, followed by an infusion of 1 g over 8 h, or a matching placebo. The risk of head injury-related mortality at 28 days was lower with tranexamic acid; the effect was more pronounced after exclusion of patients with a GCS of 3 and unreactive pupils. Tranexamic acid was significantly more effective in reducing mortality among patients with mild to moderate TBI. Disability among survivors was similar in both groups. Tranexamic acid administration did not result in an increase in the incidence of vascular occlusive events. The CRASH 3 trial was a highly impactful clinical trial that carried the potential to influence clinical practice among patients with TBI.

References

1. Oertel M, Kelly DF, McArthur D, Boscardin WJ, Glenn TC, Lee JH, et al. Progressive hemorrhage after head trauma: predictors and consequences of the evolving injury. J Neurosurg. 2002;96(1):109–16.
2. Zhang J, He M, Song Y, Xu J. Prognostic role of D-dimer level upon admission in patients with traumatic brain injury. Medicine (Baltimore). 2018;97(31):e11774.
3. Edwards P, Arango M, Balica L, Cottingham R, El-Sayed H, Farrell B, et al. Final results of MRC CRASH, a randomised placebo-controlled trial of intravenous corticosteroid in adults with head injury-outcomes at 6 months. Lancet Lond Engl. 2005;365(9475):1957–9.
4. Cooper DJ, Nichol AD, Bailey M, Bernard S, Cameron PA, Pili-Floury S, et al. Effect of early sustained prophylactic hypothermia on neurologic outcomes among patients with severe traumatic brain injury: the POLAR randomized clinical trial. JAMA. 2018;320(21):2211–20.
5. CRASH-2 trial collaborators, Shakur H, Roberts I, Bautista R, Caballero J, Coats T, et al. Effects of tranexamic acid on death, vascular occlusive events, and blood transfusion in trauma patients with significant haemorrhage (CRASH-2): a randomised, placebo-controlled trial. Lancet Lond Engl. 2010;376(9734):23–32.
6. WOMAN Trial Collaborators. Effect of early tranexamic acid administration on mortality, hysterectomy, and other morbidities in women with post-partum haemorrhage (WOMAN): an international, randomised, double-blind, placebo-controlled trial. Lancet Lond Engl. 2017;389(10084):2105–16.
7. Roberts I, Belli A, Brenner A, Chaudhri R, Fawole B, Harris T, et al. Tranexamic acid for significant traumatic brain injury (the CRASH-3 trial): statistical analysis plan for an international, randomised, double-blind, placebo-controlled trial. Wellcome Open Res. 2018;3:86.
8. CRASH-3 trial collaborators. Effects of tranexamic acid on death, disability, vascular occlusive events and other morbidities in patients with acute traumatic brain injury (CRASH-3): a randomised, placebo-controlled trial. Lancet Lond Engl. 2019;394(10210):1713–23.

Part V

Corticosteroids in Sepsis

Hydrocortisone–Fludrocortisone Combination in Septic Shock: Annane et al.

29

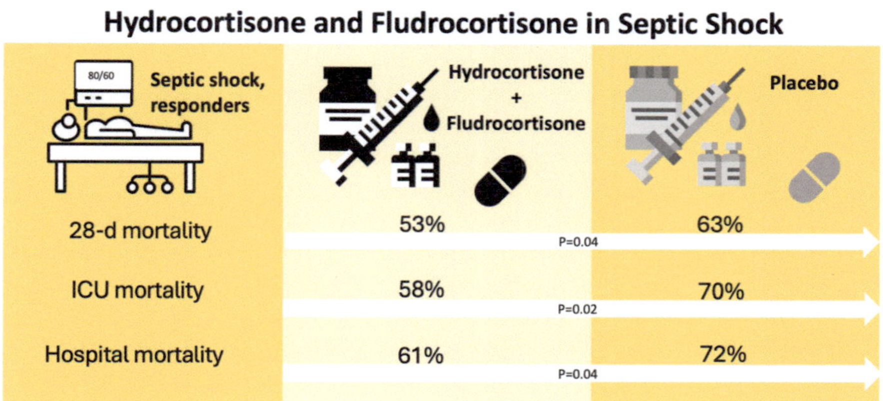

Annane et al. (JAMA, 2002)

Quick Take
Does low-dose hydrocortisone combined with fludrocortisone improve outcomes in septic shock?

The Annane et al. study was the first large randomized controlled trial (RCT) that investigated the effects of low-dose hydrocortisone and fludrocortisone on mortality in patients with septic shock. A total of 299 patients with septic shock were randomly assigned to receive either hydrocortisone and fludrocortisone or a placebo. The study found a significant reduction in 28-day mortality in the treatment group

---

Annane D, Sebille V, Charpentier C, Bollaert PE, Francois B, Korach JM, et al. Effect of Treatment with Low Doses of Hydrocortisone and Fludrocortisone on Mortality in Patients with Septic Shock.

J. Chacko et al., *Landmark Studies in Critical Care*,
https://doi.org/10.1007/978-981-95-0673-6_29

(35.4% vs. 47.2%), suggesting that low-dose corticosteroids can improve survival in patients with septic shock who exhibit signs of adrenal insufficiency. The study was a milestone in the management of septic shock, supporting the use of corticosteroids as a part of treatment for patients with shock, resistant to fluid resuscitation and vasopressors.

29.1 Introduction and Background

Historically, clinicians were often beguiled by the potent anti-inflammatory effect of corticosteroids and their putative benefits in septic patients. In the summer of 1976, William Schumer presented the tantalizing findings of his study on high-dose corticosteroid therapy in patients with septic shock at the annual meeting of the American Surgical Association. In a three-armed prospective trial, he compared methylprednisolone 30 mg/kg or dexamethasone 3 mg/kg with placebo. The author defined septic shock based on presumed "septic history" and "falling blood pressure," along with positive cultures. The mortality among patients who received such massive doses of corticosteroids appeared to be incredibly low. In the control group, the mortality was nearly three times as much compared to corticosteroid-treated patients. The study was conducted over a protracted period, between 1967 and 1975, during which the author conceded that "the use of new antibiotics, respirators, and better methods of diagnosis could have reduced mortality…" Nevertheless, high-dose corticosteroids appeared to dramatically impact sepsis-related mortality.

Almost predictably, the compelling findings of Schumer were never reproduced.

Years later, Sprung et al. conducted a similar study among patients with septic shock [1]. In this RCT, patients in septic shock were treated with methylprednisolone 30 mg/kg or dexamethasone 6 mg/kg, and compared with a control group that did not receive corticosteroids. Earlier shock reversal was observed among corticosteroid-treated patients; however, improved blood pressures did not result in a significant impact on hospital survival. Two further RCTs confirmed the lack of beneficial effect of high-dose methylprednisolone on survival in septic shock [1, 2].

The early 1990s witnessed a revival of interest in lower doses of corticosteroids over a longer duration, based on the concept of relative adrenal insufficiency in sepsis. Two RCTs of a relatively small sample size evaluated the effect of low-dose hydrocortisone on shock reversal during this period. The study by Bollaert et al. revealed a higher rate of shock reversal with hydrocortisone 100 mg administered 8 hourly intravenously compared with placebo [3]. These findings were reproduced in a later study by Briegel et al., using a loading dose of hydrocortisone 100 mg followed by 0.18 mg/kg/h. Hydrocortisone administration resulted in earlier cessation of vasopressor support, with no increase in the incidence of adverse events [4].

The integrity and activation of the hypothalamic-pituitary-adrenal axis evolved as an important factor determining outcomes in sepsis. A short corticotrophin test measuring cortisol levels at baseline, 30 and 60 min was commonly employed to test the adequacy of the stress response in sepsis. In a prospective observational study, a failure of serum cortisol levels to rise by >9 μg/dL in response to 0.25 mg of tetracosactrin (a synthetic peptide comprised of the first 24 amino acids of adrenocorticotrophic hormone) was one of the independent predictors of mortality in septic shock [5]. The stage was set for testing the concept of relative adrenal insufficiency in septic shock and the impact of low-dose corticosteroids on clinical outcomes, in contrast to the unfavorable outcomes associated with the mega-doses used previously.

29.2 Population and Design

The randomized, placebo-controlled trial was conducted in 19 French ICUs [6]. Adult patients were enrolled if they had a documented or strongly suspected focus of infection, the temperature was >38.3 °C or <35.6 °C, tachycardia >90/min, systolic BP <90 mm Hg for more than 1 h despite fluid resuscitation, and dopamine >5 μg/kg/min or any dose of norepinephrine or epinephrine, urine output <0.5 ml/kg/h, a PaO_2/FiO_2 ratio <280 mm Hg, or lactate levels >2 mmol/L, and the need for mechanical ventilation.

29.2.1 Excluded

Patients with acute myocardial infarction, pulmonary embolism, advanced malignancy, acquired immunodeficiency syndrome, and contraindications for steroid use were excluded. So were patients with a definite indication for steroids and pregnant patients. Patients who were on etomidate in the 6 h prior to randomization were also excluded.

29.2.2 Corticosteroid Group

Patients received hydrocortisone 50 mg 6 hourly, intravenously as a bolus dose, combined with one tablet of 9-α-fludrocortisone 50 μg once daily administered through the nasogastric tube. Corticosteroids were administered for 7 days.

29.2.3 Control Group

In the control group, identical placebos were administered.

A short corticotrophin test was performed to identify patients with relative adrenal insufficiency. Cortisol levels were measured at baseline and following 30 and 60 min after a 250 μg intravenous dose of tetracosactrin, an analogue of adrenocorticotrophic hormone (ACTH). Relative adrenal insufficiency was diagnosed if the serum cortisol levels failed to rise by >9 μg/dL after tetracosactrin administration; these patients were classified as *non-responders*. Patients in whom the cortisol levels rose by >9 μg/dL were classified as *responders*.

29.3 Sample Size

The authors assumed that 40% of patients would be non-responders. They also assumed 95% mortality in the control group among non-responders. A sample size of 270 patients was meant to detect a 20% difference between groups in the 28-day mortality with a 90% probability, and a type I error of 0.05.

29.4 Results

29.4.1 Patient Characteristics

The general characteristics and severity of illness were similar in the corticosteroid and the placebo groups. Pulmonary infections were most common, followed by intra-abdominal infections. The causative organism was also similar between the two groups of patients. Appropriate antibiotic therapy was administered in most patients—nearly 95% in the placebo and 91% in the corticosteroid group.

In total, 299 patients were included in the final analysis; 229 were classified as non-responders and 70 as responders. Among the non-responders, the main focus of the study, 114 belonged to the corticosteroid and 115 to the placebo group.

29.5 The Primary Outcome: 28-Day Mortality in Non-responders

Among the non-responders, the 28-day mortality was significantly lower in the corticosteroid group. In the corticosteroid group, 60/114 (53%) had died at 28 days compared with 73/115 (63%) in the placebo group (odds ratio, 0.54; 95% CI, 0.31–0.97; $p = 0.04$). In contrast, among the responders, the 28-day mortality was not significantly different [Placebo: 18/34 (53%) vs. corticosteroid: 22/36 (61%); $p = 0.96$].

The overall 28-day mortality was 82/150 (55%) in the corticosteroid group and 91/149 (61%) in the placebo group; the difference was not statistically significant.

29.6 Secondary Outcomes

29.6.1 ICU, Hospital, and 1-Year Mortality

Among the non-responders, the ICU mortality was also significantly lower in the corticosteroid group compared to the placebo group. The ICU mortality was 66/114 (58%) in the corticosteroid group compared with 81/115 (70%) in the placebo group

($p = 0.02$). The hospital mortality was also lower in the corticosteroid group (corticosteroid vs. placebo, 61% vs. 72%; $p = 0.04$). Mortality at 1 year of follow-up was lower in the corticosteroid group; however, the difference was not statistically significant (68% vs. 77%; $p = 0.07$).

There was no difference in the 28-day, ICU, hospital, and 1-year mortality between the corticosteroid and placebo groups among responders. Analysis, including all patients (responders and non-responders), also did not show a difference in mortality at any of the above time points.

29.6.2 Time to Cessation of Vasopressors

Among non-responders, vasopressors could be withdrawn earlier in the corticosteroid group compared to the placebo group (median duration: 10 days vs. 7 days). At 28 days, more patients were off vasopressors in the corticosteroid group (57% vs. 40%). The time to cessation of vasopressors was not significantly different among responders.

29.7 Adverse Events

The incidence of superinfections, including catheter-related infection, nosocomial pneumonia, urinary infection, and surgical site infection, was similar in both groups. Gastrointestinal bleeding occurred in a similar number of patients in both groups. Adverse events attributable to vasopressors, including myocardial infarction, arrhythmias, and limb ischemia, were also similar. The main results of the study are summarized in Table 29.1.

Table 29.1 Main outcomes among patients with relative adrenal insufficiency (non-responders to the corticotrophin test)

Outcome	Corticosteroid group (114 patients)	Placebo group (115 patients)	Significance
28-d mortality	53%	63%	AOR: 0.54 (0.31–0.97) $p = 0.04$
ICU mortality	58%	70%	AOR: 0.50 (0.28–0.89) $p = 0.02$
Hospital mortality	61%	72%	AOR: 0.53 (0.29–0.96) $p = 0.04$
1-y mortality	77%	88%	AOR: 0.57 (0.31–1.04) $p = 0.07$

Abbreviations: AOR adjusted odds ratio

29.8 Study Conclusions

The authors concluded that a 7-day treatment with hydrocortisone combined with fludrocortisone reduced the 28-day mortality in patients with relative adrenal insufficiency, with no obvious adverse effects. They went on to recommend that patients with catecholamine-dependent septic shock should be commenced on this combination, pending the results of the short corticotrophin stimulation test, following which corticosteroid treatment may be ceased in non-responders.

29.9 Strengths

At the time of the Annane et al. trial, corticosteroids had been in use among patients with sepsis for several decades. However, there had been few controlled trials that systematically evaluated their efficacy, and the results were conflicting. The authors conducted the first large, multicentric RCT across 19 centers in France. The study was adequately powered and double-blinded, with a low likelihood of bias. In contrast to some earlier studies that had used higher doses of corticosteroids with adverse outcomes, a low-dose strategy was followed, based on the hypothesis of relative adrenal insufficiency. The severity of illness was high among the study population. All patients were on mechanical ventilation, were oliguric, had increased serum lactate levels, and had acute respiratory distress syndrome. Corticosteroid treatment in seven non-responders led to one additional life being saved at 28 days. The study was the harbinger of future clinical trials on steroids in septic shock, including the CORTICUS and the ADRENAL trials.

29.10 Limitations

The study excluded a large number of patients—1326 patients were screened; only 300 were randomized. The overall mortality (58%) was high by present-day standards, even considering the high severity of illness in the study population. The mean time to administration of antibiotics was 7.1 h in the corticosteroid group and 6.0 h in the placebo group, which may be considered suboptimal in patients presenting with severe sepsis or septic shock. Etomidate, an inhibitor of steroid synthesis, was administered in 24% of patients and may have led to adrenal insufficiency. The protocol was amended during the study by excluding patients who had received etomidate in the 6-h period preceding randomization.

29.11 Subsequent Evidence

The CORTICUS trial was published 6 years later, including a larger sample size of 499 patients. Intravenous hydrocortisone alone was administered as (fludrocortisone was not used) and compared with a placebo among patients with septic shock [7]. The authors observed no difference in the 28-day mortality; however, a reduced time to shock reversal was observed in corticosteroid-treated patients.

The Adjunctive Corticosteroid Treatment in Critically Ill Patients with Septic Shock (ADRENAL) study [8] has been the largest RCT thus far to address this question. The study included 3800 patients in septic shock, involving 69 medical-surgical ICUs in Australia, the United Kingdom, New Zealand, Saudi Arabia, and Denmark. Hydrocortisone was administered as an intravenous infusion of 200 mg/day for 7 days and compared with a placebo. There was no significant difference in the 90-day mortality, the primary outcome. Among the secondary outcomes, the investigators observed a significant difference in the median time to shock resolution, the median time to initial discontinuation of mechanical ventilation, the median time to ICU discharge, and the number of patients who received a blood transfusion.

29.12 Summary

Considering its powerful anti-inflammatory properties, clinicians resorted to high-dose corticosteroid administration in patients with severe sepsis for over three decades from the 1950s. Some early reports suggested benefit with such high-dose therapy. However, by the 1980s, it was evident that such heavy-handed use of corticosteroids was more likely to cause harm. A resurgence of interest in low-dose therapy occurred in the 1990s, arising from the concept of relative adrenal insufficiency in sepsis. Following up on small RCTs, Annane et al. conducted their landmark trial involving multiple ICUs in France to test this hypothesis. They evaluated the efficacy of a 7-day treatment regimen, including hydrocortisone 50 mg 6 hourly combined with fludrocortisone 50 μg once daily in patients with septic shock. Failure of serum cortisol levels to rise by >9 μg/dL following tetracosactrin was considered to suggest relative adrenal insufficiency (non-responders). Among non-responders, the hydrocortisone-fludrocortisone combination resulted in significantly lower 28-day mortality, with no apparent adverse effects. This study was the first large RCT to evaluate the hypothesis of relative adrenal insufficiency in sepsis and the impact of low-dose corticosteroid therapy in septic shock.

References

1. Sprung CL, Caralis PV, Marcial EH, Pierce M, Gelbard MA, Long WM, et al. The effects of high-dose corticosteroids in patients with septic shock. A prospective, controlled study. N Engl J Med. 1984;311(18):1137–43.
2. Veterans Administration Systemic Sepsis Cooperative Study Group. Effect of high-dose glucocorticoid therapy on mortality in patients with clinical signs of systemic sepsis. N Engl J Med. 1987;317(11):659–65.
3. Bollaert PE, Charpentier C, Levy B, Debouverie M, Audibert G, Larcan A. Reversal of late septic shock with supraphysiologic doses of hydrocortisone. Crit Care Med. 1998;26(4):645–50.

4. Briegel J, Forst H, Haller M, Schelling G, Kilger E, Kuprat G, et al. Stress doses of hydrocortisone reverse hyperdynamic septic shock: a prospective, randomized, double-blind, single-center study. Crit Care Med. 1999;27(4):723–32.
5. Annane D, Sébille V, Troché G, Raphaël JC, Gajdos P, Bellissant E. A 3-level prognostic classification in septic shock based on cortisol levels and cortisol response to corticotropin. JAMA. 2000;283(8):1038–45.
6. Annane D, Sebille V, Charpentier C, Bollaert PE, Francois B, Korach JM, et al. Effect of treatment with low doses of hydrocortisone and fludrocortisone on mortality in patients with septic shock. JAMA. 2002;288(7):862–71.
7. Sprung CL, Annane D, Keh D, Moreno R, Singer M, Freivogel K, et al. Hydrocortisone therapy for patients with septic shock. N Engl J Med. 2008;358(2):111–24.
8. Venkatesh B, Finfer S, Cohen J, Rajbhandari D, Arabi Y, Bellomo R, et al. Adjunctive glucocorticoid therapy in patients with septic shock. N Engl J Med. 2018;378(9):797–808.

Hydrocortisone in Septic Shock: The CORTICUS Trial

30

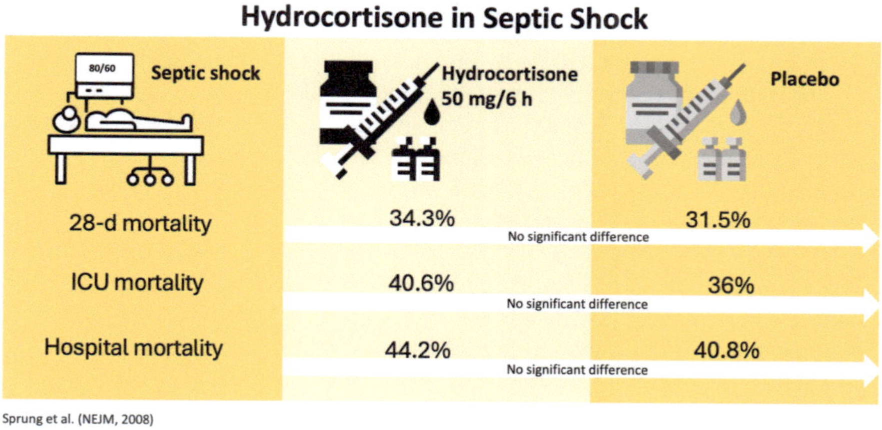

Quick Take

The CORTICUS trial asked the question: Does hydrocortisone save lives in septic shock?

This landmark trial evaluated the effect of low-dose hydrocortisone therapy on patients with septic shock who were not responding to conventional therapy. A total of 499 patients were randomized to receive either hydrocortisone or a placebo in addition to standard care. The study found that hydrocortisone administration did not significantly reduce 28-day mortality, but did improve shock reversal and the duration of vasopressor therapy.

Sprung CL, Annane D, Keh D, Moreno R, Singer M, Freivogel K, et al. Hydrocortisone therapy for patients with septic shock. N Engl J Med. 2008 Jan 10;358(2):111–24.

J. Chacko et al., *Landmark Studies in Critical Care*,
https://doi.org/10.1007/978-981-95-0673-6_30

30.1 Introduction

Historically, severe sepsis and septic shock have been associated with high mortality. Clinical trials published at the turn of the century revealed a mortality of 33–61% among patients with septic shock [1, 2]. Several adjuvant therapies had been investigated, but the results were uniformly disappointing [3]. Considering its potent anti-inflammatory effect, corticosteroids have evinced interest among clinicians since the 1970s. A two-part, prospective-retrospective study by Schumer et al., using high-dose methylprednisolone, 30 mg/kg, revealed a significantly improved survival in septic shock [4]. However, subsequent studies failed to replicate the favorable effects of high-dose corticosteroids; besides, higher mortality was noted, likely due to superinfections [5, 6].

In the 1990s, relative adrenal insufficiency secondary to suppression of the hypothalamic-adrenal-pituitary axis and was proposed as the driver of septic shock. A failure of the serum cortisol level to rise by >9 mcg/dl following corticotropin was considered to indicate relative adrenal insufficiency [7]. Annane et al. conducted a randomized controlled trial (RCT) to assess whether a combination of hydrocortisone and fludrocortisone would improve survival among patients with septic shock and relative adrenal insufficiency. They observed that a 7-day course of treatment with this combination significantly improved survival in septic shock associated with relative adrenal insufficiency, with no increase in the incidence of adverse events, including superinfections [8].

The CORTICUS (Corticosteroid Therapy of Septic Shock) trial set out to evaluate the safety and efficacy of low-dose hydrocortisone among a broad population of patients with septic shock. The study was specifically aimed to assess outcomes among patients who exhibited a normal response to corticotropin, suggesting no evidence of relative adrenal insufficiency [9].

30.2 Population and Design

The CORTICUS trial enrolled patients from 52 ICUs across nine countries (in Europe and Israel) between March 2002 and November 2002. The study population included patients with clinical evidence of infection and shock within 72 h prior to enrollment. Shock was defined as a systolic blood pressure lower than 90 mm Hg following adequate fluid resuscitation, or vasopressor requirement for at least 1 h. Eligible patients had evidence of hypoperfusion and organ dysfunction consequent to sepsis.

30.2.1 Exclusion

The study excluded patients with a poor prognosis due to underlying disease and those who were not expected to survive for >24 h. Patients who were immunosuppressed, those on long-term corticosteroid treatment within the previous 6 months, and short-term corticosteroids within 4 weeks were also excluded.

Eligible patients were randomized in a 1:1 ratio to receive hydrocortisone or placebo. Randomization was stratified based on study center in blocks of four.

30.3 Hydrocortisone Group

Hydrocortisone hemisuccinate, 50 mg 6 hourly, was administered intravenously as a bolus dose initially for 5 days. From day 6, the dose was tapered down to 50 mg twice daily until day 8, 50 mg once daily from day 9 to day 11, and ceased thereafter.

30.4 Placebo Group

Patients allocated to the control group received a placebo from identical vials.

30.5 Both Groups

Evidence-based management of sepsis and septic shock was encouraged based on standard guidelines [10]. A short corticotropin test was performed with an intravenous bolus dose of 250 mcg of cosyntropin (a synthetic derivative of corticotropin). The serum cortisol levels were measured at baseline and 60 min after the administration of cosyntropin. Absence of response was defined as a rise in the serum cortisol level by ≤9 mcg/dl. Shock reversal was defined as maintenance of a systolic blood pressure ≥90 mm Hg without vasopressors for at least 24 h.

30.6 Sample Size

The authors assumed a 28-day mortality of 50% among non-responders to corticotrophin. A sample size of 400 patients in each group provided the study with 80% power to detect a 10% mortality difference.

30.7 Results

The study was terminated after the recruitment of 500 patients. Slow recruitment, lack of funding, and time-expiry of the study drug led to premature cessation of the trial.

Among the 500 patients who were enrolled, all except one patient (who withdrew consent) were included in the intention-to-treat analysis, including 251 in the hydrocortisone group and 248 in the placebo group. Based on the corticotropin test,

50.9% of patients were non-responders, and 46.7% were responders; the results were unavailable in the remaining 2.7%.

Patients in both groups were well-matched at baseline. Most patients (54%) underwent emergency surgical procedures; medical patients were fewer (38%). The most common focus of infection was the gastrointestinal tract, followed by the lungs. The majority of patients were mechanically ventilated (92%). Norepinephrine was the most common agent employed for hemodynamic support, followed by epinephrine and dopamine.

30.8 The Primary Endpoint: 28-Day Mortality

Overall, the 28-day mortality was similar in the hydrocortisone and the placebo groups [86/251 (34.3%) vs. 78/248 (31.5%), $P = 0.51$].

Among non-responders to corticotropin, there was no significant difference in mortality between the hydrocortisone and placebo groups (39.2% vs. 36.1%, $P = 0.69$). The results were similar for responders with similar mortality in the hydrocortisone and placebo groups (28.8% vs. 28.7%, $P = 1.00$). There was no difference in mortality between groups based on the duration of shock before study entry. On post hoc analysis, the 28-day mortality was higher in both groups among patients who received etomidate before study entry.

There was no significant difference between the hydrocortisone and placebo groups in the ICU mortality (40.6% vs. 36.0%), the in-hospital mortality (44.2% vs. 40.7%), and the mortality at 1 year (56.6% vs. 54.0%). The results were similar among non-responders and responders to corticotropin.

30.9 Shock Reversal

Shock reversal occurred in a similar number of patients in the hydrocortisone and placebo groups among corticotropin non-responders (76% vs. 70.4%) and responders (84.7% vs. 79.7%). However, shock reversal occurred more rapidly among hydrocortisone-treated patients. The time to shock reversal was shorter in the hydrocortisone group among all patients ($P < 0.001$), corticotropin non-responders ($P < 0.001$), and responders ($P = 0.06$).

30.10 Other Outcomes

A similar number of patients underwent extubation by day 28 in both groups (hydrocortisone vs. placebo: 52% vs. 53%). Antibiotic therapy was considered appropriate in a similar proportion of patients in both groups. However, the appropriateness of antibiotic therapy did not appear to significantly impact outcomes. The main study outcomes are summarized in Table 30.1.

Table 30.1 Main study outcomes

Outcome	Hydrocortisone	Placebo	*P* value
28-day mortality			
Overall	34.3%	31.5%	0.51
Corticotropin responders	28.8%	28.7%	1.00
Corticotropin non-responders	39.2%	36.1%	0.69
ICU mortality	40.6%	36.0%	0.31
Hospital mortality	44.2%	40.8%	0.47
Shock reversal	79.7%	74.2%	0.18
Time to shock reversal	3.3 days	5.8 days	<0.001

30.11 Adverse Events

Hydrocortisone administration was associated with a higher incidence of superinfections and new-onset sepsis or septic shock. Besides, hyperglycemia and hypernatremia were more commonly observed in the hydrocortisone group. Clinical signs of neuromuscular weakness were rarely reported; however, electrophysiological evaluation was not performed.

30.12 Study Conclusions

Among patients with septic shock, hydrocortisone administration did not lead to improved survival or reversal of shock. Hydrocortisone resulted in a more rapid reversal of shock compared with placebo.

30.13 Strengths

The CORTICUS trial was a multicentric study across nine countries and, hence, lent external validity. The study was double-blinded, reducing the risk of bias. The authors evaluated clinically meaningful outcomes, including mortality. The study specifically analyzed outcomes related to non-responders compared to responders to corticotropin.

30.14 Weaknesses

Although the original sample size was 800 patients, the trial was terminated after the recruitment of 500 patients; hence, it failed to attain the statistical power that the authors had envisaged. The authors assumed 50% mortality in the control group; however, the overall 28-day mortality in the placebo group was lower (31.5%), increasing the likelihood of an underpowered trial. Open-label hydrocortisone was administered in 4.2% of patients, although this appeared unlikely to have significantly impacted outcomes. Approximately one-quarter of patients did not receive appropriate antibiotic therapy. The study enrolled patients within 72 h of septic shock; the question remains whether earlier administration of hydrocortisone would make a difference.

30.15 Subsequent Evidence

The ADRENAL trial, published a decade later, randomized 3800 patients to receive hydrocortisone 200 mg/day as an infusion, compared with placebo. The study did not reveal a significant impact of hydrocortisone treatment on the 90-day mortality, the primary outcome. Echoing the findings of the CORTICUS trial, earlier shock reversal was observed. Besides, the initial episode of mechanical ventilation was shorter with hydrocortisone, although the number of days alive and ventilator-free was not different between the two groups.

The APROCCHSS study had a smaller sample size than CORTICUS (1241 vs. 3800 patients). In this French multicentric study, the authors observed lower mortality at 90 days in the hydrocortisone group. Among the secondary outcomes, the ICU and hospital mortality were also lower in hydrocortisone-treated patients. Akin to the CORTICUS and ADRENAL trials, the earlier shock reversal was observed in the hydrocortisone group.

30.16 Summary

The CORTICUS trial was designed to evaluate the impact of hydrocortisone treatment in septic shock, considering the lack of firm evidence regarding the efficacy of corticosteroids. Patients in septic shock were randomized to receive hydrocortisone 200 mg/day or placebo for 7 days or until death or discharge from the ICU. The overall 28-day mortality, the primary outcome, was similar in both groups. Besides, the mortality rate was also similar among responders and non-responders to corticotropin. Shock reversal occurred in a similar number of patients in both groups; however, the time to shock reversal was significantly less—among all patients, non-responders, and responders to corticotropin. The incidence of superinfections, new-onset sepsis and septic shock, hypernatremia, and hyperglycemia were more common in hydrocortisone-treated patients. The findings of the trial contrasted with those of the study by Annane et al., which had shown significantly improved survival with a combination of hydrocortisone and fludrocortisone in septic shock associated with relative adrenal insufficiency. The CORTICUS trial triggered further research on the efficacy of corticosteroids in septic shock, leading to the ADRENAL and the APROCCHSS trials.

References

1. Abraham E, Reinhart K, Opal S, Demeyer I, Doig C, Rodriguez AL, et al. Efficacy and safety of tifacogin (recombinant tissue factor pathway inhibitor) in severe sepsis: a randomized controlled trial. JAMA. 2003;290(2):238–47.
2. Laterre PF, Levy H, Clermont G, Ball DE, Garg R, Nelson DR, et al. Hospital mortality and resource use in subgroups of the recombinant human activated protein C worldwide evaluation in severe sepsis (PROWESS) trial. Crit Care Med. 2004;32(11):2207–18.
3. Vincent JL, van der Poll T, Marshall JC. The end of "one size fits all" sepsis therapies: toward an individualized approach. Biomedicine. 2022;10(9):2260.
4. Schumer W. Steroids in the treatment of clinical septic shock. Ann Surg. 1976;184(3):333–41.
5. Lefering R, Neugebauer EA. Steroid controversy in sepsis and septic shock: a meta-analysis. Crit Care Med. 1995;23(7):1294–303.
6. Cronin L, Cook DJ, Carlet J, Heyland DK, King D, Lansang MA, et al. Corticosteroid treatment for sepsis: a critical appraisal and meta-analysis of the literature. Crit Care Med. 1995;23(8):1430–9.
7. Meyer NJ, Hall JB. Relative adrenal insufficiency in the ICU: can we at least make the diagnosis? Am J Respir Crit Care Med. 2006;174(12):1282–4.
8. Annane D, Sébille V, Charpentier C, Bollaert PE, François B, Korach JM, et al. Effect of treatment with low doses of hydrocortisone and fludrocortisone on mortality in patients with septic shock. JAMA. 2002;288(7):862–71.
9. Sprung CL, Annane D, Keh D, Moreno R, Singer M, Freivogel K, et al. Hydrocortisone therapy for patients with septic shock. N Engl J Med. 2008;358(2):111–24.
10. Summary of recommendations. Intensive Care Med. 2001;27(1):S128–34.

Hydrocortisone in Septic Shock: The ADRENAL Trial

31

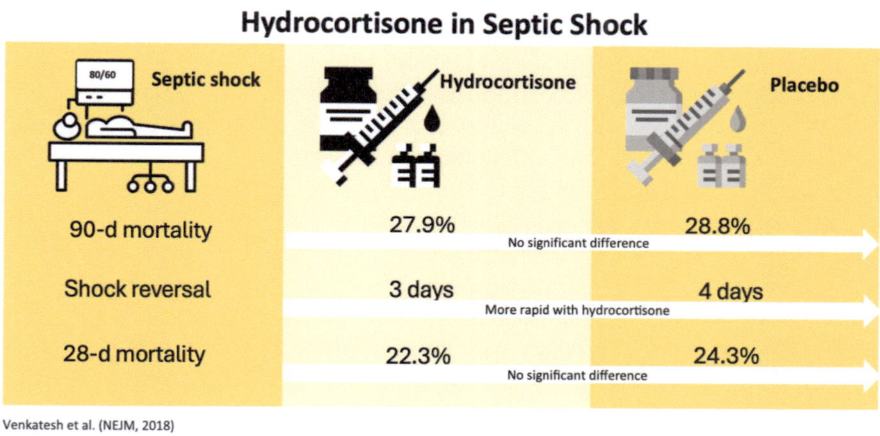

Quick Take

Do corticosteroids improve outcomes in septic shock?

The ADRENAL trial was a large-scale, randomized, double-blind study that examined the use of hydrocortisone in patients with septic shock who did not respond to fluid resuscitation and vasopressors. A total of 3800 patients were included. The study revealed no significant difference in the 90-day mortality between the hydrocortisone-treated group (53.3%) and the placebo group (54.0%).

Venkatesh B, Finfer S, Cohen J, Rajbhandari D, Arabi Y, Bellomo R, et al. Adjunctive Glucocorticoid Therapy in Patients with Septic Shock. N Engl J Med. 2018 Mar;378(9):797–808.

J. Chacko et al., *Landmark Studies in Critical Care*,
https://doi.org/10.1007/978-981-95-0673-6_31

While hydrocortisone therapy did not impact survival, it did improve hemodynamic stability and reduce the need for vasopressor support. Furthermore, the duration of the initial episode of mechanical ventilation was lower in the hydrocortisone group. The trial provided crucial evidence in assessing the role of corticosteroids in sepsis management, suggesting that while they may aid in stabilization, they may not impact overall survival.

31.1 Introduction

Corticosteroids have been used as adjuvant therapy in patients with severe sepsis and septic shock for more than four decades. Early randomized controlled trials (RCTs) from the 1980s used high-dose corticosteroids (30 mg/kg) [1]. Almost predictably, the mortality and morbidity were higher with high-dose corticosteroid administration compared with placebo [2], leading to the abandonment of such therapy. The 1990s witnessed a resurgence of interest with lower, more physiological doses, based on the hypothesis that relative adrenal insufficiency may occur in septic shock. Two RCTs were performed with hydrocortisone, 200 mg/day, based on the putative mechanism of relative adrenal insufficiency in septic shock. Annane et al. combined hydrocortisone with fludrocortisone, a mineralocorticoid, compared with placebo, in patients with septic shock [3]. The 28-day mortality was lower among patients with relative adrenal insufficiency (established with a short corticotrophin test), who received the hydrocortisone-fludrocortisone combination. The subsequent CORTICUS trial used intravenous hydrocortisone alone compared with placebo in septic shock. In contrast to the Annane et al. trial, there was no significant difference in the 28-day mortality with hydrocortisone treatment, although earlier shock reversal was observed [4]. Clinical practice varied, considering the lack of robust evidence to support adjuvant therapy with corticosteroids. The 2016 Surviving Sepsis Guidelines recommended its use among patients who remained hypotensive despite adequate fluid resuscitation and vasopressors, although the supporting evidence was weak [5].

Considering the paucity of robust evidence and conflicting results from controlled clinical trials, the Australian-New Zealand Intensive Care Society Clinical Trials Group designed a large, multinational RCT to test the hypothesis whether hydrocortisone therapy would lead to improved survival among patients with septic shock.

31.2 Population and Design

The ADRENAL trial was conducted between March 2013 and April 2017 across 69 medical-surgical ICUs in Australia, the UK, New Zealand, Saudi Arabia, and Denmark. The study included patients with septic shock on mechanical ventilation. The study subjects had documented infection or a strong clinical suspicion of infection, with ≥two criteria of the systemic inflammatory response syndrome (SIRS), and were on treatment with inotropes or vasopressors to maintain a mean arterial pressure of >60 mm Hg for at least 4 h at the time of randomization. Patients were randomized to receive intravenous hydrocortisone or placebo. Randomization was stratified by center and according to the type of admission—medical or surgical.

31.3 Excluded

Patients in whom corticosteroids might be required for indications other than septic shock and those who had received etomidate during the current hospital admission were excluded. Those who met the inclusion criteria for >24 h before randomization were excluded. Patients who were considered unlikely to survive for 90 days due to comorbidities and those in whom limitation of treatment had been decided upon were also excluded.

31.4 The Hydrocortisone Group

Intravenous hydrocortisone, 200 mg/day, was administered as a continuous infusion. The hydrocortisone solution was reconstituted at a concentration of 1 mg/ml. A total volume of 200 ml of the solution was infused over 24 h.

31.5 Placebo Group

A matching placebo was administered in identical, masked vials. The placebo solution was also administered as a continuous infusion at 200 ml/day. The trial infusion was continued for a maximum of 7 days, or until discharge from the ICU or death, whichever occurred earlier.

31.6 Sample Size

The authors assumed a baseline mortality of 33%. A sample size of 3800 patients provided the study with 90% power to detect a 5% absolute reduction in the 90-day all-cause mortality at an alpha level of 0.05, allowing for a loss to follow-up of 1%.

31.7 Results

A total of 3800 patients were enrolled—1898 were randomized to receive hydrocortisone, and 1902 to placebo. Baseline characteristics were similar in both groups. The median APACHE II score was similar in both groups (hydrocortisone: 24 vs. placebo: 23); most admissions were medical (68.8% vs. 68.2%). The most common primary focus of infection was pulmonary, followed by abdominal and blood-borne.

The median time from randomization to commencement of the study infusion was 0.8 h in both groups. The use of inotropic or vasopressor support, antimicrobial treatment, statins, and etomidate was similar in both groups. The mean arterial pressure and lactate levels were higher, and the heart rate was lower in the hydrocortisone group from days 1 to 7. Between days 1 and 14, open-label hydrocortisone was administered in 7.4% of patients in the hydrocortisone group and 8.8% in the placebo group.

31.8 The Primary Outcome: 90-Day Mortality

The 90-day all-cause mortality, the primary outcome, was similar in the hydrocortisone (27.9%) and placebo groups (28.8%) [odds ratio, 0.95; 95% confidence interval (CI), 0.82 to 1.10; $P = 0.50$]. Mortality was similar in prespecified subgroups of patients based on gender, type of admission (medical vs. surgical), dose of catecholamine (≤15 mcg/kg/min vs. more), focus of sepsis (pulmonary vs. extrapulmonary), APACHE II score ≤25 vs. more), or time from onset of shock to randomization (≤6 h vs. more). Post-hoc analysis after the exclusion of patients who had received open-label hydrocortisone yielded the same results.

31.9 Secondary Outcomes

Among the secondary outcomes, the 28-day mortality was similar in both groups. Shock resolution occurred more rapidly in the hydrocortisone group (median: 3 days vs. 4 days; $P < 0.001$). Patients who received hydrocortisone were discharged earlier from the ICU compared to placebo (median: 10 days vs. 12 days; $P < 0.001$); however, on adjusted analysis, the numbers of days alive and out of ICU were not significantly different between the two groups.

The duration of initial ventilator support was shorter in the hydrocortisone group (median 6 days vs. 7 days; $P < 0.001$). However, when episodes of re-initiation of mechanical ventilation were taken into account, the mean number of days alive and ventilator-free at 90 days was similar in both groups (61.2 days vs. 59.1 days).

The incidence of recurrent shock, re-initiation of mechanical ventilation, time to hospital discharge, days alive and out of hospital, rates of renal replacement therapy, and new-onset bacteremia or fungemia were similar in both groups. Blood transfusions were administered to fewer patients in the hydrocortisone group.

31.10 Adverse Events

Adverse events were few but higher in the hydrocortisone group (1.1% vs. 0.3%, $P = 0.009$). Among six serious adverse events, four occurred in the hydrocortisone group. The main results of the study are summarized in Table 31.1.

Table 31.1 Main study outcomes

Outcome	Hydrocortisone ($N = 1853$)	Placebo ($N = 1860$)	Significance
90-d mortality	511/1832 (27.9%)	526/1826 (28.8%)	Not significant
28-d mortality	410/1841 (22.3%)	448/1840 (24.3%)	Not significant
Time to shock resolution (median, IQR)	3 (2–5) days	4 (2–9) days	$P < 0.001$, significant
Time to cessation of initial episode of mechanical ventilation (median, IQR)	6 (3–18) days	7 (3–24) days	$P < 0.001$, significant
Days alive and ICU-free	58.2 ± 34.8 days	56.0 ± 35.4	Not significant
Days alive and ventilation-free	61.2 ± 35.6 days	59.1 ± 36.1	Not significant

31.11 Study Conclusions

Administration of hydrocortisone did not lead to a lower 90-day mortality compared with placebo in patients with septic shock. Shock reversal occurred more rapidly with hydrocortisone. The duration of ICU stay was shorter in the hydrocortisone group; moreover, the initial episode of mechanical ventilation was also shorter. Blood transfusions were administered less often in the hydrocortisone group.

31.12 Strengths

The ADRENAL trial was an international, multicentric RCT with a pragmatic design, providing external validity. The study evaluated important patient-centric clinical outcomes. Nearly 70% of eligible subjects were enrolled, in tune with other contemporaneous large-scale trials. The study was double-blinded and adequately powered to evaluate the primary outcome; analysis was by intention to treat. It remains by far the largest RCT to evaluate the effect of corticosteroids in septic shock. Pre-defined analysis was carried out, aimed at evaluating outcomes in specific subgroups of patients who might benefit from hydrocortisone. Loss to follow-up was minimal (0.7%), adding to the robustness of the trial.

31.13 Limitations

Open-label hydrocortisone was administered in 8.8% of patients in the placebo group, which may have impacted outcomes. The appropriateness of antibiotic therapy was not analyzed. The study did not evaluate neuromuscular weakness, a known complication of corticosteroid treatment. Data on nosocomial infection rates were not available (except new-onset bacteremia and fungemia). A continuous infusion of hydrocortisone was used, considering the lower likelihood of hyperglycemia and a more favorable impact on the inflammatory response [6]. However, a slower onset of action might have rendered hydrocortisone less effective compared with previous trials that used intermittent bolus dosing. Patients who had previously received etomidate, a commonly used agent in shocked patients, were excluded from the trial. Details of other aspects of care, including fluid resuscitation, were not available, although the authors state that management was based on standard guidelines.

31.14 Subsequent Evidence

The APROCCHSS trial was a multicentric RCT conducted across 34 ICUs in France. The authors evaluated a combination of hydrocortisone, 50 mg/kg intravenously, and 50 μg fludrocortisone by the enteral route once daily among patients with septic shock who were on vasopressor therapy for at least 6 h [7]. The study, originally designed to evaluate the efficacy of drotrecogin alfa combined with steroids in septic shock, took nearly 7 years to complete. Drotrecogin alfa was withdrawn from the market during the course of the study; thereafter, the hydrocortisone-fludrocortisone combination was compared with placebo. The study sample size was smaller than ADRENAL (1241 vs. 3800 patients). The APROCCHSS study revealed a significantly lower 90-day mortality among steroid-treated patients. Furthermore, the all-cause mortality was lower in the steroid group at ICU and hospital discharge, and at 180 days. Similar to the ADRENAL trial, the investigators observed more rapid shock reversal with a greater number of patients remaining vasopressor-free at day 28 in the steroid group.

31.15 Summary

Historically, corticosteroid use in severe sepsis and septic shock has been steeped in controversy. Early controlled clinical trials with high doses had revealed poor outcomes, including increased mortality. The concept of relative adrenal insufficiency and the use of more physiological doses held promise; however, conflicting findings were observed in two RCTs. Against this background, the ADRENAL trial randomized patients with septic shock to receive hydrocortisone infusion, 200 mg/day, compared with placebo. There was no significant effect of hydrocortisone administration on the 90-day mortality, the primary outcome. However, similar to the findings in other trials, the authors observed earlier shock reversal [3, 7]. Besides, the duration of the initial episode of mechanical ventilation was lower in the hydrocortisone group, although overall, the number of days alive and ventilation-free was similar in both groups. Although hydrocortisone-treated patients were discharged earlier from the ICU, the number of days alive and ICU-free did not differ between groups. Other important clinical outcomes, including the 28-day mortality, the number of days alive and out of the hospital, and the incidence of new-onset bacteremia and fungemia, were also similar. Based on the findings of the ADRENAL trial, the Surviving Sepsis Guidelines currently recommend hydrocortisone 200 mg/day in patients with septic shock and requiring a dose of 0.25 mcg/kg/min for at least 4 h to maintain target mean arterial pressures [5].

References

1. Sprung CL, Caralis PV, Marcial EH, Pierce M, Gelbard MA, Long WM, et al. The effects of high-dose corticosteroids in patients with septic shock. A prospective, controlled study. N Engl J Med. 1984;311(18):1137–43.
2. Bone RC, Fisher CJ, Clemmer TP, Slotman GJ, Metz CA, Balk RA. A controlled clinical trial of high-dose methylprednisolone in the treatment of severe sepsis and septic shock. N Engl J Med. 1987;317(11):653–8.
3. Annane D, Sébille V, Charpentier C, Bollaert PE, François B, Korach JM, et al. Effect of treatment with low doses of hydrocortisone and fludrocortisone on mortality in patients with septic shock. JAMA. 2002;288(7):862–71.
4. Sprung CL, Annane D, Keh D, Moreno R, Singer M, Freivogel K, et al. Hydrocortisone therapy for patients with septic shock. N Engl J Med. 2008;358(2):111–24.
5. Rhodes A, Evans LE, Alhazzani W, Levy MM, Antonelli M, Ferrer R, et al. Surviving sepsis campaign: international guidelines for management of sepsis and septic shock: 2016. Intensive Care Med. 2017;43(3):304–77.
6. Keh D, Boehnke T, Weber-Cartens S, Schulz C, Ahlers O, Bercker S, et al. Immunologic and hemodynamic effects of "low-dose" hydrocortisone in septic shock: a double-blind, randomized, placebo-controlled, crossover study. Am J Respir Crit Care Med. 2003;167(4):512–20.
7. Annane D, Renault A, Brun-Buisson C, Megarbane B, Quenot JP, Siami S, et al. Hydrocortisone plus fludrocortisone for adults with septic shock. N Engl J Med. 2018;378(9):809–18.

Part VI

Corticosteroids in ARDS

Methylprednisolone for Unresolving Acute Respiratory Distress Syndrome: Meduri et al.

32

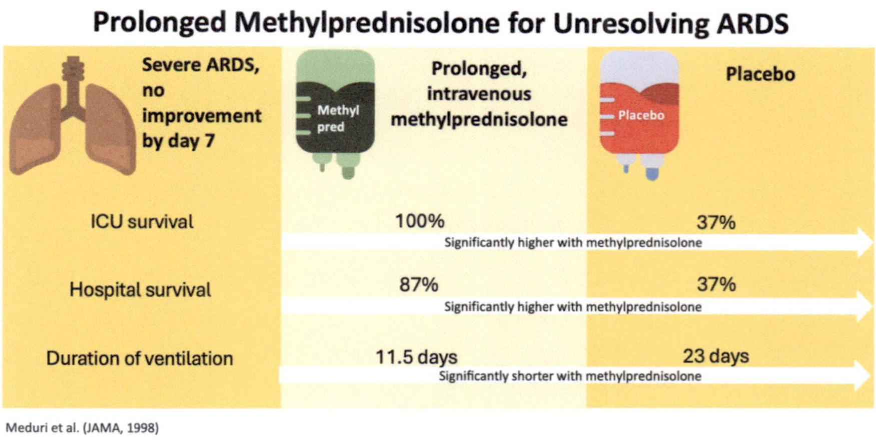

Quick Take

Could steroids offer a solution for acute respiratory distress syndrome (ARDS) that fails to resolve?

The study by Meduri et al. evaluated the use of prolonged methylprednisolone therapy in patients with unresolved acute respiratory distress syndrome (ARDS). The randomized trial found that the use of methylprednisolone in ARDS patients led to improvements in pulmonary function and a reduction in the duration of

---

Meduri GU, Headley AS, Golden E, Carson SJ, Umberger RA, Kelso T, et al. Effect of prolonged methylprednisolone therapy in unresolving acute respiratory distress syndrome: a randomized controlled trial. JAMA. 1998 Jul 8;280(2):159–65.

J. Chacko et al., *Landmark Studies in Critical Care*,
https://doi.org/10.1007/978-981-95-0673-6_32

mechanical ventilation, with no significant increase in infections. However, the potential risks of prolonged steroid use, including hyperglycemia and immunosuppression, require careful monitoring. This study highlighted the potential therapeutic benefits of corticosteroids for ARDS, especially in cases where conventional therapies failed to resolve the condition.

32.1 Introduction

Acute respiratory distress syndrome (ARDS) is characterized by hypoxemic respiratory failure secondary to diffuse, exudative pulmonary edema [1]. Although the provoking cause is adequately dealt with, no specific treatment alters the relentless trajectory of ARDS [2]. During the first week of ARDS, non-survivors often generate an intense inflammatory and fibrotic response [1]. The mortality in these patients who fail to improve within the first week remains high (>80%) [3–5]. Two meta-analyses published in 1995 had observed that high-dose, short-duration therapy with methylprednisolone appeared to offer no clinical benefit [6, 7]. However, improved lung function and survival were reported with prolonged administration of methylprednisolone [8, 9].

In their randomized controlled trial (RCT) of 1998, Meduri et al. tested the efficacy of prolonged, high-dose methylprednisolone therapy, targeting alveolar remodeling and fibrosis, the hallmark of unresolving ARDS [10].

32.2 Population and Design

The study was conducted during a 2-year period between 1994 and 1996 in four medical intensive care units in the United States. The double-blind, placebo-controlled RCT included patients with severe ARDS who had failed to improve by day 7 of acute respiratory failure. Patients were eligible if they had ARDS according to the American-European Consensus Conference criteria [11], a Lung Injury Score (LIS) $\geq$2.5 (indicating severe lung injury), had undergone 7 days of mechanical ventilation with a reduction by less than 1 point compared to day 1 of ARDS, and had no evidence of untreated infection.

32.3 Excluded

Patients with ARDS lasting >3 weeks, extensive burns, and those with a life expectancy of <3 Months due to a terminal illness, major gastrointestinal bleeding, or requiring >1 mg/kg methylprednisolone per day for a concomitant illness were excluded.

Eligible patients were randomized to receive methylprednisolone or placebo in a 2:1 ratio, stratified by center.

32.4 Methylprednisolone Group

In the intervention arm, methylprednisolone was administered in a loading dose of 2 mg/kg intravenously, with continued treatment based on the following schedule:

Day 1–14: 2 mg/kg/day
Day 15–21: 1 mg/kg/day
Day 22–28: 0.5 mg/kg/day
Days 29, 30: 0.25 mg/kg/day
Days 31, 32: 0.125 mg/kg/day

The daily dose was divided into 4 doses, administered at 6 hourly, intravenously. It was switched to a single dose when oral intake was feasible. If the patient was extubated before day 14, the dosing schedule was continued from day 15.

32.5 Control Group

Patients in the control group received a matching placebo—intravenous or oral according to schedule.

32.6 Both Groups

The ventilator management was adjusted to limit the plateau pressure to a maximum of 35 cm H_2O. Patients who did not respond to the allocated treatment (lack of improvement in the LIS by at least 1 point after 10 days of treatment) could cross-over to the other arm. Patients who developed severe gastrointestinal bleed requiring transfusion, those with candida infection at multiple sites, or with a new-onset, life-threatening condition for which methylprednisolone was indicated were withdrawn from the study. All patients underwent meticulous, daily screening for new-onset infections, including fiberoptic bronchoscopy and bronchoalveolar lavage on day 5 of ventilation and weekly thereafter to screen for ventilator-associated pneumonia.

32.7 Results

Twenty-four patients with ARDS were enrolled during the 2-year study period—16 received methylprednisolone, while 8 received a placebo. The duration of ARDS, rate of nosocomial infections, the PaO_2/FiO_2 ratio, the mean level of PEEP applied, the LIS, and the MODS score were similar in both groups at enrolment.

32.7.1 The Primary Outcomes

The primary outcomes were ICU survival and improvement in LIS by day 10. ICU survival was significantly higher in the methylprednisolone group. All 16 patients survived in the methylprednisolone group, compared to 3 of 8 (37%) patients assigned to receive placebo ($P = 0.002$). The mean LIS at 10 days was significantly better in the methylprednisolone group compared with placebo (mean: 1.7 vs. 3.0, $P < 0.001$).

32.7.2 Other Clinical Outcomes

Hospital survival was also significantly higher among patients assigned to receive methylprednisolone compared to placebo [14/16 (86%) vs. 3/8 (37%), $P = 0.03$]. Two patients developed unresolving ARDS in the methylprednisolone group; both survived. However, all five patients who developed unresolving ARDS in the placebo group died. The median duration of mechanical ventilation was shorter (11.5 days vs. 23 days, $P = 0.001$), and the number of MODS-free days by day 28 was higher (16 days vs. 6 days, $P = 0.005$) in the methylprednisolone group.

32.7.3 Physiological Endpoints by Days 5–7

A distinctive improvement was noted in physiological parameters among patients who received methylprednisolone compared to those who received a placebo. By day 5, the mean PaO_2/FiO_2 ratio and the LIS had significantly improved in the methylprednisolone group; by day 7, the MODS score was lower, and the static lung compliance was significantly higher in this group. In contrast, these parameters did not show a significant change in the placebo group.

32.7.4 Endpoints at Day 10

By day 10, all 16 patients in the methylprednisolone group were alive, including seven who were successfully extubated; in the placebo group, two had died, and the other six patients continued to be on ventilator support. Among the eight patients in the placebo group, two had improved while two had died; four patients who failed to improve were crossed over to receive methylprednisolone.

The PaO_2/FiO_2 ratio was significantly higher, the LIS, pulmonary artery pressure, and the MODS score were lower in the methylprednisolone group compared to the placebo. Although the overall incidence of nosocomial infections was similar in both groups (infections per 100 patient-days), new-onset ventilator-associated pneumonia occurred more often in the methylprednisolone group (6 vs. 1, $P = 0.70$). The main study outcomes are summarized in Table 32.1.

Table 32.1 Main study outcomes

Outcome	Methylprednisolone	Placebo	*P* value
ICU survival	16/16 (100%)	3/8 (37%)	0.002
Hospital survival	14/16 (87%)	3/8 (37%)	0.03
Median duration of ventilation	11.5 days	23 days	0.005
LIS on day 10: mean (SD)	1.7 (0.1)	3 (0.2)	<0.001
Successful extubation	7/16 (44%)	0 (0%)	0.05
Infection per 100 d of treatment	8	7	0.99

Abbreviations: LIS lung injury score, *SD* standard deviation

32.8 Study Conclusions

The authors concluded that among patients with unresolving ARDS, prolonged methylprednisolone therapy was associated with improvement in the LIS and MODS scores and lower mortality.

32.9 Strengths

The study by Meduri et al. was one of the early RCTs that evaluated the efficacy of prolonged treatment with methylprednisolone in patients with unresolving ARDS. The study was double-blinded, but crossover was permitted if there was no response to treatment. The investigators followed a diligent, protocolized approach for the early identification of nosocomial infections, including fibreoptic bronchoscopy, to diagnose ventilator-associated pneumonia.

32.10 Limitations

Although the planned sample size was 99 patients, the study was stopped early as physiological improvement was evident in the methylprednisolone group. In the final intention-to-treat analysis, the methylprednisolone group included 16 patients, compared to only eight patients assigned to receive placebo group in a 2:1 allocation. However, four patients in the placebo group crossed over to the methylprednisolone group. The relatively small sample size limited the robustness of the findings. The ventilation strategy, which could have played a pivotal role in the final outcomes, was not protocolized. The trial was conducted before the publication of the ARDSNet study [12] that established the benefits of a low tidal volume ventilation strategy, with a limitation of plateau pressure to 30 cm H_2O. (The present study allowed a maximum plateau pressure of 35 cm H_2O.)

32.11 Summary

Corticosteroids held the potential to improve outcomes in unresolving ARDS, characterized by an intense inflammatory and fibrotic response. Previous clinical trials had failed to reveal a beneficial effect of high-dose, short-duration therapy with methylprednisolone. Meduri et al. conducted an RCT that tested the efficacy of prolonged, high-dose methylprednisolone therapy in patients with unresolving ARDS. They randomized patients with ARDS who had failed to improve by day 7 to receive methylprednisolone or placebo in a 2:1 ratio. The treatment was continued for 32 days with gradual weaning of the dose after 2 weeks. Patients who received methylprednisolone revealed improved lung function, with higher PaO_2/FiO_2 ratios, and lower LIS scores by day 10. The MODS score was lower in the methylprednisolone group; moreover, the duration of mechanical ventilation was shorter compared to the placebo group. The ICU and hospital mortality were also lower among methylprednisolone-treated patients. The incidence of nosocomial infections was similar in both groups.

The Meduri et al. study emphasized the importance of prolonged therapy with methylprednisolone in unresolving ARDS and remains one of the first RCTs that revealed a potential for benefit with corticosteroids. The study paved the way for future controlled trials that tested the safety and efficacy of corticosteroids in ARDS.

References

1. Meduri GU. The role of the host defence response in the progression and outcome of ARDS: pathophysiological correlations and response to glucocorticoid treatment. Eur Respir J. 1996;9(12):2650–70.
2. Kollef MH, Schuster DP. The acute respiratory distress syndrome. N Engl J Med. 1995;332(1):27–37.
3. Bernard GR, Luce JM, Sprung CL, Rinaldo JE, Tate RM, Sibbald WJ, et al. High-dose corticosteroids in patients with the adult respiratory distress syndrome. N Engl J Med. 1987;317(25):1565–70.
4. Bone RC, Maunder R, Slotman G, Silverman H, Hyers TM, Kerstein MD, et al. An early test of survival in patients with the adult respiratory distress syndrome. The PaO2/FIo2 ratio and its differential response to conventional therapy. Prostaglandin E1 Study Group. Chest. 1989;96(4):849–51.
5. Headley AS, Tolley E, Meduri GU. Infections and the inflammatory response in acute respiratory distress syndrome. Chest. 1997;111(5):1306–21.
6. Lefering R, Neugebauer EA. Steroid controversy in sepsis and septic shock: a meta-analysis. Crit Care Med. 1995;23(7):1294–303.
7. Cronin L, Cook DJ, Carlet J, Heyland DK, King D, Lansang MA, et al. Corticosteroid treatment for sepsis: a critical appraisal and meta-analysis of the literature. Crit Care Med. 1995;23(8):1430–9.
8. Meduri GU, Belenchia JM, Estes RJ, Wunderink RG, el Torky M, Leeper KV, Fibroproliferative phase of ARDS. Clinical findings and effects of corticosteroids. Chest. 1991;100(4):943–52.
9. Hooper RG, Kearl RA. Established ARDS treated with a sustained course of adrenocortical steroids. Chest. 1990;97(1):138–43.

10. Meduri GU, Headley AS, Golden E, Carson SJ, Umberger RA, Kelso T, et al. Effect of prolonged methylprednisolone therapy in unresolving acute respiratory distress syndrome: a randomized controlled trial. JAMA. 1998;280(2):159–65.
11. Bernard GR, Artigas A, Brigham KL, Carlet J, Falke K, Hudson L, et al. The American-European Consensus Conference on ARDS. Definitions, mechanisms, relevant outcomes, and clinical trial coordination. Am J Respir Crit Care Med. 1994;149(3 Pt 1):818–24.
12. Acute Respiratory Distress Syndrome Network, Brower RG, Matthay MA, Morris A, Schoenfeld D, Thompson BT, et al. Ventilation with lower tidal volumes as compared with traditional tidal volumes for acute lung injury and the acute respiratory distress syndrome. N Engl J Med. 2000;342(18):1301–8.

33 Corticosteroids in Persistent Acute Respiratory Distress Syndrome: The LaSRS Trial

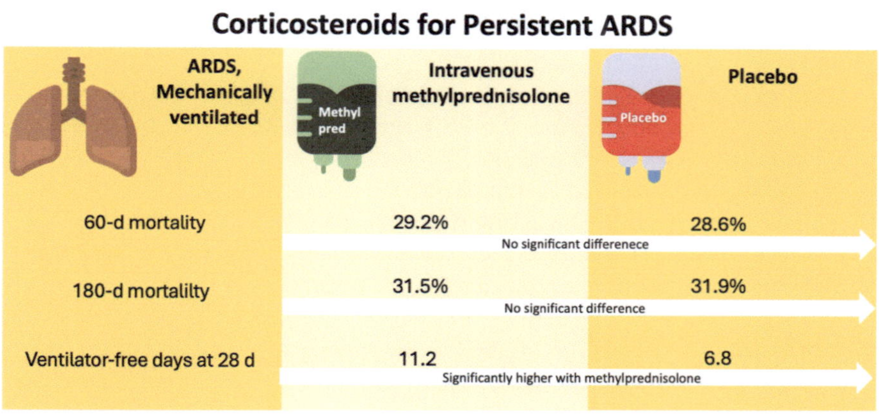

The ARDS clinical network (NEJM, 2006)

Quick Take

Could corticosteroids hold the key to improving outcomes in prolonged acute respiratory distress syndrome (ARDS)?

The LATE STEROID RESCUE STUDY (LaSRS) was a multicenter, randomized trial assessing the efficacy and safety of corticosteroid therapy in patients with persistent ARDS. The study found that corticosteroids administered to patients with ongoing ARDS improved lung function and decreased the duration of

Steinberg KP, Hudson LD, Goodman RB, Hough CL, Lanken PN, Hyzy R, et al. Efficacy and safety of corticosteroids for persistent acute respiratory distress syndrome. N Engl J Med. 2006 Apr 20;354(16):1671–84.

J. Chacko et al., *Landmark Studies in Critical Care*,
https://doi.org/10.1007/978-981-95-0673-6_33

mechanical ventilation at 28 days without increasing the risk of infections or other major adverse effects. However, mortality rates were similar in both groups. These findings did not support the routine use of methylprednisolone among patients with persistent ARDS.

33.1 Introduction and Background

Acute respiratory distress syndrome (ARDS) is characterized by an early, exudative phase with increased capillary permeability, plasma extravasation, and leukocyte infiltration. This early phase is often followed by the proliferative and fibrotic phases, with continued inflammatory reaction [1]. Considering their potent anti-inflammatory effect, corticosteroids may be an effective therapy in ARDS. Corticosteroid treatment in early ARDS had been largely disappointing [2]; treatment in the later phase of illness had shown greater promise [3]. However, the propensity to superinfections, sepsis, and neuromuscular weakness carries the potential for adverse clinical outcomes.

There was conflicting evidence regarding the efficacy of corticosteroids in ARDS at the time of the conduct of the LaSRS (Late Steroid Rescue Study) trial. In an early randomized controlled trial (RCT), Meduri et al. studied 24 patients with severe ARDS who had failed to improve by the seventh day of respiratory failure [3]. Patients were assigned in a 2:1 ratio to receive methylprednisolone or placebo. Methylprednisolone was administered in an initial dose of 2 mg/kg for 14 days, followed by gradual tapering. The total duration of treatment was 32 days. By day 10, they observed improved lung injury scores, higher PaO_2/FiO_2 ratios, and lower multiorgan dysfunction syndrome (MODS) scores among methylprednisolone-treated patients. Besides, more patients were successfully extubated in the methylprednisolone arm. All 16 patients in the methylprednisolone group had survived by day 10, compared to 6 of 8 patients in the placebo group.

The LaSRS investigators hypothesized that moderate-dose methylprednisolone would lead to improved clinical outcomes in persistent ARDS without increasing the risk of complications. They designed a multicentric RCT to determine the safety and efficacy of corticosteroids in persistent ARDS [4].

33.2 Population and Design

The trial enrolled patients between August 1997 and November 2003 from 25 US hospitals of the National Heart, Lung, and Blood Institute (NHLBI) ARDS Clinical Trials Network. The study evaluated patients who were intubated and mechanically ventilated at 7–28 days after the onset of ARDS. Patients were on mechanical ventilation with persistent, bilateral infiltrates from the onset of ARDS to study entry. The PaO_2/FiO_2 ratio had to be <200 mm Hg on the day of enrolment for study inclusion.

33.2.1 Excluded

Patients with undrained abscesses, intravascular infection, disseminated fungal infection, new-onset nosocomial pneumonia, septic shock, and burns requiring skin grafting were excluded. Other exclusion criteria were acquired immune deficiency syndrome, concurrent corticosteroid treatment, cytotoxic therapy within the past 3 weeks, post-bone marrow or lung transplant, adrenal insufficiency, chronic liver disease, severe chronic respiratory disease, and pre-existing co-morbidity with an expected 6-month mortality >60%.

Eligible patients were randomly assigned to the methylprednisolone or placebo groups. Randomization was in permuted blocks and stratified by center.

33.3 Methylprednisolone Group

Methylprednisolone sodium succinate was diluted in 50 ml 5% dextrose or distilled water. An initial dose of 2 mg/kg of predicted body weight was followed by 0.5 mg/kg every 6 hours for 14 days. Thereafter, the dose was reduced to 0.5 mg/kg every 12 hours for 7 days, followed by a tapering down of the dose. Tapering was carried out over 4 days if 21 days of treatment was complete, and the patient was unable to sustain unassisted breathing for 48 hours. Tapering was expedited over a 2-day period, if the patient was able to breathe unassisted for 48 hours, or if disseminated fungal infection or septic shock had developed.

33.4 Placebo Group

In the placebo group, patients received 50 ml of 5% dextrose in water.

33.5 Both Groups

Patients were screened regularly for evidence of new-onset infection. Bronchoalveolar-lavage fluid and blood cultures were performed at study entry and on day 7. Weaning from mechanical ventilation was protocol-based. Patients were assessed daily for readiness to wean. Weaning was commenced in the pressure support ventilation mode once the FiO_2 was down to 0.5 or less with acceptable PaO_2 levels.

33.6 Sample Size

The authors calculated the sample size based on the 60-day mortality as the primary outcome. Based on newly available data, the sample size was scaled down from 400 to 180 patients after 2 years of the study. The modified sample size assumed a mortality reduction from 40% to 20% with methylprednisolone, providing the study with 85% power at a two-sided significance level of 5%.

33.7 Results

The LaSRS study enrolled 180 patients—89 were assigned to the methylprednisolone group and 91 to receive a placebo. The baseline characteristics were similar in both groups. The median duration from the onset of ARDS to study entry was 11.3 days in both groups. The most common underlying etiology of ARDS included pneumonia, aspiration, sepsis, and trauma. Patients had severe lung involvement at baseline; the mean lung injury score (scale of 0–4, higher score indicates more severe injury) was 3.3 in the methylprednisolone group and 3.0 in the placebo group. The mean PaO_2/FiO_2 ratio was 126 in both groups, and the mean $PaCO_2$ was 53 mm Hg. The static lung compliance was poor in both groups—23.3 ml/cm H_2O in the methylprednisolone group and 24.9 ml/cm H_2O in the placebo group.

33.8 The Primary Outcome: 60-Day Hospital Mortality

Overall, there was no significant difference in the 60-day mortality between the methylprednisolone and placebo groups (29.2% vs. 28.6%, $P = 1.0$). Mortality at 180 days was also similar (31.5% vs. 31.9%, $P = 1.0$).

Among patients who had ARDS for>14 days before study enrolment, the 180-day mortality was significantly higher with methylprednisolone (44% vs. 12%).

33.9 Secondary Outcomes

Patients who received methylprednisolone experienced significantly higher ventilator-free days at 28 days (6.8 ± 8.5 vs. 11.2 ± 9.4) and 180 days (median: 159 vs. 149).

Although patients in the methylprednisolone group were able to breathe without assistance earlier, they were more likely to require re-initiation of ventilator assistance. Ventilator support had to be recommenced in a higher number of patients in the methylprednisolone group (20 vs. 6, $P = 0.008$). Neuromyopathy was a common cause for re-initiation of ventilatory assistance—a more frequent complication in the methylprednisolone group (9 vs. 2 patients). The duration of ARDS before study enrolment was not associated with re-initiation of ventilator support. Seven of these patients developed shock at the time of recommencement of ventilation; all were in the methylprednisolone group.

Methylprednisolone-treated patients showed improved cardiopulmonary physiology within 3–7 days of commencement of treatment. The PaO_2/FiO_2 ratio was significantly higher (on days 3 and 14), the plateau pressure lower (on days 4, 5, and 7), and the respiratory system compliance higher (on days 7 and 14) in the methylprednisolone group. In the first 28 days, patients in the methylprednisolone group had more shock-free days compared with placebo. The blood glucose levels tended to be higher in the methylprednisolone group.

Methylprednisolone treatment did not appear to increase the incidence of serious secondary infections compared with placebo ($P = 0.14$). Nosocomial pneumonia occurred in fewer patients in the methylprednisolone group.

33.10 Adverse Events

The overall incidence of adverse events was not significantly different in the methylprednisolone and the placebo groups (25 vs. 33, $P = 0.27$). Neuromyopathy occurred in nine patients, all in the methylprednisolone group. The use of neuromuscular blocking agents did not appear to influence the development of neuromyopathy. The main study outcomes are summarized in Table 33.1.

Table 33.1 Main study outcomes

Outcome	Methylprednisolone	Placebo	*P*-value
60-day mortality (%)	29.2	28.6	1.0
60-day mortality among those >14 days after ARDS onset (%)	35	8	0.02
180-day mortality (%)	31.5	31.9	1.0
180-day mortality among those >14 days after ARDS onset (%)	44	12	0.01
Ventilator-free days at 28 days (mean, SD)	11.2 ± 9.4	6.8 ± 8.5	<0.001
Ventilator-free days at 180 days (median, IQR)	159 (13–173)	149 (0–167)	0.04

Abbreviations: SD standard deviation, *IQR* interquartile range

33.11 Study Conclusions

Among patients with persistent ARDS, no survival benefit was noted with corticosteroid administration. Besides, commencement of methylprednisolone beyond 2 weeks of ARDS onset was associated with a higher 60- and 180-day mortality compared with placebo. Improvement in cardiopulmonary physiology was noted within 3–7 days after commencement of methylprednisolone. Ventilator-free days, shock-free days, and ICU-free days were higher in the first 28 days with methylprednisolone administration.

33.12 Strengths

The LaSRS trial remains one of the most impactful trials on corticosteroid use in ARDS. It was a well-conducted, multicentric, double-blinded RCT. The investigators evaluated important clinical outcomes, including mortality and the duration of ventilator support. The study specifically evaluated outcomes following early and late treatment with methylprednisolone. The results did not offer support for the routine use of corticosteroids in persistent ARDS, in contrast to the equivocal evidence from previous studies.

33.13 Limitations

The study randomized only 5% of eligible patients, raising questions about broader applicability. It took nearly 6 years for completion, during which new treatment modalities may have been introduced, and the overall care of critically ill patients may have improved. These include the widespread use of low tidal volumes, steroids for septic shock, and more intensive glucose control. The sample size was reduced due to a low enrolment rate and availability of new data on survival from the ARDSNet trial of low tidal volume ventilation [5]. No active screening was carried out to identify nosocomial infection. Neuromuscular weakness was not confirmed by electrophysiological testing.

33.14 Subsequent Evidence

Villar et al. performed an RCT of 277 patients with ARDS, within 1 week of the precipitating clinical insult, across 17 ICUs in Spain. They assigned patients to receive dexamethasone 20 mg once daily, intravenously, for the first 5 days and 10 mg once daily thereafter until day 10, compared to a control group that received standard care. The mean ventilator-free days were significantly higher in the dexamethasone group compared to the standard care group (12·3 vs. 7.5 days). Furthermore, the 60-day mortality was also lower in the dexamethasone group (21% vs. 36%). The incidence of adverse events was similar in both groups. Although the study was unblinded and terminated early due to low enrolment rates, it suggested that early dexamethasone administration might reduce the duration of ventilator support and improve survival in ARDS [6].

The efficacy of corticosteroids in COVID-19-related ARDS was evaluated in several studies. The RECOVERY trial revealed improved survival with dexamethasone 6 mg daily for 10 days compared with placebo [7]. The CODEX trial assigned Covid-19 patients to receive dexamethasone 20 mg per day for 5 days, followed by 10 mg, or placebo. Mechanical ventilation-free days were higher among patients who received dexamethasone, although the 28-day mortality was similar [8].

Meduri et al. published a retrospective, intention-to-treat re-analysis of the LaSRS trial in 2018. They observed that by day 28, the outcomes appeared superior in the methylprednisolone group—fewer patients had died before extubation, the rate of successful extubation was higher, and a larger number of patients were discharged alive from the ICU. They pointed out that methylprednisolone was abruptly discontinued without tapering, 3 days post-extubation. Following discontinuation of treatment, more patients in the methylprednisolone group required re-initiation of ventilatory assistance. These patients who required resumption of ventilator support carried a higher risk of adverse outcomes, including mortality, in the longer term. The authors hypothesized that adrenal suppression may have led to the resurgence of the inflammatory reaction and loss of the early outcome benefit. They suggested that gradual tapering of the methylprednisolone dose might be crucial for a sustained anti-inflammatory effect mediated by corticosteroids in patients with ARDS [9].

33.15 Summary

Persistent ARDS, characterized by continued inflammation and fibrosis, often leads to prolonged mechanical ventilation and high mortality. Corticosteroids, with their powerful anti-inflammatory effect, carry the potential to improve clinical outcomes in severe, persistent ARDS. However, corticosteroid treatment is also associated with the risk of complications, including superinfections, sepsis, and neuromuscular weakness. The evidence regarding clinical benefit was limited to studies of small sample sizes. The LaSRS investigators performed a multicenter RCT to evaluate the safety and efficacy of methylprednisolone in persistent ARDS. They randomly assigned 180 patients with persistent ARDS to receive methylprednisolone or a placebo in a 1:1 ratio. Methylprednisolone was administered in an initial dose of 2 mg/kg followed by 0.5 mg/kg every 6 hours for 14 days, followed by a tapering of the dose.

Overall, the mortality at 60 and 180 days was similar in both groups of patients. Among patients who were enrolled 14 days or more after ARDS onset, the mortality was higher with methylprednisolone. Methylprednisolone was associated with improved respiratory physiology, including better oxygenation, higher respiratory system compliance, and lower requirement for vasopressor support. Besides, methylprednisolone-treated patients experienced more ventilator-free days; however, more patients required re-initiation of ventilator support in the methylprednisolone group. The incidence of superinfections was similar in both groups; however, neuromuscular weakness was more common with methylprednisolone.

The authors concluded that their study did not support the routine use of methylprednisolone among patients with persisting ARDS. Besides, later initiation of treatment may increase the risk of mortality.

References

1. Ware LB, Matthay MA. The acute respiratory distress syndrome. N Engl J Med. 2000;342(18):1334–49.
2. Bernard GR, Luce JM, Sprung CL, Rinaldo JE, Tate RM, Sibbald WJ, et al. High-dose corticosteroids in patients with the adult respiratory distress syndrome. N Engl J Med. 1987;317(25):1565–70.
3. Meduri GU, Headley AS, Golden E, Carson SJ, Umberger RA, Kelso T, et al. Effect of prolonged methylprednisolone therapy in unresolving acute respiratory distress syndrome: a randomized controlled trial. JAMA. 1998;280(2):159–65.
4. Steinberg KP, Hudson LD, Goodman RB, Hough CL, Lanken PN, Hyzy R, et al. Efficacy and safety of corticosteroids for persistent acute respiratory distress syndrome. N Engl J Med. 2006;354(16):1671–84.
5. Acute Respiratory Distress Syndrome Network, Brower RG, Matthay MA, Morris A, Schoenfeld D, Thompson BT, et al. Ventilation with lower tidal volumes as compared with traditional tidal volumes for acute lung injury and the acute respiratory distress syndrome. N Engl J Med. 2000;342(18):1301–8.
6. Villar J, Ferrando C, Martínez D, Ambrós A, Muñoz T, Soler JA, et al. Dexamethasone treatment for the acute respiratory distress syndrome: a multicentre, randomised controlled trial. Lancet Respir Med. 2020;8(3):267–76.
7. RECOVERY Collaborative Group, Horby P, Lim WS, Emberson JR, Mafham M, Bell JL, et al. Dexamethasone in hospitalized patients with Covid-19. N Engl J Med. 2021;384(8):693–704.
8. Tomazini BM, Maia IS, Cavalcanti AB, Berwanger O, Rosa RG, Veiga VC, et al. Effect of dexamethasone on days alive and ventilator-free in patients with moderate or severe acute respiratory distress syndrome and COVID-19. JAMA. 2020;324(13):1–11.
9. Meduri GU, Bridges L, Siemieniuk RAC, Kocak M. An exploratory reanalysis of the randomized trial on efficacy of corticosteroids as rescue therapy for the late phase of acute respiratory distress syndrome. Crit Care Med. 2018;46(6):884–91.

Part VII

Nephrology and Renal Replacement Therapy

34 Low-Dose Dopamine in Early Renal Dysfunction: The ANZICS Dopamine Trial

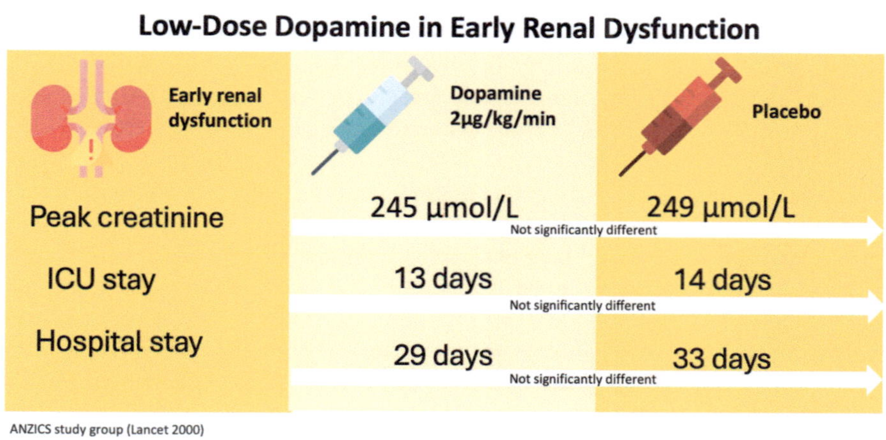

Quick Take

Is low-dose dopamine "renal protective"?

The ANZICS Dopamine trial tested the hypothesis that low-dose dopamine could prevent the progression of renal dysfunction in critically ill patients. In this large, multicenter, randomized controlled trial, 328 patients with early renal dysfunction were assigned to receive either low-dose dopamine or a placebo. The study found that low-dose dopamine did not reduce the incidence of renal failure or

---

Bellomo R, Chapman M, Finfer S, Hickling K, Myburgh J. Low-dose dopamine in patients with early renal dysfunction: a placebo-controlled randomised trial. Australian and New Zealand Intensive Care Society (ANZICS) Clinical Trials Group. Lancet. 2000 Dec 23;356(9248):2139–43.

J. Chacko et al., *Landmark Studies in Critical Care*,
https://doi.org/10.1007/978-981-95-0673-6_34

improve mortality, challenging the long-standing practice of using dopamine for renal protection. The trial provided clear evidence that low-dose dopamine has no benefit in improving renal outcomes in critically ill patients, leading to a shift away from its routine use in this context.

34.1 Introduction and Background

Nearly 60 years ago, early experimental studies on the hemodynamic and renal effects of dopamine were carried out by investigators at the Emory University, in Atlanta. In 1963, Goldberg and his co-investigators from this group published the results of a study that evaluated the effect of dopamine infusion in four patients with severe congestive cardiac failure. They observed a natriuretic effect and improved urine output, although the effect was inconsistent and appeared to be dose-dependent [1]. A year later, the same team of investigators evaluated the effect of dopamine in nine healthy volunteers and six patients with congestive cardiac failure. Similar to the findings of the preceding study, they observed a natriuretic effect. Besides, the cardiac output, measured by indocyanine green injection, increased in normal subjects. The increase in cardiac output was also associated with an increase in the glomerular filtration rate and the renal plasma flow. The authors proposed that dopamine has a unique, salutary effect on renal blood flow compared to other catecholamines [2].

Several years later, Hollenberg et al. studied the effect of dopamine infusion on 12 healthy volunteers who were being evaluated as potential kidney donors. Dopamine was administered at 3 mcg/kg/min; selective renal arteriography was carried out to assess the renal vascular response. There was no change in the arterial blood pressure at this dose; however, an increase in the renal cortical blood flow was observed, secondary to vasodilatation. This response appeared to be dose specific. A lower dose did not alter the renal blood flow; a higher dose resulted in an increase in the blood pressure without any further increase in the blood flow. They concluded that at a dose of 3 mcg/kg/min, dopamine acted as a renal cortical vasodilator and improved blood flow, without any change in the hemodynamic parameters. They went on to propose that this dose-specific effect of dopamine may enable reversal of conditions that cause renal vasoconstriction and improve renal function [3].

The favorable effects noted in normal subjects and animal studies led to a profusion in the use of dopamine over the next several decades as a catecholamine with a distinctive renal ve effect. Dopamine infusion was considered the magic bullet that would kick-start the failing kidneys, especially in patients with underlying heart failure. The presumed favorable effect of "renal dose" dopamine was attributed to its selective effect on the dopaminergic receptors in the kidneys. In a low dose of 0.5–2.5 mcg/kg/min, stimulation of the dopaminergic receptors and improved renal blood flow was considered to occur, followed by beta receptor stimulation between 2 and 5 mcg/kg/min, and alpha-adrenergic effects at higher doses. These dose-dependent effects were largely confined to human volunteers and animals [4] and were never tested in critically ill patients with multiorgan dysfunction.

By the 1990s, questions were raised, and concerns expressed regarding the dopamine-specific effect on renal blood flow. Furthermore, adverse effects were noted, including tachycardia, arrhythmias, and myocardial ischemia. A 1994 editorial suggested that the beneficial renal protective effect attributed to dopamine remained an unfulfilled dream [5]. Besides, a randomized controlled trial of 37 normovolemic patients following major vascular surgery did not reveal any effect on the urine output, serum creatinine level, or the creatinine clearance [6], leading to fervent calls to put a stop to the use of dopamine as a renal protective agent [7].

Against the background of continued widespread use, even in the face of no robust supporting evidence, the ANZICS-CTG (Australian and New Zealand Intensive Care Society Clinical Trials Group) investigators carried out a multicenter placebo-controlled RCT of low-dose dopamine infusion in critically ill patients who were at risk of acute renal failure.

34.2 Population and Design

The ANZICS-CTG dopamine study was carried out between March 1996 and April 1999 in 22 ICUs in Australia and one in Hong Kong. Patients were randomized to receive dopamine infusion or placebo [8]. Randomization was stratified according to the participating center.

34.2.1 Inclusion Criteria

Patients who met two or more criteria of the systemic inflammatory response syndrome (SIRS) over a 24-hour period were screened. At least one indicator of early renal dysfunction had to be present—a mean urine output <0.5 ml/kg for ≥4 hours, a rise in the serum creatinine level to >150 μmol/l (1.7 mg/dl), or a rise in the serum creatinine level by >80 μmol/l (0.9 mg/dl) in <24 hours, not related to rhabdomyolysis.

34.2.2 Excluded

The study excluded patients younger than 18 years of age, those with acute renal failure in the preceding 3 months, transplanted kidneys, those who received dopamine infusion during the current hospital admission, and patients with a baseline creatinine level of >300 μmol/l (3.39 mg/dl). Patients in whom dopamine could not be administered for >8 hours according to clinician judgment and those who were considered unsuitable for renal replacement therapy were also excluded.

34.3 Intervention

Dopamine was infused in a dose of 2 mcg/kg/minute using a syringe pump or a volumetric infusion pump.

34.4 Control

Normal saline was administered as a placebo in indistinguishable syringes or infusion bags.

34.5 Common Management

The dopamine or placebo infusion was continued until renal replacement therapy was commenced, or after resolution of renal dysfunction and the SIRS response for a period of at least 24 hours. The infusion was also stopped if a serious adverse event occurred.

34.6 Sample Size

The authors assumed that dopamine infusion would reduce the peak serum creatinine level, the chosen primary outcome, by 20%. After two planned interim analyses, the treatment effect was revised to a 25% decrease in the peak creatinine level with dopamine. A final sample size of 300 patients provided 90% power with an alpha level of 0.05.

34.7 Results

A total of 467 patients were screened; 328 were randomized after exclusions—163 were assigned to receive dopamine and 165 to placebo. In the final analysis, 161 patients were included in the dopamine arm and 163 in the placebo arm.

34.8 Baseline Characteristics

Patients in the dopamine and placebo groups had similar severity of illness at baseline (mean APACHE II score of 21 in both groups). The number of patients in shock (58% vs. 63%) and on mechanical ventilation (86% vs. 87%) were also similar. Dopamine was infused for a mean duration of 113 hours compared with 125 hours for placebo. After randomization, low-dose dopamine was infused for a mean of 113 hours, and placebo was infused for a mean of 125 hours.

34.9 Outcomes

34.9.1 Creatinine and Urea Levels

The peak creatinine level, the primary outcome, was similar in the dopamine and placebo groups (245 ± 144 vs. 249 ± 147 μmol/l). The rise in creatinine from baseline was also similar (62 ± 107 μmol/l vs. 66 ± 108 μmol/l). The peak serum urea levels and the rise from baseline were also similar.

34.9.2 Urine Output

The urine output rose progressively in both groups of patients after commencement of the infusion. The urine output after 24 and 48 hours of infusion was significantly higher in both groups compared to baseline. The increase in urine output was partly due to the administration of loop diuretics to 90 patients in each group. The dose of furosemide administered was similar in both groups.

34.10 Secondary Outcomes

The mean duration of mechanical ventilation was similar in the dopamine and placebo groups (10 vs. 11 days). The duration of ICU stay (13 vs. 14 days) and hospital stay (29 vs. 33 days) was also similar. Arrhythmias were common in both groups and were mostly supraventricular arrhythmias or atrial fibrillation. ICU survival was similar in the dopamine and placebo groups (67% vs. 64%); survival to hospital discharge was also similar (57% vs. 53%). Renal replacement therapy was performed in 35 patients in the dopamine group (22%) compared with 40 in the placebo group (25%); the difference was not statistically significant. The main study outcomes are summarized in Table 34.1.

Table 34.1 Main study outcomes

Outcome	Dopamine (161 patients)	Placebo (163 patients)	Significance
Peak serum creatinine (μmol/L)	245	249	Not significantly different
Peak serum urea (mmol/L)	20	23	Not significantly different
Requirement for RRT	21.7%	24.5%	Not significantly different
Mean duration of ventilation (days)	10	11	Not significantly different
ICU stay (days)	13	14	Not significantly different
Hospital stay (days)	29	33	Not significantly different
Survival to hospital discharge	57%	59.5%	Not significantly different

Abbreviations: RRT renal replacement therapy

34.11 Adverse Events

Arrhythmias were observed in seven patients in each arm and led to cessation of the infusion.

34.12 Study Conclusion

The ANZICS study did not identify any impact of dopamine on the peak serum creatinine level, the primary outcome, compared with placebo infusion. No difference was observed in clinical outcomes following the infusion of dopamine in patients at high risk of acute renal failure. The study confirmed the lack of beneficial effect of the so-called "renal dose" of dopamine in critically ill patients who were at risk of renal failure.

34.13 Strengths

The strong points of the study included its randomized controlled design and double blinding, with an adequate sample size to evaluate the primary outcome. The study included critically ill patients who were at high risk of renal failure in whom dopamine was hypothesized to improve outcomes. The multicenter design also provided generalizability.

34.14 Limitations

The peak serum creatinine level as the primary outcome measure may be debatable; it could be argued that clinical outcomes, including mortality, may have been more relevant. A possible dopamine-related protective effect in patients with normal renal function at baseline could not be ruled out. Would a higher dose of dopamine (compared to a fixed dose) produce a beneficial impact? However, the aim of the study was specifically to evaluate the use of low-dose dopamine, considering the purported effect on the renal blood flow specifically at this dose. Would dopamine impart beneficial effects among patients who are not critically ill, but nevertheless are at risk of renal dysfunction? The study could not answer this question, being confined to patients admitted to the ICU. Although the hospital mortality was high (42%), it was lower than predicted by the severity score at baseline. The effect of other vasoactive drugs, e.g., norepinephrine, on outcomes could not be discerned; however, such evaluation is rarely feasible in real-world practice. The use of loop diuretics, although similar in both groups, may also have impacted outcomes.

34.15 Later Studies

Nearly a decade after publication of the ANZICS dopamine study, De Backer et al. compared dopamine with norepinephrine as a first-line vasopressor in patients with shock, aiming to restore blood pressure [9]. This large RCT included 1679 patients, with 858 randomized to receive dopamine and 821 to norepinephrine. Alternatively, open-label vasopressors were permitted if blood pressure could not be maintained. The 28-day mortality was similar in both groups of patients. The incidence of arrhythmias was significantly higher with dopamine compared with norepinephrine. Contrary to traditional belief, dopamine use was associated with significantly higher 28-day mortality in the subgroup of patients with cardiogenic shock.

Avni et al. performed a systematic review with meta-analysis to assess the safety and efficacy of vasopressors in septic shock [10]. The review included 3544 patients from 32 trials. Norepinephrine use was associated with a significantly lower mortality compared with dopamine in this meta-analysis [RR 0.89 (95% CI 0.81–0.98)]. The risk of major adverse events, including cardiac arrhythmias, was also lower with norepinephrine compared with dopamine.

These studies further underlined the lack of evidence of a favorable effect of dopamine on renal function or other important clinical outcomes. The Surviving Sepsis Guidelines also recommend norepinephrine as the vasopressor of choice in septic shock [11].

34.16 Summary

Historically, dopamine was considered to impart beneficial effects on renal function, attributed to its effect on the dopaminergic receptors in the kidneys at low doses. Dopamine infusion was found to exert a natriuretic effect and improve the urine output; however, this effect was largely confined to normal human volunteers and in animal studies. The findings from these experimental studies led to decades of dopamine use for its presumed "renal-protective" effect, especially in patients with congestive cardiac failure, who were at high risk of renal dysfunction. However, the salutary effect on renal function was never tested in a large clinical trial including critically ill patients who were at high risk of acute kidney injury. The findings of the ANZICS dopamine trial established beyond doubt that the favorable effects attributed to low-dose dopamine do not translate to a measurable improvement in renal function, or impact clinical outcomes among critically ill patients. Subsequent studies have corroborated these findings. Furthermore, adverse events may be higher with the use of dopamine compared with norepinephrine. The unequivocal findings from these studies have confined the use of dopamine as a renal-protective agent to a handful of ardent believers.

References

1. Goldberg LI, Mcdonald RH, Zimmerman AM. Sodium diuresis produced by dopamine in patients with congestive heart failure. N Engl J Med. 1963;269:1060–4.
2. Mcdonald RH, Goldberg LI, Mcnay JL, Tuttle EP. Effect of dopamine in man: augmentation of sodium excretion, glomerular filtration rate, and renal plasma flow. J Clin Invest. 1964;43(6):1116–24.
3. Hollenberg NK, Adams DF, Mendell P, Abrams HL, Merrill JP. Renal vascular responses to dopamine: haemodynamic and angiographic observations in normal man. Clin Sci Mol Med. 1973;45(6):733–42.
4. Dasta JF, Kirby MG. Pharmacology and therapeutic use of low-dose dopamine. Pharmacotherapy. 1986;6(6):304–10.
5. Vincent JL. Renal effects of dopamine: can our dream ever come true? Crit Care Med. 1994;22(1):5–6.
6. Baldwin L, Henderson A, Hickman P. Effect of postoperative low-dose dopamine on renal function after elective major vascular surgery. Ann Intern Med. 1994;120(9):744–7.
7. Thompson BT, Cockrill BA. Renal-dose dopamine: a siren song? Lancet Lond Engl. 1994;344(8914):7–8.
8. Bellomo R, Chapman M, Finfer S, Hickling K, Myburgh J. Low-dose dopamine in patients with early renal dysfunction: a placebo-controlled randomised trial. Australian and New Zealand Intensive Care Society (ANZICS) Clinical Trials Group. Lancet Lond Engl. 2000;356(9248):2139–43.
9. De Backer D, Biston P, Devriendt J, Madl C, Chochrad D, Aldecoa C, et al. Comparison of dopamine and norepinephrine in the treatment of shock. N Engl J Med. 2010;362(9):779–89.
10. Avni T, Lador A, Lev S, Leibovici L, Paul M, Grossman A. Vasopressors for the treatment of septic shock: systematic review and meta-analysis. PLoS One. 2015;10(8):e0129305.
11. Evans L, Rhodes A, Alhazzani W, Antonelli M, Coopersmith CM, French C, et al. Surviving sepsis campaign: international guidelines for management of saepsis and septic shock 2021. Crit Care Med. 2021;49(11):e1063.

35 Continuous Venovenous Hemodiafiltration Versus Intermittent Hemodialysis for Acute Kidney Injury in the Critically Ill: The HEMODIAFE Trial

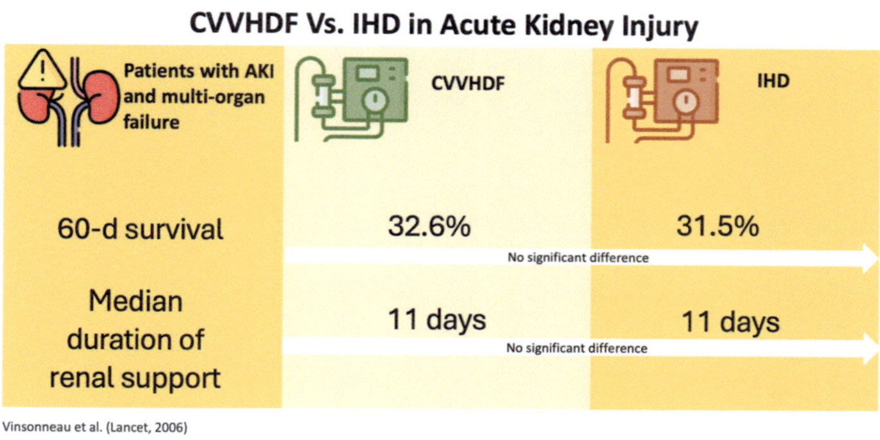

Quick Take

Which modality of renal replacement therapy may be preferred in patients with acute renal failure and multiorgan dysfunction syndrome?

The HEMODIAFE trial was a multicenter, randomized controlled trial comparing continuous veno-venous hemodiafiltration (CVVHDF) to intermittent hemodialysis (IHD) for the treatment of acute renal failure in patients with multiple organ

---

Vinsonneau C, Camus C, Combes A, Costa de Beauregard MA, Klouche K, Boulain T, et al. Continuous venovenous haemodiafiltration versus intermittent haemodialysis for acute renal failure in patients with multiple-organ dysfunction syndrome: a multicentre randomised trial. Lancet Lond Engl. 2006 Jul 29;368(9533):379–85.

J. Chacko et al., *Landmark Studies in Critical Care*,
https://doi.org/10.1007/978-981-95-0673-6_35

dysfunction syndrome (MODS). The study aimed to evaluate the impact of these two renal replacement therapies on survival rates, organ function, and complications. The results demonstrated no significant difference in mortality or other major outcomes between the two treatment strategies. Both modalities provided similar benefits in terms of renal recovery and overall clinical improvement, suggesting that either CVVHDF or IHD could be used effectively in patients with acute renal failure and MODS.

35.1 Introduction

Until the early 1980s, intermittent hemodialysis (IHD) was the standard modality of renal replacement therapy (RRT) in critically ill patients with acute renal failure. Hemodialysis effectively cleared potassium, urea, creatinine, and other molecules that accumulate in renal failure; however, hemodynamic instability was common. Besides acute shifts in the intravascular volume, the non-biocompatible, cellulose-based membranes of that era often triggered a profound inflammatory response, leading to severe hypotension. Perhaps due to fear of potential complications, clinicians were reluctant to perform dialysis in acutely ill patients until it seemed inevitable. Hemodialysis was delayed until the blood urea nitrogen level rose to well above 100 mg/dl, or the ominous appearance of "uremic frost"—deposition of urea crystals on the skin—during the late phase of renal failure. Outcomes were predictably poor with this approach, and mortality remained unacceptably high. It was abundantly clear that critically ill patients tolerated conventional hemodialysis poorly.

The concept of continuous renal replacement therapy (CRRT) arose at the 1982 meeting of the American Society for Artificial Internal Organs (ASAIO). Peter Kramer, a German physician, presented his observations when he interposed a microporous filter between the femoral artery and vein. Driven by the femoral arterial pressure, large volumes of a yellow-tinged fluid—the ultrafiltrate—poured out through the filter. Kramer replaced the ultrafiltrate with an intravenous electrolyte solution devoid of potassium, creatinine, urea, and other molecules that are excreted by the kidney. He went on to explain that this technique could be performed continuously, thereby facilitating solute clearance and fluid removal at a constant rate [1]. His words were prophetic, triggering a paradigm shift in the technique of renal replacement therapy in the critically ill.

Decades later, Robert Bartlett, widely regarded as the pioneer of extracorporeal membrane oxygenation, described his early experience with the technique of continuous arterio-venous hemofiltration that Kramer had described, among patients who remained anuric despite industrial doses of diuretics. "I wept with joy," he reminisced; most of the problems of hemodialysis were eliminated, and they could feed patients without the fear of fluid overload [2].

35.2 Background to the Hemodiafe Trial

Until the early 1990s, IHD remained the mainstay of RRT in most parts of the world. However, ICUs were generally ill-equipped to perform IHD, with special requirements including reverse osmosis-enabled water purification. ICU nurses were not trained to perform hemodialysis; the nephrologist had to prescribe and supervise treatment—all leading to a tedious process. The concept of convection-based continuous therapy led to the introduction of automated machines that were less cumbersome to operate and relatively easy to perform by the bedside. The learning curve was short, the process simpler, and nephrologist supervision was no longer required. It was apparent that continuous therapies carried several advantages, including hemodynamic stability and superior control over fluid and solute removal. IHD-related rapid solute removal often led to a drastic drop in serum osmolality, with fluid shift from the intravascular to the interstitial compartment, leading to life-threatening cerebral edema in patients with neurological injury. CRRT, with slow, controlled solute removal, held the potential to avert this devastating complication. Recovery of renal function was also considered to occur more often with continuous compared with intermittent therapies. Unsurprisingly, ICUs around the world embraced the new technique with unbridled enthusiasm.

Despite the widespread use of the technique, the question of whether CRRT resulted in improved clinical outcomes compared with IHD in critically ill patients remained unanswered. Early, non-randomized studies had suggested improved outcomes with CRRT, although patients were more severely ill at baseline [3, 4]. A randomized controlled trial (RCT) reported higher mortality with CRRT compared with IHD, although patients in the CRRT group had adverse predictors of mortality, including more profound organ dysfunction [5]. Two other RCTs [6, 7] and a meta-analysis [8] did not demonstrate any significant difference in clinical outcomes between the two modalities of therapy. These studies did not employ standardized methods of therapy in either arm, making it difficult to draw definitive conclusions. The Hemodiafe trial aimed to compare CRRT with IHD using standard polyacrylonitrile membranes and evaluate the impact on mortality in patients with acute renal failure as part of multiorgan failure [9]. The study was pertinent to many French ICUs, including that of the lead investigator, Christophe Vinsonneau, who employed both modalities of treatment.

35.3 Population and Design

The Hemodiafe trial was conducted between October 1999 and March 2003 across 21 French ICUs among patients with acute renal failure as part of multiorgan dysfunction syndrome. Acute renal failure was defined as a serum urea level of 36 mmol/l or a serum creatinine level of 310 μmol/l (3.5 mg/dl). A logistic dysfunction score ≥ represented multiorgan dysfunction syndrome. Patients were randomly allocated to receive CRRT or IHD. Randomization was stratified by center.

35.3.1 Excluded

Patients with chronic renal failure and acute renal failure due to obstructive or vascular etiology were excluded. Patients on angiotensin-converting-enzyme inhibitor, those with coagulopathies, uncontrolled bleeding, a SAPS II score ≤ 37, a moribund state, and those not expected to survive beyond 8 days were also excluded.

35.4 The CRRT Group

CRRT was commenced in the continuous veno-venous hemodiafiltration mode (CVVHDF) at a blood flow rate of ≥120 ml/min, a dialysate flow of 500 ml/hour, and an ultrafiltration rate of ≥1000 ml/hour. Prisma machines were used in the predilution mode with a bicarbonate-based replacement fluid. The filter was routinely changed every 48 hours. The settings were adjusted depending on the clinical condition, aiming to maintain the serum urea level at <30 mmol/l. Once multiorgan dysfunction had resolved and hemodynamic stability was attained, patients could be switched over to hemodialysis.

35.5 The IHD Group

In the IHD group, the initial settings included a blood flow rate of 250 ml/min, and a dialysate flow of 500 ml/min. The dialysate was cooled to 35 °C, and the sodium level in the dialysate fluid was set at 150 mmol/l for improved hemodynamic stability. Dialysis was performed for at least 4 hours once in 48 hours in the presence of continued anuria or oliguria. The frequency was customized to maintain a serum urea level of <40 mmol/l. Therapy was individualized, aiming for a urea reduction ratio of >65% during each session. IHD was carried out using machines available at the study center. All treatment was performed using the same membrane polymer with a large surface area (2 m^2), with a bicarbonate-based dialysate.

35.6 Common Management

Other therapies, including fluid resuscitation, pharmacological support of the circulation, mechanical ventilation, and antibiotic therapy, were left to the clinician judgment. Anticoagulation was carried out using unfractionated or low molecular-weight heparin based on a standard protocol.

According to the study protocol, a switch of treatment modality was not allowed until after discussion with the coordinating center. The possible reasons for a change of treatment modality were predefined, including persisting hypotension in the absence of hypovolemia, unfavorable fluid balance or poor metabolic control, technique-related adverse events, and technical problems that prevented continued treatment with the allocated modality.

35.7 Sample Size

The 60-day mortality, the primary endpoint, was assumed to be 45% in the IHD group. Assuming a 15% lower mortality in the CRRT group, the authors calculated a sample size of 240 patients in each group, allowing for a 10% dropout, providing 90% power at an alpha level of 0.05.

35.8 Results

35.8.1 Baseline Characteristics

A total of 360 patients were randomized; 184 patients from the IHD group and 175 from the CRRT group were included in the final analysis. Patients were well-matched at baseline. Most patients (70%) were medical; 96% were on mechanical ventilation, and 87% were on catecholamine support at baseline.

35.8.2 Intensity of Therapy

The mean dose of CVVHDF was 29 (±11) ml/kg/hour. IHD was performed for a mean of 3.6 (±2) sessions during the first week of treatment; seven patients underwent daily IHD during this period. IHD was carried out for a median duration of 5.2 (5.1–5.3) hours per session. The median net fluid daily fluid removal was similar in the IHD and CRRT groups [2213 ml (2141–2285) vs. 2107 ml (2011–2203)]. The efficacy of treatment, based on the mean daily urea level, did not differ between the two groups.

35.9 Outcomes

35.9.1 Primary and Secondary Outcomes

There was no difference in the 60-day survival, the primary outcome, between the IHD and the CRRT groups (31.5% vs. 32.6%, $p = 0.98$). Among the secondary outcomes, the 28-day (41.8% vs. 38.9%) and the 90-day survival (27.2% vs. 28.5%) were also similar between the two groups. The median duration of renal support was 11 days in both groups. The duration of ICU stay (20 vs. 19 days) and hospital stay (30 vs. 32 days) was also not significantly different.

35.9.2 Renal Recovery

Recovery of renal function was similar in both groups, with 6/61 (10%) in the IHD group and 4/61 (7%) patients in the CRRT group remaining dialysis-dependent

Table 35.1 Main study outcomes

Outcomes	IHD	CVVHDF	Significance
28-day survival	41.8%	38.9%	$P = 0.65$
60-day survival	31.5%	32.6%	$P = 0.98$
90-day survival	27.2%	28.5%	$P = 0.95$
Median duration of RRT	11 days	11 days	$P = 0.84$
Median ICU days	20 days	19 days	$P = 0.73$
Median hospital days	30 days	32 days	$P = 0.66$
Renal recovery	10%	7%	$P = 0.5$

Abbreviations: IHD intermittent hemodialysis, *CVVHDF* continuous veno-venous hemodiafiltration, *RRT* renal replacement therapy

following discharge from the ICU. There was a solitary patient in the CRRT group who remained on dialysis at the time of hospital discharge. The main study outcomes are summarized in Table 35.1.

35.9.3 Adverse Events and Switch of Therapy

Contrary to expectations, the incidence of hypotensive episodes, defined as a systolic BP ≤80 mm Hg or a fall by >50 mm Hg from baseline, was similar between the IHD and CRRT groups (39% vs. 35%, $p = 0.47$). The incidence of arrhythmias was also similar.

Hypothermia was less commonly observed with IHD compared with CRRT. Six patients in the IHD group were switched to CRRT—three for hemodynamic instability and two due to technical problems. Seventeen patients in the CRRT group were switched to IHD due to contraindications to anticoagulant administration, a high risk of bleeding, and recurrent clotting of the filter despite adequate anticoagulation.

35.10 Study Conclusion

The authors concluded that IHD might be feasible in nearly all critically ill patients with acute renal failure as part of multiorgan dysfunction.

35.11 Strengths of the Study

The Hemodiafe trial was conducted during an era in which CRRT was in widespread use in critically ill patients. However, the outcome benefits of CRRT compared with IHD remained uncertain. This landmark RCT compared IHD with CRRT in a sick cohort of ICU patients; most were on mechanical ventilation and required circulatory support with catecholamines. The severity of illness in both groups was well matched at baseline. The treatment protocol was standardized in both arms, and crossover was not allowed unless it was approved by the coordinating center. Among the 360 patients who were randomized, all except one were followed up and included in the final analysis.

35.12 Weaknesses

Although one of the largest RCTs that compared continuous vs. intermittent modalities of renal replacement therapy, the study was underpowered. It fell short of the calculated sample size was 480, enrolling only 360 patients. Criticisms were directed towards likely underdosing with CRRT, contrasting with a more balanced approach with IHD. The duration and frequency of IHD were greater compared to contemporaneous practice; this may have led to improved outcomes with IHD. The study may have been influenced by the findings of the Schiffl et al. trial of 2002, which showed improved survival with daily compared with alternate-day IHD [10]. In fact, the frequency of IHD was noted to increase during the course of the study. The increase in the frequency of IHD sessions may have resulted in the progressively lower mortality observed during the course of the study in the IHD group. In contrast, the mortality in the CRRT group remained stable during the entire course of the study. The recommended dose of CRRT was 35 ml/kg/hour during the period that the study was conducted [11]; however, the delivered dose was lower at 29 ml/kg/hour.

An unclear "moribund" state was one of the exclusion criteria. Did the investigators exclude patients who were on high-dose vasopressors, who may have benefited the most with CRRT?

Furthermore, the investigators modified IHD to enable therapy in hemodynamically unstable patients. The dialysate was cooled to 35 °C; cooling the dialysate has been shown to improve hemodynamic stability during high-efficiency hemodialysis [12]. The sodium level of the dialysate fluid was also set at 150 mmol/l to improve hemodynamic stability.

35.13 The Aftermath

RRT in the ICU has undergone considerable refinement since the publication of the Hemodiafe trial. This landmark trial provided the impetus for modifications of conventional hemodialysis to adapt to the specialized requirements of critically ill patients who were at risk of hemodynamic instability. Currently, prolonged, intermittent renal replacement therapies (PIRRT) carried out over an extended duration are being increasingly employed in patients who are at high risk of hemodynamic instability [13]. Hybrid therapies, variably described as sustained low-efficiency dialysis (SLED), extended daily dialysis (EDD), or slow, continuous dialysis (SCD), have evolved and are the preferred modality of RRT in many ICUs [14].

35.14 Summary

The Hemodiafe trial addressed the long-debated question of clinical outcomes following CRRT compared with IHD in critically ill patients. The trial was conducted against a background of inconclusive findings from preceding studies. IHD was already being carried out in many ICUs in France as the standard modality of RRT. Modifications were made to the technique of IHD to reduce hemodynamic instability by cooling the dialysate to 35 °C and maintaining the sodium level at 150 mmol/l. As the study progressed, the frequency of IHD also seemed to have increased, probably related to newly available evidence. The study was criticized for comparing a modified, optimized adaptation of IHD with a suboptimal dose of CRRT. However, this landmark trial spurred the development of further refinements to IHD that culminated in several modes of PIRRT employed in many ICUs today. Hence, their conclusion that "virtually all patients can be treated with intermittent hemodialysis" remains valid.

References

1. Kramer P, Böhler J, Kehr A, Gröne HJ, Schrader J, Matthaei D, et al. Intensive care potential of continuous arteriovenous hemofiltration. Trans - Am Soc Artif Intern Organs. 1982;28:28–32.
2. Bartlett RH. The origins of continuous renal replacement therapy. ASAIO J Am Soc Artif Intern Organs 1992. 2018;64(3):427–30.
3. Guérin C, Girard R, Selli JM, Ayzac L. Intermittent versus continuous renal replacement therapy for acute renal failure in intensive care units: results from a multicenter prospective epidemiological survey. Intensive Care Med. 2002;28(10):1411–8.
4. Bellomo R, Farmer M, Parkin G, Wright C, Boyce N. Severe acute renal failure: a comparison of acute continuous hemodiafiltration and conventional dialytic therapy. Nephron. 1995;71(1):59–64.
5. Mehta RL, McDonald B, Gabbai FB, Pahl M, Pascual MT, Farkas A, et al. A randomized clinical trial of continuous versus intermittent dialysis for acute renal failure. Kidney Int. 2001;60(3):1154–63.
6. Uehlinger DE, Jakob SM, Ferrari P, Eichelberger M, Huynh-Do U, Marti HP, et al. Comparison of continuous and intermittent renal replacement therapy for acute renal failure. Nephrol Dial Transplant Off Publ Eur Dial Transpl Assoc - Eur Ren Assoc. 2005;20(8):1630–7.
7. Augustine JJ, Sandy D, Seifert TH, Paganini EP. A randomized controlled trial comparing intermittent with continuous dialysis in patients with ARF. Am J Kidney Dis Off J Natl Kidney Found. 2004;44(6):1000–7.
8. Kellum JA, Angus DC, Johnson JP, Leblanc M, Griffin M, Ramakrishnan N, et al. Continuous versus intermittent renal replacement therapy: a meta-analysis. Intensive Care Med. 2002;28(1):29–37.
9. Vinsonneau C, Camus C, Combes A, Costa de Beauregard MA, Klouche K, Boulain T, et al. Continuous venovenous haemodiafiltration versus intermittent haemodialysis for acute renal failure in patients with multiple-organ dysfunction syndrome: a multicentre randomised trial. Lancet Lond Engl. 2006;368(9533):379–85.
10. Schiffl H, Lang SM, Fischer R. Daily hemodialysis and the outcome of acute renal failure. N Engl J Med. 2002;346(5):305–10.
11. Ronco C, Bellomo R, Homel P, Brendolan A, Dan M, Piccinni P, et al. Effects of different doses in continuous veno-venous haemofiltration on outcomes of acute renal failure: a prospective randomised trial. Lancet Lond Engl. 2000;356(9223):26–30.

12. Kaufman AM, Morris AT, Lavarias VA, Wang Y, Leung JF, Glabman MB, et al. Effects of controlled blood cooling on hemodynamic stability and urea kinetics during high-efficiency hemodialysis. J Am Soc Nephrol JASN. 1998;9(5):877–83.
13. Schwenger V, Weigand MA, Hoffmann O, Dikow R, Kihm LP, Seckinger J, et al. Sustained low efficiency dialysis using a single-pass batch system in acute kidney injury—a randomized interventional trial: the REnal Replacement Therapy Study in Intensive Care Unit PatiEnts. Crit Care Lond Engl. 2012;16(4):R140.
14. Berbece AN, Richardson RMA. Sustained low-efficiency dialysis in the ICU: cost, anticoagulation, and solute removal. Kidney Int. 2006;70(5):963–8.

36 Timing of Renal Replacement Therapy in Critically Ill Patients with Acute Kidney Injury: The AKIKI Trial

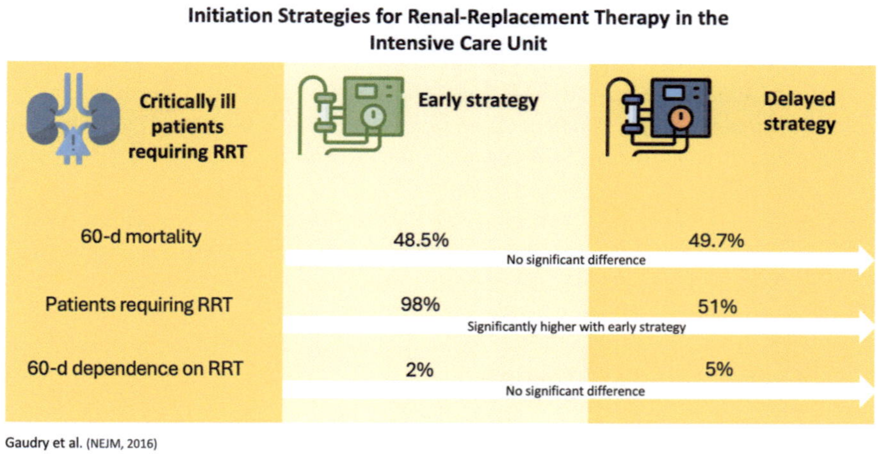

Quick Take

In critically ill patients with severe acute kidney injury (AKI), does delaying renal replacement therapy (RRT) improve survival compared to early initiation?

This pivotal randomized controlled trial evaluated early versus delayed initiation strategies for RRT in ICU patients with severe AKI. The early-strategy group received RRT within 6 hours of randomization, while in the delayed group, RRT

Gaudry S, Hajage D, Schortgen F, Martin-Lefevre L, Pons B, Boulet E, et al. Initiation Strategies for Renal-Replacement Therapy in the Intensive Care Unit. N Engl J Med. 2016 Jul 14;375(2):122–33.

J. Chacko et al., *Landmark Studies in Critical Care*,
https://doi.org/10.1007/978-981-95-0673-6_36

was initiated only if specific criteria were met, such as persistent oliguria or severe metabolic derangements. The trial enrolled 620 patients across 31 French ICUs. The study found no significant difference in 60-day mortality between the early and delayed groups. However, 49% of patients in the delayed group avoided RRT altogether, with fewer catheter-related bloodstream infections compared to the early group. Recovery of renal function, marked by increased urine output, occurred earlier in the delayed group. These findings suggest that a delayed RRT strategy can safely reduce the need for intervention in critically ill patients without compromising survival, emphasizing the importance of individualized decision-making in AKI management.

36.1 Introduction

The timing of initiating RRT in AKI continued to remain a subject of intense debate. The AKIKI (Artificial Kidney Initiation in Kidney Injury) trial was the second large randomized controlled trial (RCT) on the subject, published in *The New England Journal of Medicine* in July 2016 [1], and followed the ELAIN trial published in the *Journal of the American Medical Association* earlier in the year [2]. It aimed to evaluate the clinical dilemma of the ideal timing of commencement of renal replacement therapy (RRT) in critically ill patients.

The existing evidence on the timing of RRT was largely from observational studies and meta-analyses. The possibility of spontaneous renal recovery among those with delayed initiation of RRT had not been evaluated.

36.2 Population and Design

The AKIKI trial was a multicenter, randomized controlled trial conducted across 31 ICUs in France. It included critically ill adult patients (aged ≥18 years) who developed severe AKI, defined as Kidney Disease: Improving Global Outcomes (KDIGO) stage 3. The study population included patients on invasive mechanical ventilation or catecholamine infusions for hemodynamic support.

The primary objective was to assess whether an early RRT initiation strategy improved 60-day survival compared to a delayed approach. The trial employed a pragmatic design to reflect real-world clinical practice.

36.3 Exclusions

- A blood urea nitrogen (BUN) level of >112 mg/dl (>40 mmol/L)
- Serum potassium >6 mmol/L
- pH <7.15
- Pulmonary edema due to fluid overload with severe hypoxia
- Chronic kidney disease

- Patients who remained comatose post-cardiac arrest
- Chronic dialysis dependency
- Acute life-threatening conditions requiring immediate RRT: Severe hyperkalemia, metabolic acidosis, or pulmonary edema necessitating urgent intervention were exclusion criteria.
- Severe chronic kidney disease: Individuals with an estimated glomerular filtration rate (eGFR) <30 ml/min/1.73 m^2 were excluded.
- Post-renal AKI: Patients with obstructive uropathy were not included to avoid confounding from reversible causes.

36.4 Study Groups

Participants were randomized into two groups:

36.4.1 Early RRT Group

RRT was initiated within 6 hours of meeting KDIGO stage 3 criteria.

36.4.2 Delayed RRT Group

RRT was initiated only if patients exhibited absolute indications for dialysis, including severe hyperkalemia, metabolic acidosis, pulmonary edema, or oliguria/anuria persisting for more than 72 hours (dialysis was commenced if any of the aforementioned criteria developed after enrolment).

36.5 Common Management

Patients in both groups received standardized ICU care to ensure consistency aside from the timing of RRT initiation. The choice of the modality of RRT, duration, and frequency was at the discretion of the clinician. Fluid administration and vasopressor support were carried out to maintain adequate tissue perfusion. RRT was discontinued based on pre-defined criteria. Adherence to strict aseptic protocols and judicious use of antibiotics were employed to minimize infections.

36.6 Sample Size

A total of 620 patients were enrolled in the trial, with 311 assigned to the early RRT group and 308 to the delayed RRT group. The sample size was calculated to detect a 15% difference in 60-day mortality between the two groups, assuming a baseline mortality rate of 50%, with a power of 80% and a significance level of 0.05.

36.7 Results

36.7.1 Primary Outcome

The primary outcome of 60-day all-cause mortality revealed no significant difference between the groups (early vs. delayed: 48.5% vs. 49.7%, $P = 0.79$). The 28-day mortality was also similar in both groups (41.6% vs. 43.5%). These results indicated that early RRT initiation did not confer a survival benefit compared to a delayed approach. RRT-dependence at 28 days was also similar in both groups.

36.7.2 Secondary Outcomes

Among the secondary outcomes, RRT was utilized in only 51% of patients in the delayed group; this finding highlighted the potential for spontaneous recovery if dialysis is delayed. The proportion of patients achieving RRT independence by day 28 was similar between groups. The ICU and hospital length of stay was also similar in both groups. Complications, including infection, bleeding, and hemodynamic instability, were not significantly different.

36.7.3 Other Outcomes

On post-hoc analysis, the 60-day mortality among patients in the delayed group who never received RRT was significantly lower compared to those in the early group (37.1% vs. 48.5%, $P < 0.0001$).

The incidence of fluid overload at RRT initiation was higher in the delayed group, though this did not translate to worse outcomes. Dialysis dependency at hospital discharge was similar in both groups. The main study outcomes are summarized in Table 36.1.

Table 36.1 Main study outcomes

Outcome	Early RRT	Delayed RRT	Significance
60-day mortality	48.5%	49.7%	$P = 0.79$
28-day mortality	41.6%	43.5%	
Patients actually receiving RRT	98%	51%	$P < 0.001$
Median ventilation-free days	7	6	$P = 0.76$
Median RRT-free days	17	19	$P < 0.001$
RRT dependence, day 60	2%	5%	$P = 0.12$

Abbreviations: RRT renal replacement therapy

36.8 Study Conclusions

A delayed strategy did not increase mortality and reduced the need for RRT. The findings of the study suggested that a more conservative approach may be preferable in the absence of urgent indications.

36.9 Strengths

The AKIKI trial had several notable strengths. The pragmatic trial design reflected real-world clinical practice, enhancing the generalizability of its findings. The study included a broad ICU population encompassing a wide spectrum of critical illness. The robust randomization process ensured that baseline characteristics were balanced between the two groups at baseline. The outcomes evaluated were clinically relevant.

36.10 Limitations

The modality of dialysis—intermittent or continuous—was left to the clinician discretion, which could have led to bias. Globally, the general trend is to perform continuous renal replacement therapy in patients who are on vasopressor support. Hence, the findings may have limited applicability in other healthcare settings. The study population included patients with more severe stages of AKI and may not apply to less severe cases. Blinding was not feasible, which could have resulted in bias.

36.11 Subsequent Evidence

The findings of the AKIKI trial need to be viewed in light of other studies on the timing of initiation of RRT in critically ill patients. The ELAIN trial reported improved survival with early RRT initiation, contrasting with the AKIKI findings, possibly due to differences in study populations and protocols. The IDEAL-ICU trial focussed on patients with septic shock; no mortality benefit was observed with initiation of early RRT [3]. SRARRT-AKI, a large, multicentric international study, also demonstrated no difference in mortality between early and delayed RRT strategy, supporting the findings of the AKIKI trial [4].

36.12 Summary

The AKIKI trial provided valuable evidence that delaying RRT until the onset of absolute indications does not adversely affect mortality in critically ill patients with severe AKI. By highlighting the potential for spontaneous renal recovery, the trial underscored the importance of individualized decision-making in RRT timing. While early RRT may be warranted in select cases, a delayed strategy can effectively balance the risks and benefits, minimizing unnecessary interventions without compromising outcomes.

References

1. Gaudry S, Hajage D, Schortgen F, Martin-Lefevre L, Pons B, Boulet E, et al. Initiation strategies for renal-replacement therapy in the intensive care unit. N Engl J Med. 2016;375(2):122–33.
2. Zarbock A, Kellum JA, Schmidt C, Van Aken H, Wempe C, Pavenstädt H, et al. Effect of early vs delayed initiation of renal replacement therapy on mortality in critically ill patients with acute kidney injury: the ELAIN randomized clinical trial. JAMA. 2016;315(20):2190.
3. Barbar SD, Clere-Jehl R, Bourredjem A, Hernu R, Montini F, Bruyère R, et al. Timing of renal-replacement therapy in patients with acute kidney injury and sepsis. N Engl J Med. 2018;379(15):1431–42.
4. STARRT-AKI Investigators, Canadian Critical Care Trials Group, Australian and New Zealand Intensive Care Society Clinical Trials Group, United Kingdom Critical Care Research Group, Canadian Nephrology Trials Network, Irish Critical Care Trials Group, et al. Timing of initiation of renal-replacement therapy in acute kidney injury. N Engl J Med. 2020;383(3):240–51.

Comparing Two Delayed Strategies for Renal Replacement Therapy Initiation in Severe Acute Kidney Injury: The AKIKI 2 Trial

37

Comparison of two delayed strategies for RRT initiation for severe AKI (AKIKI 2)

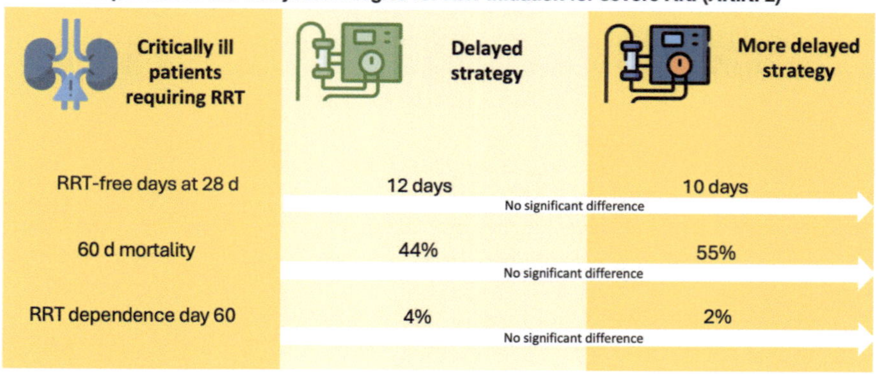

Gaudry et al. (Lancet, 2021)

Quick Take

In critically ill patients with severe acute kidney injury (AKI), does a "more delayed" renal replacement therapy (RRT) strategy provide additional benefits compared to a delayed strategy?

This pivotal multicenter, randomized controlled trial evaluated two delayed RRT initiation strategies in ICU patients with severe AKI. Patients in the delayed group began RRT after meeting specific criteria (oliguria >72 hours or blood urea

---

Gaudry S, Hajage D, Martin-Lefevre L, Lebbah S, Louis G, Moschietto S, et al. Comparison of two delayed strategies for renal replacement therapy initiation for severe acute kidney injury (AKIKI 2): a multicentre, open-label, randomised, controlled trial. Lancet. 2021 Apr 3;397(10281):1293–300.

J. Chacko et al., *Landmark Studies in Critical Care*,
https://doi.org/10.1007/978-981-95-0673-6_37

nitrogen >112 mg/dL), while those in the more-delayed group had RRT postponed further unless severe complications arose or blood urea nitrogen exceeded 140 mg/dL. The study found no significant difference in the primary outcome of RRT-free days at 28 days between the delayed and more-delayed groups. However, a prespecified multivariable analysis revealed higher 60-day mortality in the more-delayed group.

These findings suggest that extending the delay for RRT initiation does not confer additional benefits and may increase mortality risk in critically ill patients with severe AKI.

37.1 Introduction

Acute kidney injury (AKI) is a significant concern in critically ill patients, often requiring renal replacement therapy (RRT). However, the optimal timing for initiating RRT remains debatable. The AKIKI 2 trial, published in *The Lancet* in 2021, aimed to build on the findings of the earlier AKIKI trial by exploring the outcomes of two delayed strategies for RRT initiation in patients with severe AKI [1].

The original AKIKI trial, conducted by the same group of researchers, compared early RRT initiation with a delayed strategy, wherein RRT was initiated only when absolute indications arose or after a predefined delay [2]. The findings revealed no significant mortality difference between the two approaches, with nearly half of the patients in the delayed group not requiring RRT; the renal function had recovered spontaneously among these patients. However, the AKIKI trial left unanswered questions about the potential risks and benefits of further delaying RRT initiation to allow additional time for renal recovery. These gaps motivated the AKIKI 2 trial, which aimed to refine the delayed approach by comparing two delayed strategies: a standard delay versus a "more delayed" strategy.

37.2 Population and Design

The AKIKI 2 trial was a multicenter, open-label, randomized controlled trial conducted across 39 ICUs in France [1]. Critically ill adults (≥18 years old) with acute kidney injury, KDIGO stage 3, who were on mechanical ventilation, or catecholamine infusion, were eligible. The primary aim was to compare the outcomes of two delayed RRT initiation strategies and determine whether a more delayed strategy would improve patient survival and reduce the need for RRT.

37.3 Exclusions

To focus on the appropriate patient population, the AKIKI 2 trial applied the following exclusion criteria:

- Patients receiving maintenance dialysis before ICU admission.
- Conditions such as severe hyperkalemia, metabolic acidosis, or pulmonary edema necessitate urgent RRT.
- Patients with an estimated glomerular filtration rate (eGFR) <30 mL/min/1.73 m^2 were excluded.
- Obstructive uropathy was an exclusion criterion to eliminate potentially reversible causes.
- Patients with refractory shock were excluded due to their higher likelihood of requiring immediate RRT.

37.4 Study Groups

Participants were randomized into two groups.

37.4.1 Delayed RRT Group

RRT was initiated based on the criteria used in the original AKIKI trial—KDIGO stage 3 with oliguria or anuria (urine output less than 0·3 mL/kg per h or less than 500 mL/day for more than 3 days) or blood urea nitrogen (BUN) of 112–140 mg/dL.

37.4.2 More Delayed RRT Group

RRT was initiated if the blood urea nitrogen concentration exceeded 140 mg/dL (serum urea concentration of 50 mmol/L). RRT was also performed if patients had persistent oliguria/anuria for 96 hours or if they developed absolute indications, including serum potassium >6 mmol/L or >5.5 mmol/L despite medical treatment, metabolic acidosis with arterial pH <7.15, or fluid overload with hypoxia.

37.5 Common Management

The choice of therapy—continuous vs. intermittent—was left to the clinician discretion. Both groups received standardized ICU care to ensure consistency aside from the timing of RRT initiation. This included fluid resuscitation and administration of vasopressors or inotropes to maintain adequate perfusion. Fluid overload was carefully monitored to avoid overload. Serum electrolyte levels, including potassium and bicarbonate, were monitored at regular intervals. The choice of RRT modality, anticoagulation, and duration was left to the discretion of the treating physician, but adhered to national guidelines to maintain consistency across centers. RRT was carried out in both groups if an absolute indication arose.

Discontinuation of RRT was considered if the spontaneous urine output was 500 mL/24 h or more, and highly recommended if >2000 mL/24 h among those on diuretics. Spontaneous drop in the serum creatinine level mandated cessation of RRT.

37.6 Sample Size Calculation

The sample size calculation was based on the assumption that extending the delay in RRT initiation would increase the number of RRT-free days from 17 (in the delayed group) to 21 days (in the more delayed group). A total of 278 patients were needed to achieve 80% power to detect this difference with a two-sided significance level of 5%, accounting for a 5% dropout rate. This robust calculation ensured the trial was adequately powered to assess its primary endpoint while allowing for variability in patient outcomes.

37.7 Results

37.7.1 Primary Outcome

The primary endpoint was the number of RRT-free days between randomization and day 28. The results showed no significant difference between the two groups. In the delayed strategy group, the median RRT-free days were 12 (IQR 0–25) compared with 10 (IQR 0–24) in the more delayed group ($P = 0.93$). These findings indicated that extending the delay in RRT initiation did not result in a meaningful increase in RRT-free days.

37.7.2 Secondary Outcomes

Among the secondary outcomes, the 60-day mortality was 44% (60/137) vs. 55% (77/141) in the more delayed group. Although this difference was not statistically significant, on multivariable analysis, a more delayed strategy was one of the significant risk factors for mortality (HR 1·65; 95% CI 1·09–2.50, $P = 0.018$).

More patients underwent RRT in the delayed strategy group compared to the more delayed group (98% vs. 79%, $P < 0.0001$). RRT dependence at day 60 was similar in both groups. The rate of renal recovery was similar in both groups, suggesting that further delay in RRT did not impact recovery. ICU and hospital lengths of stay, ventilator-free days, and vasopressor-free days were similar between the two groups. Complication rates, including infections, bleeding, and electrolyte imbalances, were also comparable between groups. The main study outcomes are summarized in Table 37.1.

Table 37.1 Main study outcomes

Outcome	Delayed group	More delayed group	Significance
Median RRT-free days at 28 days	12 (0–25)	10 (0–24)	$P = 0{\cdot}93$
Number of patients who underwent RRT	98%	79%	$P < 0.0001$
60-day mortality	60%	77%	$P = 0.071$
RRT-dependence at 28 days	16%	11%	$P = 0.33$

Abbreviations: RRT renal replacement therapy

37.8 Study Conclusions

The AKIKI 2 trial demonstrated that extending the delay in RRT initiation for critically ill patients with severe AKI did not significantly increase RRT-free days and was associated with higher 60-day mortality on multivariable analysis. While the more delayed strategy reduced RRT utilization, the increased mortality underscores the potential risks of pushing the delay threshold too far. These findings highlight the need for careful patient selection and monitoring when considering extended delays in RRT initiation.

37.9 Strengths

The multicenter design and rigorous randomization ensured the generalizability and robustness of the findings. The pragmatic approach mirrored real-world clinical practice, enhancing the applicability of results. The study focused on critically ill patients with severe AKI, a population with high morbidity and mortality.

37.10 Weaknesses

The open-label design could have introduced bias in decision-making and outcome assessment. Generalizability may be limited outside France due to the single-country setting. The relatively small sample size restricted the ability to detect differences among patient subgroups or secondary outcomes.

37.11 Other Evidence

The AKIKI 2 findings align and contrast with previous RCTs exploring RRT timing:

1. *AKIKI Trial:* Demonstrated the safety of delaying RRT initiation until absolute indications arose. AKIKI 2 built on these findings, revealing that further delays might increase mortality [2].

2. *ELAIN Trial:* Reported improved survival with early RRT initiation [3]. Differences between ELAIN and AKIKI 2 likely reflect variations in patient populations, with ELAIN including less critically ill patients.
3. *IDEAL-ICU Trial:* Found no survival benefit with early RRT in septic shock patients, aligning with the findings of the AKIKI 2 trial that delayed RRT may be safe in selected patients [4].
4. *STARRT-AKI Trial:* Showed no significant mortality difference between early and delayed RRT but emphasized the risks of unnecessary RRT, supporting the focus of the AKIKI 2 trial on reducing RRT utilization [5].

37.12 Summary

The AKIKI 2 trial provides valuable insights into the timing of RRT initiation in severe AKI. While extending the delay in RRT initiation reduced RRT utilization, it did not improve RRT-free days and was associated with higher mortality. These findings underscore the importance of balancing the benefits of allowing spontaneous renal recovery with the risks of delayed intervention. Compared to other major RCTs, AKIKI 2 highlights the potential harms of excessive delays, contributing to the evolving evidence base for individualized RRT timing strategies in critically ill patients.

References

1. Gaudry S, Hajage D, Martin-Lefevre L, Lebbah S, Louis G, Moschietto S, et al. Comparison of two delayed strategies for renal replacement therapy initiation for severe acute kidney injury (AKIKI 2): a multicentre, open-label, randomised, controlled trial. Lancet. 2021;397(10281):1293–300.
2. Gaudry S, Quenot JP, Hertig A, Barbar SD, Hajage D, Ricard JD, et al. Timing of renal replacement therapy for severe acute kidney injury in critically ill patients. Am J Respir Crit Care Med [Internet]. 2019 [cited 2019 Mar 21]. Available from: https://www.atsjournals.org/doi/10.1164/rccm.201810-1906CP
3. Zarbock A, Kellum JA, Schmidt C, Van Aken H, Wempe C, Pavenstädt H, et al. Effect of early vs delayed initiation of renal replacement therapy on mortality in critically ill patients with acute kidney injury: the ELAIN randomized clinical trial. JAMA. 2016;315(20):2190.
4. Barbar SD, Clere-Jehl R, Bourredjem A, Hernu R, Montini F, Bruyère R, et al. Timing of renal-replacement therapy in patients with acute kidney injury and sepsis. N Engl J Med. 2018;379(15):1431–42.
5. STARRT-AKI Investigators, Canadian Critical Care Trials Group, Australian and New Zealand Intensive Care Society Clinical Trials Group, United Kingdom Critical Care Research Group, Canadian Nephrology Trials Network, Irish Critical Care Trials Group, et al. Timing of initiation of renal-replacement therapy in acute kidney injury. N Engl J Med. 2020;383(3):240–51.

Early Versus Late Initiation of Renal Replacement Therapy in Acute Kidney Injury: The ELAIN Trial

38

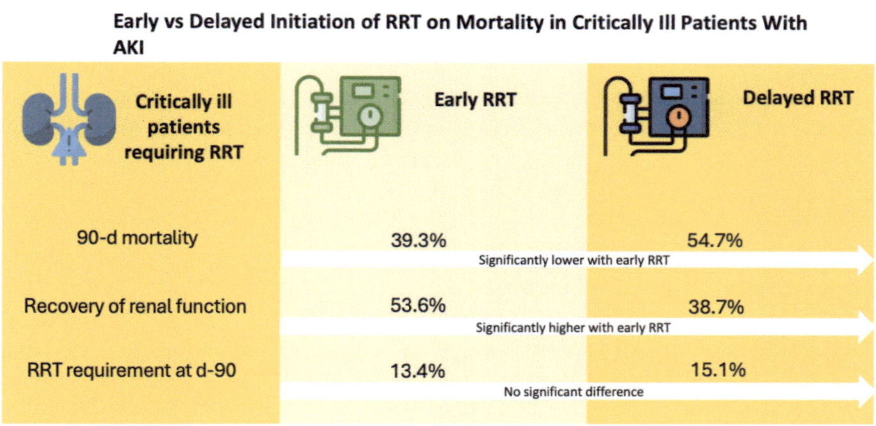

Zarbock et al. (JAMA, 2016)

Quick Take

In critically ill patients with acute kidney injury (AKI), does early initiation of renal replacement therapy (RRT) improve outcomes compared to delayed initiation?

This pivotal randomized controlled trial evaluated the impact of early versus delayed initiation of RRT in ICU patients with AKI. The early initiation group, where RRT was started within 8 hours of fulfilling KDIGO stage 2 AKI criteria,

---

Zarbock A, Kellum JA, Schmidt C, Van Aken H, Wempe C, Pavenstädt H, et al. Effect of Early vs Delayed Initiation of Renal Replacement Therapy on Mortality in Critically Ill Patients With Acute Kidney Injury: The ELAIN Randomized Clinical Trial. JAMA. 2016 May 24;315(20):2190.

J. Chacko et al., *Landmark Studies in Critical Care*,
https://doi.org/10.1007/978-981-95-0673-6_38

experienced significantly lower 90-day mortality compared to the delayed group, in which RRT was initiated only after meeting stage 3 AKI criteria or severe complications. Additionally, early RRT was associated with improved renal recovery and shorter duration of RRT dependency. Importantly, there was no significant increase in adverse events, such as hemodynamic instability, in the early RRT group. The findings highlighted the potential benefits of early intervention in critically ill patients with AKI to improve survival and long-term renal outcomes.

38.1 Introduction

Acute kidney injury (AKI) is a common and severe complication in critically ill patients, with a high risk of mortality and long-term morbidity. Among the pivotal clinical questions in the management of AKI is the timing of initiating renal replacement therapy (RRT). Early initiation may pre-empt complications such as metabolic derangements and fluid overload, potentially improving outcomes. On the other hand, delaying RRT might allow for spontaneous renal recovery, sparing patients from unnecessary intervention and its associated risks. The ELAIN (Early vs. Late Initiation of Renal Replacement Therapy in Critically Ill Patients with Acute Kidney Injury) trial, conducted by Zarbock et al., aimed to address the critical issue of the optimal time to commence RRT in critically ill patients with AKI.

38.2 Population and Design

The ELAIN trial was a prospective, single-center, randomized controlled trial conducted in a tertiary care hospital in Germany [1]. The study enrolled critically ill adult patients (aged ≥18 years) who developed AKI categorized as KDIGO stage 2, a phase associated with moderate kidney dysfunction. The primary objective of the trial was to compare the early initiation of RRT versus a delayed strategy to evaluate the impact on the 90-day all-cause mortality. The trial was conducted with strict adherence to randomization and blinding protocols to minimize bias.

38.3 Exclusions

The study excluded patients with pre-existing chronic kidney disease and already on RRT. Patients with renal artery lesions, glomerulonephritis, interstitial nephritis, obstructive uropathy, hemolytic uremic syndrome, and thrombotic thrombocytopenic purpura were excluded. Patients with AIDS with a low CD4 count, hematological malignancy with reduced neutrophil count, and those who had undergone a renal transplant were also excluded.

38.4 Study Groups

Participants were randomized into two groups.

Early RRT Group: Patients initiated RRT within 8 hours of meeting KDIGO stage 2 AKI criteria. This stage includes serum creatinine levels 2–3 times the baseline or urine output of <0.5 mL/kg/hour for more than 12 hours.

Delayed RRT Group: RRT was initiated only if patients progressed to KDIGO stage 3 AKI (serum creatinine ≥3 times baseline, anuria for ≥12 hours, or other clinical indications such as severe hyperkalemia or refractory acidosis).

The protocol emphasized using continuous renal replacement therapy (CRRT) in the veno-venous hemodiafiltration mode to ensure hemodynamic stability in the ICU setting.

38.5 Common Management

Patients in both groups received standardized management protocols to ensure consistency in care aside from the timing of RRT initiation. Vasopressors and inotropes were administered as appropriate. Fluid balance was meticulously managed using crystalloids, with diuretics administered where indicated to promote urine output.

38.6 Sample Size

A total of 231 patients were enrolled in the study, with 112 allocated to the early RRT group and 119 to the delayed RRT group. The sample size was calculated to detect a statistically significant difference in 90-day all-cause mortality between the two groups, with an alpha level of 0.05 and a power of 80%.

38.7 Results

38.7.1 Primary Outcome

The primary outcome was 90-day all-cause mortality. The trial reported a significantly lower mortality rate in the early RRT group compared to the delayed group [early vs. delayed RRT: 39.3% vs. 54.7%; hazard ratio 0.66 (95% CI: 0.45–0.97; $p = 0.03$)]. This finding suggested the potential survival benefits of initiating RRT early in patients with KDIGO stage 2 AKI.

Table 38.1 Main study outcomes

Outcomes	Early group	Delayed group	Significance
90-day mortality	39.3%	54.7%	$P = 0.03$
90-day RRT independence	53.6%	38.7%	$P = 0.02$
Median ICU stay	15.5 days	16.0 days	$P = 0.0$
Median hospital stay	33 days	43 days	$P = 0.05$
Duration of mechanical ventilation	125.5 hours	181 hours	$P = 0.002$

Abbreviation: RRT renal replacement therapy

38.7.2 Secondary Outcomes

The trial also evaluated several secondary outcomes. A higher proportion of patients in the early RRT group achieved independence from RRT by day 90 compared to the delayed group. This suggests that early intervention might facilitate renal recovery. The duration of mechanical ventilation was significantly shorter in the early group. Both groups had comparable lengths of stay in the ICU and hospital. The incidence of complications, including infections, bleeding, and hemodynamic instability, was similar in both groups.

38.7.3 Other Outcomes

Among the exploratory outcomes, the levels of inflammatory markers were similar in both groups. Both groups of patients achieved effective control of electrolyte imbalance and metabolic disturbances. The main study findings are summarized in Table 38.1.

38.8 Study Conclusions

In critically ill patients with AKI, a strategy of early initiation of RRT was associated with a lower 90-day mortality. Besides, it reduced the duration of RRT and reduced the length of stay in the hospital.

38.9 Strengths

The study followed a rigorous, randomized controlled design. The definition of early vs. delayed initiation was clear cut. CRRT was used in all patients, ensuring uniformity across patient groups. Outcomes, complications, and recovery parameters were meticulously recorded, adding to the reliability of the findings.

38.10 Limitations

Despite its strengths, the ELAIN trial carried certain limitations. Being a single-center study, the findings may not be extrapolable to a broader patient population in different healthcare settings. The study enrolled mainly surgical ICU patients—the results may not apply to medical patients. Besides, the study had a low fragility index—if a change in the primary outcome of just three patients would have made the results non-significant.

38.11 Subsequent Evidence

The ELAIN trial's findings sparked significant interest and debate in the nephrology and critical care communities. However, subsequent trials such as AKIKI (Artificial Kidney Initiation in Kidney Injury) [2] and IDEAL-ICU (Initiation of Dialysis Early Versus Delayed in Intensive Care Unit) [3] provided contrasting results, emphasizing the complexity involved in the appropriate timing of RRT in the critically ill.

The AKIKI trial was conducted in a more heterogenous ICU population; the investigators found no significant difference in mortality between early and delayed RRT initiation, challenging the ELAIN results.

The IDEAL-ICU Trial focused on septic shock patients; this study also reported no clear mortality benefit with early RRT initiation.

The variability in findings underscores the importance of individualized decision-making, considering patient-specific factors such as comorbidities, underlying AKI etiology, and hemodynamic stability.

38.12 Summary

The ELAIN trial provided compelling evidence supporting early RRT initiation in critically ill patients with KDIGO stage 2 AKI, demonstrating significant survival benefits and better renal recovery without increasing complications. However, its findings must be interpreted in the context of subsequent studies and the nuances of real-world clinical practice. While the trial underscored the potential advantages of early intervention, it also highlighted the need for a personalized approach, balancing the risks and benefits of RRT timing for each patient.

References

1. Zarbock A, Kellum JA, Schmidt C, Van Aken H, Wempe C, Pavenstädt H, et al. Effect of early vs delayed initiation of renal replacement therapy on mortality in critically ill patients with acute kidney injury: the ELAIN randomized clinical trial. JAMA. 2016;315(20):2190.
2. Gaudry S, Hajage D, Schortgen F, Martin-Lefevre L, Pons B, Boulet E, et al. Initiation strategies for renal-replacement therapy in the intensive care unit. N Engl J Med. 2016;375(2):122–33.
3. Barbar SD, Clere-Jehl R, Bourredjem A, Hernu R, Montini F, Bruyère R, et al. Timing of renal-replacement therapy in patients with acute kidney injury and sepsis. N Engl J Med. 2018;379(15):1431–42.

39 Timing of Renal Replacement Therapy in Septic Shock with Acute Kidney Injury: The IDEAL-ICU Trial

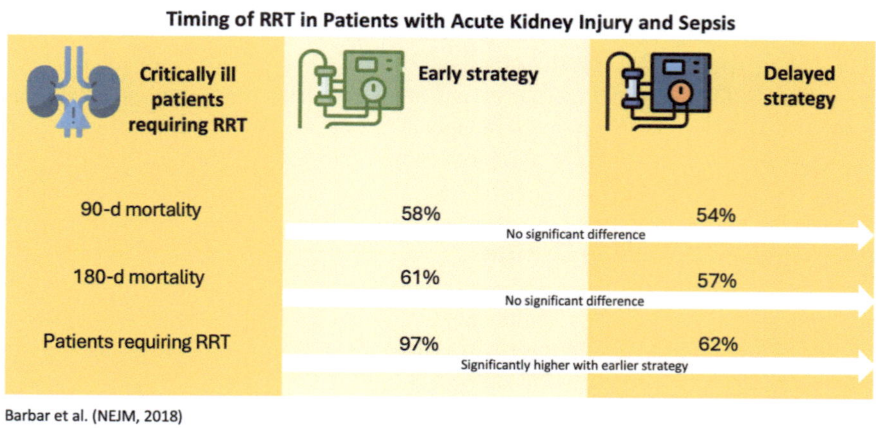

Quick Take

In critically ill patients with severe acute kidney injury (AKI), does delaying renal replacement therapy (RRT) improve survival compared to early initiation?

This pivotal randomized controlled trial evaluated early versus delayed initiation strategies for RRT in ICU patients with severe AKI. The early-strategy group received RRT within 6 hours of randomization, while the delayed group only initiated RRT if specific criteria, such as persistent oliguria or severe metabolic derangements, were met. The trial enrolled 620 patients across 31 French ICUs. The study

---

Barbar SD, Clere-Jehl R, Bourredjem A, Hernu R, Montini F, Bruyère R, et al. Timing of Renal-Replacement Therapy in Patients with Acute Kidney Injury and Sepsis. New England Journal of Medicine. 2018 Oct 11;379(15):1431–42.

J. Chacko et al., *Landmark Studies in Critical Care*,
https://doi.org/10.1007/978-981-95-0673-6_39

found no significant difference in 60-day mortality between the early and delayed groups. However, 49% of patients in the delayed group avoided RRT altogether, with fewer catheter-related bloodstream infections compared to the early group. Recovery of renal function, marked by increased urine output, occurred earlier in the delayed group. These findings suggest that a delayed RRT strategy can safely reduce the need for intervention in critically ill patients without compromising survival, emphasizing the importance of individualized decision-making in AKI management.

39.1 Introduction

The timing of renal replacement therapy (RRT) in patients with acute kidney injury (AKI) complicated by septic shock remains a contentious issue. Early initiation of RRT may mitigate the metabolic and hemodynamic consequences of AKI, but delaying RRT could reduce unnecessary interventions and associated complications by allowing spontaneous renal recovery. The IDEAL-ICU (Initiation of Dialysis Early Versus Delayed in the Intensive Care Unit) trial, published in *The New England Journal of Medicine* in 2018, specifically evaluated the optimal timing of RRT initiation among critically ill patients with septic shock [1].

39.2 Population and Design

The IDEAL-ICU trial was a multicenter, randomized controlled trial conducted across 29 ICUs in France. It focused on adult patients (aged ≥18 years) with septic shock, who required vasopressor support despite adequate volume resuscitation. Patients were enrolled within 48 hours of the commencement of vasopressors. Patients who were in the "failure" stage of the RIFLE classification were eligible. The primary aim was to determine whether early RRT initiation improved 90-day survival compared to a delayed strategy.

39.3 Exclusions

Key exclusion criteria were pre-defined to target the relevant population:

- Chronic dialysis dependency: Patients already on maintenance dialysis were excluded.
- Life-threatening complications of AKI: Severe hyperkalemia, metabolic acidosis, or pulmonary edema necessitating urgent RRT were excluded.
- End-stage renal disease: Individuals with a history of severe chronic kidney disease (eGFR <30 mL/min/1.73 m^2) were not included.

- Post-renal AKI: Patients with obstructive uropathy or reversible causes of AKI were excluded.
- Patients who were considered moribund and unlikely to survive for 28 days.

39.4 Study Groups

Participants were randomized into two groups.

39.4.1 Early RRT Group

In the early group, RRT was initiated within 12 hours of meeting KDIGO stage 3 criteria.

39.4.2 Delayed RRT Group

In patients randomized to the late group, RRT initiation was deferred until the development of absolute indications, including severe hyperkalemia, metabolic acidosis, pulmonary edema, or persistent oliguria/anuria for more than 48 hours.

39.5 Common Management

Patients in both groups received standardized ICU care to ensure consistency of care. The modality of RRT—intermittent vs. continuous—was left to the clinician discretion. RRT was commenced expeditiously if life-threatening complications arose—including hyperkalemia ($K^+ > 6.5$ mmol/L), severe metabolic acidosis (pH <7.15), and refractory pulmonary edema. If the renal function improved within 48 hours after randomization, RRT was withheld based on the clinician judgment. Antibiotics were administered, and source control measures were carried out as appropriate in both groups. A balanced fluid resuscitation strategy was followed to avoid overload. Electrolyte, acid-base, and metabolic parameters were monitored regularly.

39.6 Sample Size

The trial enrolled 488 patients, with 246 assigned to the early RRT group and 242 to the delayed RRT group. The sample size was powered to detect a 15% absolute difference in 90-day mortality between groups. The authors assumed a baseline mortality rate of 50%; the sample size provided 80% power at a significance level of 0.05.

39.7 Results

39.7.1 Primary Outcome

The primary outcome, the 90-day all-cause mortality, showed no significant difference between the two groups: At 90 days, 138 of 239 (58%) patients in the early group had died compared with 128 of 238 (54%) patients in the delayed group ($P = 0.38$). Mortality at 28 and 180 days was also similar in both groups.

These results indicated that early RRT initiation did not improve survival compared to a delayed approach.

39.7.2 Secondary Outcomes

In the delayed group, 38% of patients never required RRT, suggesting spontaneous renal recovery. The median time from the diagnosis of AKI to initiation of RRT was longer in the late group (51.5 hours vs. 7.6 hours, $P < 0.001$). RRT-free days were higher in the late group (16 vs. 12 days, $P < 0.001$). Similar proportions of patients in both groups achieved independence from RRT by day 28.

Other important outcomes were similar in the early and late groups, including the median ventilation-free days (2 vs. 3 days), vasopressor-free days (16 vs. 17 days), hospital length of stay (23 days in both groups), RRT-dependence at day 90 (2% vs. 3%), and complications, including severe bleeding episodes, infections, and hemodynamic instability. The main study outcomes are summarized in Table 39.1.

Table 39.1 Main study outcomes

Outcomes	Early RRT	Delayed RRT	Significance
90-day mortality	58%	54%	$P = 0.38$
28-day mortality	45%	42%	$P = 0.48$
180-day mortality	61%	57%	$P = 0.37$
Patients receiving RRT	97%	62%	$P < 0.001$
Median RRT days	4	2	$P < 0.001$
Median RRT-free days	12	16	$P = 0.006$
Median ventilation-free days	2	3	$P = 0.19$
Median vasopressor-free days	16	17	$P = 0.87$
Median ICU days	11	10	$P = 0.91$
Median hospital days	23	23	$P = 0.34$

Abbreviation: RRT renal replacement therapy

39.8 Study Conclusions

Among patients with early septic shock with AKI, early initiation of RRT was not associated with a lower 90-day mortality, compared to a delayed strategy of initiation after 48 hours. Besides, the use of RRT was lower with a delayed strategy.

39.9 Strengths

The IDEAL-ICU trial focused on patients with septic shock, a high-risk group of patients in the ICU. A robust randomization process was followed, ensuring balanced baseline characteristics. The trial design reflected real-world practices, enhancing external validity. The authors evaluated relevant patient-centered outcomes; there was minimal loss to follow-up.

39.10 Limitations

The study allowed the choice of therapy—continuous vs. intermittent—based on clinician discretion. However, in other healthcare systems, patients in septic shock may be treated exclusively with continuous modalities. The mortality rate was high, which may have overshadowed potential differences in outcomes. The study was stopped early for futility, which may have led to a lack of power to evaluate important outcomes; besides, the limited sample size precluded detailed subgroup analysis. Blinding of the study was not feasible, which may have led to bias.

39.11 Subsequent Evidence

The IDEAL-ICU trial findings are consistent with other contemporaneous randomized controlled trials. The AKIKI Trial also revealed no survival benefit with early RRT in a heterogeneous ICU population [2]. The findings of the STARRT-AKI trial were also along similar lines, supporting a delayed RRT strategy, while highlighting the potential for spontaneous renal recovery [3].

39.12 Summary

The IDEAL-ICU trial concluded that early initiation of RRT in patients with AKI and septic shock does not confer a survival advantage compared to a delayed approach. Delaying RRT until the development of absolute indications can avoid unnecessary interventions and complications with no significant difference in patient-centered outcomes. These findings underscore the importance of individualized clinical decision-making in the management of septic shock-related AKI.

References

1. Barbar SD, Clere-Jehl R, Bourredjem A, Hernu R, Montini F, Bruyère R, et al. Timing of renal-replacement therapy in patients with acute kidney injury and sepsis. N Engl J Med. 2018;379(15):1431–42.
2. Gaudry S, Quenot JP, Hertig A, Barbar SD, Hajage D, Ricard JD, et al. Timing of renal replacement therapy for severe acute kidney injury in critically ill patients. Am J Respir Crit Care Med [Internet]. 2019 [cited 2019 Mar 21]. Available from: https://www.atsjournals.org/doi/10.1164/rccm.201810-1906CP
3. STARRT-AKI Investigators, Canadian Critical Care Trials Group, Australian and New Zealand Intensive Care Society Clinical Trials Group, United Kingdom Critical Care Research Group, Canadian Nephrology Trials Network, Irish Critical Care Trials Group, et al. Timing of initiation of renal-replacement therapy in acute kidney injury. N Engl J Med. 2020;383(3):240–51.

40 Timing of Initiation of Renal Replacement Therapy in Acute Kidney Injury: The STARRT-AKI Trial

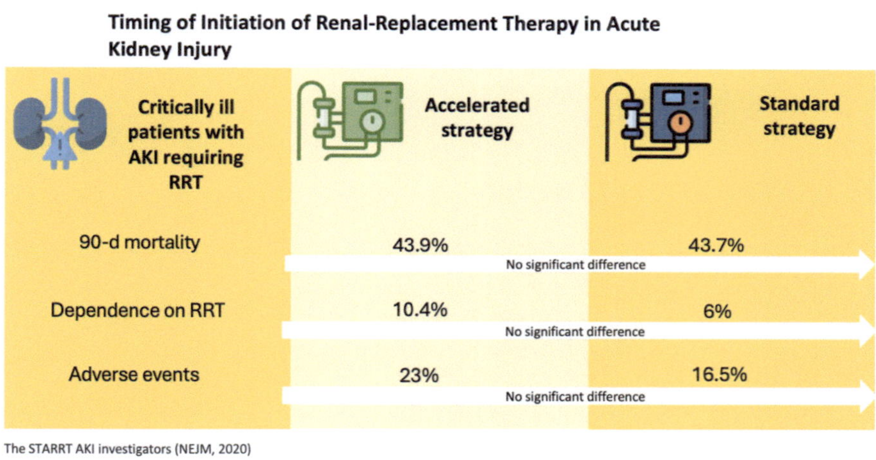

Quick Take

Can early renal replacement therapy (RRT) improve outcomes in ICU patients with acute kidney injury (AKI)?

The STARRT-AKI trial, a multicenter RCT across 15 countries, assessed whether early RRT initiation improves survival compared to a delayed approach in critically ill patients with severe AKI. Over 3000 patients were randomized to either an accelerated strategy (RRT within 12 hours of eligibility) or a standard strategy (RRT only

---

STARRT-AKI Investigators; Canadian Critical Care Trials Group; Australian and New Zealand Intensive Care Society Clinical Trials Group; Timing of Initiation of Renal-Replacement Therapy in Acute Kidney Injury. N Engl J Med. 2020 Jul 16;383(3):240–51.

J. Chacko et al., *Landmark Studies in Critical Care*,
https://doi.org/10.1007/978-981-95-0673-6_40

for severe complications or persistent AKI beyond 72 hours). The trial found no difference in 90-day mortality between the groups. However, 38% of patients in the standard strategy group never required RRT, suggesting unnecessary dialysis was avoided. The delayed approach also led to fewer RRT days and lower dialysis dependence at 90 days.

40.1 Introduction

Despite older observational studies and more recent randomized controlled trials (RCTs), the initiation timing of renal replacement therapy (RRT) in acute kidney injury (AKI) still remained a critical and unresolved question in critical care. The STARRT-AKI trial, an international, multicenter study, was designed to provide robust evidence on whether an early RRT initiation strategy improves outcomes compared to a delayed strategy. Published in *The New England Journal of Medicine* in 2020, this trial included diverse populations from multiple countries and offered insights into the benefits and risks of early versus delayed RRT initiation in critically ill patients with severe AKI [1].

40.2 Population and Design

The STARRT-AKI trial was an RCT conducted across 168 hospitals in 15 countries. It enrolled adult patients (aged ≥18 years) in the ICU who developed severe AKI and met the Kidney Disease: Improving Global Outcomes (KDIGO) stage 2 or 3 criteria. At least one of the three criteria had to be met:

- Rise of serum creatinine to more than twice the baseline level
- Serum creatinine level of >4 mg/dl (354 μmol/L) or more with an increase of 0.3 mg/dl (27 μmol/L) from baseline
- Urine output <6 ml/kg in the previous 12 hours

The trial sought to compare an accelerated strategy with a standard strategy of RRT initiation in terms of survival and other patient-centered outcomes. The investigators employed an open-label design with concealed allocation to ensure unbiased randomization while allowing practical implementation in busy ICU settings.

40.3 Exclusions

To focus on patients where the timing of RRT initiation was a clinical decision rather than an absolute necessity, the trial excluded:

- Patients requiring immediate RRT: Those with life-threatening complications such as hyperkalemia ($K^+ > 5.5$ mmol/L), severe acidosis ($HCO_3 < 15$ mmol/L, or pulmonary edema)
- End-stage renal disease with eGRF <20 ml/min/1.73m^2
- RRT was performed in the preceding 2 months
- Renal transplant in the preceding year
- Pre-existing conditions: Patients with chronic kidney disease expected to require dialysis soon or with an expected poor prognosis due to underlying diseases. Obstructive uropathy, rapidly progressive glomerulonephritis, and thrombotic microangiopathy
- Uncontrolled infections or bleeding disorders
- $K > 5.5$ mmol/L
- $HCO_3 < 15$ mmol/L
- Drug overdose necessitating dialysis

40.4 Study Groups

Participants were randomized into two groups:

40.4.1 Accelerated Strategy

RRT was initiated within 12 hours of meeting the inclusion criteria.

40.4.2 Standard Strategy

RRT was initiated only if patients developed severe complications necessitating RRT (hyperkalemia, metabolic acidosis, pulmonary edema, or oliguria/anuria lasting beyond 72 hours). Dialysis was discouraged unless persistent AKI occurred with serum creatinine >50% of the level at randomization, with an absolute indication, including serum $K^+ > 6$ mmol/L, pH < 7.2, or $HCO_3 < 12$ mmol/L, or fluid overload.

40.5 Common Management

Standardized care was provided to patients in both groups to minimize bias from non-RRT-related interventions. The hemodynamic status was optimized with fluid resuscitation and the use of vasopressors as appropriate. Electrolyte and acid-base levels were regularly monitored to identify urgent indications for RRT. Stringent aseptic measures were followed with the timely use of antibiotics in case of infection. Enteral or parenteral nutrition was tailored to meet nutritional requirements. The modality of RRT—continuous or intermittent—was left to the clinician discretion; citrate anticoagulation was commonly used for continuous renal replacement therapy. RRT was continued until recovery of kidney function, death, or withdrawal of active life support measures.

40.6 Sample Size

A total of 3019 patients were enrolled, with 1515 assigned to the early RRT group and 1504 to the delayed RRT group. The large sample size provided adequate power to detect a modest but clinically significant difference in 90-day mortality between the groups.

40.7 Results

40.7.1 Primary Outcome

The primary outcome, the 90-day all-cause mortality, was not significantly different between the two groups. In the accelerated significant strategy group, 643/1465 (43.9%) patients died, compared with 639/1462 (43.7%) in the standard strategy group (Relative Risk: 1.00 (0.93–1.09). This finding indicated that early RRT initiation did not confer a survival advantage over a delayed strategy.

40.7.2 Secondary Outcomes

The study analyzed several secondary outcomes. In the standard group, 38% of patients did not require RRT, suggesting potential avoidance of unnecessary dialytic intervention. The number of RRT-free days at 90 days was higher in the standard strategy group (64 vs. 50 days). RRT-dependence at 90 days was lower with the standard compared with the accelerated strategy (6% vs. 10.4%). The ICU stay was shorter in the accelerated strategy group by 1 day (9 vs. 10 days).

There was no significant difference in the composite outcome of all-cause mortality and RRT-dependence at 90 days. The incidence of major adverse kidney events at 90 days was similar. The ICU mortality, 28-day mortality, and hospital mortality were similar between the two groups. Mechanical ventilation-free days and vasopressor-free days did not differ significantly between the two groups. The main study outcomes are summarized in Table 40.1.

Table 40.1 Main study outcomes

Outcome	Accelerated strategy	Standard strategy	Significance
90-day mortality	43.9%	43.7%	RR: 1.00 (0.93 to 1.09)
90-day RRT-dependence	10.4%	6%	RR: 1.74 (1.24 to 2.43)
90-day death or RRT dependence	50%	47.3%	RR: 1.06 (0.98 to 1.14)
90-day major adverse kidney events	76.7%	77.1%	RR: 0.99 (0.95 to 1.04)
Median RRT-free days at 90 days	50	64	Difference: −2.62 (−5.66 to 0.42)

Abbreviations: RRT renal replacement therapy, *RR* risk ratio

40.8 Study Conclusions

Among critically ill patients with AKI, an accelerated strategy of RRT compared with a standard strategy did not reduce the 90-day mortality. The standard strategy was also associated with more RRT-free days. RRT-dependence at 90 days was also lower with the standard strategy compared to an accelerated strategy.

40.9 Strengths

The STARRT-AKI trial enrolled over 3000 patients, providing sufficient power for detecting meaningful differences in important clinical outcomes. It followed a pragmatic design, reflecting real-world clinical practices. Hence, the trial adds relevance to everyday ICU practice. Recording of outcomes was comprehensive, enabling robust analyses. Analysis was by intention-to-treat, and follow-up nearly complete, adding to the robustness of the trial. There was a clear separation between groups regarding the creatinine levels and fluid balance at the time of commencement of RRT, adding relevance to the findings.

40.10 Limitations

Blinding was not feasible; the open-label design may have introduced bias; however, outcome assessors were blinded to the study arm. The study included a heterogeneous population, with diverse underlying conditions that may have diluted subgroup-specific effects. The delayed strategy allowed for significant clinician discretion, potentially influencing the timing of RRT initiation. Assessment of quality-of-life, long-term functional outcomes, and cost-effectiveness may have been relevant endpoints.

40.11 Other Evidence

The findings of the STARRT-AKI trial align with other major studies on RRT timing.

- *AKIKI Trial:* Demonstrated no mortality difference between early and delayed RRT strategies, with a significant proportion of patients in the delayed group avoiding RRT [2].
- *ELAIN Trial:* Suggested a survival benefit with early RRT initiation, though differences in patient populations and methodologies complicate direct comparisons [3].
- *IDEAL-ICU Trial:* Focused on septic shock patients and found no mortality advantage with early RRT initiation, echoing the conclusions of the STARRT-AKI trial [4].

40.12 Summary

The STARRT-AKI trial reinforced the notion that a delayed RRT initiation strategy is safe and effective for most critically ill patients with AKI. By highlighting the potential for spontaneous renal recovery in the delayed group, the trial emphasized the importance of individualized decision-making and judicious use of RRT. While early initiation may be appropriate in select clinical scenarios, a delayed approach can reduce unnecessary interventions without compromising patient outcomes.

References

1. STARRT-AKI Investigators, Canadian Critical Care Trials Group, Australian and New Zealand Intensive Care Society Clinical Trials Group, United Kingdom Critical Care Research Group, Canadian Nephrology Trials Network, Irish Critical Care Trials Group, et al. Timing of initiation of renal-replacement therapy in acute kidney injury. N Engl J Med. 2020;383(3):240–51.
2. Gaudry S, Quenot JP, Hertig A, Barbar SD, Hajage D, Ricard JD, et al. Timing of renal replacement therapy for severe acute kidney injury in critically ill patients. Am J Respir Crit Care Med [Internet]. 2019 [cited 2019 Mar 21]. Available from: https://www.atsjournals.org/doi/10.1164/rccm.201810-1906CP
3. Zarbock A, Kellum JA, Schmidt C, Van Aken H, Wempe C, Pavenstädt H, et al. Effect of early vs delayed initiation of renal replacement therapy on mortality in critically ill patients with acute kidney injury: the ELAIN randomized clinical trial. JAMA. 2016;315(20):2190.
4. Barbar SD, Clere-Jehl R, Bourredjem A, Hernu R, Montini F, Bruyère R, et al. Timing of renal-replacement therapy in patients with acute kidney injury and sepsis. N Engl J Med. 2018;379(15):1431–42.

41 Intensity of Renal Support in Critically Ill Patients with Acute Kidney Injury: The VA/NIH Trial

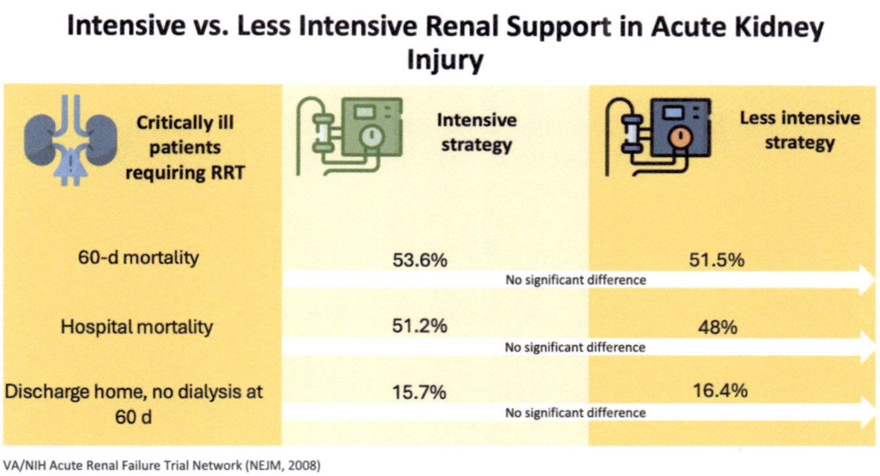

Quick Take

How does the intensity of renal support influence outcomes in critically ill patients with acute kidney injury (AKI)?

The VA/NIH Acute Renal Failure Trial Network study addressed this by comparing two levels of renal support: intensive and less-intensive treatment strategies. This multicenter, randomized controlled trial involved 1124 patients with severe AKI who were randomly assigned to receive either an intensive treatment strategy or a less-intensive strategy. In the intensive treatment group, patients underwent

---

VA/NIH Acute Renal Failure Trial Network. Intensity of renal support in critically ill patients with acute kidney injury. N Engl J Med. 2008 Jul 3;359(1):7–20.

J. Chacko et al., *Landmark Studies in Critical Care*,
https://doi.org/10.1007/978-981-95-0673-6_41

intermittent hemodialysis (IHD) or sustained low-efficiency dialysis (SLED) six times per week; hemodynamically unstable patients underwent continuous venovenous hemodiafiltration (CVVHDF) was carried out at a rate of 35 ml per kilogram of body weight per hour. In contrast, the less-intensive treatment group received IHD or SLED three times per week; CVVHDF was delivered at a rate of 20 ml per kilogram per hour in hemodynamically unstable patients. The results showed no significant difference in 60-day mortality between the two groups. Furthermore, there was no significant difference in the recovery of kidney function or other secondary outcomes. The study concluded that more intensive renal support did not result in improved survival or kidney recovery compared to less-intensive strategies. These findings suggest that less aggressive renal replacement therapies may be sufficient for critically ill patients with severe AKI.

41.1 Introduction

Critical illness often leads to acute kidney injury. Besides treating the underlying cause, renal replacement therapy may be required in a substantial number of patients. The hospital mortality among patients with acute kidney injury who undergo renal replacement therapy remains high, between 50% and 80%. Although renal replacement therapy was first introduced several decades ago, questions remain regarding the timing, modality of support, and, importantly, the optimal dose of therapy.

Results of clinical trials that evaluated the intensity of renal replacement therapy in critically ill patients have been conflicting. Ronco et al., in a randomized controlled trial (RCT), compared three doses of continuous renal replacement therapy in critically ill patients at 20, 35, and 45 ml/kg/hour. They observed improved survival with higher doses of 35 and 45 ml/kg/hour compared with 20 ml/kg/hour. Survival rates were similar with the higher doses of 35 or 45 ml/kg/hour [1]. Schiffl et al. compared daily hemodialysis with conventional intermittent therapy in patients with acute kidney injury. Uremic control was more effective, the incidence of hypotension was lower, and the resolution of renal failure occurred earlier among patients who underwent daily hemodialysis [2]. However, another study that compared standard (20 ml/kg/hour) with high-volume continuous venovenous hemodiafiltration (35 ml/kg/hour) did not reveal a significant difference in the 30-day survival (56% vs. 49%, $P = 0.32$) [3].

Considering the equipoise relating to the optimal dose of renal replacement therapy in the critically ill with acute kidney injury, the Veterans Affairs/National Institutes of Health (VA-NIH) study group in the US designed an RCT that compared two different intensities of therapy. In contrast to previous studies that evaluated a single treatment modality (continuous or intermittent), the authors allowed an integrated approach. The modality of treatment, continuous or intermittent, could be chosen based on the hemodynamic status, determined by the cardiovascular Sequential Organ Failure Assessment (SOFA) score, which is consistent with usual practice in many centers.

41.2 Population and Design

The VA-NIH trial was conducted between November 2003 and July 2007 across 27 centers in the US [4]. The study population included critically ill patients with acute kidney injury requiring renal replacement therapy. Failure of one or more non-renal organ systems or the presence of sepsis was required for eligibility. Organ failure was defined as a non-renal SOFA score of ≥2. The other inclusion criteria were the presence of oliguria (≤20 mL/hour for >24 hours) and a rise in serum creatinine level to ≥2 mg/dl in men and ≥1.5 mg/dl in women.

Patients were randomized to a strategy of intensive or less intensive renal replacement therapy. Randomization was stratified based on site, the cardiovascular SOFA score (0–2 vs. 3–4), and the presence of oliguria (urine output <20 ml/hour for >24 hours).

41.3 Exclusion

Patients who had undergone more than one session of intermittent hemodialysis, or sustained low-efficiency dialysis, or who had been treated with >24 hours of continuous renal replacement therapy were excluded. Other exclusion criteria were chronic kidney disease with a creatinine level of ≥2 mg/dl in men and ≥1.5 mg/dl in women, post renal transplant, and patients who were moribund or considered unlikely to survive 28 days due to an underlying terminal disease.

41.4 Choice of the Modality of Renal Replacement Therapy

Patients who were hemodynamically stable with a cardiovascular SOFA score of 0–2 received intermittent hemodialysis. If hemodynamically unstable (cardiovascular SOFA score of 3–4), they underwent sustained low-efficiency dialysis or continuous renal replacement therapy, based on local practice. Patients who were commenced on intermittent hemodialysis were switched to sustained low-efficiency dialysis or continuous renal replacement therapy if they developed hemodynamic instability. Contrariwise, those who were on sustained low-efficiency dialysis or continuous renal replacement therapies could be transitioned to intermittent hemodialysis once they had attained hemodynamic stability.

41.5 Intensive Strategy

Intermittent therapies (intermittent hemodialysis or sustained low-efficiency dialysis) were performed 6 days per week. Among patients who underwent continuous renal replacement therapy in the intensive strategy group, the effluent rate was set at 35 ml/kg/hour.

41.6 Less Intensive Strategy

Intermittent therapies were carried out thrice a week; among patients who underwent continuous renal replacement therapy, the effluent rate was set at 20 ml/kg/hour.

41.7 Both Groups

Intermittent hemodialysis or sustained low-efficiency dialysis was prescribed, aiming for a single-pool Kt/V_{urea} of 1.2–1.4 per session. If severe volume overload was present, patients who received intermittent therapies were provided with isolated ultrafiltration and fluid removal as appropriate. The assigned modality of therapy was continued for up to 28 days, recovery of renal function, ICU discharge, withdrawal of therapy, or death.

41.8 Sample Size

The sample size was calculated based on the 60-day mortality, the primary outcome. Identification of an absolute reduction in mortality by 10% (from 55% in the less intensive to 45% in the intensive strategy group) required a sample size of 1164 patients, allowing for 10% loss to follow-up. This sample size provided the study with 90% power to detect the difference at a two-sided significance level of 0.05.

41.9 Results

A total of 1124 patients underwent randomization—per protocol analysis was carried out among 563 who were assigned to receive intensive therapy and 561 assigned to less-intensive therapy.

The baseline characteristics were similar in both groups. The mean age of the study population was 59.7 ± 15.3 years, and the majority were male patients (70.6%). The etiology of acute kidney injury was multifactorial in most patients (59%). The most common cause of acute kidney injury was attributed to ischemia (80.9%), followed by sepsis (54.9%), and nephrotoxins (28%). Overall, 80.6% of patients received mechanical ventilation, 63% had sepsis, and 78% were oliguric.

41.9.1 Characteristics of Therapy

Patients in the intensive-therapy group who received intermittent therapies underwent an average of 5.4 sessions of treatment per week, compared with 3 sessions per week in the less-intensive therapy group. Continuous renal replacement therapy was performed in a dose of 36.2 ± 3.8 ml/kg in the intensive-therapy group compared with 21.5 ± 4.3 ml/kg body weight in the less-intensive therapy group.

41.9.2 The Primary Outcome—60-Day Mortality

The 60-day mortality was similar in both groups of patients. At 60 days, 302/563 (53.6%) of patients in the intensive therapy group had died compared to 289/561 (51.5%) in the less-intensive therapy group (odds ratio:1.09; 95% CI: 0.86–1.40; $P = 0.47$). Mortality was similar among prespecified subgroups of patients based on gender, the SOFA score, the presence of oliguria, and sepsis.

41.9.3 Secondary Outcomes

There was no significant difference in secondary outcomes between the intensive and less-intensive therapy groups. These included in-hospital mortality (51.2% vs. 48%), discharged home without requirement for continued renal replacement therapy at day 60 (15.7% vs. 16.4%), complete (15.4% vs. 18.4%) or partial (8.9% vs. 9.0%) renal recovery, renal replacement therapy-free days at day 28 (6 vs. 7 days), hospital-free days at day 60 (11 vs. 13 days), and ICU-free days at 60 days (18.7 vs. 20.1 days). The organ failure-free days at day 14, based on the SOFA scores of each system (cardiovascular, respiratory, liver, coagulation, and the central nervous system), were also similar in both groups.

41.9.4 Complications

When all modalities of renal replacement therapy were considered, the incidence of hypotension requiring vasopressor support was significantly higher among patients who received intensive compared with less-intensive therapies (14.4% vs. 10%, $P = 0.02$). However, the modality of support did not appear to impact hemodynamic stability during renal replacement therapy. Intensive therapy resulted in a higher incidence of hypophosphatemia (17.6% vs. 10.9%, $P = 0.001$) and hypokalemia (7.5% vs. 4.5%, $P = 0.03$). Other adverse events, including catheter-related and treatment-related complications, were similar in both groups. The main study outcomes are summarized in Table 41.1.

41.10 Study Conclusions

Among critically ill patients with AKI, intensive renal support compared with a less intense strategy did not result in lower mortality or lead to improved recovery of renal function. The incidence of non-renal organ failures was also similar in both groups of patients.

Table 41.1 Main study outcomes

Outcome	Intense strategy	Less intense strategy	
60-day mortality (number, %)	302 (53.6)	289 (51.5)	0.47
In-hospital mortality (number, %)	288 (51.2)	269 (48.0)	0.27
Discharge home, with no RRT at 60 days (%)	15.7	16.4	0.75
RRT-free days at 28 days	6.0 ± 0.4	7.0 ± 0.4	0.07
ICU-free days at 60 days	18.7 ± 0.9	20.1 ± 0.9	0.25
Hospital-free days at 60 days	11.0 ± 0.7	13.0 ± 0.7	0.053
Complete renal recovery at 28 days	15.4%	18.4%	
Partial renal recovery at 28 days	8.9%	9.0%	
No renal recovery at 28 days	75.8%	72.6%	

Abbreviation: RRT renal replacement therapy

41.11 Strengths

The VA-NIH trial was an adequately powered, multicentric RCT designed to answer the clinical question regarding outcomes from two different intensities of renal replacement therapy among critically ill patients with acute renal failure. Unlike previous studies, the study compared two treatment doses that could be considered adequate. The less-intensive approach reflected real-world practice based on a pre-trial survey [5]. Transition between modalities was allowed based on hemodynamic stability—a common practice followed in many centers. The intensity of therapy was based on clearance of small solutes, including urea; besides, if volume overload was a problem, isolated ultrafiltration was allowed based on clinician assessment.

41.12 Limitations

Three different modalities of renal replacement therapy were employed, including intermittent hemodialysis, sustained low-efficiency dialysis, and continuous renal replacement therapy. Hence, it is unclear whether the type of therapy influenced outcomes. This is particularly relevant in ICUs that do not commonly resort to intermittent modalities of treatment. Transition between modalities was allowed; however, equivalence of dosing when switching modalities may have contributed to the complexity of the approach. The timing of therapy was not standardized, and hence could have impacted outcomes. Patients with high baseline creatinine were excluded; hence, the results cannot be extrapolated to patients with chronic kidney disease. The study population included predominantly male patients (25% of patients were enrolled from Veterans Affairs hospitals, with a predominantly male population); generalizability to the female population may be limited.

41.13 Subsequent Evidence

The RENAL study, published a year later, evaluated continuous venovenous hemodiafiltration at two effluent doses—40 ml/kg/hour (higher intensity) and 25 ml/kg/hour (lower intensity) in an RCT conducted across 35 ICUs in Australia and New Zealand [6]. The study enrolled 1508 patients—721 in the higher-intensity and 743 in the lower-intensity group. The 90-day mortality was similar (44.7% in both groups). Besides, a similar number of patients continued to receive renal replacement therapy at 90 days in both groups (higher intensity: 6.8%, lower intensity: 4.4%). Hypophosphatemia occurred more often with higher-intensity therapy. Based on the findings of the VA-NIH and the RENAL trials, the KDIGO (Kidney Disease: Improving Global Outcomes) guidelines went on to recommend an effluent dose of 20–25 ml/kg/hour with continuous renal replacement therapy and a weekly Kt/V of 3.9 when intermittent therapies are employed [7].

41.14 Summary

The VA-NIH RCT compared the clinical impact of an intensive with a less-intensive strategy of renal replacement therapy among critically ill patients with acute renal failure. The investigators did not observe improved clinical outcomes with a conventional, less-intensive approach compared with an intensive strategy. Among the important clinical outcomes, no significant difference was observed in the 60-day or in-hospital mortality. Furthermore, they observed a similar rate of renal recovery in both groups; progression to non-renal organ failures was also similar. Hemodynamic instability occurred more often with intensive therapy but appeared to be unrelated to the modality of treatment—whether continuous or intermittent. As expected, electrolyte abnormalities, including hypophosphatemia and hypokalemia, were observed more commonly in the intensive therapy group. Against the background of uncertainty, the VA-NIH trial went a long way in establishing the efficacy of a less-intensive strategy of renal replacement therapy in critically ill patients with acute renal failure.

References

1. Ronco C, Bellomo R, Homel P, Brendolan A, Dan M, Piccinni P, et al. Effects of different doses in continuous veno-venous haemofiltration on outcomes of acute renal failure: a prospective randomised trial. Lancet. 2000;356(9223):26–30.
2. Schiffl H, Lang SM, Fischer R. Daily hemodialysis and the outcome of acute renal failure. N Engl J Med. 2002;346(5):305–10.
3. Tolwani AJ, Campbell RC, Stofan BS, Lai KR, Oster RA, Wille KM. Standard versus high-dose CVVHDF for ICU-related acute renal failure. J Am Soc Nephrol. 2008;19(6):1233–8.
4. VA/NIH Acute Renal Failure Trial Network, Palevsky PM, Zhang JH, O'Connor TZ, Chertow GM, Crowley ST, et al. Intensity of renal support in critically ill patients with acute kidney injury. N Engl J Med. 2008;359(1):7–20.

5. Overberger P, Pesacreta M, Palevsky PM, VA/NIH Acute Renal Failure Trial Network. Management of renal replacement therapy in acute kidney injury: a survey of practitioner prescribing practices. Clin J Am Soc Nephrol. 2007;2(4):623–30.
6. RENAL Replacement Therapy Study Investigators, Bellomo R, Cass A, Cole L, Finfer S, Gallagher M, et al. Intensity of continuous renal-replacement therapy in critically ill patients. N Engl J Med. 2009;361(17):1627–38.
7. Khwaja A. KDIGO clinical practice guidelines for acute kidney injury. Nephron Clin Pract. 2012;120(4):c179–84.

Part VIII

Trauma

Immediate Versus Delayed Resuscitation in Penetrating Torso Injury: Bickell et al.

42

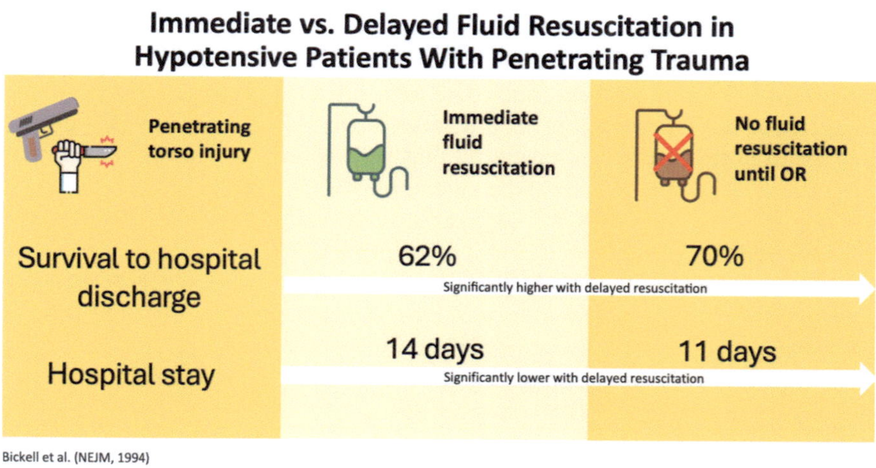

Quick Take

Could delaying fluid resuscitation improve survival in penetrating trauma?

This randomized controlled trial compared the effects of immediate vs. delayed fluid resuscitation in patients with hypotension following penetrating torso injuries. The study enrolled 598 patients and found that early fluid resuscitation did not improve survival rates. In fact, the delayed resuscitation group, which received fluids only after reaching the hospital, showed a slightly better survival rate (20% vs. 16%) compared to the immediate resuscitation group. The trial challenged

---

Bickell WH, Wall MJ, Pepe PE, Martin RR, Ginger VF, Allen MK, et al. Immediate versus delayed fluid resuscitation for hypotensive patients with penetrating torso injuries. N Engl J Med. 1994 Oct 27;331(17):1105–9.

J. Chacko et al., *Landmark Studies in Critical Care*,
https://doi.org/10.1007/978-981-95-0673-6_42

traditional trauma care protocols, suggesting that immediate fluid resuscitation may not always be beneficial in the management of hypotensive trauma patients, particularly in those with penetrating injuries.

42.1 Introduction

Early, aggressive fluid administration was long considered to be the key to the resuscitation of patients who suffered major hemorrhage following trauma. However, experience from the battlefield suggested that too much fluid in patients with continued bleeding may be associated with adverse outcomes. During World War I, Walter Cannon, a well-renowned physiologist of the time, collaborated with John Fraser, a senior surgeon at the Harvard Base Hospital, to take care of soldiers injured on the battlefield. From their first-hand experience of hypotensive, wounded soldiers, they noted that intravenous fluids aimed to increase blood pressure might be detrimental. They proposed that hemorrhage may arrest spontaneously as the blood pressure drops to levels too low to dislodge the newly formed clot. In their treatise titled "The preventive treatment of wound shock" published in the Journal of the American Medical Association (JAMA) of 1918, they asserted that "Injection of a fluid that will increase blood pressure carries danger in itself." They proposed that attempting to raise the blood pressure prior to achieving hemostasis through surgical intervention leads to "loss of blood that is sorely needed" [1].

The experience during World War II echoed these findings. Henry Beecher, Harvard's first chief anesthesiologist, served in the US army during the war. He often encountered the harrowing experience of resuscitating wounded soldiers in "shock tents" on the battlefields of Italy and North Africa. From his own experience, he recommended a systolic BP of no more than 80 mm Hg if there was a good pulse and the peripheries were warm. He suggested that blood transfusion may be withheld until definitive surgical intervention is carried out to arrest the bleeding [2].

The Vietnam war blew a wind of change in resuscitation practice. Large-volume resuscitation was often resorted to with the emerging concept of 3:1 volume replacement with crystalloids [3]. The recommendations of the Advanced Trauma Life Support (ATLS) guidelines followed, advocating the rapid infusion of 2 L of crystalloid in hemorrhagic shock [4]. However, the harmful effects of excessive crystalloid resuscitation were soon evident, with the development of acute respiratory distress syndrome, bowel and myocardial edema, and abdominal and extremity compartment syndrome [5]. There was also growing concern based on animal models of traumatic hemorrhage that an aggressive crystalloid resuscitation strategy might lead to clot disruption and increase the risk of hemorrhage, thereby leading to reduced survival [6].

42.2 The Landmark Bickell et al.'s Paper (1994)

Against this background, Bickell et al. sought to test the hypothesis that in hypotensive patients with penetrating torso injuries, delaying fluid resuscitation until surgical intervention and arrest of bleeding would lead to improved outcomes [7].

42.3 Population and Design

The study was conducted through the Houston Emergency Medical Services system during a 3-year period between November 1989 to December 1992. Patients 16 years or older who sustained a stab or gunshot injury to the torso with a systolic BP of ≤90 mm Hg were eligible. The victims were transferred by paramedics to the major trauma center at the Ben Taub General Hospital in Houston, Texas. Patients with fatal gunshot wounds to the head and those with minor injuries that did not require surgical intervention were excluded from the outcome analysis.

Study patients were treated based on an immediate or a delayed resuscitation protocol. The immediate resuscitation strategy was followed on even-numbered and a delayed strategy on odd-numbered calendar days.

42.4 Immediate Resuscitation Group

In the immediate resuscitation group, two or more 14 G intravenous cannulae were inserted; fluid resuscitation was commenced with Ringer's acetate solution before surgical intervention in the pre-hospital and trauma care setting. Patients who arrived at the emergency department with a systolic BP of ≤100 mm Hg continued to receive crystalloid resuscitation. Packed red cells were administered according to the criteria of the American College of Surgeons trauma committee.

42.5 Delayed Resuscitation Group

Intravenous cannulae were inserted in the delayed resuscitation group, but no fluid was administered. Fluids and blood products were administered once the patient was in the operating room and after induction of anesthesia.

42.6 Common Management in Both Groups

Endotracheal intubation was carried out, and mechanical ventilation commenced as appropriate, followed by rapid transfer to the trauma center. After arrival in the operating room and induction of anesthesia, crystalloids and packed red cells were administered to both groups to maintain a systolic BP of 100 mm Hg, a hematocrit of ≥25%, and a urine output of at least 50 ml/hour. Hetastarch was occasionally used for intravascular volume expansion.

42.7 Sample Size

The sample size was calculated based on an expected mortality of 35% in patients with penetrating torso injuries. The authors assumed a 10–15% improvement in survival with a delayed resuscitation strategy. Six hundred patients were required for a two-tailed p-value of 0.05 with 80% power. Analysis was based on intention to treat.

42.8 Results

A total of 1069 patients with penetrating torso injuries and hypotension were transferred to the trauma center during the study period. Among these, 172 patients who suffered cardiopulmonary arrest and 299 patients who did not require major surgical intervention were excluded. Of the remaining patients, 309 were assigned to the immediate resuscitation group and 289 to the delayed resuscitation group. The patients were well-matched at baseline; the most common site of injury was the abdomen, followed by chest and neck injuries. The injury severity score (ISS) was 26 ± 14 in both groups. The systolic BP was significantly higher, and the hemoglobin level significantly lower in the immediate resuscitation group upon arrival to the trauma center.

Seventy patients died before they reached the operating room. Among the remaining 528 patients who underwent surgical intervention, 268 were in the immediate resuscitation group and 260 in the delayed resuscitation group. On arrival to the operating room and before the induction of anesthesia, the blood pressures, the venous pH, and bicarbonate levels were similar in both groups.

42.8.1 The Volume of Fluids Administered

The delayed resuscitation group received fluids along with administration of antibiotics, contrast media, and a minimum flow was maintained to ensure venous patency. In the pre-hospital phase, the immediate resuscitation group received a mean volume of 870 ml of fluid compared with 92 ml in the delayed group. At the trauma center, the corresponding volumes administered were 1608 ml and 283 ml. There was no significant difference in the volume of fluid administered intraoperatively between the two groups. Similar volumes of packed red cells, autologous transfusions, fresh frozen plasma, and platelets were administered to both groups.

42.8.2 Outcomes

Survival to hospital discharge, the primary outcome, was significantly higher with the delayed resuscitation strategy. In the immediate resuscitation group, 193/309 (62%) patients survived, compared with 203/289 (70%) in the delayed resuscitation group ($p = 0.04$). The results remained significant after adjustment for the time interval spent at the scene and at the hospital prior to arrival in the operating room. Intraoperative blood loss was similar in both groups, although there was a non-significant increase in the immediate resuscitation group. The duration of ICU stay was similar between the two groups; however, the duration of hospital stay was significantly longer in the immediate resuscitation group.

The beneficial effect of a delayed resuscitation strategy seemed more pronounced among patients with more severe injury. The survival rate in patients with an Injury Severity Scores of ≥25 or higher was 61% in the delayed resuscitation group compared with 48% in the immediate resuscitation group ($P = 0.02$).

Based on these findings, the authors proposed that fluid resuscitation should be delayed in hypotensive patients with penetrating torso injuries until they were ready for operative intervention aimed at achieving hemostasis. The lower hemoglobin level in the immediate resuscitation group could likely have been due to continued bleeding; besides, excessive fluid administration may also have resulted in the coagulopathy observed in this group. The authors suggested that their study did not support the practice of aggressive fluid resuscitation for all patients with trauma and hypotension, presumably related to hemorrhage. They contended that although the necessity of fluid resuscitation remained unquestioned, the timing and the volume need to be reconsidered in light of their findings. They recommended future studies to explore the concept of delayed resuscitation in blunt trauma. The main study outcomes are summarized in Table 42.1.

Table 42.1 Main study outcomes

Outcome	Immediate resuscitation ($N = 309$)	Delayed resuscitation ($N = 289$)	*P* value
Survived to hospital discharge	62%	70%	0.04
Hospital LOS	14 ± 24 days	11 ± 19 days	0.11
ICU LOS	8 ± 16	7 ± 11	0.3
Mean intraoperative blood loss	3127 ± 4937 ml	2555 ± 3546 ml	0.006

Abbreviation: LOS length of stay

42.9 Study Conclusions

The findings of the study suggested that excessive early resuscitation may be detrimental, probably related to exacerbation of bleeding before definitive hemorrhage control. The authors concluded that in hypotensive patients with penetrating trauma to the torso, an aggressive fluid resuscitation strategy should be delayed until definitive operative intervention.

42.9.1 Strengths

The Bickell et al. study was among the first controlled trials that evaluated the concept of hypotensive resuscitation in bleeding trauma patients. The study was adequately powered to estimate a survival benefit with the delayed resuscitation strategy. Analysis was based on intention to treat. The study confirmed a physiologically plausible hypothesis that excessive fluid administration in the face of continued bleeding could lead to harm emanating from potential clot dislodgement and coagulopathy.

42.9.2 Limitations

Patients were assigned to the study group using a quasi-randomized, alternate-day method. According to the authors, this design was chosen to avoid delays in resuscitation that may have occurred with conventional methods of randomization. Questions were raised about Ringer's acetate, the resuscitation fluid used by the investigators, which could potentially cause hypotension due to the release of adenosine and vasodilatation. The volume of fluid administered in the immediate resuscitation group was lower than expected, with a mean volume of 133 ml of packed red cells and 1.6 L of crystalloid. In the delayed resuscitation group, 22 patients received early resuscitation fluid, which could have affected outcomes. The single-center study was conducted in an established trauma system; patients were ready in the operating room within an average duration of 79 minutes of the trauma call. Surgical intervention was carried out expeditiously, within 40–50 minutes of arrival at the trauma center. Similar timelines may be difficult to achieve in other healthcare settings. Hence, these results may not be generalizable to less experienced trauma systems.

42.10 Later Studies That Explored the Concept of Limited Resuscitation

The Bickell et al. study triggered considerable research and many controlled trials to further explore the concept of limited early resuscitation of trauma victims.

Following this landmark trial, the Fluid Resuscitation in Trauma (FRT) study was undertaken between 1996 and 1999 [8]. The FRT study included patients with blunt or penetrating injury who were actively bleeding with a systolic BP of less than 90 mm Hg recorded within an hour of injury. Unlike the Bickell et al. study, patients were randomized to receive resuscitation fluids titrated to a systolic BP of >100 mm Hg or 70 mm Hg. Once the target BP was achieved, a policy of fluid restriction was followed, with the appropriate use of sedative or analgesic drugs aimed at maintaining blood pressure within the target range. The resuscitation strategy was continued until hemostasis was achieved. The study included 110 patients, with 55 in each group; mortality was low, with four deaths in each group. Although the target of 70 mm Hg was aimed for in the low BP arm, the mean systolic BP was 100 mm Hg compared with 114 mm Hg in the high BP group. The authors concluded that a strategy aimed at deliberate hypotension did not lead to higher mortality in the trauma patient with active bleeding.

A later pilot study by Schreiber et al. evaluated the safety and feasibility of a controlled compared with a standard resuscitation strategy in hypotensive trauma patients [9]. Patients included in this study had a systolic BP ≤90 mm Hg. In the controlled resuscitation group, a 250 ml bolus of fluid was administered if there was no palpable radial pulse or if the systolic BP was <70 mm Hg. Additional boluses of 250 ml were administered to maintain the systolic BP ≥70 mm Hg. In the standard resuscitation group, an initial bolus of 2 L of fluid was administered, followed by additional boluses to maintain the systolic BP ≥110 mm Hg. The protocol was followed until hemostasis was achieved or until 2 hours after arrival at the hospital. The mean volume of intravenous fluid administered was 1 L in the controlled resuscitation group compared with 2 L in the standard group. At 24 hours post-admission, a trend towards lower mortality was observed in the controlled resuscitation group, although the difference was not statistically significant (5% vs. 15%). In blunt trauma victims, the 24-hour survival was significantly higher with a controlled compared with a standard resuscitation strategy (3% vs. 18%). The authors suggested that a controlled resuscitation strategy may improve early survival in trauma patients with ongoing hemorrhage.

In contrast to the above studies, Carrick et al. did not observe a 30-day survival advantage with a hypotensive strategy among patients who underwent thoracotomy or laparotomy for hemorrhage control. In this study, a target mean arterial pressure (MAP) target of 50 mm Hg was compared with a higher MAP of 65 mm Hg [10].

42.11 Summary

Conventional resuscitation practice in severe trauma was based on the administration of large volumes of intravenous fluid with the aim of restoring hemodynamic stability and preserving organ function. This dictum was largely based on animal studies from the 1950s that suggested improved outcomes in traumatic hemorrhage with the normalization of hemodynamic parameters. However, in the clinical setting, there was increasing concern that attempts to restore intravascular volume before hemorrhage control was attained could lead to deleterious effects arising from clot dislodgement and continued bleeding. Besides, excessive administration of intravenous fluids in the bleeding patient could lead to dilutional coagulopathy and reduce blood viscosity, contributing to secondary hemorrhage. These mechanisms could entail reduced survival in patients who were subjected to overzealous fluid resuscitation. The Bickell et al. study challenged conventional wisdom and contemporaneous guidelines of the era that recommended large-volume fluid resuscitation among all hypotensive trauma patients, irrespective of the attainment of hemorrhage control. Although the study had several limitations, including a suboptimal, quasi-randomized design, it led to a rethink among clinicians regarding the appropriateness of aggressive resuscitation measures in the bleeding trauma patient. Over the years, permissive hypotension came to be incorporated as a basic tenet of "damage control" resuscitation along with control of life-threatening hemorrhage and prevention of contamination arising from visceral injury [11]. Continued resuscitation with definitive measures to correct physiologic derangements follows the initial phase of damage control. This paper underlined the importance of avoiding an aggressive fluid resuscitation strategy in hypotensive patients following penetrating torso trauma. The overriding emphasis lies in the control of hemorrhage through timely surgical intervention. A harbinger of change, this landmark trial reasserted the "less is more" concept in critical care practice.

References

1. WB Cannon: a trauma pioneer—ST Horne; 2004 [Internet]. [cited 2023 Jan 31]. Available from: https://journals.sagepub.com/doi/abs/10.1191/1460408604ta301oa
2. Beecher HK. Preparation of battle casualties for surgery. Ann Surg. 1945;121(6):769–92.
3. Shires GT, Canizaro PC. Fluid resuscitation in the severely injured. Surg Clin North Am. 1973;53(6):1341–66.
4. Bell RM, Krantz BE, Weigelt JA. ATLS: a foundation for trauma training. Ann Emerg Med. 1999;34(2):233–7.
5. Maxwell RA, Fabian TC, Croce MA, Davis KA. Secondary abdominal compartment syndrome: an underappreciated manifestation of severe hemorrhagic shock. J Trauma. 1999;47(6):995–9.
6. Stern SA, Dronen SC, Birrer P, Wang X. Effect of blood pressure on hemorrhage volume and survival in a near-fatal hemorrhage model incorporating a vascular injury. Ann Emerg Med. 1993;22(2):155–63.
7. Bickell WH, Wall MJ, Pepe PE, Martin RR, Ginger VF, Allen MK, et al. Immediate versus delayed fluid resuscitation for hypotensive patients with penetrating torso injuries. N Engl J Med. 1994;331(17):1105–9.
8. Dutton RP, Mackenzie CF, Scalea TM. Hypotensive resuscitation during active hemorrhage: impact on in-hospital mortality. J Trauma. 2002;52(6):1141–6.
9. Schreiber MA, Meier EN, Tisherman SA, Kerby JD, Newgard CD, Brasel K, et al. A controlled resuscitation strategy is feasible and safe in hypotensive trauma patients: results of a prospective randomized pilot trial. J Trauma Acute Care Surg. 2015;78(4):687–95; discussion 695–697.
10. Carrick MM, Morrison CA, Tapia NM, Leonard J, Suliburk JW, Norman MA, et al. Intraoperative hypotensive resuscitation for patients undergoing laparotomy or thoracotomy for trauma: early termination of a randomized prospective clinical trial. J Trauma Acute Care Surg. 2016;80(6):886–96.
11. Shapiro MB, Jenkins DH, Schwab CW, Rotondo MF. Damage control: collective review. J Trauma. 2000;49(5):969–78.

43 Tranexamic Acid in Bleeding Trauma Patients: The CRASH-2 Trial

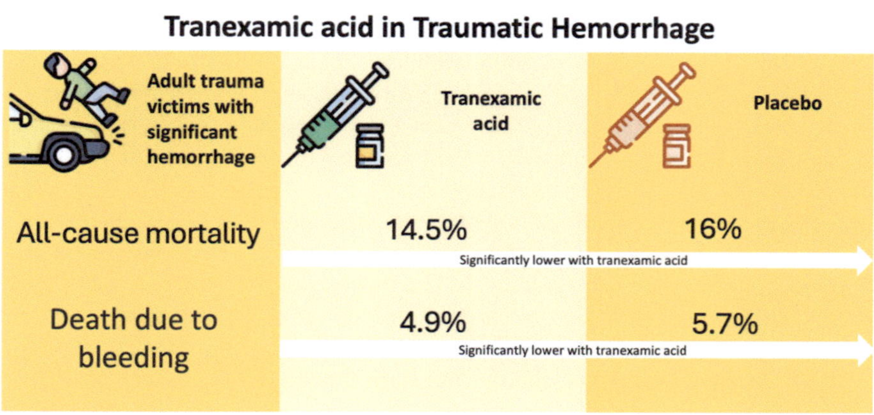

CRASH-2 trial collaborators (Lancet, 2010)

Quick Take

Can tranexamic acid save lives in bleeding trauma victims?

The CRASH-2 trial investigated the use of tranexamic acid, an antifibrinolytic, in trauma patients with significant hemorrhage. A total of 20,211 patients were randomized to receive either tranexamic acid or a placebo within 8 hours of injury. The study found that tranexamic acid significantly reduced the risk of death due to bleeding, with no increase in vascular occlusive events. These results provided strong evidence for the use of tranexamic acid in trauma patients with severe

CRASH-2 trial collaborators. Effects of tranexamic acid on death, vascular occlusive events, and blood transfusion in trauma patients with significant haemorrhage (CRASH-2): a randomized, placebo-controlled trial. Lancet Lond Engl. 2010 Jul 3;376(9734):23–32.

J. Chacko et al., *Landmark Studies in Critical Care*,
https://doi.org/10.1007/978-981-95-0673-6_43

bleeding, leading to its adoption as a life-saving treatment in trauma protocols globally. The trial also demonstrated that early administration is crucial for optimal outcomes.

43.1 Introduction

Back in the 1950s, in war-torn Japan, a husband-and-wife team of researchers, Shosuke and Utako Okamoto, were scripting medical history. They were passionately focused on identifying an antagonist of clot breakdown that might arrest severe hemorrhage. Exsanguinating postpartum hemorrhage was a leading cause of maternal mortality in Japan during this period. They realized that the clot became "liquified", often leading to unrelenting hemorrhage—the process we know today as fibrinolysis. Plasmin was later identified as the enzyme that led to clot breakdown. The couple spent tireless hours in their laboratory in pursuit of an agent that could inhibit plasmin and thus, prevent clot breakdown. They finally zeroed in on the amino acid lysine as a likely plasmin inhibitor. An analog of lysine, aminocaproic acid, was soon introduced as a potent inhibitor of plasmin. Aminocaproic acid was clinically effective, but relatively less potent and required large doses, often leading to side effects. The search for a more potent agent led to the discovery of tranexamic acid, 27 times as powerful as aminocaproic acid.

Shosuke and Utako Okamoto first reported tranexamic acid as a potent inhibitor of fibrinolysis in The Keio Journal of Medicine in September 1962 [1]. However, their discovery was received with icy disdain by the male-dominated research community in Japan. Obstetricians, too, seemed largely uninterested; use was confined to reducing heavy menstrual bleeding and following tooth extraction. Utako Okamoto went on to become chair at the Kobe Gakuin University in Japan from 1966 to 1990. She died on 21 April 2016, just a year before the publication of the WOMAN trial that conclusively demonstrated improved survival with tranexamic acid in severe postpartum hemorrhage. Today, tranexamic acid features in the World Health Organization's list of essential medicines.

43.2 Background to the CRASH-2 Trial

The hemostatic system plays a key role in maintaining circulation following vascular injury due to major surgery or trauma. The coagulation cascade is activated to control bleeding. The clotting mechanism is countered by the fibrinolytic system, which prevents excessive clotting. In some situations, the fibrinolytic mechanism appears to evoke a pathological response leading to uncontrolled hemorrhage [2]. Antifibrinolytic agents appear to decrease blood loss following surgery, with no greater risk of complications [3].

A Cochrane review of 2007, including 53 randomized controlled trials (RCTs), had revealed a reduced requirement for blood transfusion with tranexamic acid use among patients undergoing elective surgery, although it had no impact on mortality [3]. The CRASH-2 investigators searched for clinical trials of tranexamic acid in severe trauma, but none seemed to exist.

Considering the similar hemostatic response following major surgery and trauma, the authors of the CRASH-2 trial hypothesized that tranexamic acid might reduce hemorrhage-related mortality in victims of major trauma [4].

43.3 Population and Design

The CRASH-2 RCT compared the effect of tranexamic acid with placebo among trauma patients who were bleeding or were at risk of significant hemorrhage. The study was conducted in 274 hospitals across 40 countries and commenced recruitment in May 2005. Randomization was in blocks of eight and stratified by center.

43.4 Inclusion Criteria

Adult trauma victims with evidence of significant hemorrhage, defined as a systolic blood pressure of less than 90 mm Hg, or a heart rate of >110/min, or considered to be at risk of significant hemorrhage, within 8 hours of injury, were considered for enrolment. Patients were eligible for randomization if the treating clinician was unsure whether to treat with tranexamic acid.

43.5 Exclusion Criteria

Patients who were considered likely to benefit from tranexamic acid according to clinician judgment received the drug anyway and were not included in the study. Patients who had a clear contraindication to tranexamic acid were also excluded.

43.6 Intervention

Tranexamic acid was administered as an initial loading dose of 1 g over 10 minutes, followed by 1 g over 8 hours as an infusion. Each treatment pack contained four ampoules of tranexamic acid, 500 mg.

43.7 Control

The control group received normal saline as a placebo. The treatment packs of tranexamic acid and placebo were identical and ensured blinding.

43.8 Sample Size

The risk of death in study patients was assumed to be around 20%. The authors considered a 2% improvement in survival among tranexamic acid-treated patients as a clinically important benefit. The sample size required to identify this difference was estimated to be 20,000 patients, allowing an 85% chance of attaining a two-sided p value of <0.01, and a 95% chance of a two-sided p value of <0.05. Analysis was on an intention-to-treat basis.

43.9 Results

A total of 20, 211 were randomized—10,096 patients were assigned to receive tranexamic acid and 10,015 patients to receive placebo. After exclusion of patients who withdrew consent and those who were lost to follow-up, in the final analysis, 10,060 patients were included in the tranexamic acid arm, and 10,060 patients in the placebo arm.

Patients in the tranexamic acid and placebo arms were well-matched at baseline; more patients suffered blunt (67.5% vs. 67.7%) compared to penetrating injury. The median time from injury to enrolment was 2.8 vs. 2.9 hours.

43.10 The Primary Outcome: All-Cause Hospital Mortality at 4 Weeks

The all-cause mortality was significantly lower in the tranexamic acid group; 1463/10,060 (14.5%) patients died in the tranexamic acid group compared with 1613/10,067 (16.0%) patients in the placebo group. The relative risk of mortality with tranexamic acid was 0.91, 95% CI: (0.85–0.97), $p = 0.0035$. Based on these figures, 67 patients required tranexamic acid treatment to save one life (the number needed to treat, NNT). The fragility index (the minimum number of patients who need to change from survivor to non-survivor status to make the result non-significant) was 48, larger than most contemporary landmark studies. On subgroup analysis, there was no difference in the all-cause mortality in subgroups of patients based on systolic blood pressures, the Glasgow coma score, blunt vs. penetrating injury, and those who received early compared to late treatment with tranexamic acid.

43.11 Secondary Outcomes

Death due to bleeding was also lower in the tranexamic acid group (4.9% vs. 5.7%, $p = 0.0077$). Mortality associated with vascular occlusion (a potential complication of tranexamic acid use), including myocardial infarction, stroke, and pulmonary embolism, was similar between the two groups. Similarly, deaths due to multiorgan failure and traumatic brain injury were also similar. Transfusion of blood products

Table 43.1 Main study outcomes

Outcome	Tranexamic acid (%)	Placebo (%)	Significance
All-cause mortality	14.5	16	$P = 0.0035$
Death due to bleeding	4.9	5.7	$P = 0.0077$
Dependent	12.9	12.6	$P = 0.63$
Blood product transfusion	50.4	51.3	$P = 0.21$

and the number of surgical interventions performed were also similar between the two groups. The number of patients who were dead or dependent at discharge or 28 days, and those who were asymptomatic at 28 days, were also not significantly different between the two groups. The main study outcomes are summarized in Table 43.1.

43.12 Study Conclusions

The CRASH-2 trial concluded that tranexamic acid significantly reduces the risk of death in trauma patients with significant bleeding, particularly when administered within 3 hours of injury. The study found no significant increase in vascular occlusive events, making TXA a safe and effective intervention for bleeding trauma patients.

43.13 Strengths of the Study

The CRASH-2 trial was one of the largest RCTs in critical care and was powered to detect a 2% difference in mortality. Being multicentric, involving 274 centers in 40 countries, it had robust external validity. The study was blinded, minimizing the risk of bias. The loss to follow-up was minimal. The primary outcome was mortality, an important and clinically appropriate endpoint.

43.14 Limitations

One of the criteria for study inclusion was a risk of significant bleeding as judged by the clinician; the subjectivity in decision-making could have led to selection bias. The treating clinicians could decide to use tranexamic acid if they considered it to be clinically indicated, and thus exclude the patient from the trial. The number of patients excluded by this criterion is unclear. Considering the relatively low incidence of occlusive events, definitive conclusions cannot be drawn regarding whether tranexamic acid administration may lead to such events. The fibrinolytic activity was not evaluated, casting doubts over the mechanism of action of tranexamic acid. Although the authors hypothesized that the efficacy of tranexamic acid might be due to its inhibitory effect on pathological hyperfibrinolytic activity that may occur in bleeding trauma patients, there is no substantive evidence to support this theory. The use of blood products was not different between groups. The lack of an effect on transfusions may be because decisions on blood product administration are usually made in the early phase of trauma, much earlier than the 8-hour window during which tranexamic acid was administered. Furthermore, it is quite likely that survival alone could have resulted in a greater window of opportunity to receive transfusions (competing risks). There was no stratification based on the severity of injury, hence it is unclear whether the efficacy of tranexamic acid may be confined to subgroups of patients with severe injury.

43.15 Subsequent Evidence

43.15.1 Exploratory Analysis

In an exploratory analysis published a year later, the investigators evaluated the effect of the timing of tranexamic acid administration on outcomes [5]. Overall, 1063 deaths (35%) occurred due to bleeding. Early treatment saved more lives. Death due to bleeding among patients who were administered tranexamic acid within the first hour of injury was significantly lower compared with placebo (5.3% vs. 7.7%; RR: 0.68, 95% CI 0.57–0.82). Administration between 1 and 3 hours also led to reduced bleeding-related mortality (4.8% vs. 6.1%; RR 0.79, 95% CI 0.64–0.97). In contrast, tranexamic acid administration after 3 hours of injury appeared to increase mortality. This exploratory analysis strongly suggested that early treatment, within the first 3 hours, saves lives; later treatment may, in fact, lead to harm. The systolic blood pressure, Glasgow coma score, or type of injury had no impact on the effect of tranexamic acid on death due to bleeding.

43.15.2 The MATTERS Study

The Military Application of Tranexamic Acid in Trauma Emergency Resuscitation (MATTERS) study evaluated the use of tranexamic acid in the combat setting to assess the impact on coagulopathy and survival following battlefield injury. This retrospective observational study compared tranexamic administration to a control group that received standard care alone; patients included in the study had received at least one unit of packed red cells. The study was conducted at a single surgical center at Camp Bastion in Southern Afghanistan. Patients who received tranexamic acid revealed lower mortality compared to the control group (17.4% vs 23.9%; $p = 0.03$). Improved survival was particularly evident among the most severely injured, in penetrating trauma, and those requiring more than 10 units of red cell transfusion (14.4% vs 28.1%; $p = 0.004$). The authors concluded that tranexamic acid administration combined with resuscitation based on blood products leads to improved survival and alleviation of coagulopathy. The most profound benefit was observed among patients who underwent massive transfusion. They went on to recommend tranexamic acid as part of the resuscitation strategy in severe wartime injury and hemorrhage [6]. A later study by the same group found that cryoprecipitate in combination with tranexamic acid may enhance survival benefit among victims of combat injuries who required red cell transfusion [7].

43.16 The Impact of the Study

The CRASH-2 trial, despite limitations, generated a cascading impact in clinical practice, leading to widespread acceptance and adoption by the British and American armies. The British army introduced its use in the battlefields of Afghanistan; the WHO added tranexamic acid to its list of essential medicines. However, ambivalence and inertia with the routine use of tranexamic acid in severe trauma were evident in some healthcare settings, perhaps due to the indifference of pharmaceutical companies in promoting a cheap, generic drug. As Ian Roberts, one of the CRASH-2 collaborators, surmised, "if pharma is not interested, it's not done." The CRASH-2 trial also stimulated research on tranexamic administration in other types of bleeding. The WOMAN trial, published in 2017, included more than 20,000 patients, revealed that it is highly effective in postpartum hemorrhage; tranexamic acid significantly reduced death due to bleeding with no apparent adverse effects [8].

43.17 Summary

Exsanguinating hemorrhage from severe trauma is a monumental health problem across the globe. The CRASH-2 trial revealed that an inexpensive, widely available, and easily administered drug could save lives in patients at risk of bleeding following severe trauma. It was a large, pragmatic, real-world study conducted across several continents, thus establishing the generalizability of the results. Although the mechanism of action is unsubstantiated, tranexamic acid represents an affordable method of improving survival in trauma-related hemorrhage, with no apparent increase in thrombosis-related complications. Pre-hospital administration of tranexamic acid to all trauma victims as a single bolus appears pragmatic and easy to apply in clinical practice. The CRASH-2 trial turned out to be a truly pivotal study with the potential to save lives through a simple intervention.

References

1. Okamoto S, Okamoto U. Amino-methyl-cyclohexane-carboxylic acid: Amcha. Keio J Med. 1962;11(3):105–15.
2. Lawson JH, Murphy MP. Challenges for providing effective hemostasis in surgery and trauma. Semin Hematol. 2004;41(1 Suppl 1):55–64.
3. Henry DA, Carless PA, Moxey AJ, O'Connell D, Stokes BJ, McClelland B, et al. Anti-fibrinolytic use for minimising perioperative allogeneic blood transfusion. Cochrane Database Syst Rev. 2007;(4):CD001886.

4. CRASH-2 trial collaborators, Shakur H, Roberts I, Bautista R, Caballero J, Coats T, et al. Effects of tranexamic acid on death, vascular occlusive events, and blood transfusion in trauma patients with significant haemorrhage (CRASH-2): a randomised, placebo-controlled trial. Lancet Lond Engl. 2010;376(9734):23–32.
5. CRASH-2 collaborators, Roberts I, Shakur H, Afolabi A, Brohi K, Coats T, et al. The importance of early treatment with tranexamic acid in bleeding trauma patients: an exploratory analysis of the CRASH-2 randomised controlled trial. Lancet Lond Engl. 2011;377(9771):1096–101. 1101.e1–2
6. Morrison JJ, Dubose JJ, Rasmussen TE, Midwinter MJ. Military Application of Tranexamic Acid in Trauma Emergency Resuscitation (MATTERs) Study. Arch Surg Chic Ill 1960. 2012;147(2):113–9.
7. Morrison JJ, Ross JD, Dubose JJ, Jansen JO, Midwinter MJ, Rasmussen TE. Association of cryoprecipitate and tranexamic acid with improved survival following wartime injury: findings from the MATTERs II Study. JAMA Surg. 2013;148(3):218–25.
8. WOMAN Trial Collaborators. Effect of early tranexamic acid administration on mortality, hysterectomy, and other morbidities in women with post-partum haemorrhage (WOMAN): an international, randomised, double-blind, placebo-controlled trial. Lancet Lond Engl. 2017;389(10084):2105–16.

Part IX

Extracorporeal Support

44 Extracorporeal Membrane Oxygenation in Acute Respiratory Failure: The CESAR Trial

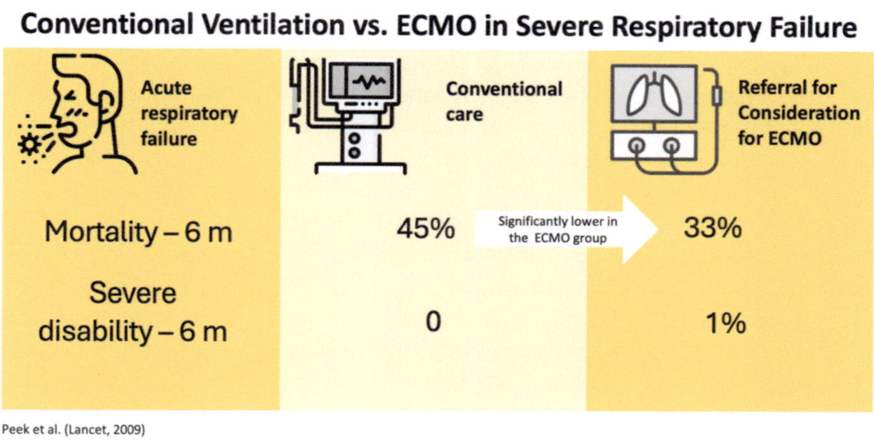

Quick Take

Does extracorporeal membrane oxygenation (ECMO) improve outcomes in patients with severe adult respiratory failure?

The CESAR trial compared the efficacy and cost-effectiveness of ECMO vs. conventional ventilatory support in patients with severe adult respiratory failure. A total of 180 patients were randomized to receive either conventional care or ECMO. The trial found that ECMO was associated with a significant reduction in 6-month survival without major disability. However, the study also highlighted the

---

Peek GJ, Mugford M, Tiruvoipati R, Wilson A, Allen E, Thalanany MM, et al. Efficacy and economic assessment of conventional ventilatory support versus extracorporeal membrane oxygenation for severe adult respiratory failure (CESAR): a multicentre randomised controlled trial. Lancet Lond Engl. 2009 Oct 17;374(9698):1351–63.

J. Chacko et al., *Landmark Studies in Critical Care*,
https://doi.org/10.1007/978-981-95-0673-6_44

substantial costs associated with ECMO, which raises important considerations for resource allocation in critical care. The trial established ECMO as a viable option for patients with severe, refractory respiratory failure.

44.1 Introduction

By the turn of the millennium, refinements in ventilation strategies, including the use of low tidal volumes and optimal application of positive end-expiratory pressure (PEEP), led to improved outcomes in patients with acute respiratory distress syndrome (ARDS). However, the mortality in severe ARDS remained between 34% and 58% [1, 2].

Ventilator-induced lung injury (VILI) may lead to worsening of lung damage in ARDS [3]. Volutrauma occurs due to injury related to alveolar overdistension, while the use of high ventilation pressures leads to dissection of air along the facial planes and accumulation in the pleural space. Repeated opening and closing of unstable lung units during each respiratory cycle leads to atelectrauma, characterized by increased stress at the junction between open and closed alveoli. Injurious ventilation patterns provoke biotrauma—a massive surge of inflammatory mediators, including cytokines and chemokines, that trigger lung edema, migration of neutrophils, and capillary vasodilatation. Besides, pulmonary toxicity related to high FiO_2 levels may add insult to injury in the severely damaged lung [4].

Considering the inevitable worsening of lung injury induced by suboptimal ventilation strategies, extracorporeal gas exchange was regarded as a viable option for several decades. The concept of venovenous extracorporeal membrane oxygen (VV-ECMO) arose from the basic design of cardiopulmonary bypass, which had been long established for open heart surgery. VV-ECMO involves the drainage of venous blood through a pump into an oxygenator where gas exchange occurs. The oxygenated blood is returned into the venous system. Extracorporeal gas exchange enables using less injurious ventilation techniques while "resting" the lung and allowing it time to heal.

The first-ever randomized controlled trial (RCT) on ECMO for acute respiratory failure by Zapol et al. was published in the *Journal of American Medical Association* in November 1979 [5]. They included patients between 12 and 65 years of age. The study followed two different protocols—a "fast" and a "slow" entry. Patients with a PO_2 below 50 mm Hg while on an FiO_2 of 1.0 and PEEP of 5 cm H_2O for more than 2 hours were assigned to the fast protocol. Patients who underwent optimal medical therapy for 48 hours, with a PaO_2 of less than 50 mm Hg while on FiO_2 0.6 and a PEEP of 5 cm H_2O, were assigned to the "slow" entry protocol. Pneumonia was the most common cause of acute respiratory failure (66%). Venoarterial bypass was carried out based on contemporary practice, using roller pumps in vogue during the study period. Four types of membrane oxygenators were employed, with intravenous heparin for anticoagulation. If stability was attained, the bypass flow was weaned at 0.5 l every 12 hours. Both groups of patients received mechanical ventilation and adjustment of PEEP based on clinician judgment; no standard protocol was followed. Sedatives, muscle relaxants, and antibiotics were administered as appropriate. ECMO could be weaned off based on the discretion of the clinician if the PaO_2 remained consistently >70 mm Hg on an FiO_2 <0.6. The clinician, in their best judgment, could also terminate ECMO support if no improvement was observed after 5 days of therapy.

The results of this early RCT were disheartening. Overall, there were just eight survivors, four in each group, with no discernible benefit from ECMO. The authors hypothesized that a shorter duration of mechanical ventilation before initiation of ECMO may improve survival—seven of the eight survivors had been on ventilation for less than a week before the commencement of ECMO.

Several years later, Morris et al. evaluated the impact of extracorporeal CO_2 removal combined with low-frequency positive pressure ventilation in another RCT. The results of this study were equally disappointing, with no apparent beneficial effect of extracorporeal CO_2 removal on the 30-day survival. The design and devices employed in these early studies were modifications of the heart-lung machine, primarily used during open heart surgery. Considering the major advancements in mechanical ventilation and ECMO technology since these early studies, the CESAR trial investigators aimed to evaluate the safety, efficacy, and cost-effectiveness of ECMO compared with conventional mechanical ventilation in a rigorous RCT.

44.2 Population, Setting, and Design

The CESAR trial was conducted between July 2001 and August 2006 across multiple centers in the UK [6]. The study population included patients aged 18–65 years with potentially reversible acute respiratory failure. Patients with a Murray Score ≥3, or uncompensated hypercapnia with a pH <7.2, were eligible. Patients who were being ventilated with a peak inspiratory pressure of >30 cm H_2O, or on an FiO_2 >0.8 for 7 days, those who had intracranial hemorrhage, contraindication to anticoagulation with heparin, and those in whom limitation of care was planned were excluded. A total of 180 patients were randomized—90 each to the ECMO and conventional ventilation arms.

Conventional mechanical ventilation was carried out in 92 tertiary centers. Patients from 11 other hospitals were transferred to either the ECMO center or the tertiary center, depending on the assigned modality of care—ECMO or conventional mechanical ventilation. Eligible patients were randomized in a 1:1 ratio. In the intervention group, patients were transferred to the specialist center for consideration of ECMO therapy. In the control group, conventional mechanical ventilation or high-frequency oscillation ventilation was carried out as appropriate.

44.3 The ECMO Group

Patients randomized to the ECMO group were transferred to the specialist center at Glenfield Hospital, Leicester. A standardized ventilation protocol was commenced if they were hemodynamically stable. This included restriction of ventilation pressure to 30 cm H_2O, and PEEP titrated to oxygen saturation. The FiO_2 was adjusted to maintain oxygen saturation >90%. Other modalities of care included the use of prone ventilation, diuretics, and a target packed cell volume of 40%. ECMO was carried out if there was no satisfactory response within 12 hours of protocolized care, with an FiO_2 requirement of >0.9 or acidosis with pH >7.2, or if hemodynamic instability occurred.

ECMO was carried out in the venovenous mode, following percutaneous cannulation. Ventilation during ECMO was performed in the pressure-controlled mode, at peak pressures of 20–25 cm H_2O, PEEP of 10–15 cm H_2O, respiratory rate of 10/minute, and FiO_2 of 0.3. ECMO was continued until clinical improvement or if irreversible multiorgan failure was deemed to have occurred.

44.4 The Control Group

Patients randomized to the control group were offered the best available care at the tertiary center. A tidal volume of 4–8 ml/kg and plateau pressure <30 cm H_2O was recommended; however, considering the pragmatic nature of the trial, a strict protocol was not mandated. Crossover to ECMO was not allowed.

44.5 Sample Size

The primary outcome was death or severe disability at 6 months. Severe disability represented confinement to bed and inability to wash or dress independently. The initial sample size of 120 patients per group was based on a reduction in the primary outcome from 73% to 55% with ECMO. The sample size was reduced to 90 patients per group after review by the data monitoring committee during the course of the study.

44.6 Results

During the study period, 766 patients were screened for eligibility, of whom 180 were randomized—for consideration for ECMO or conventional management. One hundred and three patients were excluded because ECMO beds were unavailable. Among the 90 patients allocated to the ECMO group, five died before they reached the ECMO center. From among the remaining 85 patients, 68 underwent ECMO, while 17 received the standardized ventilation protocol at the ECMO center.

44.6.1 Primary Composite Outcome: Alive and Disability-Free at 6 Months

Overall, 57/90 patients (63%) allocated to the ECMO arm were alive and free of severe disability at 6 months—among these were 43/68 who actually received ECMO and 14/17 patients who received protocolized ventilation strategy at the ECMO center. In the conventional ventilation arm, 41 of 87 (47%) patients on whom full information was available were alive and free of severe disability at 6 months. Thus, patients allocated for the consideration of ECMO at the specialized center had a significantly reduced risk of death or severe disability at 6 months (relative risk: 0.69; 95% CI: 0.05–0.97, $p = 0.03$).

44.6.2 Mortality at 6 Months

Thirty-three patients (37%) had died before discharge or at 6 months in the ECMO group compared with 45 (45%) in the control group; the difference was not statistically significant ($p = 0.07$).

44.6.3 Severe Disability at 6 Months

None of the survivors in the ECMO group experienced severe disability at 6 months, compared to one with severe disability in the conventional group.

Respiratory failure was the cause of death in more patients in the control group compared to the ECMO group (60% vs. 24%). Multiorgan failure leading to death was more common in the ECMO group compared to the control group (42% vs. 33%). The ICU and hospital length of stay were longer among patients assigned to the ECMO arm compared to the control group.

44.6.4 Healthcare Costs

Treatment with ECMO came at a price—mean healthcare costs were more than twice as high compared with the control group. All patients underwent initiation of ECMO at the specialist center. The authors hypothesized that if ECMO could be initiated at the referring hospital prior to transfer, it might further improve outcomes. The main study outcomes are summarized in Table 44.1.

Table 44.1 Main study outcomes

Outcome at 6 months	ECMO group ($N = 90$) (%)	Control group ($N = 90$) (%)	Significance
Death or severe disability	37	53	$P = 0.03$
Death	37	45	$P = 0.07$
Severe disability	0	1	

Abbreviation: ECMO extracorporeal membrane oxygenation

44.7 Study Conclusions

At 6 months, survival without disability was significantly better in the group of patients who were transferred to a specialist center for consideration of ECMO compared with conventional mechanical ventilation. The 6-month mortality was also lower in the former group; however, the difference was not significant.

44.7.1 Strengths

The two RCTs that preceded the CESAR trial were conducted using outdated technology during an era when the lung protective ventilation strategy had not been established. The CESAR trial was a pragmatic RCT that compared conventional ventilation with transfer to a specialist center for consideration of ECMO. At the specialist center, ECMO was initiated if there was no improvement within a 12-hour period. This strategy is in tune with real-world practice. Patients were randomized at an early stage of illness; transfer to the assigned center was carried out by an expert team, with due consideration of the associated risks. The 6-month follow-up, as part of the primary outcome, was conducted by trained members of the research team, who were blinded to the assigned treatment.

44.7.2 Weaknesses

Twenty-two of 90 patients assigned to the ECMO arm did not receive ECMO. This included five patients who died before ECMO could be considered. The specialist center where patients were transferred for consideration of ECMO employed a protocolized ventilation strategy; however, no strict ventilation protocol was followed among patients in the control group who were treated at the 92 tertiary centers. Hence, it could be argued that the improved outcomes may have been at least partly due to a standardized ventilation strategy and perhaps better overall care at the ECMO center. The high survival rate (14/17) of patients who were assigned to ECMO, but managed with conventional ventilation at the specialist center may also point towards such an effect.

The primary outcome was a composite of death and severe disability at 6 months. Composite outcomes may be less preferred; the 6-month mortality, although lower in the ECMO arm, was not significantly different compared to the control group. On analysis based on the assigned treatment (in contrast to intention-to-treat), the mortality difference between groups was still less.

Recruitment was slow and took nearly twice as long as originally planned. The study ultimately took 5 years—a fairly long duration, over which outcomes may have generally improved.

44.7.3 Subsequent Studies

The H1N1 pandemic swept through Australia and New Zealand in the winter of 2009. Among 722 patients who were infected and admitted to ICUs, 68 patients underwent ECMO. These patients had a median PaO_2/FiO_2 ratio of 56 mm Hg and a median PEEP level of 18 cm H_2O. They were more severely ill than those in the CESAR trial based on the median acute lung injury score. The hospital survival of 75% in this observational study further bolstered the evidence to support the use of ECMO among the most severely hypoxic patients [7].

The EOLIA RCT compared ECMO with conventional ventilation in patients with a PaO_2/FiO_2 ratio of <50 mm Hg for >3 hours, or <80 mm Hg for >6 hours, or an arterial pH of <7.25 with PCO_2 >60 mm Hg for >6 hours [8]. Patients in the conventional ventilation arm were allowed to cross over to receive ECMO if they had refractory hypoxemia with oxygen saturation <80% for >6 hours. The 60-day mortality, the primary endpoint, was not significantly different between the ECMO and control groups (35% vs. 46%, $p = 0.09$). However, the key secondary endpoint was treatment failure, defined as death or crossover to ECMO in the control group and death in the ECMO group. Treatment failure was significantly higher in the control group compared to the ECMO group (58% vs. 35%, $p < 0.001$).

When COVID-19 pneumonia spread across the globe in the recent past, leaving in its trail wave after wave of severely hypoxemic patients, ECMO was widely used by many healthcare systems. In a meta-analysis of 58,472 patients, 4044 patients underwent ECMO therapy. The mortality was higher with COVID-19 compared to patients with influenza pneumonia who were treated with ECMO (44% vs. 38%) [9]. However, ECMO therapy probably saved many lives among patients with severe COVID-19 pneumonia who did not respond to conventional therapies.

The cumulative evidence overwhelmingly supports the use of ECMO in patients with refractory hypoxia when conventional ventilation strategies fail. However, conducting yet another RCT to cement the evidence in favor of ECMO may remain an elusive goal considering its ubiquitous use in specialized centers across the world.

44.8 Summary

After long years of disappointing results, the CESAR trial represented the first RCT that evaluated the use of a technologically advanced ECMO design. Although there were shortcomings, it was a pragmatic trial that reflected real-world practice. Patients in the ECMO arm had significantly higher disability-free survival at 6 months compared to a conventional ventilation strategy. The observational trials during the H1N1 pandemic and the subsequent EOLIA trial support the use of ECMO in patients with refractory hypoxia.

References

1. Rubenfeld GD, Herridge MS. Epidemiology and outcomes of acute lung injury. Chest. 2007;131(2):554–62.
2. Bersten AD, Edibam C, Hunt T, Moran J, Australian and New Zealand Intensive Care Society Clinical Trials Group. Incidence and mortality of acute lung injury and the acute respiratory distress syndrome in three Australian States. Am J Respir Crit Care Med. 2002;165(4):443–8.
3. Gattinoni L, Tonetti T, Cressoni M, Cadringher P, Herrmann P, Moerer O, et al. Ventilator-related causes of lung injury: the mechanical power. Intensive Care Med. 2016;42(10):1567–75.
4. Hochberg CH, Semler MW, Brower RG. Oxygen toxicity in critically ill adults. Am J Respir Crit Care Med. 2021;204(6):632–41.
5. Zapol WM. Extracorporeal membrane oxygenation in severe acute respiratory failure: a randomized prospective study. JAMA. 1979;242(20):2193.
6. Peek GJ, Mugford M, Tiruvoipati R, Wilson A, Allen E, Thalanany MM, et al. Efficacy and economic assessment of conventional ventilatory support versus extracorporeal membrane oxygenation for severe adult respiratory failure (CESAR): a multicentre randomised controlled trial. Lancet Lond Engl. 2009;374(9698):1351–63.
7. ANZIC Influenza Investigators, Webb SAR, Pettilä V, Seppelt I, Bellomo R, Bailey M, Cooper DJ, Cretikos M, Davies AR, Finfer S, Harrigan PWJ, Hart GK, Howe B, Iredell JR, McArthur C, Mitchell I, Morrison S, Nichol AD, Paterson DL, Peake S, Richards B, Stephens D, Turner A, Yung M. Critical care services and 2009 H1N1 influenza in Australia and New Zealand. N Engl J Med. 2009;361(20):1925–34.
8. Combes A, Hajage D, Capellier G, Demoule A, Lavoué S, Guervilly C, et al. Extracorporeal membrane oxygenation for severe acute respiratory distress syndrome. N Engl J Med. 2018;378(21):1965–75.
9. Bertini P, Guarracino F, Falcone M, Nardelli P, Landoni G, Nocci M, et al. ECMO in COVID-19 patients: a systematic review and meta-analysis. J Cardiothorac Vasc Anesth. 2022;36(8):2700–6.

45 Extracorporeal Membrane Oxygenation in Severe Acute Respiratory Distress Syndrome: The EOLIA Trial

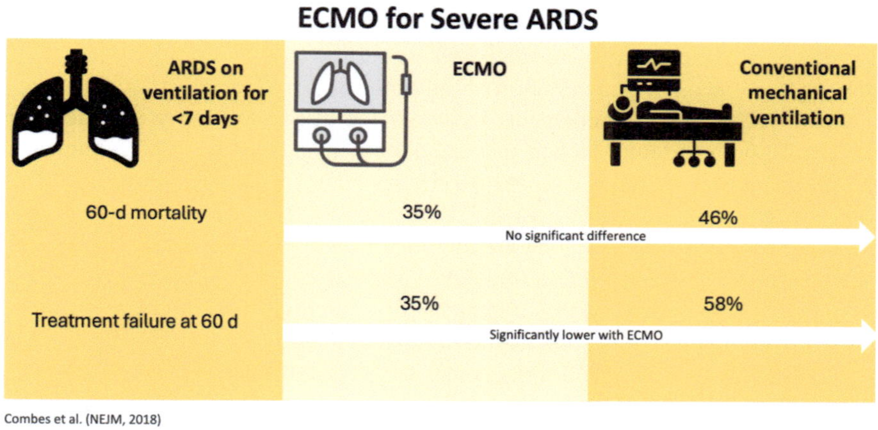

Quick Take

Can extracorporeal membrane oxygenation (ECMO) turn the tide and save lives in severe acute respiratory distress syndrome (ARDS)?

The EOLIA trial investigated the use of ECMO in patients with severe ARDS. This multicenter, randomized trial compared ECMO to conventional mechanical ventilation strategies in ARDS patients who were not responding to standard treatments. The study found that ECMO did not significantly improve 60-day mortality compared to conventional management. However, ECMO was associated with a lower incidence of death due to refractory hypoxemia, and there

---

Combes A, Hajage D, Capellier G, Demoule A, Lavoué S, Guervilly C, et al. Extracorporeal Membrane Oxygenation for Severe Acute Respiratory Distress Syndrome. N Engl J Med. 2018 May 24;378(21):1965–75.

J. Chacko et al., *Landmark Studies in Critical Care*,
https://doi.org/10.1007/978-981-95-0673-6_45

was a trend toward improved long-term outcomes. The trial suggests that ECMO may be beneficial in specific subsets of ARDS patients, but it also highlights the need for further research to identify which patients are most likely to benefit from this intensive therapy.

45.1 Introduction

Despite advancements in ventilation strategy, ARDS carries high mortality [1]. In 1979, Zapol et al. conducted the first-ever randomized controlled trial (RCT) of ECMO in patients with severe acute respiratory failure [2]. They included patients between 12 and 65 years of age; most patients had severe community-acquired pneumonia leading to respiratory failure. ECMO therapy turned out to be hugely disappointing in this early trial, with mortality exceeding 90% in the ECMO and the control arms. However, ECMO technology was in its infancy; the study employed a veno-arterial strategy using roller pumps. Furthermore, the ventilation strategy was not standardized and was conducted well before the benefits of a lung-protective strategy were recognized by the turn of the century.

Major technological refinements have evolved in the ensuing years since this early RCT with the introduction of veno-venous bypass, centrifugal pumps, and membrane oxygenators [3]. During the H1N1 pandemic of 2009, many researchers reported improved outcomes with ECMO therapy in observational studies [4, 5]. The CESAR RCT evaluated the efficacy of ECMO among patients with severe ARDS who were randomized to transfer to a specialist center for consideration of ECMO or receive conventional treatment [6]. Patients in the intervention group experienced improved clinical outcomes in this trial. However, the comparison was between transfer to a single referral center for consideration of ECMO and a non-protocolized management strategy at multiple centers, limiting the robustness of the findings. Considering the lack of firm evidence for the use of ECMO in severe ARDS, the Rescue Lung Injury in Severe ARDS (EOLIA) trial was designed to evaluate the impact of early ECMO initiation on clinical outcomes among patients with severe ARDS [7].

45.2 Population and Design

The EOLIA trial was an international trial conducted over a 6-year period across 64 centers, predominantly in France. Patients who met the American–European Consensus definition for ARDS and were on invasive mechanical ventilation for less than 7 days were eligible if they met the following severity criteria despite an optimal ventilation strategy, including $FiO_2 \geq 0.8$, tidal volume of 6 ml/kg, and PEEP of ≥ 10 cm H_2O.

- PaO_2/FiO_2 ratio of <50 mm Hg for >3 hours
- PaO_2/FiO_2 ratio of <80 mm Hg for >6 hours
- Arterial pH <7.25 with $PaCO_2$ of ≥60 mm Hg for >6 hours with a respiratory rate of 35/minute and Pplat ≤32 cm H_2O

The use of neuromuscular blockade and prone positioning were encouraged before study entry. Rescue therapies, including inhaled nitric oxide, recruitment maneuvers, and high-frequency oscillation ventilation, were left to the clinician's discretion, based on local practices.

45.2.1 Excluded

The study excluded patients with a body weight of >1 kg/cm of height or a body mass index of >45, those with chronic respiratory insufficiency on home oxygen therapy or non-invasive ventilation, cardiac failure necessitating veno-arterial ECMO, a Simplified Acute Physiology Score (SAPS II) of >90, and those with heparin-induced thrombocytopenia. Patients who remained comatose after cardiac arrest, those with irreversible neurological injury, and those in whom life-sustaining therapies were withheld or withdrawn were also excluded.

Eligible patients were randomized to undergo ECMO or conventional mechanical ventilation (control group). Randomization was stratified by center and based on the duration of ventilation before randomization.

45.3 ECMO Group

Veno-venous cannulation was performed by the percutaneous route. Anticoagulation was carried out with unfractionated heparin, titrated to an activated partial thromboplastin time of 40–55 seconds or anti-Xa activity 0.2–0.3 IU/ml.

45.4 Control Group

Patients were ventilated using the increased recruitment strategy employed in the EXPRESS trial [8]. The PEEP was titrated as high as possible while maintaining the plateau pressure below 28–30 cm of H_2O, regardless of the effect on oxygenation. Neuromuscular blockade and prone ventilation for extended durations were encouraged. If oxygenation targets were not met, recruitment maneuvers, inhaled nitric oxide, or intravenous almitrine were allowed based on the clinician's discretion.

Patients in the control group who experienced refractory hypoxemia despite conventional measures (saturation <80% for >6 hours) could crossover to receive ECMO, provided irreversible multiorgan failure had not set in according to clinical judgment.

45.5 Sample Size

The sample size was calculated based on the 60-day mortality, the primary endpoint. The use of ECMO therapy was assumed to result in an absolute reduction in mortality by 20% (from 60% in the control group). The authors calculated a sample size of 331 patients, which provided the study with 80% power at an alpha level of 5%.

45.6 Results

The trial was ceased for futility after enrolment of 249 patients when the fourth interim analysis revealed no significant difference between groups in the 60-day mortality. Among the 1015 patients screened, 124 were randomized to undergo ECMO, while 125 were included in the control group.

Patients were well-matched at baseline. The mean SOFA score and PaO_2/FiO_2 ratio were similar in both groups. The most common etiology of ARDS was bacterial pneumonia. The ventilation parameters and arterial blood gases were also similar at baseline. Rescue therapies, including prone ventilation, the use of neuromuscular blockade, inhaled nitric oxide, and prostacyclin, were not significantly different between the two groups.

ECMO was commenced at 3.3 ± 2.8 hours after randomization. The mean duration of ECMO support was 15 ± 13 days.

The tidal volume, plateau pressure, driving pressure, and respiratory rate decreased from baseline in the ECMO group. Among patients in the control group, 90% underwent prone ventilation, and 83% were treated with inhaled nitric oxide or prostacyclin; neuromuscular blockers were administered to all patients.

45.7 The Primary Endpoint: 60-Day Mortality

The 60-day mortality was lower among patients who received ECMO, although the difference fell short of statistical significance. Among 124 ECMO-treated patients, 44 (35%) had died at 60 days, compared with 57 of 125 (46%) patients in the control group (hazard ratio, 0.7; 95% CI, 0.47 to 1.04; $P = 0.07$). The results remained unchanged after adjustment for prognostic factors.

45.7.1 Key Secondary Endpoint—Treatment Failure

Treatment failure at 60 days—death in the ECMO group and death or crossover to ECMO in the control group—was significantly higher in the control group. At

60 days, 72 of 125 (58%) experienced treatment failure in the control group—significantly higher compared to 44 of 124 (35%) patients in the ECMO group ($P < 0.001$).

45.8 Other Secondary Endpoints at 60 Days

At 60 days, patients in the ECMO group experienced more prone ventilation-free days compared to the control group (median: 59 vs. 64 days). Based on the Sequential Organ Failure Assessment (SOFA score), renal failure-free days (median: 46 vs. 21 days) and cardiac failure-free days (median: 48 vs. 41 days) were higher in the ECMO group. Patients in the ECMO group also underwent significantly fewer days of renal replacement therapy.

On subgroup analysis, the 60-day mortality was not associated with baseline demographic characteristics, severity of ARDS, or type of center (ECMO centers vs. non-ECMO centers).

45.9 Crossover from the Control Group to ECMO

Thirty-five patients (28%) received ECMO in the control group for refractory hypoxemia. The characteristics of patients who crossed over from the control group to receive ECMO were strongly suggestive of more severe ARDS—they had higher plateau pressure, driving pressure, lower respiratory system compliance, and more extensive infiltrates on the chest radiograph. The median PaO_2/FiO_2 ratio was a low 51 mm Hg, and the oxygen saturation was 77% at the time of crossover. At 60 days, 20 of 35 patients (57%) who crossed over from the control group to receive ECMO had died.

45.10 Adverse Events

Two deaths occurred due to complications that arose following ECMO cannulation. Severe thrombocytopenia (platelet count <20,000/cu mm) and episodes of bleeding requiring transfusion occurred more often in the ECMO group. There was a similar incidence of pneumothorax, ventilator-associated pneumonia, and massive hemorrhage in both groups. Among ECMO-treated patients, the incidence of bleeding was 53%, hematoma at the cannula site, 6%, infection at the cannula site 14%, and intravascular hemolysis, 5%. The main study results are summarized in Table 45.1.

Table 45.1 Main study results

Outcome	ECMO (124 patients)	Control (125 patients)	Relative risk or difference (95% CI)	*P* value
60-d mortality	44 (35%)	57 (46%)	0.76 (0.55–1.04)	0.09
Treatment failure at 60 days	44 (35%)	72 (58%)	0.62 (0.47–0.82)	<0.001
Renal failure-free days at 60 days	46	21	Median difference: 25 (6–53) days	
RRT-free days at 60 days	50	32	Median difference 18 (0–51)	
Cardiac failure-free days at 60 days	48	41	Median difference 7 (0–51) days	

Abbreviations: CI confidence interval, *RRT* renal replacement therapy

45.11 Study Conclusions

In patients with severe ARDS and refractory hypoxia, the 60-day mortality was similar between rescue ECMO therapy and continued conventional mechanical ventilation. Crossover to the ECMO arm occurred in 28% of patients in the conventional ventilation group. Treatment failure at 60 days, defined as death in the ECMO group and death over crossover to ECMO in the control group, was significantly lower in the ECMO group. The frequency of complications did not differ, except for a higher incidence of bleeding requiring transfusion in the ECMO group.

45.12 Strengths

Although ECMO had been in use for hypoxemic respiratory failure for decades with favorable results, no controlled trial had specifically evaluated clinical outcomes compared with standard ventilatory management. To date, the EOLIA trial is the largest multicentric RCT to date that assessed the efficacy of ECMO in severe ARDS. The inclusion criteria were clearly defined; crossover was allowed among control patients for persisting refractory hypoxemia. Mechanical ventilation and the conduct of ECMO were carried out based on a standardized protocol.

45.13 Limitations

The study was ceased before attaining the calculated sample size following an interim analysis that revealed no significant mortality difference at 60 days. The premature cessation of the trial probably resulted in a small sample size and could have led to a type II error (false negative result). The sample size was calculated based on 60% mortality in the control group; however, the actual mortality was only 46%, which may also have led to an inadequate sample size. Furthermore, the authors assumed a 20% mortality reduction with ECMO, which may have reflected an unrealistic treatment effect. A substantial number of patients (28%) in the control group received ECMO as crossover was allowed, which may have resulted in favorable outcomes in the control group on intention-to-treat analysis. The decision to initiate ECMO among patients in the control group was largely based on clinician judgment. Patients were included from both ECMO centers and non-ECMO referral centers, which could have led to bias. However, patients at non-ECMO centers required initiation of ECMO by a retrieval team within 2 hours of randomization, followed by transfer to the ECMO center. The trial took nearly 6 years to complete, during which refinements in practice could have impacted outcomes. Although prone ventilation, proven to improve survival in ARDS, was encouraged, it was not part of a standardized protocol; only 56% of patients underwent prone ventilation prior to initiation of ECMO. A trial of prone ventilation is generally recommended before consideration of ECMO in severe ARDS with refractory hypoxia.

45.14 Subsequent Analysis

Goligher et al. performed a post hoc Bayesian analysis of the EOLIA trial, specifying statistical prior distributions [9]. In contrast to the findings of the EOLIA trial, their re-analysis suggested improved survival with ECMO compared with conventional mechanical ventilation. They estimated the probability of a clinically important mortality benefit ranging from a relative risk (RR) <1 to <0.67 (0.67 was the RR assumed in sample size calculation in the EOLIA trial) and absolute risk reduction from 2% to 20% (20% absolute risk reduction was assumed in the sample size calculation of the EOLIA trial). They estimated a 96% posterior probability of RR <1 for 60-day mortality in the ECMO group. Furthermore, in the ECMO group, the posterior probability of RR <0.67 was 18%; the probability of absolute risk reduction of 2% or more was 92%, while the probability of absolute risk reduction of ≥20% was 2%.

Although subject to the inherent weaknesses of such analysis, the Bayesian approach suggested a high probability of improved survival with ECMO in patients with severe ARDS. However, the benefit may not be as large as assumed in the design of the EOLIA trial.

45.15 Summary

In 1979, the first RCT that evaluated the efficacy of ECMO in severe acute respiratory failure did not reveal improved survival compared with a control group that received conventional mechanical ventilation. However, major advancements in the ECMO circuitry and technique have evolved since then. Later observational studies, particularly during the 2009 H1N1 pandemic, had revealed favorable clinical outcomes in patients with severe ARDS. Although the CESAR RCT revealed significantly lower mortality or severe disability at 6 months in the ECMO group, the study had methodological limitations. Considering the equipoise, the EOLIA trial group conducted an RCT to test the efficacy of ECMO compared with a control group that received conventional mechanical ventilation in severe ARDS.

The trial was terminated for futility after enrolment of 240 patients compared to the planned sample size of 331 patients. At this stage, the investigators observed an 11% absolute reduction in the 60-day mortality with ECMO; however, the difference was not statistically significant. One of the secondary outcomes was treatment failure at 60 days—death or crossover to ECMO in the control group and death in the ECMO group. Treatment failure was significantly higher in the control group. Those who experienced treatment failure in the control group included 28 patients (35%) who crossed over to receive ECMO.

Although the EOLIA trial did not reveal a significant difference in the primary endpoint of 60-day mortality, among the 35 patients who crossed over from the control group, 20 (43%) survived. The survival of these patients, who carried a dismal prognosis otherwise, suggested that ECMO is likely to be an effective rescue intervention among hypoxemic patients with severe ARDS. This finding assumes importance considering the ethical dilemma of conducting an adequately sized RCT in the future.

References

1. Bellani G, Laffey JG, Pham T, Fan E, Brochard L, Esteban A, et al. Epidemiology, patterns of care, and mortality for patients with acute respiratory distress syndrome in intensive care units in 50 countries. JAMA. 2016;315(8):788–800.
2. Zapol WM, Snider MT, Hill JD, Fallat RJ, Bartlett RH, Edmunds LH, et al. Extracorporeal membrane oxygenation in severe acute respiratory failure. A randomized prospective study. JAMA. 1979;242(20):2193–6.
3. Combes A, Brodie D, Bartlett R, Brochard L, Brower R, Conrad S, et al. Position paper for the organization of extracorporeal membrane oxygenation programs for acute respiratory failure in adult patients. Am J Respir Crit Care Med. 2014;190(5):488–96.
4. Noah MA, Peek GJ, Finney SJ, Griffiths MJ, Harrison DA, Grieve R, et al. Referral to an extracorporeal membrane oxygenation center and mortality among patients with severe 2009 influenza A(H1N1). JAMA. 2011;306(15):1659–68.
5. Australia and New Zealand Extracorporeal Membrane Oxygenation (ANZ ECMO) Influenza Investigators, Davies A, Jones D, Bailey M, Beca J, Bellomo R, et al. Extracorporeal membrane oxygenation for 2009 influenza A(H1N1) acute respiratory distress syndrome. JAMA. 2009;302(17):1888–95.
6. Peek GJ, Mugford M, Tiruvoipati R, Wilson A, Allen E, Thalanany MM, et al. Efficacy and economic assessment of conventional ventilatory support versus extracorporeal membrane oxygenation for severe adult respiratory failure (CESAR): a multicentre randomised controlled trial. Lancet. 2009;374(9698):1351–63.
7. Combes A, Hajage D, Capellier G, Demoule A, Lavoué S, Guervilly C, et al. Extracorporeal membrane oxygenation for severe acute respiratory distress syndrome. N Engl J Med. 2018;378(21):1965–75.
8. Mercat A, Richard JCM, Vielle B, Jaber S, Osman D, Diehl JL, et al. Positive end-expiratory pressure setting in adults with acute lung injury and acute respiratory distress syndrome: a randomized controlled trial. JAMA. 2008;299(6):646–55.
9. Goligher EC, Tomlinson G, Hajage D, Wijeysundera DN, Fan E, Jüni P, et al. Extracorporeal membrane oxygenation for severe acute respiratory distress syndrome and posterior probability of mortality benefit in a post hoc Bayesian analysis of a randomized clinical trial. JAMA. 2018;320(21):2251–9.

Part X
Infections

Duration of Antibiotic Therapy for Ventilator-Associated Pneumonia: The PNEUMA Trial

46

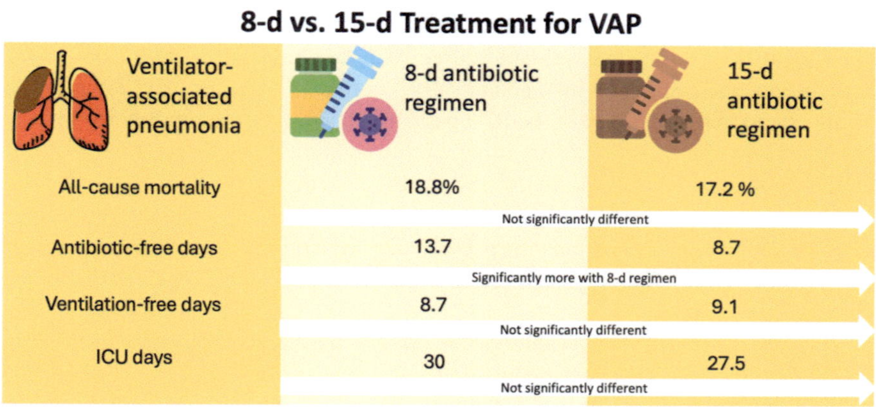

Chastre et al. (JAMA, 2003)

Quick Take

Are shorter antibiotic courses adequate for ventilator-associated pneumonia (VAP)?

This randomized controlled trial compared the duration of antibiotic therapy (8 days vs. 15 days) for VAP. A total of 1015 patients with VAP were randomized to receive either 8 or 15 days of antibiotics. The study found no significant difference in clinical outcomes, including mortality, between the two groups. However, the shorter duration of therapy (8 days) led to reduced antibiotic use, lower costs, and fewer adverse effects related to prolonged antibiotic treatment. The trial provided

---

Chastre J, Wolff M, Fagon JY, Chevret S, Thomas F, Wermert D, et al. Comparison of 8 vs 15 days of antibiotic therapy for ventilator-associated pneumonia in adults: a randomized trial. JAMA. 2003 Nov 19;290(19):2588–98.

J. Chacko et al., *Landmark Studies in Critical Care*,
https://doi.org/10.1007/978-981-95-0673-6_46

strong evidence that shorter courses of antibiotics are equally effective in treating VAP, supporting a shift toward more conservative antibiotic strategies to reduce resistance and complications.

46.1 Introduction

The occurrence of pneumonia has been a known complication among mechanically ventilated patients for more than half a century. In a report of cases from the 1950s, a disturbingly high incidence of necrotizing pneumonia due to gram-negative organisms was noted. The authors attributed the high incidence of nosocomial pneumonia to the use of mainstream reservoir nebulizers connected to the mechanical ventilators in use during this period [1]. In 1986, Craven et al. evaluated risk factors for ventilator-associated pneumonia among 233 patients. They observed that frequent changes of the ventilator circuit and the use of cimetidine, an H2-receptor antagonist, were among the important risk factors for VAP [2]. In an observational study, ICUs were by far the predominant source of nosocomial infections (53%), with most infections occurring in mechanically ventilated patients. Antibiotics were administered in the majority of the ICU patients (61%), most commonly for respiratory tract infections [3]. VAPs are often caused by multidrug-resistant bacteria [4]; effective therapy may be limited or even non-existent [5] in many cases. A more focused antibiotic strategy, with emphasis on better utilization, may confer benefits in dealing with resistant organisms. In particular, reducing the duration and number of antibiotics employed may curb the emergence and spread of multidrug-resistant organisms [6].

In the era preceding the conduct of the present study, the usual recommendation was to continue antibiotic treatment for 14–21 days among patients with VAP [7]. The risk of relapse after a shorter duration of therapy was considered high. However, in susceptible bacteria, the risk of relapse is likely to be low, in contrast to some species, such as *Pseudomonas aeruginosa*, which may take a longer duration of therapy for eradication. Adding to the problem was the poorly defined patient cohort in most trials and the non-standardized diagnostic approach.

The authors of the PNEUMA randomized controlled trial (RCT) sought to clear the ambiguity in the diagnosis and optimal duration of treatment of VAP. They confirmed the diagnosis of VAP by quantitative culture of bronchoscopic specimens and compared outcomes among patients treated with an 8- or 15-day course of antibiotics [8].

46.2 Population and Design

The trial was carried out between May 1999 and June 2002 across 51 ICUs in France. Patients who were on invasive mechanical ventilation were eligible if:

1. There was clinical suspicion of VAP, defined as a new, persistent, radiographic infiltrate with one of (a) purulent tracheal secretions, (b) white blood cell count of >10,000/μL, (c) temperature of ≥38.3 °C
2. Positive quantitative cultures from secretions obtained by bronchoscopy
3. Appropriate antibiotic therapy was commenced within 24 hours of bronchoscopy based on the sensitivity pattern

46.2.1 Excluded

Patients were excluded if they had a poor chance of survival, were neutropenic, had acquired immunodeficiency syndrome, were on steroids or long-term immunosuppressive agents. Those with extrapulmonary infection and onset of pneumonia within 5 days of mechanical ventilation who were not receiving antibiotics in the preceding 15 days were also excluded.

46.3 Randomization

Patients were randomized to receive antibiotics for 8 or 15 days once the quantitative cultures confirmed that the initial empirical treatment was appropriate.

The choice of antibiotic was at the discretion of the clinician. However, the protocol encouraged an initial empirical regimen that combined a broad-spectrum beta-lactam with an aminoglycoside or fluoroquinolone. Therapy was narrowed down based on the bronchoscopic cultures. Therapy was continued for 8 or 15 days based on the study arm unless more prolonged treatment was specifically indicated.

46.4 Sample Size

The investigators aimed to demonstrate noninferiority in terms of mortality and recurrence rates with the 8-day regimen compared to the 15-day regimen. Two hundred patients in each group provided the study with 90% power, assuming 40% mortality and 25% recurrence rates with the 15-day regimen. Besides, the sample size was appropriate to detect a 20% reduction in antibiotic-free days with the 8-day regimen, assuming a mean duration of 10 (±5) antibiotic-free days with the 15-day regimen.

46.5 Results

The trial enrolled 402 patients over a 3-year period. All except one patient who withdrew consent were included in the final analysis—197 were randomized to the 8-day regimen and 204 to the 15-day regimen. The baseline characteristics were similar in both groups of patients. During the initial 8 days of therapy, the antibiotics used in both groups were similar.

46.6 The Primary Outcomes

46.6.1 28-day Mortality After VAP Onset

At 28 days after the onset of VAP, the mortality was similar in both groups—18.8% in the 8-day regimen compared with 17.2% in the 15-day regimen (risk difference 1.6; 95% CI −3.7 to 6.9).

46.6.2 Recurrence Rates

Recurrence rates, based on quantitative cultures, were also similar in both groups (28.9% vs. 26%). The incidence of recurrent infection, considered to be relapses vs. superinfections, was similar.

46.6.3 Antibiotic-Free Days

Patients who received an 8-day regimen revealed significantly more antibiotic-free days (13.1 ± 7.4 vs. 8.7 ± 5.2 days, $P < 0.001$). The number of days of broad-spectrum antibiotic-free days was also lower with the 8-day regimen.

46.6.4 Analysis Adjusted for Baseline Variables

The risk ratio for mortality was similar between groups after adjustment for baseline variables, including age, gender, type of admission, duration of ventilation before VAP onset, severity of organ dysfunction, bacteremia, and type of pathogen.

46.7 Secondary Outcomes

Among the secondary outcomes, the duration of ventilation-free days was similar in the 8- and 15-day groups (8.7 vs. 9.1 days). The mean ICU length of stay was 30 days vs. 27.5 days—the difference was not statistically significant. Furthermore, the number of organ failure-free days did not differ significantly between the two groups (7.5 vs. 8.0 days).

Unfavorable outcomes, defined as death, recurrence of infection, or initiation of new antibiotic therapy, were also similar in both groups during the study period.

Table 46.1 Main study outcomes

Outcomes	8-day regimen	15-day regimen	Significance
All-cause mortality 28 days after VAP onset	18.8%	17.2%	Not significant
Mean antibiotic-free days	13.7 ± 7.4	8.7 ± 5.2	Significantly higher with the 8-day regimen
Mean ventilation-free days	8.7 ± 9.1	9.1 ± 9.4	Not significant
Mean organ failure-free days	7.5 ± 8.7	8.0 ± 8.9	Not significant
Mean ICU LOS	30 ± 20	27.5 ± 17.5	Not significant

Abbreviations: *VAP* ventilator-associated pneumonia, *LOS* length of stay

Among patients with VAP due to non-fermenting gram-negative bacilli, including *Pseudomonas aeruginosa*, outcomes were similar, except for a higher rate of recurrent pulmonary infection with an 8-day compared with a 15-day regimen. The main study outcomes are summarized in Table 46.1.

46.8 Study Conclusions

The study found no significant difference in clinical outcomes, including mortality among patients with VAP who were treated for 8 vs.15 days of antibiotic therapy. A shorter duration of therapy led to was associated with less antibiotic use, lower costs, and fewer adverse effects. Among patients infected with non-fermenting gram-negative bacilli, the authors noted a higher rate of recurrence with a shorter duration of treatment.

46.9 Strengths

The PNEUMA trial was a multicentric RCT with an adequate sample size to address the question of the duration of treatment of VAP. The diagnosis was confirmed by quantitative cultures, ensuring that the appropriate study population was included. The outcome measures, including mortality, recurrence rates, and antibiotic-free days, were clinically relevant. Recurrence rates were addressed based on the pathogen involved—including non-fermenting gram-negative bacilli. The study clearly demonstrated that a shorter duration of antibiotic therapy of 8 days was non-inferior to 15-day therapy.

46.10 Weaknesses

A shorter duration of treatment was associated with higher recurrence rates in non-fermenting gram-negative bacilli, raising concerns regarding the generalizability of the findings. The study excluded high-risk populations, including those who were immunosuppressed and had high severity scores, thus limiting its applicability to these subgroups of patients. Although the investigators followed a standard protocol, the choice of antibiotics and local resistance patterns may have influenced outcomes. Patients were followed up for 28 days—longer-term outcomes were not evaluated. The impact of the duration of antibiotic therapy on the emergence of resistant bacteria was not evaluated. Besides, the cost-effectiveness of a shorter duration of therapy was not analyzed.

46.11 Subsequent Evidence

In a re-analysis of the PENUMA trial, Combes et al. evaluated predictors of VAP recurrence [9]. Using a logistic regression model, they observed that the predictors of recurrent VAP on day 8 were the SAPS II score, radiological score, temperature, causation by gram-negative bacilli or methicillin-resistant *Staphylococcus aureus*, and dependence on mechanical ventilation. The predictors of 28-day mortality on day 8 were female gender, the SOFA score, and nonfermenting gram-negative bacilli as the underlying pathogen. The duration of therapy was not associated with adverse outcomes.

Bouglé et al. evaluated the efficacy of short-duration antibiotic therapy (8 days) compared with longer duration (15 days) in patients with VAP due to *Pseudomonas Aeruginosa*. Patients were randomized in a 1:1 ratio to short- or long-duration therapy. The study was stopped prematurely after the enrolment of 190 patients (the planned sample size was 600) due to slow recruitment. The composite primary endpoint of ICU mortality and recurrent VAP within 90 days was not significantly different between shorter and longer duration therapy (35.2% vs. 25.5%). Recurrent pneumonia occurred in nearly twice as many patients in the 8-day therapy group (17% vs. 9.2%). The duration of mechanical ventilation and ICU stay was similar in both groups. Due to premature cessation, the trial lacked adequate power to demonstrate a difference between the two groups [10].

46.12 Summary

At the time of the conduct of the PNEUMA trial, the usual practice was administration of antibiotics for typically around 15 days for VAP, based on the contention that a longer course was more effective in eradicating infection and preventing recurrence. There was a lack of high-quality evidence to guide the duration of antibiotic therapy, with recommendations based on expert opinion and observational studies. However, this practice was contentious and carried an increased risk of antibiotic resistance with the likelihood of adverse clinical outcomes. The PNEUMA trial aimed to address these concerns by evaluating whether a shorter course of antibiotics could be equally effective in the treatment of VAP, with similar clinical outcomes.

Patients with VAP, according to pre-defined criteria, were randomized to receive appropriate antibiotic therapy for 8 or 15 days.

A shorter duration of treatment was not associated with higher mortality or an increase in the incidence of recurrent pneumonia. Antibiotic-free days were significantly more with a shorter duration of treatment.

The authors observed a marginally higher rate of recurrence among patients infected with nonfermenting gram-negative bacilli who were assigned to the 8-day regimen. Despite the higher recurrence rate, the 8-day regimen was not associated with increased mortality or other unfavorable outcomes among this subgroup of patients. They concluded that an 8-day antibiotic regimen was non-inferior to a longer, 15-day regimen.

The study supports a shorter, 8-day antibiotic regimen for most patients diagnosed with VAP, providing treatment comparable with a longer, 15-day regimen that was recommended during the period of the study. Furthermore, a shorter duration of treatment offers the potential for enhanced antibiotic stewardship.

References

1. Reinarz JA, Pierce AK, Mays BB, Sanford JP. The potential role of inhalation therapy equipment in nosocomial pulmonary infection. J Clin Invest. 1965;44(5):831–9.
2. Craven DE, Kunches LM, Kilinsky V, Lichtenberg DA, Make BJ, McCabe WR. Risk factors for pneumonia and fatality in patients receiving continuous mechanical ventilation. Am Rev Respir Dis. 1986;133(5):792–6.
3. Bergmans DC, Bonten MJ, Gaillard CA, van Tiel FH, van der Geest S, de Leeuw PW, et al. Indications for antibiotic use in ICU patients: a one-year prospective surveillance. J Antimicrob Chemother. 1997;39(4):527–35.
4. Kollef MH, Fraser VJ. Antibiotic resistance in the intensive care unit. Ann Intern Med. 2001;134(4):298–314.
5. Mahgoub S, Ahmed J, Glatt AE. Completely resistant Acinetobacter baumannii strains. Infect Control Hosp Epidemiol. 2002;23(8):477–9.
6. Goldmann DA, Weinstein RA, Wenzel RP, Tablan OC, Duma RJ, Gaynes RP, et al. Strategies to prevent and control the emergence and spread of antimicrobial-resistant microorganisms in hospitals. A challenge to hospital leadership. JAMA. 1996;275(3):234–40.
7. Hospital-acquired pneumonia in adults: diagnosis, assessment of severity, initial antimicrobial therapy, and preventive strategies. A consensus statement, American Thoracic Society, 1995. Am J Respir Crit Care Med. 1996;153(5):1711–25.
8. Chastre J, Wolff M, Fagon JY, Chevret S, Thomas F, Wermert D, et al. Comparison of 8 vs 15 days of antibiotic therapy for ventilator-associated pneumonia in adults: a randomized trial. JAMA. 2003;290(19):2588–98.
9. Combes A, Luyt CE, Fagon JY, Wolff M, Trouillet JL, Chastre J. Early predictors for infection recurrence and death in patients with ventilator-associated pneumonia. Crit Care Med. 2007;35(1):146–54.
10. Bouglé A, Tuffet S, Federici L, Leone M, Monsel A, Dessalle T, et al. Comparison of 8 versus 15 days of antibiotic therapy for Pseudomonas aeruginosa ventilator-associated pneumonia in adults: a randomized, controlled, open-label trial. Intensive Care Med. 2022;48(7):841–9.

Duration of Hypotension Before Effective Antibiotic Therapy and Survival in Septic Shock: Kumar et al.

47

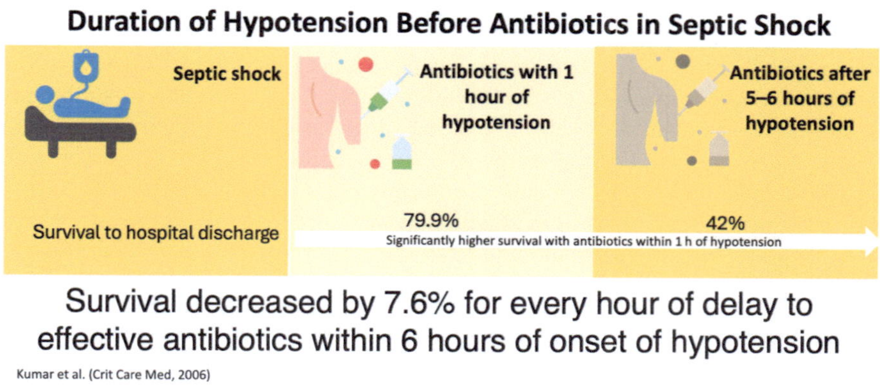

Quick Take

In septic shock, how does delay in commencement of antimicrobial therapy correlate with mortality?

Kumar et al. conducted a pivotal observational study to determine the impact of delayed antimicrobial therapy in patients with septic shock. The study found that each hour of delayed antimicrobial therapy after the onset of hypotension significantly increased the risk of death. The critical finding was that the duration of hypotension before starting effective therapy was the most important factor determining survival, highlighting the urgent need for timely administration of antibiotics in septic shock to improve patient outcome.

Kumar A, Roberts D, Wood KE, Light B, Parrillo JE, Sharma S, et al. Duration of hypotension before initiation of effective antimicrobial therapy is the critical determinant of survival in human septic shock. Crit Care Med. 2006 Jun;34 (6):1589–96.

J. Chacko et al., *Landmark Studies in Critical Care*,
https://doi.org/10.1007/978-981-95-0673-6_47

47.1 Introduction

In the summer of 1928, Alexander Fleming, on his return from holidays, was disconcerted by a mold that had contaminated his Petri dishes. On examination under the microscope, he noted that the mold had suppressed the growth of staphylococci all around. Little did he realize that he had stumbled upon one of the most groundbreaking discoveries in the history of medicine. In less than three decades since the discovery of penicillin, life expectancy had risen by nearly 8 years; patients suffering from seemingly minor injuries or severe illnesses like pneumonia no longer had to languish, hoping for a miracle.

Although sepsis was recognized from time immemorial, considerable discordance existed in the interpretation. Roger Bone and colleagues came up with a consensus definition at the Society of Critical Care Medicine (SCCM)—American College of Chest Physicians (ACCP) meeting of 1991 [1]. A bundled approach towards the expeditious care of septic patients was proposed by the Surviving Sepsis Guidelines in 2004 [2]. The 3- and 6-hour bundles were revamped to a 1-hour bundle in 2018 [3]. One of the key elements of the 1-hour bundle was the administration of broad-spectrum antibiotics. Timely administration of antibiotics is intuitive in patients with sepsis; however, no robust evidence has supported a timeframe for the initiation of therapy. In contrast, hemodynamic stabilization with fluid resuscitation and vasopressors were firmly entrenched in the initial management of sepsis. Kumar et al. in their landmark study of 2004, asked the question—does a delay in antimicrobial administration lead to increased mortality in septic shock?

47.2 Setting and Design

The retrospective cohort study included patients who were admitted to 14 ICUs in Canada and the US [4]. Three patient cohorts were included—two between 1999 and 2004 and one between 1989 and 1999. Patients were screened to confirm septic shock based on the 1991 SCCM/ACCP consensus statement [1]. Hypotension was defined as a mean arterial pressure of <65 mm Hg, a systolic BP <90 mm Hg, or a decrease in systolic BP by >40 mm Hg from the baseline. Septic shock was deemed to have occurred if hypotension persisted despite fluid resuscitation or improved transiently, for less than 1 hour. Antimicrobial therapy was considered *effective* if it was appropriate for the pathogen isolated. In culture-negative septic shock, antimicrobial therapy was considered effective if it was in concordance with accepted national guidelines. Besides, antimicrobial therapy had to be administered within 6 hours of the onset of septic shock to be considered effective.

47.3 Results

47.3.1 Patient Characteristics

The study included 2731 patients who fulfilled the criteria for septic shock. All three patient cohorts had a similar distribution of infections, APACHE II scores, and time to effective antimicrobial therapy following hypotension; hence, the data were combined and analyzed. The mean age of the cohort was 62.7 ± 16.4 years, and 54.3% were male patients. The mean APACHE II score was 26 ± 8.6. Community-acquired infections occurred in 58.1% of patients, while the infection was considered nosocomial in 41.9%.

Infections were documented in 77.9% of cases; in the rest, infection was *suspected*—no pathogens were isolated on cultures, nor could infection be confirmed otherwise. The most common foci of infection were the lungs (37.2%), followed by the abdomen (29.3%), and genitourinary (10.7%). Gram-negative infections were more common, with *E. coli* being the most frequently isolated organism (22.4%).

In the whole cohort of 2731 patients, 19 did not receive effective antimicrobial therapy until death; 558 patients received effective therapy before the onset of hypotension. The remaining 2154 patients received effective antimicrobial therapy only after the onset of hypotension; the mortality among this group was 58.0%. The median time to effective antimicrobial therapy following the onset of hypotension was 6 (2.0–15.0) hours.

47.3.2 Outcomes

The time interval between recurrent or persistent hypotension and commencement of effective antimicrobial therapy was a critical determinant of survival to ICU or hospital discharge. Increasing delays with the initiation of effective therapy was associated with higher mortality. The mortality rate with initiation of effective antimicrobial therapy at 2 hours after the onset of hypotension was significantly higher compared with initiation of therapy within the first hour (adjusted odds ratio 1.67; 95% confidence interval, 1.12–2.48). There was a continuous increase in the odds ratio of death with increasing delay—to a maximum level at 36 hours after the onset of hypotension. Each 1-hour delay in the commencement of effective antimicrobials was associated with a decrease in survival by 7.6% during the first 6 hours after the onset of hypotension.

The authors performed multivariate analysis, including effectiveness of antimicrobial therapy, the volume and type of initial fluid resuscitation, monotherapy vs. combination antibiotic therapy, and vasopressor support. Among all these variables, the time to effective antibiotic therapy was most strongly associated with survival. The strong association between time to effective therapy and survival persisted after inclusion of the APACHE II score, the number of organ failures, and the site of

Table 47.1 Main study outcomes

Outcome	Survival%
Survival when antibiotics administered within 30 min of hypotension	82.7
Survival when antibiotics administered in the second half hour after onset of hypotension	77.2
Survival when antibiotics administered in the 6th h after onset of hypotension	42.0

There was a decrease in survival by 7.6% for each hour of delay in antibiotic administration in the first 6 hours after the onset of hypotension.

infection in the model. On subgroup analysis, the increase in hospital mortality associated with longer delays in antimicrobial administration was evident regardless of the focus of infection, and whether the infection was documented or suspected. The findings were also consistent across patients with positive or negative cultures, gram-positive, negative, or fungal infections, and regardless of community-acquired or nosocomial infection. The main study outcomes are summarized in Table 47.1.

47.4 Study Conclusions

In patients with septic shock, the administration of effective antibiotics within an hour of the onset of hypotension was associated with improved survival. Delayed administration led to increased mortality by 7.6% for every hour in the ensuing 6 hours.

47.5 Strengths

The importance of timely antimicrobial therapy in conjunction with source control as appropriate, cannot be overemphasized. However, a key clinical conundrum lies in the definitive diagnosis of sepsis within a reasonable time frame, considering the paucity of information available at an early stage. In their desperation to conform to a bundled approach, clinicians may often be under pressure to administer antibiotics even if the diagnosis of sepsis is uncertain. This approach may lead to an inappropriate overuse of antibiotics, leading to an adverse impact on the gut microbiome, overgrowth with resistant organisms, and superinfections, including *Clostridium difficile* diarrhea. A randomized controlled trial comparing early with delayed antimicrobial therapy is unrealistic considering the ethical implications of such a study. Kumar et al. embarked upon their retrospective study based on information from databases involving three cohorts of patients. Their landmark study conveyed the powerful message that the key to survival may lie in the time interval between the onset of septic shock and antibiotic administration. Every hour of delay following the onset of hypotension led to an increase in mortality. The study was highly impactful and led to the bundled approach to sepsis recommended by the Surviving Sepsis Guidelines, with early antibiotic administration being pivotal [3].

47.6 Limitations

The study was based on retrospective data of three patient cohorts from Canada and the US. It was a long, drawn-out period of data collection—between 1989 and 2004, during which many aspects of care among critically ill patients may have undergone far-reaching changes. Infection was just "suspected" in 22.1% of cases, with neither a plausible pathogen grown on culture, nor was the presence of infection confirmed by any other modality of investigation. The likelihood of non-infectious mimics (e.g., cardiogenic shock) as a confounding variable was not considered. The timing and effectiveness of antimicrobial therapy were based on predefined rules; however, in doubtful scenarios, the decision was based on physician review and judgment, which could have led to bias. In the absence of a positive culture, appropriateness of therapy was based on available guidelines, casting ambiguity on the effectiveness of the agents used. No information was available on the performance of source control interventions and their timing, often more important than punctilious antibiotic administration in severe sepsis. The study did not consider the use of sedative agents in mechanically ventilated patients as a possible cause for hypotension. Information was not available on the incidence and severity of organ dysfunction, a major determinant of mortality in critically ill patients. Antibiotics were commenced prior to the onset of hypotension in 558 patients; however, inexplicably, survival in this subgroup of patients was lower than those who received antimicrobial agents within 5 hours of the onset of hypotension. The study was also supported by grants from pharmaceutical companies, leading to conflicts of interest.

47.7 Subsequent Evidence

A prospective observational study included 2796 patients with severe sepsis; the hospital mortality was 41.6% among the cohort. Early broad-spectrum antibiotics resulted in lower hospital mortality [5]. Seymour et al. evaluated patients with septic shock reported to the New York health department. Among this cohort, 82.5% of patients revealed adherence to the 3-hour bundle, including blood cultures, administration of broad-spectrum antibiotics, and measurement of lactate levels. Among those who completed the bundle in 12 hours, a delay in commencement of antibiotics was associated with a higher risk-adjusted in-hospital mortality. Intriguingly, a longer time to completion of an intravenous fluid bolus was not associated with higher mortality [6]. Liu et al. retrospectively studied 35,000 randomly selected patients with sepsis who received antibiotics within 6 hours of registration in the emergency department. Each hour of delay in antibiotic administration resulted in an increase in absolute mortality by 0.4% in patients with severe sepsis and 1.8% in those with septic shock [7]. Another prospective observational study evaluated in-hospital mortality among patients who presented to the emergency department with sepsis. In patients with septic shock who received antibiotics within 3 hours of presentation, every hour of delay was associated with an increased risk of mortality. The association was not observed in patients with sepsis without shock [8].

47.8 Summary

Although guidelines recommended antimicrobial therapy within an hour of presentation in patients with severe sepsis and septic shock, no clinical studies had been carried out to support this recommendation. Specifically, the likely adverse outcomes consequent to delayed administration of antibiotics had not been rigorously evaluated during the period when Kumar et al. embarked upon their landmark study. The authors had previously demonstrated that the onset of septic shock is a key determinant of outcome in a murine model. Against this background, they conducted a retrospective study including data from ICUs in the USA and Canada. They set out to evaluate the impact of delays in effective antimicrobial therapy among patients with septic shock. Among patients with septic shock, effective antimicrobial therapy was administered in approximately 50% of patients within 6 hours of onset of hypotension. The authors observed a strong association between delays in the initiation of effective antimicrobials and in-hospital mortality. Survival was highest when effective antimicrobials were commenced within an hour of the onset of hypotension; mortality increased with every hour of delay. The findings of this retrospective study underlined the urgency of effective antibiotic administration in patients with septic shock and provided the impetus for further research.

References

1. Bone RC, Balk RA, Cerra FB, Dellinger RP, Fein AM, Knaus WA, et al. Definitions for sepsis and organ failure and guidelines for the use of innovative therapies in sepsis. The ACCP/SCCM Consensus Conference Committee. American College of Chest Physicians/Society of Critical Care Medicine. Chest. 1992;101(6):1644–55.
2. Dellinger RP, Carlet JM, Masur H, Gerlach H, Calandra T, Cohen J, et al. Surviving Sepsis Campaign guidelines for management of severe sepsis and septic shock. Crit Care Med. 2004;32(3):858–73.
3. Levy MM, Evans LE, Rhodes A. The surviving sepsis campaign bundle: 2018 update. Crit Care Med. 2018;46(6):997–1000.
4. Kumar A, Roberts D, Wood KE, Light B, Parrillo JE, Sharma S, et al. Duration of hypotension before initiation of effective antimicrobial therapy is the critical determinant of survival in human septic shock. Crit Care Med. 2006;34(6):1589–96.
5. Ferrer R, Artigas A, Suarez D, Palencia E, Levy MM, Arenzana A, et al. Effectiveness of treatments for severe sepsis: a prospective, multicenter, observational study. Am J Respir Crit Care Med. 2009;180(9):861–6.
6. Seymour CW, Gesten F, Prescott HC, Friedrich ME, Iwashyna TJ, Phillips GS, et al. Time to treatment and mortality during mandated emergency care for sepsis. N Engl J Med. 2017;376(23):2235–44.
7. Liu VX, Fielding-Singh V, Greene JD, Baker JM, Iwashyna TJ, Bhattacharya J, et al. The timing of early antibiotics and hospital mortality in sepsis. Am J Respir Crit Care Med. 2017;196(7):856–63.
8. Im Y, Kang D, Ko RE, Lee YJ, Lim SY, Park S, et al. Time-to-antibiotics and clinical outcomes in patients with sepsis and septic shock: a prospective nationwide multicenter cohort study. Crit Care. 2022;26(1):19.

48 Diagnostic Techniques for Ventilator-Associated Pneumonia

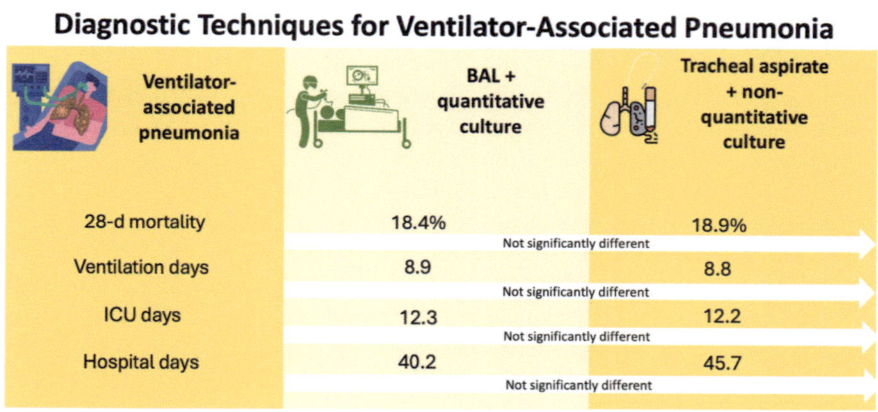

Canadian Critical Care Trials Group (NEJM, 2006)

Quick Take

Which diagnostic strategy is most effective for ventilator-associated pneumonia (VAP) in critically ill patients?

This multicenter trial by the Canadian Critical Care Trials Group randomized 740 patients on mechanical ventilation for at least 4 days, with suspected VAP, to undergo either bronchoalveolar lavage with quantitative cultures or endotracheal aspiration with nonquantitative cultures. Patients colonized or infected with methicillin-resistant *Staphylococcus aureus* or *Pseudomonas* species were excluded. Empirical antibiotics were initiated in all patients and later tailored based on culture results. The primary outcome, 28-day mortality, showed no significant

---

Canadian Critical Care Trials Group. A randomized trial of diagnostic techniques for ventilator-associated pneumonia. N Engl J Med. 2006 Dec 21;355(25):2619–30.

J. Chacko et al., *Landmark Studies in Critical Care*,
https://doi.org/10.1007/978-981-95-0673-6_48

difference between the bronchoalveolar lavage group and the endotracheal aspiration group. Secondary outcomes, including rates of targeted therapy, antibiotic-free days, maximum organ dysfunction scores, and ICU or hospital stay lengths, were also similar between the groups. This study demonstrated that, despite theoretical advantages of bronchoalveolar lavage in pathogen identification, it did not result in superior clinical outcomes compared to the less invasive endotracheal aspiration. The findings suggest that endotracheal aspiration, which is simpler and less invasive, may be an equally effective diagnostic strategy for suspected VAP in critically ill patients.

48.1 Introduction

VAP is among the most common nosocomial infections and may occur in up to 10% of patients who undergo invasive mechanical ventilation [1]. The development of VAP is associated with adverse clinical outcomes, including a longer duration of mechanical ventilation, ICU stay, and higher mortality [2, 3].

The proximal airway of the ventilated patient is usually colonized by potentially pathogenic bacteria. Hence, secretions aspirated from the endotracheal or tracheostomy tube do not consistently distinguish between colonization of the proximal airway and true infection of the lower respiratory tract. Hence, dependence on endotracheal aspirate cultures often leads to a misdiagnosis of VAP [4, 5]. Sampling techniques that enable focused collection of specimens from the distal airways without contamination by colonizers from the proximal airways through bronchoscopic techniques offer the potential for a more precise diagnosis and classification; besides, such techniques may enable selection of appropriate antibiotic therapy. On the other hand, caregivers skilled in bronchoscopy may not always be readily available, leading to delays in diagnosis and treatment.

An observational study had previously evaluated mechanically ventilated patients with a clinical suspicion of VAP. Ninety-two patients who underwent bronchoscopic sampling of secretions were compared with 49 who did not. The duration of mechanical ventilation and ICU length of stay were similar in both groups; however, mortality was lower among patients who underwent bronchoscopic evaluation. Furthermore, greater physician confidence in the diagnosis of VAP allowed limitation or early discontinuation of antibiotic treatment [6]. However, the results from randomized controlled trials (RCTs) were discordant; three studies did not reveal any advantage with an invasive diagnostic strategy [7–9], while a lone RCT found significantly lower mortality at 14 days with a bronchoscopic strategy [10]. Against the background of uncertainty regarding the optimal diagnostic strategy in VAP, the Canadian Critical Care Trials Group conducted an RCT comparing quantitative culture of bronchoalveolar lavage fluid and nonquantitative endotracheal aspirate culture in VAP.

48.2 Population and Design

The Canadian Critical Care Group Trials study was conducted between May 2000 and February 2005 across 28 ICUs in Canada and the United States [11]. The investigators aimed to compare clinical outcomes between quantitative culture of bronchoalveolar lavage fluid and endotracheal aspirate cultures in critically ill patients with VAP. They hypothesized that quantitative culture of bronchoalveolar lavage fluid would be associated with lower mortality and reduced use of antibiotics.

The eligible study population included consecutive adult patients who had undergone mechanical ventilation for at least 5 days, with suspected VAP, defined as new or persistent radiological infiltrates with two or more of the following features:

- Fever > 38 °C
- Leukocytosis > 11.0×10^3 per cu mm or neutrophil count < 3500 per cu mm
- Purulent endotracheal secretions
- Pathogenic bacteria isolated from endotracheal aspirates
- Increasing FiO_2 requirement

48.3 Excluded

The study excluded immunocompromised patients and those who were considered unsuitable to undergo bronchoscopy. Patients who were colonized with *Pseudomonas* species or methicillin-resistant *Staphylococcus aureus* were excluded. Also excluded were patients who were allergic to penicillins, cephalosporines, carbapenems, and ciprofloxacin, and those who had received meropenem within 7 days or ciprofloxacin within 24 hours (the study drugs) before study inclusion. Pregnant patients were excluded.

Patients were randomly assigned to undergo bronchoscopy and quantitative culture of bronchoalveolar lavage fluid or nonquantitative culture of the endotracheal aspirate. The 2-by-2 factorial design also compared empirical combination vs. monotherapy with antibiotics. Patients were stratified by center and by severity of illness—an APACHE II score ≤24 was defined as less severe, and >24 as severe illness.

48.4 Bronchoalveolar Lavage Group

Bronchoalveolar lavage was performed in the region of the lung involved, as identified on the chest radiograph. The bronchoscope was passed into the pre-identified zone of the lung, avoiding suction of secretions from the proximal airways. Gram stain and quantitative cultures were performed on the collected sample.

48.5 Endotracheal Aspiration Group

A sterile suction catheter was passed, and secretions collected on a suction trap. Normal saline, 3–5 ml could be instilled if secretions were scanty. Gram stain and culture were carried out on the sample.

48.6 Randomization of Antibiotic Therapy

After completion of the diagnostic procedure, patients were randomized to receive empirical antibiotic therapy with either meropenem alone or a combination of meropenem and ciprofloxacin. Meropenem was administered in a dose of 1 g 8 hourly intravenously, and ciprofloxacin, 400 mg 12 hourly, intravenously. If a positive culture was obtained, a single antibiotic with the narrowest spectrum was administered. If the culture was negative, antibiotics were discontinued unless physician judgment suggested otherwise, based on a high pre-test probability of VAP. The final decision whether to treat or not was thus left to the clinician discretion.

48.7 Sample Size

The authors assumed a mortality of 40%, which entailed enrollment of 740 patients to detect an absolute risk reduction of 10%, with 80% power and a two-sided significance level of 0.049. The study design assumed that the two different interventions—diagnostic modality and antibiotic treatment—would not interact.

48.8 Results

Among the 1144 patients who met the eligibility criteria, 740 were enrolled; one patient who withdrew consent was excluded from the analysis. Baseline characteristics were similar between the bronchoalveolar lavage and the endotracheal aspiration groups. Antibiotics prescribed within 24 hours before enrollment and the total number of antibiotics administered before enrollment were similar in both groups. Patients who underwent bronchoalveolar lavage were more likely to be culture positive compared to those who underwent endotracheal aspiration. Meropenem and ciprofloxacin were used for a median duration of 3 days among patients in both groups. Empirical antibiotic administration was appropriate in similar numbers of patients in both groups. The number of patients who were identified as not having VAP was also similar in both groups.

48.9 The Primary Endpoint: 28-Day Mortality

The 28-day mortality was similar in both groups of patients; in the bronchoalveolar lavage group 69/374 (18.4%) patients had died at 28 days compared with 69/365 (18.9%) in the endotracheal aspiration group. The relative risk of death at 28 days in the endotracheal aspiration group was 1.01 (95% confidence interval, 0.75 to 1.37; $P = 0.94$). On subgroup analysis, the mortality was similar among patients with a high pre-test likelihood of VAP, severe or less severe illness based on the APACHE II score, duration of ICU stay before randomization, receipt of antibiotics within 3 days before randomization, and the type of organism cultured (high risk vs. not high risk).

There was no significant difference in mortality between patients who received monotherapy with meropenem and those who received combination therapy with meropenem and ciprofloxacin. The treatment effect of the two diagnostic modalities was the same regardless of the antibiotic therapy; besides, the treatment effect of the two antibiotic regimens was also the same, irrespective of the diagnostic modality employed.

48.10 Secondary Outcomes

The duration between the time of randomization to discontinuation of mechanical ventilation, ICU discharge, and hospital discharge was similar in both groups of patients. Patients who experienced clinical and microbiological cure or failure were also similar. By day 6, all antibiotics were discontinued in 21.1% and the study antibiotics were ceased in 59.9% of all patients, with no significant difference between groups. The number of days alive and without antibiotics and the maximum organ dysfunction scores were similar. The rates of targeted therapy were also similar in both groups. The main study outcomes are presented in Table 48.1.

Table 48.1 Main study outcomes

Outcome	Bronchoalveolar lavage	Endotracheal aspiration	*P* value
28-day mortality	69/374 (18.4%)	69/365 (18.9%)	0.94
Median ventilation days	8.9	8.8	0.31
ICU days	12.3	12.2	0.22
Hospital days	40.2	45.7	0.13
Days alive with no antibiotics	10.4	10.6	0.86
Maximum organ dysfunction score (0–24)	8.3	8.6	0.26

48.11 Study Conclusions

This study found no significant difference in clinical outcomes, including mortality, between invasive (bronchoalveolar lavage) and noninvasive (endotracheal aspiration) diagnostic techniques for VAP. Both approaches led to similar antibiotic use and clinical cure rates, suggesting that less invasive methods may be sufficient for diagnosing VAP.

48.12 Strengths

The RCT was adequately powered to evaluate the clinical question. Randomization was concealed, and all patients were followed up for the primary endpoint. Analysis was by intention to treat, and key aspects of care were protocolized, adding to the strength of the study. The multicentric nature of the study also suggested generalizability.

48.13 Limitations

Clinicians were aware of the diagnostic intervention. The pretest likelihood and clinical classification of VAP were based on clinician judgment; subjective assessment could have led to treatment bias.

Patients who were colonized with *Pseudomonas* species and methicillin-resistant *Staphylococcus aureus* were excluded, thus limiting the applicability of the study findings, especially considering the predominance of infection with these organisms in many clinical settings. Furthermore, the study revealed a low incidence of infection with *Pseudomonas* species and methicillin-resistant *Staphylococcus aureus*—again, limiting extrapolation to ICUs, which have a higher incidence of VAP due to these organisms. Immunocompromised patients, those with chronic disease, and those who had already received one of the study drugs were also excluded. Thus, the majority of instances of VAP generally encountered in most units may involve a patient population that was excluded from the study. Presumably, bronchoalveolar lavage and quantitative cultures may be more beneficial in these difficult-to-treat infections.

48.14 Subsequent Studies

In a 2020 meta-analysis, Fernando et al. evaluated the precision of commonly used parameters in the diagnosis of VAP, including physical examination, chest radiography, endotracheal aspirate culture, and bronchoscopic sampling by protected brush specimen or bronchoalveolar lavage. The meta-analysis included 1639 patients from 25 studies. They observed that although endotracheal aspirate culture had a higher sensitivity compared with bronchoalveolar lavage (75.7 vs. 71.1%), it had much less specificity (67.9 vs 79.6%) [12]. Currently, the guidelines of the American Thoracic Society/Infectious Diseases Society of America (ATS/IDSA) recommend endotracheal aspirates to diagnose VAP [13]. Rapid diagnostic tests, including quantitative and multiplex polymerase chain reaction, are being increasingly used to test endotracheal aspirates and bronchoalveolar lavage specimens, allowing rapid identification of respiratory pathogens. Reducing the time to accurately identify the micro-organisms involved and the institution of appropriate treatment carries the potential to improve clinical outcomes in VAP. However, there is a paucity of prospective controlled studies that confirm their superiority compared with conventional techniques.

48.15 Summary

VAP is among the commonest of nosocomial infections among critically ill patients. The cornerstone of care involves the identification of the culprit organism and appropriately tailored treatment. Endotracheal aspiration is easy to perform at the bedside; however, there is a high likelihood of contamination with organisms from the proximal airways with this strategy. Bronchoscopy requires skilled personnel and may be time-consuming, although culture of the lavage fluid can potentially enhance specificity by sampling secretions from areas of the lung that are involved. Evidence regarding the relative efficacy of these techniques and their impact on clinical outcomes remained inconclusive. The Canadian Critical Care Trials group compared tracheal aspiration and nonquantitative cultures with quantitative culture of bronchoalveolar fluid, and their relative efficacy on clinical outcomes. The authors observed no significant difference in important clinical outcomes, including the 28-day mortality, antibiotic use, the severity of organ dysfunction, and the duration of stay in the ICU or hospital. The study excluded a large number of patients, including immunocompromised patients and those colonized with *Pseudomonas* species or methicillin-resistant *Staphylococcus aureus*. Bronchoscopic techniques will clearly have a role in the microbiological diagnosis of these high-risk patients and will enable de-escalation of antibiotic treatment, an important facet in preventing antibiotic resistance.

References

1. Wang Y, Eldridge N, Metersky ML, Verzier NR, Meehan TP, Pandolfi MM, et al. National Trends in patient safety for four common conditions, 2005–2011. N Engl J Med. 2014;370(4):341–51.
2. Heyland DK, Cook DJ, Griffith L, Keenan SP, Brun-Buisson C. The attributable morbidity and mortality of ventilator-associated pneumonia in the critically ill patient. The Canadian Critical Trials Group. Am J Respir Crit Care Med. 1999;159(4 Pt 1):1249–56.
3. Rello J, Ollendorf DA, Oster G, Vera-Llonch M, Bellm L, Redman R, et al. Epidemiology and outcomes of ventilator-associated pneumonia in a large US database. Chest. 2002;122(6):2115–21.

4. Andrews CP, Coalson JJ, Smith JD, Johanson WG. Diagnosis of nosocomial bacterial pneumonia in acute, diffuse lung injury. Chest. 1981;80(3):254–8.
5. Fagon JY, Chastre J, Hance AJ, Guiguet M, Trouillet JL, Domart Y, et al. Detection of nosocomial lung infection in ventilated patients. Use of a protected specimen brush and quantitative culture techniques in 147 patients. Am Rev Respir Dis. 1988;138(1):110–6.
6. Heyland DK, Cook DJ, Marshall J, Heule M, Guslits B, Lang J, et al. The clinical utility of invasive diagnostic techniques in the setting of ventilator-associated pneumonia. Canadian Critical Care Trials Group. Chest. 1999;115(4):1076–84.
7. Sanchez-Nieto JM, Torres A, Garcia-Cordoba F, El-Ebiary M, Carrillo A, Ruiz J, et al. Impact of invasive and noninvasive quantitative culture sampling on outcome of ventilator-associated pneumonia: a pilot study. Am J Respir Crit Care Med. 1998;157(2):371–6.
8. Ruiz M, Torres A, Ewig S, Marcos MA, Alcón A, Lledó R, et al. Noninvasive versus invasive microbial investigation in ventilator-associated pneumonia: evaluation of outcome. Am J Respir Crit Care Med. 2000;162(1):119–25.
9. Solé Violán J, Fernández JA, Benítez AB, Cardeñosa Cendrero JA, Rodríguez de Castro F. Impact of quantitative invasive diagnostic techniques in the management and outcome of mechanically ventilated patients with suspected pneumonia. Crit Care Med. 2000;28(8):2737–41.
10. Fagon JY, Chastre J, Wolff M, Gervais C, Parer-Aubas S, Stéphan F, et al. Invasive and noninvasive strategies for management of suspected ventilator-associated pneumonia. A randomized trial. Ann Intern Med. 2000;132(8):621–30.
11. Canadian Critical Care Trials Group. A randomized trial of diagnostic techniques for ventilator-associated pneumonia. N Engl J Med. 2006;355(25):2619–30.
12. Fernando SM, Tran A, Cheng W, Klompas M, Kyeremanteng K, Mehta S, et al. Diagnosis of ventilator-associated pneumonia in critically ill adult patients-a systematic review and meta-analysis. Intensive Care Med. 2020;46(6):1170–9.
13. Kalil AC, Metersky ML, Klompas M, Muscedere J, Sweeney DA, Palmer LB, et al. Management of Adults with Hospital-acquired and Ventilator-associated Pneumonia: 2016 Clinical Practice Guidelines by the Infectious Diseases Society of America and the American Thoracic Society. Clin Infect Dis. 2016;63(5):e61–111.

Procalcitonin and Antibiotic Exposure in the ICU: The PRORATA Trial

49

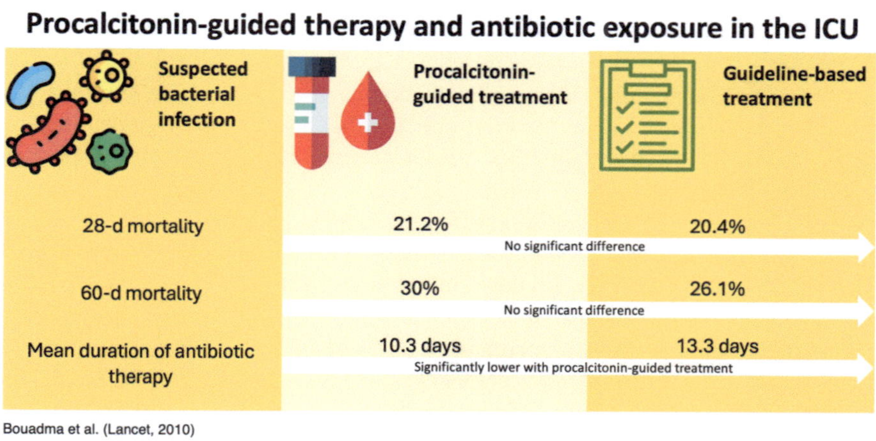

Quick Take

Can procalcitonin guidance reduce antibiotic consumption in ICU patients?

The PRORATA trial investigated whether procalcitonin levels could guide antibiotic therapy to reduce inappropriate exposure in critically ill patients. This multicenter, randomized controlled trial enrolled ICU patients with suspected or confirmed infections and compared two strategies: procalcitonin-guided therapy versus standard care. The results showed that the procalcitonin group had a significantly shorter duration of antibiotic treatment without compromising patient outcomes, such as mortality or infection-related complications. The trial concluded

---

Bouadma L, Luyt CE, Tubach F, Cracco C, Alvarez A, Schwebel C, et al. Use of procalcitonin to reduce patients' exposure to antibiotics in intensive care units (PRORATA trial): a multicentre randomised controlled trial. 2010;375.

J. Chacko et al., *Landmark Studies in Critical Care*,
https://doi.org/10.1007/978-981-95-0673-6_49

that using procalcitonin as a biomarker to guide antibiotic therapy can safely reduce antibiotic exposure in the ICU, offering an effective strategy to combat antibiotic overuse and resistance. Procalcitonin levels alone have little value in the diagnosis of infection and deciding on the commencement of antibiotic therapy; however, it is likely to guide the clinician regarding the duration of therapy.

49.1 Introduction

The inappropriate use of antibiotics has led to the widespread emergence of antibiotic resistance [1]. Critically ill patients with sepsis experience high mortality [2]; however, less than 60% of patients initially diagnosed with sepsis are later confirmed to have a focus of infection [3]. The use of antibiotics in the ICU may be curtailed by restricting therapy to those with true infection and by shortening the duration of treatment. Biomarkers may, along with clinical parameters and microbiological evidence, carry the potential to guide appropriate antibiotic therapy. Serial levels of a biomarker may especially enable guidance to cessation of antibiotic therapy at the appropriate time. Procalcitonin, a precursor of the hormone calcitonin, is a marker of severe bacterial infection [4]. Procalcitonin-guided therapy has been shown to reduce antibiotic use in patients with lower respiratory tract infections [5].

A previous randomized controlled trial (RCT) had evaluated the usefulness of procalcitonin among patients with severe sepsis and septic shock. The median duration of antibiotic therapy was 3.5 days shorter among patients who received procalcitonin-guided therapy compared to the control group [6]. Another RCT employed procalcitonin-guided antibiotic therapy in surgical ICU patients [7]. Antibiotics were ceased if there were signs of clinical improvement, with a drop in the procalcitonin level to <1 ng/ml, or 25–30% of initial levels over 3 days. The mean duration of antibiotic therapy was shorter with procalcitonin-guided therapy (5.9 +/− 1.7 versus 7.9 +/− 0.5 days) compared to a control group, with no adverse impact on clinical outcomes.

The PRORATA trial group embarked upon a large RCT to evaluate the utility of procalcitonin levels to guide commencement, continuation, or cessation of antibiotics in ICU patients with suspected bacterial infection. The main aim of the study was to assess whether a procalcitonin-guided strategy would reduce antibiotic consumption [8].

49.2 Population and Design

The PRORATA trial was conducted between June 2007 and May 2008 across seven ICUs in France. Adult patients (>18 years) with suspected bacterial infection who had not received antibiotics or were treated with antibiotics for <24 hours were eligible. The duration between admission and study inclusion had to be <12 hours. Patients who developed sepsis during ICU stay were also eligible.

49.2.1 Exclusion

Patients with an expected ICU length of stay of <3 days, those following bone marrow transplant or chemotherapy-induced neutropenia, and specific infections that required long-term antibiotic therapy (e.g., infective endocarditis, bone and joint infection) were excluded. Patients who were not expected to survive and those with do-not-resuscitate orders were also excluded.

Patients were randomized in a 1:1 ratio to the procalcitonin or control group. Randomization was stratified by center, in blocks of 2, 4, or 6.

49.3 Procalcitonin Group

The investigators employed a predefined, procalcitonin-based algorithm to guide antibiotic therapy. The baseline procalcitonin level was used to encourage or discourage the commencement of antibiotics. If antibiotics were not commenced, clinical assessment and procalcitonin levels were repeated in 6–12 hours for a delayed rise in procalcitonin concentration, and antibiotic administration if appropriate. Procalcitonin levels were measured daily until cessation of antibiotic treatment and for each new episode of suspected infection.

The procalcitonin algorithm for the commencement of antibiotics was as follows:

Procalcitonin level	Recommendation for antibiotics
<0.25 μg/L	Strongly discouraged
≥0.25 and <0.5 μg/L	Discouraged
≥0.5 and <1.0 μg/L	Encouraged
≥1.0 μg/L	Strongly encouraged

Discontinuation of antibiotic therapy was recommended when the procalcitonin level declined to <80% of the peak level, or when an absolute level of <0.5 μg/L was reached. The procalcitonin algorithm for discontinuation of antibiotics was as follows:

Procalcitonin level	Recommendation for antibiotics
<0.25 μg/L	Discontinuation strongly encouraged
≥0.25 and <0.5 μg/L or ≥80% decrease from peak level	Discontinuation encouraged
≥0.5 μg/L and <80% decrease from peak level	Continuation encouraged
≥0.5 μg/l and increase from peak	Changing antibiotics strongly encouraged

The procalcitonin-based algorithm was employed for the first and subsequent infections until day 28, or discharge from ICU, whichever occurred earlier. The final decision on antibiotic administration was left to the clinician discretion.

49.4 Control Group

The duration of antimicrobial treatment was based on recommendations derived from international and local guidelines. The duration of antibiotic treatment was based on the clinician judgment.

49.5 Both Groups

The choice of antibiotic was left to the clinician's discretion. Broad-spectrum antibiotics were recommended for initial treatment of severe infections, including septic shock. De-escalation of antibiotic therapy was strongly encouraged based on culture reports. Every episode of infection was classified as follows: microbiologically documented infection (presence of a focus with identification of the pathogen); clinically documented infection (presence of a focus with no pathogen identified); absence of infection (absence of a focus and antibiotics administered for <2 days); possible infection (other situations).

49.6 Sample Size

The authors assumed a mean of 12 ± 7.5 antibiotic-free days at day 28 in the control group. An increase in the antibiotic-free days by 3 days in the procalcitonin group required 133 patients per group for 90% power and a two-sided alpha of 0.05. They aimed to demonstrate non-inferiority in mortality with a procalcitonin-guided approach. Six hundred patients were required to achieve 80% power to exclude a 10% difference in mortality between groups, assuming 35% mortality in the control group. Accounting for loss to follow-up, they planned to enroll 630 patients.

49.7 Results

Among 1315 patients who were screened, 630 were enrolled—311 were assigned to the procalcitonin group, and 319 to the control group. In the final analysis, there were 307 patients in the procalcitonin group and 314 in the control group. Patients were well-matched in both groups. Approximately 90% of patients were medical; the severity of illness based on the SOFA score was also similar. Septic shock was present in a similar proportion of patients (procalcitonin: 17% vs. control: 18%). A similar proportion of patients were classified as having microbiologically documented or clinically documented infection, possible or absent infection. The empirical antibiotic therapy employed was considered adequate in most patients—91% in the procalcitonin group and 93% in the control group.

Recommendations regarding the duration of antibiotic therapy were not followed in 219 episodes in the procalcitonin group. Of these, antibiotics were commenced in 65 patients based on clinician judgment despite procalcitonin levels being low

(<0.5 μg/L); in contrast, four patients were not commenced on antibiotics although the procalcitonin levels were high (>0.5 μg/L), as a non-infectious illness was suspected. In 39 patients, antibiotics were discontinued early, although the procalcitonin levels remained high (>0.5 μg/L). On the other hand, 111 patients continued to receive antibiotics although their procalcitonin had come down (<0.5 μg/L); 32 of these patients had been transferred out of the ICU where the algorithm was not followed, while 79 were deemed to be clinically unstable, necessitating continued antibiotic therapy.

In the control group, the recommendation on the duration of therapy was not adhered to in 146 episodes. These included 15 episodes when antibiotic therapy was initially withheld as infection was judged to be unlikely, prematurely stopped on 46 occasions as the infection was considered cured, and 85 occasions when the duration of therapy was extended as cure was not considered to have occurred. Overall, the recommended algorithm was not adhered to in 45% of patients in the control group.

49.8 Primary Outcomes

Mortality at 28 days [procalcitonin: 65/207 (21.2%) vs. control: 64/214 (20.4%)] and 60 days (30% vs. 26.1%) was non-inferior in the procalcitonin group compared with the control group. The odds ratio for death in the procalcitonin group at 28 days was 0.89 (90% CI 0.62–1.28), and 1.09 (0.79–1.51) at 60 days.

The mean duration of antibiotic therapy was significantly lower in the procalcitonin group at 28 days (10.3 ± 0.7.7 days vs. 13.3 ± 7.6 days, $p < 0.0001$). Besides, there was a 23% relative reduction in antibiotic exposure among patients in the procalcitonin group. Fewer patients received antibiotics throughout the study in the procalcitonin group. The difference between groups in the proportion of patients receiving antibiotics increased steadily from 5.6% on day 1 to 37•6% on day 7.

49.9 Secondary Outcomes

Between the procalcitonin and the control groups, the number of ventilation-free days (16.2 ± 11.1 vs. 16.9 ± 10.9 days), the ICU length of stay (15.9 ± 16.1 vs.14.4 ± 14.1 days), and the hospital length of stay (26.1 ± 19.3 vs. 26.4 ± 18.3 days) were not significantly different. The emergence of multidrug-resistant bacteria was similar in both groups (17.6% vs. 16.6%). Relapse or superinfections were also similar.

The duration of initial antibiotic therapy was shorter in the procalcitonin group overall. The duration was shorter, specifically in patients with community- and ventilator-acquired pneumonia, and urinary infection; the duration was similar in patients with intra-abdominal infection and infections with positive blood culture.

Table 49.1 Main study outcomes

Outcome	Procalcitonin group	Control group	Significance
28-day mortality	21.2%	20.4%	OR: 0.89 (90% CI 0.62–1.28) (NS)
60-day mortality	30%	26.1%	OR: 1.09 (0.79–1.51) (NS)
Mean duration of antibiotic therapy	10.3 ± 0.7.7 days	13.3 ± 7.6 days	*P* = 0.0001 (S)
Ventilator-free days	16.2 ± 11.1 days	16.9 ± 10.9 days	*P* = 0.47 (NS)
ICU stay	15.9 ± 16.1 days	14.4 ± 14.1 days	*P* = 0.23 (NS)
Hospital stay	26.1 ± 19.3 days	26.4 ± 18.3 days	*P* = 0.87 (NS)

Abbreviations: *OR* odds ratio, *CI* confidence interval, *S* significant, *NS* non-significant

49.10 Subgroup Analysis

Antibiotic exposure was lower in the procalcitonin group in predefined subgroups, including community-acquired infection, hospital-acquired infection, patients who were immunocompromised, and patients who were managed with strict adherence to the study algorithms. Mortality at 28 days was non-inferior in most subgroups; there was insufficient evidence in some subgroups to support non-inferiority. The main study outcomes are depicted in Table 49.1.

49.11 Study Conclusions

The study demonstrated that among patients with suspected infection at admission or during subsequent stay in the ICU, procalcitonin guidance significantly reduced exposure to antibiotics. Clinical outcomes were comparable in both groups.

49.12 Strengths

The PRORATA trial was the first large, multicentric RCT that demonstrated the efficacy and non-inferiority of procalcitonin-guided antibiotic therapy.

The study population included severely ill patients with a broad range of infections; two-thirds required mechanical ventilation, and 40% had septic shock. The study thus reinforced a procalcitonin-guided strategy among the critically ill.

49.13 Weaknesses

The investigators were not blinded to individual patient allocation, which may have led to bias. The authors calculated the sample size for non-inferiority based on a 10% difference in mortality, which may be considered too high, although suggested by guideline recommendations. If the difference for non-inferiority was set at 5%, the 60-day mortality would have been significantly higher in the procalcitonin group. Only 10% were surgical patients; the impact of a procalcitonin-guided strategy remains unclear among this population, in whom source control assumes priority. The results may not be extrapolatable to patients who are immunosuppressed, neutropenic, or infected with high-risk pathogens (e.g., Pseudomonas aeruginosa). In 53% of patients assigned to the procalcitonin group, the algorithm was not followed—either based on clinician discretion or because they were transferred out of ICU. The study did not demonstrate the utility of procalcitonin-guided therapy in the emergence of multidrug-resistant organisms—one of the purported benefits of reducing the duration of antibiotic therapy. Besides, clinical endpoints, including the duration of mechanical ventilation and ICU length of stay, were similar in both groups of patients. Relapse and superinfection in the later course of illness may not have been adequately followed up once the patient was transferred out of the ICU.

49.14 Subsequent Evidence

A meta-analysis by Pap et al. evaluated the usefulness of procalcitonin-guided antibiotic therapy compared to standard of care [9]. The authors included 9048 patients from 26 RCTs in their analysis. They observed a significantly shorter duration of antibiotic therapy with procalcitonin and a lower 28-day mortality. The mortality benefit was more evident among patients who fulfilled the Sepsis-3 criteria. The odds of recurrent infection were higher in the procalcitonin group; the incidence of secondary infection was similar in both groups. The ICU and hospital length of stay were also similar in both groups.

49.15 Summary

The PRORATA investigators evaluated the impact of a procalcitonin-guided antibiotic strategy on the duration of antibiotic therapy in critically ill patients with suspected infection. Procalcitonin-guided therapy resulted in significantly greater antibiotic-free days compared to a control group, who were managed according to local and international guidelines. However, no significant difference was observed in clinical endpoints—including the 28- and 60-day mortality, mechanical ventilation-free days, or ICU length of stay. The incidence of relapse and superinfection was also similar in both groups. Procalcitonin levels do not appear to have reduced the frequency of initial commencement of antibiotic therapy; on the contrary, the duration of therapy could be reduced. Clearly, procalcitonin levels alone have little value in the diagnosis of infection, and deciding upon the commencement of antibiotic therapy—it is more likely to guide the clinician regarding the duration of therapy.

References

1. Dellit TH, Owens RC, McGowan JE, Gerding DN, Weinstein RA, Burke JP, et al. Infectious Diseases Society of America and the Society for Healthcare Epidemiology of America guidelines for developing an institutional program to enhance antimicrobial stewardship. Clin Infect Dis. 2007;44(2):159–77.
2. Vincent JL, Rello J, Marshall J, Silva E, Anzueto A, Martin CD, et al. International study of the prevalence and outcomes of infection in intensive care units. JAMA. 2009;302(21):2323–9.
3. Klein Klouwenberg PMC, Cremer OL, van Vught LA, Ong DSY, Frencken JF, Schultz MJ, et al. Likelihood of infection in patients with presumed sepsis at the time of intensive care unit admission: a cohort study. Crit Care Lond Engl. 2015;19(1):319.
4. Tang BMP, Eslick GD, Craig JC, McLean AS. Accuracy of procalcitonin for sepsis diagnosis in critically ill patients: systematic review and meta-analysis. Lancet Infect Dis. 2007;7(3):210–7.
5. Christ-Crain M, Jaccard-Stolz D, Bingisser R, Gencay MM, Huber PR, Tamm M, et al. Effect of procalcitonin-guided treatment on antibiotic use and outcome in lower respiratory tract infections: cluster-randomised, single-blinded intervention trial. Lancet Lond Engl. 2004;363(9409):600–7.
6. Nobre V, Harbarth S, Graf JD, Rohner P, Pugin J. Use of procalcitonin to shorten antibiotic treatment duration in septic patients: a randomized trial. Am J Respir Crit Care Med. 2008;177(5):498–505.
7. Hochreiter M, Köhler T, Schweiger AM, Keck FS, Bein B, von Spiegel T, et al. Procalcitonin to guide duration of antibiotic therapy in intensive care patients: a randomized prospective controlled trial. Crit Care. 2009;13(3):R83.
8. Bouadma L, Luyt CE, Tubach F, Cracco C, Alvarez A, Schwebel C, et al. Use of procalcitonin to reduce patients' exposure to antibiotics in intensive care units (PRORATA trial): a multicentre randomised controlled trial. Lancet. 2010;375:463–74.
9. Papp M, Kiss N, Baka M, Trásy D, Zubek L, Fehérvári P, et al. Procalcitonin-guided antibiotic therapy may shorten length of treatment and may improve survival—a systematic review and meta-analysis. Crit Care. 2023;27(1):394.

Part XI

Cardiology, Cardiac Surgery

Rate Versus Rhythm Control for Atrial Fibrillation Following Post-Cardiac Surgery: The CTSN Trial

50

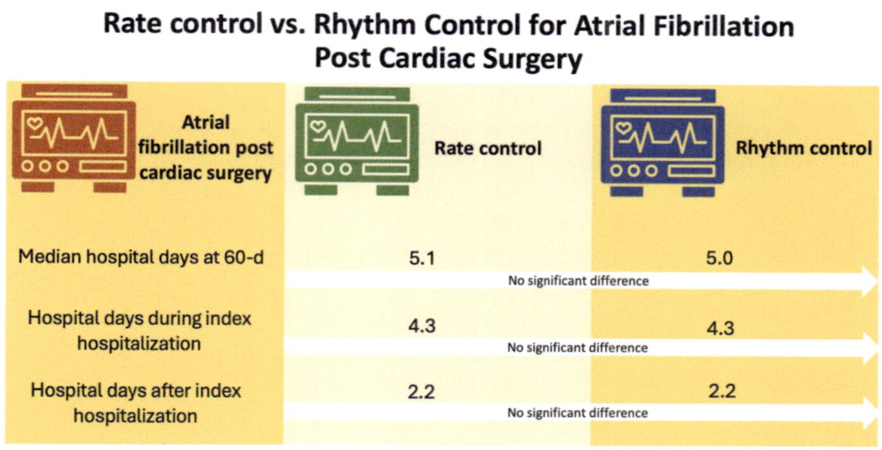

Gillinov et al. (NEJM, 2016)

Quick Take

Which is better for post-cardiac surgery atrial fibrillation (AF)—rate control or rhythm control?

This randomized trial compared rate control to rhythm control for the management of AF after cardiac surgery. A total of 1500 patients who developed new-onset AF following cardiac surgery were randomized to receive either a rate-control strategy (using beta-blockers or calcium channel blockers) or a rhythm-control strategy (using antiarrhythmic drugs or electrical cardioversion). The study found no

Gillinov AM, Bagiella E, Moskowitz AJ, Raiten JM, Groh MA, Bowdish ME, et al. *Rate Control* versus *Rhythm Control for Atrial Fibrillation after Cardiac Surgery. N Engl J Med. 2016 May 19;374(20):1911–21.*

J. Chacko et al., *Landmark Studies in Critical Care*,
https://doi.org/10.1007/978-981-95-0673-6_50

significant difference in clinical outcomes, including mortality or stroke, between the two strategies. The incidence of adverse events was similar in both groups. These findings suggest that both treatment strategies are equally effective.

50.1 Introduction and Background

Atrial fibrillation is common following cardiac surgery, occurring in approximately 25–50% of patients [1]. Postoperative atrial fibrillation carries an increased risk of complications and may be associated with higher mortality [2]. Furthermore, new-onset atrial fibrillation in the postoperative period often leads to prolongation of ICU and hospital stay [3, 4]. The management of postoperative atrial fibrillation revolves around two basic strategies—control of the heart rate or maintenance of sinus rhythm by electrical cardioversion or using anti-arrhythmic drugs as appropriate.

The AFFIRM trial had previously evaluated the two treatment strategies among non-surgical patients with atrial fibrillation and a high risk of stroke or death. The study enrolled 4060 patients. In this study, rhythm control did not offer a survival advantage compared with rate control alone. The 5-year mortality was 23.8% in the rhythm control vs. 21.3% in the rate control group [hazard ratio, 1.15 (95% confidence interval, 0.99–1.34); $P = 0.08$]. Hospitalization was required more often with rhythm control; furthermore, adverse effects due to anti-arrhythmic drugs were also more common in this group. The authors concluded that a rhythm control strategy offers no advantages over a rate control approach; besides, potential harm may ensue from adverse effects related to anti-arrhythmic drugs [5].

The efficacy of a rhythm control compared to a rate control strategy among post-cardiac surgical patients was also evaluated in a few studies of small sample size. In a randomized controlled trial (RCT), Lee et al. failed to demonstrate a difference between the two strategies in the time taken for conversion to sinus rhythm. The duration of hospital stay was shorter among patients who received anti-arrhythmic therapy; however, at the time of study completion, most patients were in sinus rhythm, with no significant difference between the two groups [6]. The PREVENT-IV trial examined the management of atrial fibrillation following coronary artery bypass surgery. Most patients were treated with a rhythm control strategy (81%). The 30-day mortality was higher in patients who had atrial fibrillation compared to those who maintained sinus rhythm [7].

The debate over the relative merits compared with the potential harmful effects of a rhythm vs. rate control strategy remained unresolved. Clinicians who espoused a rhythm control strategy highlighted advantages, including a reduced risk of thromboembolism, minimization of the anticoagulant dose, and earlier restoration of functional capacity. However, advocates of rate control argued that the adverse effects of anti-arrhythmic drugs and cardioversion-related complications might offset any potential benefit. In light of contrasting viewpoints, the Cardiothoracic Surgical Trials Network (CTSN) undertook an RCT to evaluate the safety and efficacy of a rate control compared with a rhythm control strategy among patients with new-onset atrial fibrillation or atrial flutter following cardiac surgery [8].

50.2 Population and Design

The CTSN trial was conducted across 23 sites in the United States and Canada over a 1-year period between May 2014 and May 2015. Patients who underwent elective coronary artery bypass graft or valve replacement surgery and remained hemodynamically stable were eligible for inclusion. Patients who developed postoperative atrial fibrillation that persisted for >60 minutes or experienced recurrent atrial fibrillation during the index hospitalization within 7 days of surgery were randomized.

50.2.1 Excluded

Patients who had experienced episodes of atrial fibrillation in the past were excluded to avoid changes to medications they may have already been on. Patients who had undergone ablation for atrial fibrillation, those with contraindications to amiodarone, changes on the ECG that increased vulnerability to arrhythmias and heart blocks, and those with active or high risk of bleeding were among those excluded.

50.3 Rate Control Group

In the rate control group, patients were administered medication to slow down the heart rate, aiming to achieve a resting heart rate of <100/min. Those who did not revert to sinus rhythm after rate control measures could receive interventions aimed at rhythm control if deemed appropriate to attain hemodynamic stability or symptomatic improvement.

50.4 Rhythm Control Group

In the rhythm control group, patients received amiodarone combined with rate control agents as appropriate. Electrical cardioversion was recommended if atrial fibrillation persisted for longer than 24–48 hours after medical treatment. The recommended dose of amiodarone was a total dose of 3 g before hospital discharge, with a maintenance dose of ≤200 mg/day if electrical cardioversion was successful. The recommended duration of treatment with amiodarone was 60 days; however, treatment could be discontinued in case of adverse events, including symptomatic bradycardia, QTc >480 msec, or neuropathy.

50.5 Both Groups

If atrial fibrillation persisted or recurred at 48 hours after randomization, anticoagulation with warfarin was commenced with a bridging period of low-molecular-weight heparin. The recommended duration of anticoagulant therapy was 60 days unless complications developed in the interim. The authors specified criteria for hospital discharge from the perspective of atrial fibrillation; this was meant to control for non-cardiovascular reasons for continued hospitalization. In the rate control group, a target heart rate of <100/min met the criteria for discharge. In the rhythm control group, discharge criteria included a full loading dose of amiodarone, an atrial fibrillation-free period of 24 hours, and no atrial fibrillation at the time of discharge. Patients who remained in atrial fibrillation despite at least 48 hours of amiodarone treatment and those who underwent electrical cardioversion could be discharged if their heart rate was adequately controlled.

50.6 Sample Size Calculation

The primary outcome was the total number of days in hospital (including visits to the emergency department) within 60 days of randomization. The null hypothesis assumed no difference between groups in the primary outcome. The authors calculated a sample size of 520 patients, which provided the study with 90% power to detect a 2-day difference between groups.

50.7 Results

Among 695 of 2109 eligible patients who developed postoperative atrial fibrillation, 523 were randomized—262 patients to rate control and 261 to rhythm control. Patient characteristics were similar at baseline. Coronary artery bypass surgery was performed in 40%, valve surgery in 40%, and a combination of both procedures in 20% of patients. Atrial fibrillation occurred in the postoperative period in 28.1% of patients who underwent coronary artery bypass surgery, 33.7% of those who underwent valve surgery, and in 47.3% of those who underwent both procedures. In 24% of patients randomized to the rhythm control group, the full course of amiodarone was not completed; they received beta-blockers, calcium-channel blockers, or a combination of both. Contrariwise, 26.7% of patients assigned to rate control received rhythm control measures, including electrical cardioversion. Overall, 9.2% of patients assigned to rate control and 13.8% in the rhythm control group underwent electrical cardioversion.

50.8 The Primary Outcome

There was no difference in the primary outcome, the number of hospital days from randomization until day 60, between the rate and rhythm control groups [median: 5.1 (3.0–7.4) vs. 5.0 (3.2–7.5), $P = 0.76$]. The results were similar for all types of surgery—be it coronary artery bypass graft, valve surgery, or a combination of both procedures. Besides, the duration of hospital stay during the index hospitalization, and the number of days in hospital after discharge from the index hospitalization did not differ between groups. The length of hospital stay considering discharge readiness based on the status of atrial fibrillation was also similar.

50.9 Readmissions

There were 159 readmissions reported during the study period, including visits to the emergency department; the readmission rates were similar in both groups. Readmissions within 30 days of hospital discharge occurred in 22.8% in the rate control group and 21.4% in the rhythm control group.

50.10 Onset and Resolution of Atrial Fibrillation

The average time of onset of atrial fibrillation was 2.4 days after surgery. At hospital discharge, atrial fibrillation had resolved with a stable, sustained rhythm in most patients—93.5% in the rhythm control and 89.9% in the rate control group. Patients in the rhythm control group attained a stable rhythm without atrial fibrillation earlier compared to those in the rate control group. Furthermore, significantly more patients were free of atrial fibrillation between 30 and 60 days of randomization in the rhythm control group.

At the time of discharge, 42.7% of patients in the rate control and 43.3% of patients in the rhythm control group were on anticoagulation with warfarin. The main outcomes are summarized in Table 50.1.

Table 50.1 Main study outcomes. Median hospital days (interquartile range)

Outcome	Rate control (262 patients)	Rhythm control (261 patients)	*P* value
Hospital days at day-60	5.1 (3.0–7.4)	5.0 (3.2–7.5)	0.76
Hospital days during index hospitalization	4.3 (2.9–6.6)	4.3 (3.0–7.0)	0.88
Hospital days after index hospitalization	2.2 (0.6–5.0)	2.1 (1.0–4.7)	0.82

50.11 Adverse Events

At the 60-day follow-up, three patients in the rate control group and two in the rhythm control group had died. The incidence of serious adverse events did not differ significantly between the rate control and the rhythm control groups (24.8 per 100 patient months vs. 26.4 per 100 patient-months). The incidence of thromboembolism, cerebrovascular or otherwise, was also similar. Serious bleeding occurred at similar rates in both groups.

50.12 Study Conclusion

The authors concluded that a rate control strategy compared with a rhythm control strategy did not significantly impact clinical outcomes among patients who developed postoperative atrial fibrillation following elective cardiac surgery. The duration of hospitalization, complications, and persistent atrial fibrillation at 60 days remained similar with both strategies.

50.13 Strengths

The study was by far the largest RCT that compared a rate vs. rhythm control strategy in atrial fibrillation among postoperative cardiac surgical patients. The study was adequately powered to evaluate the primary endpoint of the number of days of hospitalization at 60 days post-randomization. The multicentric design offered external validity. Loss to follow-up was minimal at the end of the study period; analysis was carried out by intention-to-treat.

50.14 Limitations

The primary outcome, the duration of hospitalization, was used as a surrogate for important clinical endpoints, including stroke and serious bleeding, considering the unrealistically large sample size that would have been necessary to evaluate more specific outcomes. The trial enrolled hemodynamically stable patients who underwent elective cardiac surgery before they developed atrial fibrillation. Patients with postoperative atrial fibrillation that persisted for >60 minutes were randomized. It is plausible that spontaneous reversion to sinus rhythm (without specific treatment) may have occurred in many patients.

Patients with additional risk factors (poor left ventricular function) and a longer duration of atrial fibrillation could have benefited from rhythm control measures, including amiodarone and electrical cardioversion.

Crossover occurred in a significant number of patients in both groups—24% of those assigned to rhythm control did not complete the full course of amiodarone, while 26.7% who were randomized to rate control received amiodarone or underwent electrical cardioversion. Crossover to the alternate treatment strategy could have impacted outcomes.

The overall management was not protocolized; no data were available on ancillary care, including preventive measures, e.g., maintenance of electrolyte levels within a specific range. The authors did not evaluate quality-of-life measures; besides, continuous home monitoring was not employed to assess the incidence of postoperative atrial fibrillation, leading to a possible underestimate of the true incidence.

There have been conflicting reports on the incidence and duration of atrial fibrillation with concomitant use of statins [9, 10]. The study did not provide data on the possible impact of statin use. Details of preoperative medication may have been useful to understand the influence of drugs on postoperative atrial fibrillation—especially regarding the possible protective effect on the nearly 67% of patients who did not develop the arrhythmia.

50.15 Summary

The Gillinov et al. study confirmed that atrial fibrillation is common following cardiac surgery; overall, more than 30% of patients experienced persistent or recurrent atrial fibrillation. The incidence was higher (nearly 50%) among patients who underwent coronary artery bypass graft combined with valve replacement surgery. The investigators observed no difference between a rate control compared with a rhythm control strategy in the duration of hospital stay within 60 days of randomization. The incidence of adverse events was similar in both groups. Persistent atrial fibrillation at 60 days occurred in relatively few patients in both groups. Patients in the rhythm control group attained a stable heart rhythm earlier compared to the rate control group. Besides, more patients were atrial fibrillation-free between 30 and 60 days after randomization in the rhythm control group.

References

1. Bessissow A, Khan J, Devereaux PJ, Alvarez-Garcia J, Alonso-Coello P. Postoperative atrial fibrillation in non-cardiac and cardiac surgery: an overview. J Thromb Haemost JTH. 2015;13(Suppl 1):S304–12.
2. Eikelboom R, Sanjanwala R, Le ML, Yamashita MH, Arora RC. Postoperative atrial fibrillation after cardiac surgery: a systematic review and meta-analysis. Ann Thorac Surg. 2021;111(2):544–54.
3. Nair SG. Atrial fibrillation after cardiac surgery. Ann Card Anaesth. 2010;13(3):196–205.
4. Chelazzi C, Villa G, De Gaudio AR. Postoperative atrial fibrillation. ISRN Cardiol. 2011;2011:203179.
5. Wyse DG, Waldo AL, DiMarco JP, Domanski MJ, Rosenberg Y, Schron EB, et al. A comparison of rate control and rhythm control in patients with atrial fibrillation. N Engl J Med. 2002;347(23):1825–33.

6. Lee JK, Klein GJ, Krahn AD, Yee R, Zarnke K, Simpson C, et al. Rate-control versus conversion strategy in postoperative atrial fibrillation: trial design and pilot study results. Card Electrophysiol Rev. 2003;7(2):178–84.
7. Al-Khatib SM, Hafley G, Harrington RA, Mack MJ, Ferguson TB, Peterson ED, et al. Patterns of management of atrial fibrillation complicating coronary artery bypass grafting: results from the PRoject of ex-vivo vein graft ENgineering via transfection IV (PREVENT-IV) trial. Am Heart J. 2009;158(5):792–8.
8. Gillinov AM, Bagiella E, Moskowitz AJ, Raiten JM, Groh MA, Bowdish ME, et al. Rate control versus rhythm control for atrial fibrillation after cardiac surgery. N Engl J Med. 2016;374(20):1911–21.
9. Kuhn EW, Slottosch I, Wahlers T, Liakopoulos OJ. Preoperative statin therapy for patients undergoing cardiac surgery. Cochrane Database Syst Rev. 2015;8:CD008493.
10. Zheng Z, Jayaram R, Jiang L, Emberson J, Zhao Y, Li Q, et al. Perioperative rosuvastatin in cardiac surgery. N Engl J Med. 2016;374(18):1744–53.

51 Optimal PCI Strategy in Cardiogenic Shock Following Acute Myocardial Infarction: The CULPRIT-SHOCK Trial

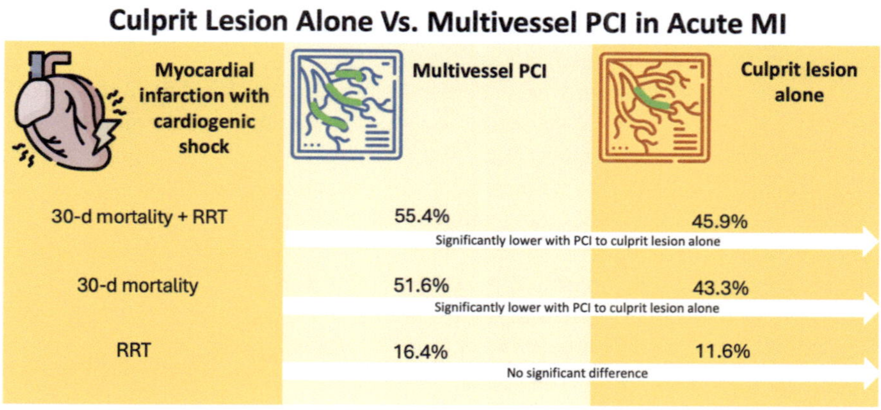

Thiele et al. (NEJM, 2017)

Quick Take

In patients with cardiogenic shock following acute myocardial infarction (MI), should revascularization be initially confined to the culprit lesion alone, or should concurrent, non-culprit lesions also be addressed?

This randomized trial evaluated different percutaneous coronary intervention (PCI) strategies in patients with acute MI complicated by cardiogenic shock. A total of 706 patients were randomly assigned to undergo either immediate PCI with complete revascularization or a more selective strategy of PCI involving the culprit lesion alone. The study found that complete revascularization did not improve

---

Thiele H, Akin I, Sandri M, Fuernau G, De Waha S, Meyer-Saraei R, et al. *PCI Strategies in Patients with Acute Myocardial Infarction and Cardiogenic Shock. N Engl J Med. 2017 Dec 21;377(25):2419–32.*

J. Chacko et al., *Landmark Studies in Critical Care*,
https://doi.org/10.1007/978-981-95-0673-6_51

survival or reduce the incidence of death or severe complications when compared to selective PCI. However, the complete revascularization strategy did result in better outcomes in terms of left ventricular function and fewer repeat revascularization procedures. These results challenged the prevailing belief that complete revascularization is always superior in this population and suggested that a more selective PCI approach may be just as effective in improving survival in the short term.

51.1 Introduction

Cardiogenic shock following acute myocardial infarction carries high mortality; besides, long-term outcomes remain poor among survivors [1]. The SHOCK trial, the first systematic study that evaluated the efficacy of emergency revascularization in patients with cardiogenic shock, was published nearly a quarter or a century ago. In a randomized controlled trial (RCT), emergency revascularization by angioplasty or coronary artery bypass grafting within 36 hours after acute myocardial infarction was compared with initial medical stabilization. Mortality at 6 months was significantly lower among patients who underwent emergency revascularization (50.3% vs. 63.1%) [2]. In a follow-up study, long-term outcomes were evaluated over 1–11 years [3]. Early revascularization was associated with a 67% improvement in the 6-year survival compared with initial medical stabilization. The survival benefit of early revascularization persisted through the entire follow-up period of up to 11 years.

Apart from the culprit vessel lesion, cardiogenic shock following acute myocardial infarction is often associated with chronic occlusion of other vessels [4]. Besides, the presence of multivessel disease is associated with higher mortality compared to single-vessel disease [5, 6]. In this scenario, should revascularization be confined to the infarct-related vessel alone or include other vessels with clinically important stenoses? Emergency revascularization of all affected vessels may potentially enhance overall myocardial perfusion and augment cardiac function. However, a multivessel revascularization strategy could be hazardous too—it may lead to worsening of ischemia, volume overload, and renal dysfunction related to a higher dose of contrast administration.

In the SHOCK trial, percutaneous coronary intervention (PCI) of the culprit lesion alone was the most common initial intervention. Intuitively, more complete revascularization might be expected to offer additional benefit; however, the subgroup of patients who underwent initial multivessel PCI revealed higher mortality compared to the subgroup that underwent revascularization of the culprit lesion alone [2].

A meta-analysis including 10 cohort studies compared immediate multivessel intervention with revascularization of the culprit lesion alone in patients with cardiogenic shock following acute myocardial infarction. Most patients (80.3%) underwent revascularization of the culprit lesion alone. The short-term mortality was significantly lower in those who underwent revascularization of the culprit lesion alone (28.8% vs. 37.5%). The long-term mortality, reinfarction rates, new-onset stroke, and acute renal failure did not differ significantly between the two groups.

The DANAMI-3—PRIMULTI trial studied patients with ST-elevation myocardial infarction (STEMI) who had additional, clinically significant coronary stenosis in vessels other than the infarct-related artery [7]. Patients were randomly allocated to undergo primary percutaneous coronary intervention of the infarct-related artery alone or to complete revascularization guided by the fractional flow reserve. The composite primary outcome, including all-cause mortality, non-fatal myocardial infarction, and later revascularization of lesions in non-infarct-related arteries, was significantly lower with complete revascularization. However, this study had excluded patients with cardiogenic shock.

Considering the lack of firm evidence, there were no strong recommendations from guidelines. While the European guidelines recommended consideration of PCI to non-culprit lesions in the presence of cardiogenic shock [8], the US guidelines suggested revascularization of non-culprit vessels if cardiogenic shock persisted [9]. Against the background of clinical equipoise, the CULPRIT-SHOCK trial was conceived [10]. The investigators hypothesized that PCI of the culprit lesion alone, with revascularization of concurrent lesions at a later stage as appropriate, would lead to more favorable clinical outcomes compared with immediate, multivessel PCI in patients with cardiogenic shock following acute myocardial infarction.

51.2 Population and Design

The CULPRIT-SHOCK trial was conducted between April 2013 and April 2017 and included 706 patients from 83 centers across Europe. Patients with acute myocardial infarction (ST-segment elevation or non-ST-segment elevation) complicated by cardiogenic shock, with an identified culprit lesion, were eligible. Patients had multivessel disease, defined as involving at least two major vessels with more than 70% stenosis. Cardiogenic shock was defined as a systolic BP of <90 mm Hg for >30 min or the requirement for catecholamine support to maintain systolic BP >90 mm Hg, with clinical signs of pulmonary congestion and diminished organ perfusion including one the following: altered sensorium, cold and clammy extremities, urine output of <30 ml/hour, and arterial lactate level of >2.0 mmol/L.

51.2.1 Excluded

Patients who had undergone cardiopulmonary resuscitation for >30 min, those with no intrinsic myocardial activity, fixed dilated pupils, indication for primary coronary artery bypass grafting, cardiogenic shock due to a mechanical cause, duration of shock >12 hours, massive pulmonary embolism, pre-existing severe renal dysfunction, age > 90 years, and comorbidities with a life expectancy of <6 months were excluded.

51.2.2 Randomization

Immediately following angiography, patients were randomized, in a 1:1 ratio, to PCI of the culprit lesion alone or immediate multivessel PCI.

51.2.3 PCI of the Culprit Lesion Alone

Following randomization, PCI was performed on the culprit lesion alone. Staged revascularization of non-culprit lesions was carried out later, as deemed clinically appropriate. The requirement for later revascularization was based on the presence of residual ischemic lesions and the overall clinical and neurological status. Residual ischemia was assessed by measurement of the fractional flow reserve (FFR). FFR is defined as the ratio of the maximum achievable flow through a stenotic segment to the maximum achievable flow with the hypothetical absence of blockage.

FFR = Pressure distal to the blockage/pressure proximal to the blockage. The normal FFR is 1.0. A low FFR indicates reduced flow; e.g., an FFR of 0.70 indicates a maximum flow through a blocked artery of 70% of the flow achievable had there been no blockage [11].

51.2.4 Multivessel PCI

In the multivessel group, PCI of the culprit lesion was performed first, followed by PCI of all major coronary arteries with >70% stenosis. All chronic total occlusions were meant to be recanalized during the acute phase. The maximum dose of contrast material recommended was 300 ml.

51.2.5 Common Management

Other therapeutic interventions were carried out as clinically appropriate, including mechanical circulatory support and renal replacement therapy, based on accepted ICU guidelines. Renal replacement therapy was considered in the presence of intractable volume overload, a potassium level of >6.0 mmol/L, a blood urea level of >50 mg/dl, or persistent metabolic acidosis with a pH of <7.2.

51.2.6 Sample Size Calculation

The sample size was calculated based on the event rate of the composite primary outcome—the all-cause mortality and severe acute kidney injury requiring renal replacement therapy at 30 days post-randomization. The investigators assumed an event rate of 50% in the multivessel group and 38% in the culprit-lesion-only group. A sample size of 684 patients provided the trial with 80% power to disprove the null hypothesis at a two-sided alpha level of 0.048. Seven hundred and six patients were recruited, allowing for a withdrawal rate of 3%.

51.3 Results

Among the 706 patients included, 351 were assigned to culprit-lesion-only PCI and 355 to multivessel PCI. In the final analysis, there were 344 patients in the culprit-lesion-only group and 341 patients in the multivessel PCI group. Crossover occurred both ways; culprit-lesion-only to multivessel in 43 patients (12.5%) and contrariwise in 32 patients (9.4%). Staged revascularization of concurrent, non-culprit lesions was performed in 17.7% of patients in the culprit-lesion-only group. As expected, the total contrast dose was significantly higher in the multivessel group. Mechanical circulatory support and adjunctive medications were used at similar rates in both groups.

51.3.1 The Primary Outcome

The primary outcome, a composite of all-cause mortality and severe acute kidney injury requiring renal replacement therapy at 30 days post-randomization, was significantly lower in the culprit-lesion-only group compared with the multivessel group [45.9% vs. 55.4%; relative risk: 0.83 (0.71–0.96); $P = 0.01$)]. Per-protocol analysis revealed similar outcomes, favoring the culprit-lesion-only strategy. The composite primary outcome was similar in predefined subgroups of patients based on age, gender, presence of diabetes, hypertension, type of infarct (STEMI vs. NSETMI), location of infarct, previous infarct, the number of affected vessels, and the presence of chronic total occlusion.

51.3.2 Secondary Outcomes

The secondary outcomes included individual components of the composite primary outcome. The 30-day all-cause mortality was significantly lower with a culprit-lesion-only strategy compared to multivessel intervention [43.3% vs. 51.6%; relative risk, 0.84; (0.72–0.98); $P = 0.03$]. The requirement for renal replacement therapy did not differ significantly between the two groups. The incidence of recurrent myocardial infarction, stroke, rehospitalization for cardiac failure, and bleeding complications was similar in both groups. Among other secondary outcomes, the median time to attain hemodynamic stability (2 days in both groups), duration of catecholamine support (2 days in both groups), duration of ICU stay (5 days in both groups), and the duration of mechanical ventilation (3 days in both groups) were also similar in both groups. The main study outcomes are summarized in Table 51.1.

Table 51.1 Main study outcomes

Outcomes	PCI of culprit lesion alone	Multivessel PCI	Significance
All-cause mortality and AKI requiring RRT at 30 d	45.9%	55.4%	$P = 0.01$
All-cause mortality	43.3%	51.6%	$P = 0.03$
AKI requiring RRT	11.6%	16.4%	$P = 0.07$
Death, recurrent MI, rehospitalization CCF	43.9%	52.3%	$P = 0.03$

Abbreviations: *PCI* percutaneous coronary intervention, *AKI* acute kidney injury, *RRT* renal replacement therapy, *MI* myocardial infarction, *CCF* congestive cardiac failure

51.4 Study Conclusions

The study compared immediate multivessel PCI with PCI of the culprit lesion alone among patients with acute myocardial infarction and cardiogenic shock. The authors found that the composite outcome of death or renal failure requiring renal replacement therapy was lower in patients who initially underwent PCI of the culprit lesion alone. The 30-day all-cause mortality was also lower in those who underwent PCI of the culprit lesion alone.

51.5 Why Did Multivessel PCI Lead to Worse Outcomes?

The authors hypothesized that the higher 30-day mortality may have occurred due to the higher mean dose of contrast used in the multivessel PCI group (250 ml vs. 190 ml), leading to a more profound decline in renal function. However, the requirement for renal replacement therapy was not significantly different between the two groups. Acute left ventricular volume overload may also have arisen from the increased dose of contrast, adversely impacting myocardial function and recovery. The longer procedural time associated with multivessel intervention may also have jeopardized outcomes in an unstable clinical situation, through increased bleeding and inflammation. Furthermore, attempting PCI in stable lesions may have provoked further damage to the already compromised myocardium [12].

51.6 Strengths

The CULPRIT-SHOCK trial was a well-conducted RCT, with the sole participant being lost to follow-up. Risk estimates for the primary endpoint were consistent on per-protocol, intention-to-treat, and as-treated analysis, adding to the robustness of the findings. The study findings challenged conventional wisdom and the limited antecedent evidence that suggested improved clinical outcomes with a more complete revascularization strategy.

51.7 Weaknesses

Blinding of the treatment strategy was technically not feasible and, hence, may have led to bias, especially in the assessment of secondary outcomes. The management of cardiogenic shock revolves around many complex interventions; it is plausible that some bias may have occurred during the conduct of the study due to the lack of blinding. Due to the absence of a final informed consent, some patients could not be included in the final analysis. Crossover occurred from the culprit-lesion-only to the multivessel strategy arm in 43 patients (12.5%) and contrariwise in 32 patients (9.4%). Crossovers underline the importance of individualization of care and clinical judgment in the setting of multivessel involvement. The study protocol mandated revascularization of chronic total occlusions; would such a strategy have contributed to adverse outcomes in the multivessel strategy group? Considering a substantial number of patients who underwent cardiopulmonary resuscitation before PCI (54%), evaluation of the neurological status may have been relevant.

51.8 One-Year Outcomes

Although immediate multivessel PCI, including non-culprit lesions, may be associated with adverse outcomes at 30 days, how does it impact long-term outcomes? A follow-up of the CUPRIT-SHOCK subjects evaluated clinical outcomes at 1 year [13]. Data of all patients who had at least 30 days of follow-up were included; analysis was based on intention-to-treat. All except one patient were followed up between 30 days and 1 year. The overall mortality between 30 days and 1 year was 6.6%. Although the all-cause mortality remained higher in the multivessel PCI group at 1 year, the difference was no longer statistically significant [50.0% vs. 56.9%; relative risk, 0.88; (0.76–1.01)]. Death due to cardiovascular causes was also not significantly different between the two groups at the 1-year follow-up. At the end of 1 year, repeat procedures for revascularization were performed more often in the culprit-lesion-only group (32.3% vs. 9.4%). The rehospitalization rate for congestive cardiac failure was low in both groups, although it was significantly higher with the culprit-lesion-only strategy (5.2% vs. 1.2%).

This follow-up study did not support the hypothesis that a multivessel revascularization strategy may improve longer-term outcomes among patients presenting with cardiogenic shock.

51.9 Summary

The CULPRIT-SHOCK trial addressed an important clinical question with contrasting evidence and viewpoints. The study evaluated a culprit-vessel-only approach compared with a multivessel PCI among patients with cardiogenic shock following acute myocardial infarction. PCI of the culprit lesion alone led to a lower incidence of the composite outcome—the 30-day all-cause mortality and the requirement for renal replacement therapy, compared to a multivessel strategy. The favorable primary outcome was driven almost entirely by improved 30-day survival in the culprit-lesion-only group; the need for renal replacement therapy was similar in both groups. This well-conducted RCT with near complete follow-up offered convincing evidence that it may be more appropriate to direct intervention initially to the culprit lesion alone in patients with acute myocardial infarction complicated by cardiogenic shock. It is important to emphasize that the patient population included were severely ill—81% underwent mechanical ventilation, 90% required catecholamine support, and 54% had undergone cardiopulmonary resuscitation prior to PCI. Hence, the findings of the study may not be extrapolable to those who are less severely ill. Besides, as the authors pointed out, one size may not fit all, and the type of intervention requires adaptation to the clinical setting.

References

1. Hochman JS, Sleeper LA, White HD, Dzavik V, Wong SC, Menon V, et al. One-year survival following early revascularization for cardiogenic shock. JAMA. 2001;285(2):190–2.
2. Hochman JS, Sleeper LA, Webb JG, Sanborn TA, White HD, Talley JD, et al. Early revascularization in acute myocardial infarction complicated by cardiogenic shock. N Engl J Med. 1999;341(9):625–34.
3. Hochman JS, Sleeper LA, Webb JG, Dzavik V, Buller CE, Aylward P. Early revascularization improves long-term survival for cardiogenic shock complicating acute myocardial infarction. JAMA. 2007;295(21):2511–5.
4. Conde-Vela C, Moreno R, Hernández R, Pérez-Vizcayno MJ, Alfonso F, Escaned J, et al. Cardiogenic shock at admission in patients with multivessel disease and acute myocardial infarction treated with percutaneous coronary intervention: related factors. Int J Cardiol. 2007;123(1):29–33.
5. Webb JG, Lowe AM, Sanborn TA, White HD, Sleeper LA, Carere RG, et al. Percutaneous coronary intervention for cardiogenic shock in the SHOCK trial. J Am Coll Cardiol. 2003;42(8):1380–6.
6. Sanborn TA, Sleeper LA, Webb JG, French JK, Bergman G, Parikh M, et al. Correlates of one-year survival inpatients with cardiogenic shock complicating acute myocardial infarction: angiographic findings from the SHOCK trial. J Am Coll Cardiol. 2003;42(8):1373–9.
7. Engstrøm T, Kelbæk H, Helqvist S, Høfsten DE, Kløvgaard L, Holmvang L, et al. Complete revascularisation versus treatment of the culprit lesion only in patients with ST-segment elevation myocardial infarction and multivessel disease (DANAMI-3—PRIMULTI): an open-label, randomised controlled trial. Lancet Lond Engl. 2015;386(9994):665–71.
8. Ibánez B, James S, Agewall S, Antunes MJ, Bucciarelli-Ducci C, Bueno H, et al. 2017 ESC Guidelines for the management of acute myocardial infarction in patients presenting with ST-segment elevation. Rev Esp Cardiol Engl Ed. 2017;70(12):1082.
9. Patel MR, Calhoon JH, Dehmer GJ, Grantham JA, Maddox TM, Maron DJ, et al. ACC/AATS/AHA/ASE/ASNC/SCAI/SCCT/STS 2016 appropriate use criteria for coronary revascularization in patients with acute coronary syndromes: a report of the American College of Cardiology Appropriate Use Criteria Task Force, American Association for Thoracic Surgery, American Heart Association, American Society of Echocardiography, American Society of Nuclear Cardiology, Society for Cardiovascular Angiography and Interventions, Society of Cardiovascular Computed Tomography, and the Society of Thoracic Surgeons. J Nucl Cardiol. 2017;24(2):439–63.

10. Thiele H, Akin I, Sandri M, Fuernau G, De Waha S, Meyer-Saraei R, et al. PCI strategies in patients with acute myocardial infarction and cardiogenic shock. N Engl J Med. 2017;377(25):2419–32.
11. Pijls NH, De Bruyne B, Peels K, Van Der Voort PH, Bonnier HJ, Bartunek J, Koolen JJ, et al. Measurement of fractional flow reserve to assess the functional severity of coronary-artery stenoses. N Engl J Med. 1996;334(26):1703–8.
12. Thiele H, Desch S. CULPRIT-SHOCK (Culprit Lesion Only PCI Versus Multivessel Percutaneous Coronary Intervention in Cardiogenic Shock): implications on guideline recommendations. Circulation. 2018;137(13):1314–6.
13. Thiele H, Akin I, Sandri M, De Waha-Thiele S, Meyer-Saraei R, Fuernau G, et al. One-year outcomes after PCI strategies in cardiogenic shock. N Engl J Med. 2018;379(18):1699–710.

Coronary Angioplasty Versus Fibrinolytic Therapy in Acute Myocardial Infarction: The DANAMI-2 Trial

52

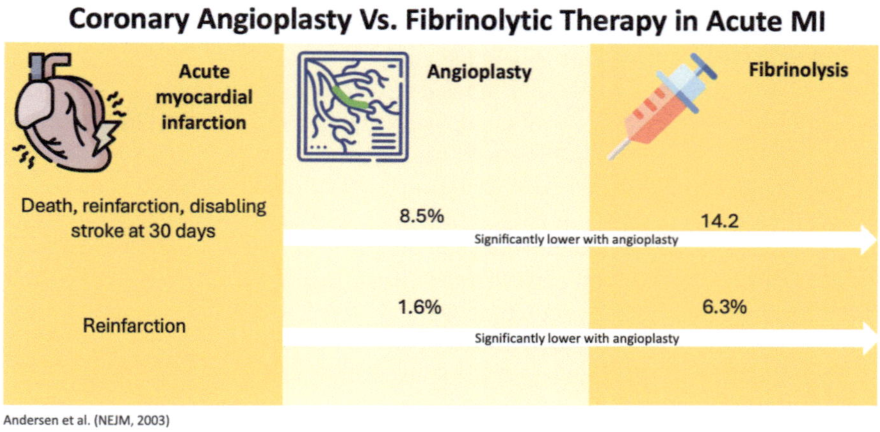

Quick Take

Which is better in acute myocardial infarction (MI)—Percutaneous Coronary Intervention (PCI) or fibrinolytic therapy?

The DANAMI II trial PCI with fibrinolytic therapy in patients with acute MI presenting within 12 hours of symptom onset. Patients were randomized to receive either PCI or fibrinolysis. The study found that PCI was superior to fibrinolytic therapy in reducing the risk of death, recurrent myocardial infarction, and the need for repeat revascularization. Patients who underwent PCI also had better long-term survival outcomes. The results from this trial reinforced the benefit of

Andersen HR, Nielsen TT, Rasmussen K, Thuesen L, Kelbaek H, Thayssen P, et al. A comparison of coronary angioplasty with fibrinolytic therapy in acute myocardial infarction. N Engl J Med. 2003 Aug 21;349 (8):733–42.

J. Chacko et al., *Landmark Studies in Critical Care*,
https://doi.org/10.1007/978-981-95-0673-6_52

PCI over fibrinolysis in STEMI patients, especially those presenting early, and provided strong evidence for early angioplasty as the preferred strategy in this patient group.

52.1 Introduction

In September 1977, a 38-year-old man presented to the University Hospital in Zurich, Switzerland, with acute myocardial infarction. The likely culprit was a discrete occlusion of the left anterior descending coronary artery. By then, coronary artery bypass surgery had already been established as one of the treatment modalities available for atherosclerotic occlusion. Considering the patient's reluctance to undergo an operative procedure that cut through the middle of the chest, Andreas Grüntzig, his physician, offered him the option of opening the blocked vessel using a balloon catheter. Grüntzig had previously demonstrated the efficacy of this technique in peripheral arterial occlusions; the atheroma could be compressed, leaving behind a smooth lumen. As his patient lay awake, Grüntzig passed the balloon catheter into the stenotic segment and inflated it with consummate ease. The results were spectacular, as evident on follow-up angiography. Subsequently, he performed the procedure on four more patients with equally good results. He predicted that this new technique may offer a viable therapeutic modality for patients with angina pectoris in the years to come [1].

By the 1980s, several studies were published demonstrating the efficacy of intravenous fibrinolysis, an alternative therapy. Most coronary care units adopted this treatment modality, allowing for a time window of 6 hours after the onset of symptoms [2, 3]. The GUSTO IIb randomized controlled trial (RCT) compared primary angioplasty with fibrinolytic therapy using recombinant tissue plasminogen activator in patients who presented within 12 hours of ST-segment elevation myocardial infarction (STEMI). Primary angioplasty was superior, with a significantly lower incidence of the composite outcome of death, nonfatal reinfarction, and disabling stroke at 30 days [4].

At the time of the conduct of the DANAMI-2 trial, most patients with acute myocardial infarction presented to hospitals that did not have the facility for angioplasty. The standard practice was expeditious intravenous fibrinolysis or transfer to a center with the facility to perform primary angioplasty. Although primary angioplasty had been shown to be superior, the requirement for transfer from the local hospital to an angioplasty center presented a significant bottleneck on its widespread implementation. The DANAMI-2 trial investigated outcomes with on-site fibrinolysis compared to transfer to an invasive-treatment center for primary angioplasty in patients with STEMI.

52.2 Population and Design

The DANAMI-2 randomized controlled trial (RCT) was conducted between 1997 and 2001 in patients with ST-elevation myocardial infarction [5]. Adult patients, 18 years or older, who experienced symptoms for ≥30 minutes and < 12 hours with a cumulative ST-segment elevation of ≥4 mm in two contiguous leads were included. Patients were initially evaluated at 24 referral hospitals or five invasive-treatment centers in Denmark. They were randomized to undergo fibrinolytic therapy or primary angioplasty. Patients who were initially evaluated at the referral center and randomized to primary angioplasty were transferred to one of five invasive treatment centers. Patients were taken directly to the coronary care unit of the referral hospital by ambulance personnel (not via the emergency department); transfer to the invasive-treatment center was carried out by the same ambulance staff, thus avoiding delays.

52.2.1 Exclusion

Patients with contraindications to fibrinolysis, left bundle branch block, those who had sustained acute myocardial infarction and underwent fibrinolysis in the previous 30 days, those with pulseless femoral arteries, previous coronary artery bypass surgery, renal dysfunction with creatinine level > 2.83 mg/dl, diabetes on metformin, non-ischemic heart disease, and a life expectancy of <12 months were excluded. Patients deemed to be at high risk for transfer due to cardiogenic shock, severe heart failure, persistent life-threatening arrhythmias, and those on mechanical ventilation were also excluded.

52.3 The Fibrinolysis Group

Patients randomized to the fibrinolysis group received aspirin 300 mg and an intravenous beta-blocker equivalent to 20 mg of metoprolol. They received tissue plasminogen activator (alteplase) as the fibrinolytic agent—an initial bolus dose of 15 mg was followed by an infusion of 0.75 mg/kg over 30 minutes, and 0.5 mg/kg over 60 minutes. Unfractionated heparin was administered as a bolus dose of 5000 units, followed by a continuous infusion for 48 hours, aiming to maintain an activated partial thromboplastin time (APTT) between 70 and 90 seconds. Repeat fibrinolysis or rescue angioplasty was considered if failed reperfusion was suspected, or reinfarction or recurrent ischemia occurred.

52.4 The Angioplasty Group

The management protocol in the angioplasty group consisted of aspirin 300 mg, a similar dose of beta-blocker, and 10,000 U of unfractionated heparin, with further doses aiming for an APTT level of 350–450 seconds during the procedure. Platelet glycoprotein IIb/IIIa (GP IIb/IIIa) inhibitors were administered at the clinician's discretion. Angioplasty was performed on the infarct-related artery if it was totally occluded, >30% of the lumen was occluded, or if the flow grade was <3 based on the Thrombolysis in Myocardial Infarction (TIMI) classification. Stenting was attempted unless the arterial diameter was <2.0 mm. Patients were given ticlopidine, 500 mg, or clopidogrel, 75 mg daily for a month after the procedure. Repeat angioplasty was performed if reinfarction or recurrent ischemia occurred.

52.5 Sample Size

The authors calculated the sample size based on the composite primary outcome of all-cause mortality, clinical reinfarction, or disabling stroke at 30 days of follow-up. The incidence of the composite primary outcome was assumed to be 16% with fibrinolysis, 10% among those randomized to angioplasty and transferred to invasive-treatment centers, and 9% among those who were initially evaluated at the invasive-treatment center and randomized to undergo angioplasty. The sample size required 1100 patients to be treated at referral hospitals and 800 at invasive treatment centers.

52.6 Results

The study was terminated after the third interim analysis revealed superior outcomes with primary angioplasty compared to fibrinolysis in the subgroup of patients randomized at the referral hospitals. A total of 1129 patients had undergone randomization at the referral hospitals and 443 at the invasive-treatment centers at the time of termination of the study. All except eight of 567 patients (99%) who were randomized to angioplasty at the referral hospitals were transferred to invasive-treatment centers. The baseline characteristics were similar between patients assigned to fibrinolysis or primary angioplasty.

The median transfer time, defined as the time from randomization at the referral hospital to arrival in the catheterization laboratory, was 67 minutes (interquartile range, 50–85). Nearly all patients (96%) reached the catheterization laboratory at the invasive-care center within 2 hours of randomization at the referral hospital.

Complications during transfer were uncommon—atrial fibrillation occurred in 14, intermittent atrioventricular block in 13, and ventricular fibrillation in eight patients. No deaths occurred during transfer.

Seven hundred and seventy-five of 782 (99%) patients randomized to the fibrinolysis arm received the assigned treatment. In the angioplasty group, 777/790 (98%) received the assigned treatment. The left anterior descending artery was the culprit vessel in 46% of patients; the right coronary artery was involved in 35%, and the left circumflex artery in 12% of patients.

52.7 Outcomes

52.7.1 The Primary Outcome

The composite primary outcome of all-cause mortality, reinfarction, and disabling stroke at 30 days was significantly lower with primary angioplasty compared to fibrinolysis [107/782 (13.7%) vs. 63/790 (8%); $p < 0.001$]. The superior primary outcome was observed among patients enrolled at the referral hospitals and at invasive-treatment centers. The relative reduction in the composite outcome was 40% among patients enrolled at referral hospitals and 45% among those enrolled at invasive-treatment centers. The primary composite outcome was superior among prespecified subgroups of patients treated with angioplasty based on age (63 years vs. older), gender, duration of symptoms, anterior vs. non-anterior myocardial infarction, and smoking status. The outcome benefit related to angioplasty over fibrinolysis was evident regardless of the duration of symptoms (less than 2 hours, between 2 and 4 hours, more than 4 hours).

The number needed to treat with primary angioplasty to prevent one death, reinfarction, or disabling stroke was 17.5 patients in the overall cohort.

Among the individual components of the primary outcome, the reinfarction rate was significantly lower with angioplasty compared to fibrinolysis. The beneficial effect of angioplasty over fibrinolysis was mainly due to a 75% reduction in the incidence of reinfarction (1.6% vs. 6.3%). Among patients who suffered reinfarction, the 30-day mortality was significantly higher compared to those who did not (24.2% vs. 6.5%).

The 30-day all-cause mortality was lower with angioplasty compared with fibrinolysis, although the difference was not statistically significant (6.6 vs. 7.8%, $p = 0.35$). The incidence of disabling stroke was also not significantly different between groups. The main study outcomes are summarized in Table 52.1.

Table 52.1 Main study outcomes

30-day outcome	Fibrinolysis (782 patients)	Angioplasty (790 patients)	Significance (p-value)
All-cause mortality	61 (7.8%)	52 (6.6%)	NS (0.35)
Reinfarction	49 (6.3%)	13 (1.6%)	S (<0.001)
Disabling stroke	16 (2%)	9 (1.1%)	NS (0.15)
The composite outcome	*107 (13.7%)*	*63 (8%)*	*S (<0.001)*

Abbreviations: *NS* not significant, *S* significant

52.7.2 Repeat Revascularization

At 30 days of follow-up, in the fibrinolysis group, 20 patients had undergone coronary artery bypass surgery, while 129 underwent angioplasty. In the angioplasty group, 30 patients underwent coronary artery bypass surgery, while 45 underwent repeat angioplasty. Repeat revascularization was significantly lower with angioplasty compared to fibrinolysis.

52.8 Study Conclusions

The DANAMI II trial demonstrated that primary angioplasty is superior to fibrinolysis for patients with STEMI, even when they are initially evaluated at a community hospital and have to be transferred to an invasive-treatment center, provided the transport time is less than 2 hours. The primary study end point, a composite of death, clinical evidence of reinfarction, or disabling stroke at 30 days, was significantly lower in the angioplasty group. Among the individual components of the primary outcome, the reinfarction rate was lower with primary angioplasty; however, mortality and the incidence of disabling stroke did not differ significantly.

52.9 Limitations

Although 4278 patients were screened, following exclusions, only 1572 (37%) were randomized. Patients with diabetes on metformin, peripheral vascular disease, previous coronary artery bypass surgery, and renal dysfunction were all excluded—these represent subgroups of patients who may have poor outcomes with angioplasty. In the angioplasty group, clopidogrel was administered in >80% of patients, which may have reduced the incidence of reinfarction. The time to transfer to the invasive-treatment center appears crucial; nearly all patients arrived within 2 hours of randomization. Expeditious transfer to a center with a facility for angioplasty may hold the key to improved outcomes. Among patients who underwent fibrinolysis, rescue angioplasty was performed sparingly (15 patients); this may be at variance with contemporary practice.

52.10 Subsequent Studies

The findings of the PRAGUE-2 RCT echoed those of the DANAMI II trial [6]. The investigators randomized 850 patients with STEMI within <12 hours of symptom onset at a community hospital to undergo fibrinolysis ($n = 421$) or transfer to a center with the facility for primary angioplasty ($n = 429$). Thirty-day mortality, the primary endpoint, was lower among patients who underwent primary angioplasty compared with those who underwent fibrinolysis (6.0% vs 10.4%, $p < 0.05$). The improved survival was largely confined to patients who were randomized >3 hours after the onset of symptoms. The composite endpoint of death, reinfarction, and stroke at 30 days was also lower among patients who underwent primary angioplasty (8.4% vs. 15.2%, $p < 0.003$). The European and American guidelines currently recommend primary percutaneous coronary intervention (pPCI) if the duration between STEMI diagnosis or first medical contact to reperfusion is expected to be less than 120 minutes [7, 8].

52.10.1 Follow-Up Studies of the DANAMI II Trial

A 3-year follow-up of the DANAMI II trial revealed sustained benefits among patients who underwent primary angioplasty [9]. The composite endpoint of death, reinfarction, or disabling stroke remained significantly lower compared to fibrinolysis (19.6 vs. 25.2%, $p = 0.006$). The results at 16 years of follow-up were published in August 2019, including the status of all except 5 of the 1572 patients originally included [10]. The primary outcome was a composite of all-cause mortality or rehospitalization for myocardial infarction. Patients who had undergone primary angioplasty revealed a lower rate of the composite endpoint compared to those who underwent fibrinolysis [58.7% vs. 62.3%; HR 0.86, 95% confidence interval (CI) 0.76–0.98]. The superiority of angioplasty was driven by a lower rate of rehospitalization in patients treated with angioplasty (19.0% vs. 24.5%; HR 0.75, 95% CI 0.60–0.93). There was no significant difference in all-cause mortality between the two groups. However, the risk of cardiac death was lower with primary angioplasty (18.3% vs. 22.7%; HR 0.78, 95% CI 0.63–0.98). This study established the sustained beneficial effects of primary angioplasty compared with fibrinolytic therapy at 16 years of follow-up.

52.11 Summary

The DANAMI-2 trial established the superiority of angioplasty compared to fibrinolysis in patients with STEMI, even among those who had to be transferred to an invasive treatment center to undergo the procedure. It remains the first and largest RCT that compared transferring patients with STEMI for primary angioplasty with administration of onsite fibrinolysis. In fact, the benefit of primary angioplasty was similar for patients who were transferred from referral hospitals compared with those who were admitted directly to the invasive-treatment centers. Complications were few, with no deaths reported during the transfer. The study provided the impetus for the establishment of routine angioplasty at community hospitals for patients with STEMI. The findings of the DANAMI-2 trial and similar findings from other studies led to the recommendation that percutaneous coronary intervention may be carried out if the duration between the diagnosis of STEMI or first medical contact to balloon time is expected to be less than 120 minutes.

References

1. Gruntzig A. Transluminal dilatation of coronary-artery stenosis. Lancet Lond Engl. 1978;1(8058):263.
2. Effectiveness of intravenous thrombolytic treatment in acute myocardial infarction. Gruppo Italiano per lo Studio della Streptochinasi nell'Infarto Miocardico (GISSI). Lancet Lond Engl. 1986;1(8478):397–402.
3. ISIS-2 (Second International Study of Infarct Survival) Collaborative Group. Randomised trial of intravenous streptokinase, oral aspirin, both, or neither among 17,187 cases of suspected acute myocardial infarction: ISIS-2. Lancet Lond Engl. 1988;2(8607):349–60.
4. A clinical trial comparing primary coronary angioplasty with tissue plasminogen activator for acute myocardial infarction. N Engl J Med. 1997;336(23):1621–8.
5. Andersen HR, Nielsen TT, Rasmussen K, Thuesen L, Kelbaek H, Thayssen P, et al. A comparison of coronary angioplasty with fibrinolytic therapy in acute myocardial infarction. N Engl J Med. 2003;349(8):733–42.
6. Widimský P, Budesínský T, Vorác D, Groch L, Zelízko M, Aschermann M, et al. Long distance transport for primary angioplasty vs immediate thrombolysis in acute myocardial infarction. Final results of the randomized national multicentre trial--PRAGUE-2. Eur Heart J. 2003;24(1):94–104.
7. Neumann FJ, Sousa-Uva M, Ahlsson A, Alfonso F, Banning AP, Benedetto U, et al. 2018 ESC/EACTS Guidelines on myocardial revascularization. Eur Heart J. 2019;40(2):87–165.
8. O'Gara PT, Kushner FG, Ascheim DD, Casey DE, Chung MK, de Lemos JA, et al. 2013 ACCF/AHA guideline for the management of ST-elevation myocardial infarction: a report of the American College of Cardiology Foundation/American Heart Association Task Force on Practice Guidelines. Circulation. 2013;127(4):e362–425.
9. Busk M, Maeng M, Rasmussen K, Kelbaek H, Thayssen P, Abildgaard U, et al. The Danish multicentre randomized study of fibrinolytic therapy vs. primary angioplasty in acute myocardial infarction (the DANAMI-2 trial): outcome after 3 years follow-up. Eur Heart J. 2008;29(10):1259–66.
10. Thrane PG, Kristensen SD, Olesen KKW, Mortensen LS, Bøtker HE, Thuesen L, et al. 16-year follow-up of the Danish Acute Myocardial infarction 2 (DANAMI-2) trial: primary percutaneous coronary intervention vs. fibrinolysis in ST-segment elevation myocardial infarction. Eur Heart J. 2020;41(7):847–54.

Part XII

Sepsis—Resuscitation

53 Goal-Directed Resuscitation in Sepsis: The Rivers et al., ProCESS, ARISE, and ProMISe Trials

Quick Take

Against the background of the Rivers et al. trial on early goal-directed therapy (EGDT) in sepsis, the broad question of whether EGDT truly conferred a measurable benefit was addressed in three separate multicenter trials undertaken in three different parts of the world—the ProCESS (Protocol-Based Care for Early Septic Shock), ARISE (Australasian Resuscitation in Sepsis Evaluation), and ProMISe (Procolized Management in Sepsis) trials.

The ProCESS trial was a multicenter study conducted in 31 centers in the USA, including 1351 patients, to evaluate the effectiveness of Early Goal-Directed Therapy (EGDT) in septic shock. It compared three approaches: EGDT, protocol-based standard care, and usual care. The study found that EGDT did not improve survival rates compared to the other two approaches. It also showed that less invasive resuscitation strategies were as effective as EGDT.

This ARISE trial enrolled 1600 patients across 51 centers, primarily in Australia and New Zealand, to evaluate the efficacy of EGDT, a protocol-driven approach targeting specific hemodynamic goals, compared to usual care in the first 6 hours of septic shock management. The study found no significant difference in 90-day mortality between the EGDT and usual care groups. Similarly, there were no major differences in secondary outcomes such as organ support requirements or hospital stay duration. Importantly, the trial demonstrated that usual care, which has evolved significantly since EGDT was first proposed, is non-inferior in terms of patient outcomes.

The ProMISe trial enrolled 1260 patients from 56 centers in the United Kingdom to evaluate EGDT, a protocolized approach involving specific hemodynamic targets, compared to usual care in the first 6 hours of septic shock management. The trial found no significant difference in 90-day mortality between the EGDT and usual care groups. Additionally, no substantial differences were observed in secondary outcomes, including organ support or length of stay. The findings highlighted

J. Chacko et al., *Landmark Studies in Critical Care*,
https://doi.org/10.1007/978-981-95-0673-6_53

that usual care, incorporating early recognition and prompt treatment of sepsis, achieved comparable outcomes to EGDT.

The findings of these randomized controlled trials offered robust evidence that rigid EGDT protocols are not superior to contemporary sepsis care, emphasizing flexibility and individualized patient management in the treatment of septic shock.

53.1 Introduction

Despite an increased awareness of sepsis among healthcare providers and even the general public, sepsis nevertheless remains a major health issue, one that is associated with high morbidity, mortality, and cost [1–3]. Sepsis afflicts all populations and societies, yet it disproportionately affects those from resource-poor regions, where basic healthcare services are often substandard, and where access to medical care is frequently limited [1]. The risk for sepsis is especially high, and outcomes are usually worse among certain groups, including the very young, the elderly, and those with chronic diseases and immunocompromised conditions [1, 4, 5]. While research continues to focus on ways to attenuate and modulate the host immune response and cellular dysregulation that characterizes sepsis, management still largely depends upon prompt identification of afflicted patients, prompt pathogen identification, quick implementation of infection control, early administration of antimicrobial drugs, and hemodynamic resuscitation and restoration of organ system failures that develop [1, 6, 7, 8, 9].

53.2 Early Studies on Physiologic Goals

Early investigations into sepsis management focused on close and continuous monitoring and optimization of key physiologic targets, including heart rate, mean arterial pressure, urine output, central venous pressure, serum lactate, oxygen delivery and consumption indices, pulmonary capillary wedge pressure, and other metrics of cardiac function and evolving anaerobic metabolism [10–14]. Despite evidence from several, often small studies that assessed optimization of surrogate endpoints, the effect upon patient mortality and morbidity remained inconclusive [15, 16]. Furthermore, the incidence of sepsis remained high, an observation likely confounded by factors such as an increased clinical understanding and recognition of sepsis as a unique and serious entity, the aging of the population, and possibly even changes in sepsis definitions and diagnostic criteria [3, 15, 17]. In addition, since specifically targeted interventions for sepsis were frequently delayed and often not provided until ICU admission or even beyond, it is likely that the "golden hour" when patients were most likely to benefit was probably missed [18–20].

53.3 Early Goal-Directed Therapy: The Rivers et al. Trial [19][1]

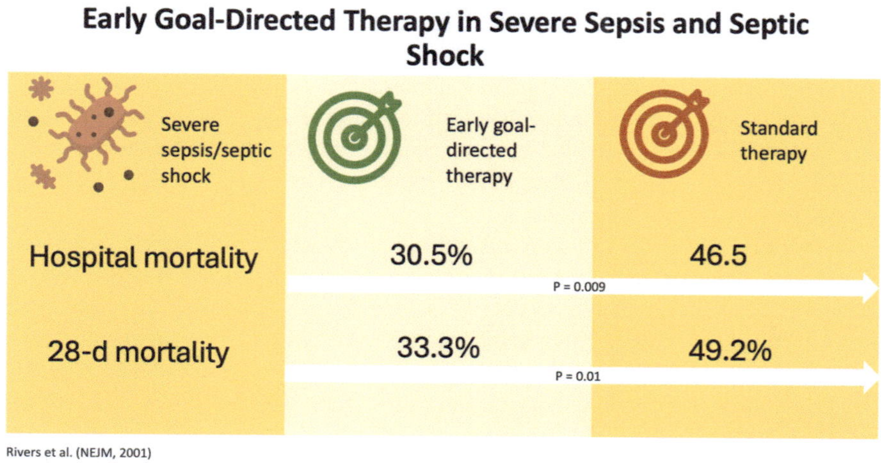

It became evident that key factors in improving sepsis care and outcomes were prompt recognition of the disease early in its course, close monitoring of afflicted patients, and rapid initiation of targeted management as soon as possible before the patient is transferred to the ICU. Along these lines, general agreement had emerged that maximization of oxygen delivery and correction of the mismatch between oxygen delivery and oxygen consumption was the likely key to sepsis care. However, no consensus existed about the best methodology to achieve this and whether these interventions in practice actually conferred a meaningful clinical benefit in terms of improved survival [10–15, 19]. Similarly, among the many physiologic parameters studied, it was not certain which parameters were the most useful, what were specific targets and thresholds to aim for, which interventions would best correct any physiologic shortfalls, what vasoactive agents worked best, which intravenous fluids one should use, and what infusion volumes were most ideal and perhaps even least harmful. Many of these questions remain topics of active investigation; yet a consensus seemed to evolve in regard to correcting the imbalance between oxygen supply and demand in septic patients, coupled with the growing awareness of the benefit of rapid diagnosis, spurred investigations into organized, systematic, and protocolized approaches for sepsis management. A further impetus was the concurrent recognition that sepsis care was quite variable, often from patient to patient, thereby hindering the ability to even garner what factors in sepsis management best contributed to better outcomes [19].

Rivers and colleagues [19], motivated by these questions and coupled with their observation that sepsis mortality exceeded 50% in their institution, developed and

[1] *Rivers E, Nguyen B, Havstad S, Ressler J, Muzzin A, Knoblich B, Peterson E, Tomlanovich M; Early Goal-Directed Therapy Collaborative Group. Early goal-directed therapy in the treatment of severe sepsis and sep-tic shock. N Engl J Med. 2001 Nov 8;345 (19):1368–77.*

implemented a protocol for sepsis management that used a targeted, carefully defined, task-based approach to manage patients diagnosed with severe sepsis and in septic shock to be activated immediately upon presentation to the emergency department (ED). Their study specifically focused not just upon early recognition, but a goal-oriented strategy comprising a bundled care protocol that consisted of, along with early antibiotic administration, aggressive intravenous fluid infusion, and vasopressor therapy guided by pre-specified targeted hemodynamic, cardiac, and oxygenation parameters designed to optimize preload, afterload, contractility, oxygenation, and acid-base status.

In this study, 263 patients with a diagnosis of severe sepsis or septic shock who presented to the ED at Henry Ford Hospital, a tertiary care, urban hospital located in Detroit, Michigan, USA, between 1997 and 2000, were enrolled and randomized in a 1:1 pattern to receive either standard therapy or what they termed early goal-directed therapy, EGDT. Patients randomized to the EGDT arm had a 16% reduction in the absolute risk of in-hospital mortality, from 46.5% to 30.5%, in addition to decreased organ system dysfunction when compared to the cohort randomized to usual care.

The findings from this study generated great interest, not just due the significant reduction in mortality in the EGDT group, but because of its paradigm shift in terms of beginning sepsis-focused care in the ED as soon as the patient presents, as opposed to the more traditional approach of waiting until ICU admission, which could be hours later, or even longer. Given the profound increase in survival and the pre-specified novelty of initiating critical care services immediately upon presentation outside of the ICU, EGDT was incorporated into the original guidelines that were issued by the Surviving Sepsis Campaign (SSC) several years later [19, 21, 22].

Yet, despite these promising findings by Rivers et al. and the inclusion into the SSC recommendations, EGDT was not readily adopted, due to several issues including concerns about the complex steps that the EGDT protocol required and the complicated and costly logistics about incorporating the actual steps that EGDT entailed, practices that were not yet standard practice—most notable being the need for SvO2 monitoring by specially designed CVP catheters, the need for dedicated staff specifically trained in EGDT practice, and the fact that the Rivers et al. study was conducted at a single center, where the baseline mortality of 46.5% in the control group appeared to many to be unusually high, and thus, not necessarily representative of the broader sepsis population [19, 21, 23, 24].

In response to these issues, and the general question of whether EGDT truly conferred an actual, measurable, and repeatable benefit, three separate but coordinated and harmonized, multicenter, publicly funded trials were undertaken and subsequently published in three different parts of the world—(1) ProCESS (Protocol-Based Care for Early Septic Shock) [25], (2) ARISE (Australasian Resuscitation in Sepsis Evaluation) [26], and (3) ProMISe (Procolized Management in Sepsis) [27]. The ProCESS study was conducted in the United States, whereas ARISE was predominantly based in centers across Australia and New Zealand (collectively Australasia), and ProMISe was undertaken in England, specifically in National Health Service (NHS) hospitals.

What follows is an overview of these three related studies, followed by an assessment of their strengths, limitations, and a discussion about the impact and ramifications of these three studies and some of the work and commentary that followed their dissemination.

53.4 A Randomized Trial of Protocol-Based Care for Early Septic Shock: The ProCESS Trial[2]

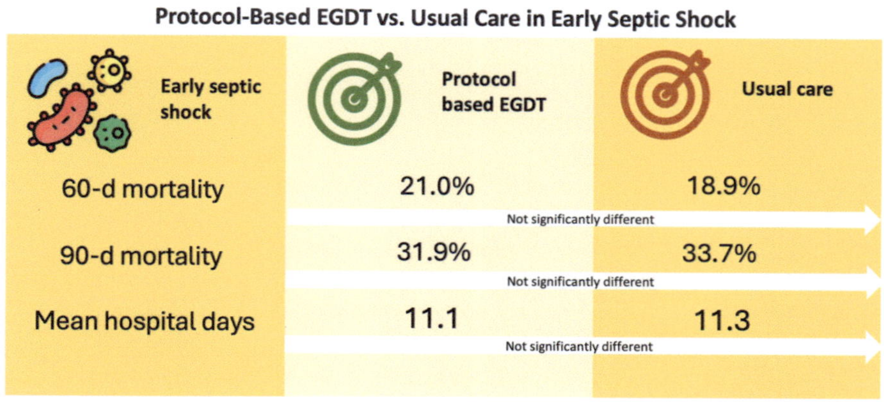

The ProCESS investigators (NEJM, 2014)

53.4.1 Study Rationale

Following the inclusion of EGDT recommendations into the Surviving Sepsis Guidelines, and questions concerning whether the findings from Rivers et al. could be replicated and whether EGDT should be broadly implemented, the ProCESS trial, like the ARISE and ProMISe trials, was designed to assess the efficacy of EGDT. Could the findings of the Rivers et al. trial be replicated in a larger multicenter randomized study and ultimately provide further quantitative insight as to whether or not EGDT confers a clinical benefit to septic patients?

53.4.2 Population and Design

The ProCESS study was conducted in 31 hospitals in the United States between March 2008 and May 2013. The study population included patients 18 years of age or older who presented to the ED with severe sepsis and septic shock. All participating hospitals were academic centers with EDs that treated more than 40,000 patients per year.

[2] *The ProCESS Investigators; New Engl J Med 2014; 370: 1683–1693*

To qualify for enrollment in ProCESS, patients were required to have a confirmed or suspected infection and two or more criteria of the systemic inflammatory response syndrome (SIRS) [28]. Patients were also eligible if they had refractory hypotension, defined as a systolic blood pressure (SBP) less than 90 mm Hg or the need for vasopressors to maintain the SBP at his threshold, or a serum lactate of 4 mmol or greater. Patients who met eligibility criteria had to be enrolled within 2 hours after shock manifested and within 12 hours after ED presentation. A fluid challenge of 20 ml per kg of body weight was initially specified for initial resuscitation due to refractory hypotension, but this was subsequently changed in April of 2010 to just 1 liter infused over 30 minutes.

53.4.3 Study Interventions

Unlike the Rivers et al. trial and two other harmonized studies (ARISE and ProMISe), ProCESS had three distinct resuscitation groups versus two: (1) protocol-based EGDT (Pro-EGDT), (2) protocol-based standard therapy (Pro-ST), or (3) usual care (UC). Patients were randomized equally into one of these three groups via block randomization of three, six, or nine patients. The Pro-EGDT group protocol closely paralleled the format used Rivers et al., whereas the Pro-ST group employed a less aggressive protocol, most notably the substitution of a peripheral intravenous (IV) line versus the requirement for central venous access (CVP) equipped with ScvO2 monitoring, unless SvO2 monitoring was deemed clinically warranted. It also had a lower red cell transfusion threshold, and the need for fluid infusion in this group was determined by bedside clinical assessment versus a specifically delineated numerical CVP threshold. For the UC group, all care that was provided was determined solely by the treating physicians caring for the patient, versus pre-specified physiologic criteria, a feature that closely aligned with the ARISE and ProMISe studies.

53.4.4 Outcome Measures and Sample Size

The primary outcome for ProCESS used to determine analytical power was the rate of all-cause, in-hospital mortality at 60 days. Some of the main secondary outcomes consisted of all-cause mortality at 90 days, cumulative mortality at both 90 days and 1 year, development of acute respiratory failure, acute renal failure, ICU and hospital lengths of stay, discharge disposition, and related outcome measures.

Data were analyzed on an intention-to-treat basis. The main comparative analyses in ProCESS were between the two protocol-based arms (i.e., Pro-EGDT and Pro-ST) as compared to UC, the combined data from the two protocol-based arms to UC, each of the protocol-based arms, or both of them combined, were superior to UC, and the comparison of Pro-EGDT to Pro-ST. All analyses were designed to test for superiority.

A sample size of 1950 patients was calculated using a power of 80% to detect a 6–7% reduction in mortality. The mortality for the UC, or control, group, was assumed to vary between 30% and 46%, which, of note, closely corresponds to the mortality observed in the EGDT and standard care groups, respectively, in the Rivers et al. trial.

53.4.5 Results

53.4.5.1 Baseline Characteristics and Protocol Adherence

A total of 1351 patients underwent randomization and were enrolled between March 2008 and May 2013, out of 12,707 who were screened. Ten of the enrolled patients withdrew during the course of the study, thereby leaving 1341 patients who were ultimately analyzed. Of those who remained, 439 were randomized to Pro-EGDT, 446 to Pro-ST, and 456 to UC. All three groups had similar baseline characteristics, and the four most common etiologies for sepsis were, in descending order, pneumonia, urinary tract infection, and intra-abdominal infection, followed by unknown pathogens and other organ systems and sites.

At baseline assessment, all three groups were largely similar. The APACHE II scores at entry were approximately 20—21, refractory hypotension was present between 53.3% and 55.6% of patients, hyperlactatemia was noted in approximately 60%, and the time to randomization from meeting all entry criteria averaged between 66 and 72 hours, and nearly three times this range when measured from the point of ED arrival. Among the two protocol-based groups, adherence to protocol requirements was quite high, with 88.1% and 95.6% adherence observed in the Pro-EGDT and Pro-ST groups, respectively.

53.4.5.2 Resuscitation, Hemodynamics, and Physiologic Parameters

Both protocol-based groups received statistically greater amounts of IV fluid in the first 6 hours than the UC group (2.8 liters Pro-EGDT, 3.3 liters Pro-ST, and 2.3 liters UC), with crystalloid administration exceeding colloid use, by far, for all 3 groups. The two protocol-based cohorts had a statistically higher level of vasopressor use than the UC patients (54.9% for Pro-EGDT, 52% for Pro-ST, and 44.1% UC, with $P = 0.003$ for the comparison of the combined protocol group patients to those randomized to UC). Antibiotic and glucocorticoid use, however, along with blood product transfusions, were similar for all three cohorts.

In the subsequent 6 to 72 hours following randomization, all three groups received comparable amounts of IV fluids for resuscitation and vasoactive agents (vasopressors plus dobutamine). The use of low-tidal volume ventilation and moderate glycemic control was also similar among all groups, although the two protocol-based cohorts had a greater percentage of patients who attained the mean arterial pressure target as compared to the UC patients, whereas the level of acidosis in the UC group was lower than for the Pro-EGDT and Pro-ST cohorts.

Table 53.1 Main study outcomes

Outcome	Pro-EGDT	Pro-ST	UC	*P*-value[a]
60-day mortality	92/439 (21.0%)	81/446 (18.2%)	86/456 (18.9%)	0.83[b]
90-day mortality	129/405 (31.9%)	128/415 (30.8%)	139/412 (33.7%)	0.66
ICU LOS (days)	5.1 ± 6.3	5.1 ± 7.1	4.7 ± 5.8	0.63

Abbreviations: *EGDT* early goal-directed therapy, *Pro-ST* protocol-based standard therapy, *UC* usual care

[a]*P*-values represent 3-group comparisons, unless otherwise indicated

[b]*P*-values compare UC to the combined EGDT groups

53.4.5.3 Clinical Outcomes

The 60-day mortality, the primary outcome measure for ProCESS, showed no significant differences between the three groups, with 21.0% mortality at day 60 for Pro-EGDT, 18.2% for Pro-ST, and 18.9% for UC, and a collective 60-day mortality of 19.5% for all study enrollees. For the secondary outcomes, no significant mortality differences were observed at either 90 days or 1 year, and no changes were noted when the data were adjusted to account for possible study site differences.

The two protocol-based cohorts observed higher rates of acute kidney injury (AKI) when compared to the UC patients and accordingly received a higher percentage of renal-replacement therapy (RRT). As for other secondary outcomes that were analyzed, respiratory and cardiovascular failure were comparable for all groups, including ICU and hospital LOS and discharge disposition. The main study outcomes are summarized in Table 53.1.

53.5 Goal-Directed Resuscitation for Patients with Early Septic Shock: (The ARISE Trial)[3]

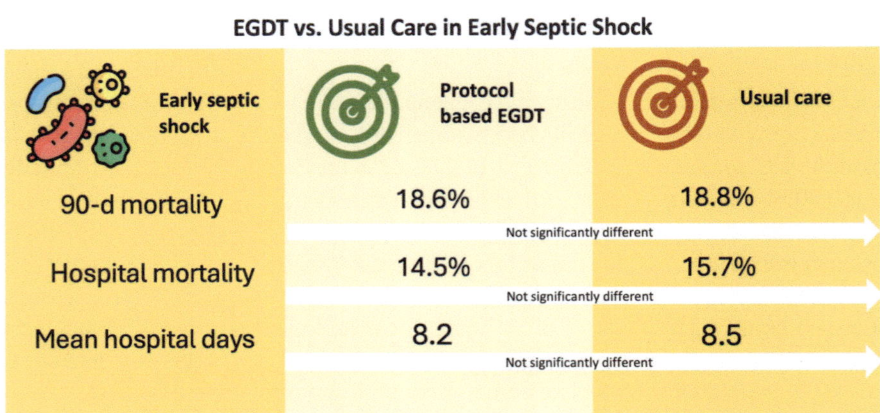

The ARISE Investigators and the ANZICS Clinical Trials Group (NEJM, 2014)

[3]*The ARISE Investigators and the ANZICS Clinical Trial Group; New Engl J Med 2014: 371: 1496–1506.*

53.5.1 Study Rationale

The ARISE trial, as with ProCESS and ProMISe, and on the heels of the inclusion of EGDT recommendations in the Surviving Sepsis Campaign, was designed to assess whether the implementation of EGDT protocols improved outcomes for patients presenting to hospital EDs with early septic shock. Furthermore, since the ProCESS study failed to demonstrate a survival benefit in a multicenter trial in a United States population, in contrast to the single-center Rivers study published 13 year earlier, ARISE studied whether a benefit for EGDT might be observed in a different part of the world and healthcare system than the US, where both Rivers et al. and ProCESS were conducted. Unlike ProCESS but similar to ProMISe, ARISE had only one group randomized to protocolized care versus two, thus resulting in two cohorts for comparison versus three.

53.5.2 Population and Design

The ARISE trial was conducted between October 2008 through April 2014 in 51 centers, with most centers located in Australasia (Australia and New Zealand), with 45 participating sites. The remaining six centers were in Finland, Hong Kong, or Ireland. Patients were recruited from both tertiary and non-tertiary centers, and hospitals in both urban and rural settings. EGDT sepsis-based protocols were not implemented in any of the participating centers before the beginning of the trial.

Patients 18 years of age or older with a suspected or confirmed infection, who exhibited two or more SIRS criteria, were eligible to participate in the study, provided they met all inclusion criteria within 6 hours after presentation to the ED. Refractory hypotension was defined, similar to ProCESS, as a mean arterial pressure (MAP) <65 mm Hg or SBP <90 after a 1-liter fluid infusion within 60 minutes. Hypoperfusion was indicated by a serum lactate of ≥4.0 mmol/L. Patients were randomized via a 1:1 ratio to either the EGDT or the usual care (UC) cohort. Randomization was stratified by center and had to take place within 2 hours after all inclusion criteria were met. The protocol further mandated the administration of antimicrobial therapy for every enrolled patient before randomization.

53.5.3 Study Interventions

As previously described, stated, ARISE patients were assigned to one of two study groups: (1) the experimental group, or those randomized to receive EGDT, or (2) the control group, or those randomized to UC. Treatment decisions for the UC patients were exclusively made by the managing bedside physicians, and it specifically disallowed ScvO2 monitoring during the first 6 hours following randomization. The EDGT protocol was standardized across and for all participating sites, and it mandated the placement of both an arterial line along a central venous catheter capable of $ScvO_2$ monitoring. As stipulated by the protocol, both lines had to be placed within 1 hour following randomization.

53.5.4 Outcome Measures and Sample Size

The primary outcome for ARISE was all-cause, in-hospital mortality at 90 days, versus 60 days for ProCESS. Some of the major secondary and tertiary outcomes were ICU and hospital mortality, ICU and hospital total length of stay, 28-day mortality, inpatient mortality at 60 days, 90-day cause-specific mortality, limitations to care (e.g., do not resuscitate orders), and the use and duration of mechanical ventilation, renal replacement therapy, and vasopressor support.

A sample size of 1600 patients was calculated to have a power of 85–90%, based on the assumption of a 28% inpatient mortality for the UC group, a rate lower than that used in ProCESS. The authors further assumed that EGDT would lead to a 7.6% reduction in the absolute risk of 90-day all-cause mortality (the primary outcome).

53.5.5 Results

53.5.5.1 Baseline Characteristics and Protocol Adherence

Of the 1600 patients who underwent randomization, 796 were assigned to the EGDT arm and 804 to UC. The final number of patients who completed the study and for whom data were available for the intention-to-treat analysis on the primary outcome variable was 1588 patients—792 from the EGDT and 796 from the UC group.

Baseline demographic and clinical data at randomization were similar for both cohorts, and there were no notable differences with respect to the percentage of patients with elevated lactate, refractory hypotension, infused fluid volume, time from ED presentation to randomization, time to initiation of antimicrobial therapy, source of infection, and the proportion of patients with positive blood cultures.

53.5.5.2 Resuscitation, Hemodynamics, and Physiologic Parameters

EGDT patients received more fluids, vasoactive therapy (vasopressors plus dobutamine), and red-cell transfusions within the first 6 hours than UC patients. Similarly, the use of vasoactive agents beyond the initial stage of care, during the subsequent 6–72 hours of care, was also higher among those randomized to EGDT.

At the end of the initial 6 hours of care, the MAP was higher in the EGDT group, but at 72 hours after randomization, no differences between groups were observed for any of the physiological and laboratory values.

53.5.5.3 Clinical Outcomes

Mortality at 90 days following randomization, the study's primary outcome, was comparable for both groups, with an 18.6% rate for the EGDT cohort versus 18.8% in the UC patients ($P = 0.90$). Survival times and between-group mortality were similar for both groups, and no changes were observed after adjusting for multiple pre-specified variables.

Table 53.2 Main study outcomes

Outcomes	EGDT ($n = 793$)	UC ($n = 798$)	P-value
90-day mortality number/total (%)	147/792 (18.6%)	150/792 (18.8%)	0.90
Death by day 28 number/total (%)	117/792 (14.8%)	127/797 (15.9%)	0.53
Death by ICU discharge number/total/ (%)	79/793 (10.9%)	125/797 (12.9%)	0.28

Abbreviations: *EGDT* early goal-directed therapy, *UC* usual care

Secondary and tertiary outcomes demonstrated few differences between the groups, except for length of stay in the ED and proportion of patients who required vasopressor therapy. Specifically, EGDT patients spent 1.4 fewer hours in the ED than the UC cohort ($P < 0.001$), and although a greater number of EGDT patients received vasopressor therapy, the mean duration for all patients who required vasopressor support did not significantly differ. No significant difference was observed between groups in the incidence of adverse events. The main study outcomes are summarized in Table 53.2.

53.6 Trial of Early, Goal-Directed Resuscitation for Septic Shock: (the The ProMISe Trial)[4]

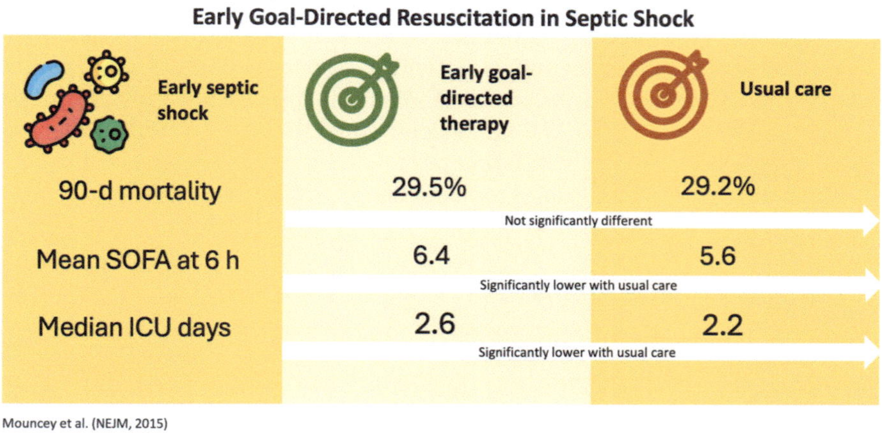

53.6.1 Study Rationale

The ProMISe trial represented the third of the three large, harmonized, multicenter studies that were conducted to determine if EGDT provided benefit for patients

[4] *Moncey, R, Osborn, TM, Power GS,* et al, *for the ProMISe Trial Investigators. New Engl J Med 2015; 372: 1301–1311*

presenting with severe sepsis or septic shock, in response to the inclusion of recommendations for implementing EGDT protocols by the SSC following the publication of the study by Rivers et al., which showed significant benefit in patients who randomized to the EGDT arm in a single center medical center. The ProMISe trial was conducted in the United Kingdom, whereas ProCESS was undertaken in United States, while ARISE was mainly studied in hospitals from Australia and New Zealand (45 sites plus six sites outside Australasia). Unlike the Rivers et al. study, ProCESS and ARISE failed to show a mortality benefit for those subjects assigned to EGDT versus usual or standard care. The mortality rates for all patients who completed both trials were similar across all groups and lower than expected.

53.6.2 Population and Design

The ProMISe trial was designed as a pragmatic, parallel-group, open, randomized controlled study conducted in National Health Service (NHS) hospitals in England that did not use EGDT protocols that included SvcO2 monitoring prior to the beginning of the study. The 56 institutions that participated in the trial included both teaching (29%) and non-teaching (71%) hospitals, and all screening took place between February 16, 2011, and July 24, 2014.

Patients 18 years or older who, within 6 hours of presenting to the ED, had a confirmed or suspected infection, two or more SIRS criteria, and either refractory hypotension (similar definitions as the ProCESS and ARISE studies) or a lactate ≥4 mmol/liter, were deemed eligible for enrollment. For those deemed eligible, randomized was mandated to take place within 2 hours of meeting all inclusion criteria, and the protocol further dictated administration of antimicrobial therapy prior to randomization. Patients were randomized via 1:1 allocation into either the EGDT or the usual care group. ProMISe was unique from the other two multicenter EGDT trials in that it also included a concurrent cost-effectiveness analysis.

53.6.3 Study Interventions

The usual care (UC) group, as with ProCESS and ARISE, was managed and monitored by the treating physicians assigned to each patient's care, and in accordance with local paradigms, standards, procedures, and policies already in place.

The EGDT group patients in the ProMISe trial were managed according to a similar protocol used by both ARISE and the protocolized EGDT cohort in ProCESS, initiated immediately after the randomization. For those randomized to the EGDT group, a central venous catheter equipped with SvO2 monitoring technology was required to be inserted. Arterial line placement was recommended in ProMISe, although not mandatory, and fluid boluses, if warranted, were infused every 30 minutes until a CVP of 8 mm Hg was attained. The blood pressure targets (90 mm Hg SBP, 65 mm Hg MAP), and red-cell transfusion thresholds were also akin to the ARISE and ProCESS targets. The EGDT protocol was adhered to for the full 6 hours following randomization, at which point all care decisions were transferred exclusively to the treating physicians assigned to each patient at each site.

53.6.4 Outcome Measures and Sample Size

The primary outcome for ProMISE was all-cause mortality at 90 days, similar to ARISE, for which the study was powered. Major secondary outcomes included Sequential Organ Failure Assessment (SOFA) Score at both 6 and 72 hours, ICU and hospital LOS, duration of stay in the ED, use of renal, cardiovascular, and respiratory support, all-cause mortality at 28 days and 1-year, and adverse events. The authors also carried out a cost-effectiveness analysis, including resource use, cost of care, and the quality-of-life (QoL) at 90 days and 1 year, using a standard QoL assessment tool.

The ProMISE investigators estimated that the 90-day mortality for the UC group would be 40%, and that, for a power of 80% to detect a 20% relative risk reduction in the EGDT patients, or an absolute risk reduction of 8%, 1260 patients would have to be enrolled. The P values were set to less than 0.05, and all analyses were based upon the principle of intention-to-treat.

53.6.5 Results

Overall, 6192 patients from the 56 participating institutions were screened, and ultimately 1251 patients were enrolled, with 625 randomized to the EGDT group and 626 to the UC group. Due to the withdrawal of eight patients before 90 days, 1243 patients (623 EGDT, 620 UC) were left for the analysis. With the exception of age (mean age = 66.4 years for EGDT vs. 64.3 for UC, $P = 0.01$), the baseline characteristics for both groups did not show any significant differences with respect to APACHE II [29] and SOFA [29] scores, site of infection, gender, blood lactate, percentage with refractory hypotension, volume of infused IV fluids, and the use of supplemental O_2.

Mortality at 90 days, the primary outcome, was also similar in both groups, with 29.5% mortality for the EGDT group versus 29.2% for those randomized to UC, or an unadjusted relative risk of death at 90 days of 1.01 for those who received EGDT ($P = 0.90$; 95% CI of 0.85 to 1.20). Most of the secondary outcomes were similar for both groups, except for a longer mean ICU LOS for the EGDT patients (2.6 to 2.2 days, $p = 0.005$), and a higher percentage of EGDT patients who were given advanced cardiovascular support (37% vs. 30.9%, $p = 0.026$).

From an economic standpoint, EGDT patients incurred higher mean total per-patient costs ($USD 17,647) than the UC group ($USD 16,239). However, this difference did not reach statistical significance ($P = 0.26$). Given that outcomes were similar, but more resources were consumed and costs were higher for the EGDT patients, UC was therefore deemed cost-effective, in that fewer resources were consumed to achieve similar levels of benefit or outcomes. Quantitatively, the marginal,

Table 53.3 Main study outcomes

Outcome	EGDT ($n = 793$)	UC ($n = 798$)	Significance
90-day mortality number /total (%)	184/623 (29.5%)	181/620 (29.2%)	$P = 0.90$
28-day mortality number/total/(%)	125/625 (24.8%)	152/621 (24.5%)	$P = 0.90$
Death at hospital discharge number/total/ (%)	160/793 (25.6%)	154/625 (24.6%)	$P = 0.74$
Cost up to 90 days (USD, mean + SD)	17,647 + 21,280	16,239 + 22,356	Incremental Effect (95% CI) 1406 (−1032–3845)

Abbreviations: *EGDT* early goal-directed therapy, *UC* usual care

or incremental net-benefit for EGDT was negative as compared to UC, for both comparisons of the entire study cohort along with prespecified subgroups. Sensitivity analysis further showed that for all possible scenarios likely to be encountered via multiple hypothetical simulations, EGDT would be cost-effective less than 20% of the time. The main study outcomes are summarized in Table 53.3.

53.7 Discussion: Study Comparisons, Collective Lessons, and Conclusions

The concordant findings from the ProCESS, ARISE, and ProMISe trials strongly indicate that EGDT or more specifically, its 6-hour sepsis bundle, is not superior to stand care and thus, does not offer measurable clinical benefit to patients in early sepsis. This argument was further strengthened by a follow-up, patient-based meta-analysis that pooled all subjects enrolled in these 3 trials and similarly showed no measurable differences as well [30], in addition to a subsequent literature-based meta-analysis that included two more EGDT studies—the initial study by Rivers et al. plus a separate 3-center EGDT clinical trial—and reached similar conclusions [31].

Given the many strengths of the ProCESS, ARISE, and ProMISe triad, one certainly could conclude that EGDT may not confer benefit and in fact, as the ProMISe cost-effectiveness analysis and other investigators suggest, EGDT may actually increase costs and reduce cost-effectiveness without changing outcomes. In the ensuing years after the results from these three studies were published and widely disseminated, the SSC revised its recommendations for inclusion of EGDT [3, 32, 33]. It needs to be reiterated that Rivers et al. was a single center study, albeit one that was randomized, derived from ED patients who presented to a busy, urban, US hospital, as opposed a multicenter randomized investigation like the other three, where the number of sites ranged from 31 centers in ProCESS to a high of 56 in ProMISe. In general, large, robust, multicenter trials are often viewed as more convincing than single-site investigations, a factor which might be enhanced by the fact that the multiple multicenter investigations reach similar conclusions.

Nevertheless, EGDT or at least certain components of the protocols that were implemented may still provide benefit to certain patient subgroups. The expected and observed mortality for the patients enrolled in the Rivers et al. trial, especially in the control group, were noticeably higher what was observed in the three studies, with an all-cause, 28-day mortality of 46.5% for UC patients and 30.5% mortality observed in the EGDT group in Rivers et al., versus a 60-day collective mortality rate of 19.5% for ProCESS, a 90-day all-cause mortality rate of just under 19% for both groups in ARISE, and a 90-day mortality rate between just under 30% for ProMISE. Since a higher percentage of patients in the Rivers et al. trial had baseline lactate levels of 4 mmol/L or higher along with higher APACHE II scores, it is possible that EGDT may have a better chance of conferring benefit in more severely ill patients, although the subgroup analyses performed in the other studies may mitigate this in part. Cecconi et al., in a systematic review of goal-directed care in critically ill surgical patients, show evidence that suggests that goal-directed therapy may provide better efficacy in high-risk surgical patients, especially those identified with an extremely high risk of death [34]. Certainly, further work should consider identifying patient groups and even different phenotypes who stand to benefit from a more personalized and tailored approach to care, with respect to EGDT, specific EGDT protocol components, and other emerging treatment paradigms.

Similarly, a significant period of time elapsed between the publication of the Rivers et al. trial in 2001 and the publication of ProCESS, ARISE, and ProMISE, all of which were published between 2014 and 2015. It is safe to say that sepsis awareness, recognition, and even treatment changed in this intervening period, including the use of low-tidal volume ventilation, more rapid and more uniform time-based antimicrobial administration, the growth in specialized sepsis teams and locally-developed sepsis protocols that are captured, activated, and tracked by electronic medical records (EMRs), and other practices that were not available or widely implemented in the in the late nineties and early 2000's may have improved overall outcomes from sepsis and septic shock. Since ProCESS, ARISE, and ProMISe all observed lower than expected mortalities in all patient groups and certainly in those patients randomized to receive usual or standard care, the possibility of underpowered studies should be considered in potential future evaluations.

Lastly, both the initial EGDT study by Rivers et al. and the three multicenter trials all evaluated a multi-step protocol that consisted of several distinct but interrelated tasks and targets. It is certainly possible that some of the protocolized steps may provide a measurable individual benefit without the others, and given concerns about the complexity, cost, and logistical barriers associated with the EGDT protocols that were studied (or for that matter, any complicated process that demands a unique set of skills or marked changes to existing procedures). Future research should consider assessing some of these individual interventions and targets in concert with treatment paradigms that may emerge in the care of sepsis patients.

53.8 Summary

Despite the enthusiasm for the EGDT bundle studied by Rivers et al., three large, harmonized multicenter studies performed over a decade later all observed that EGDT implementation may not confer a benefit to patients with sepsis. Yet all studies had lower than expected mortality, and given potential improvements in general sepsis awareness and other changes in management and treatment paradigms, it is clear that early recognition, focused attention to a more uniform approach to care and monitoring, and the initiation of care as soon as the patient presents remains key to achieving the best outcomes. Even as health care rapidly evolves with emerging technologies such as artificial intelligence and machine learning applications, personalized medicine and individually targeted therapy, and other as yet to be discovered therapies materialize for sepsis, septic shock, and for critical care and all disciplines for that matter, early identification of afflicted septic patients, coupled with focused care and attention will remain key to achieving the best overall outcomes.

References

1. Meyer NJ, Prescott HC. Sepsis and septic shock. N Engl J Med. 2024;391(22):2133–46. https://doi.org/10.1056/NEJMra2403213. PMID: 39774315.
2. Rudd KE, Johnson SC, Agesa KM, Shackelford KA, Tsoi D, Kievlan DR, Colombara DV, Ikuta KS, Kissoon N, Finfer S, Fleischmann-Struzek C, Machado FR, Reinhart KK, Rowan K, Seymour CW, Watson RS, West TE, Marinho F, Hay SI, Lozano R, Lopez AD, Angus DC, Murray CJL, Naghavi M. Global, regional, and national sepsis incidence and mortality, 1990-2017: analysis for the Global Burden of Disease Study. Lancet. 2020;395(10219):200–11. https://doi.org/10.1016/S0140-6736(19)32989-7. PMID: 31954465; PMCID: PMC6970225.
3. Angus DC, Linde-Zwirble WT, Lidicker J, Clermont G, Carcillo J, Pinsky MR. Epidemiology of severe sepsis in the United States: analysis of incidence, outcome, and associated costs of care. Crit Care Med. 2001;29(7):1303–10. https://doi.org/10.1097/00003246-200107000-00002. PMID: 11445675.
4. Carrol ED, Ranjit S, Menon K, Bennett TD, Sanchez-Pinto LN, Zimmerman JJ, Souza DC, Sorce LR, Randolph AG, Ishimine P, Flauzino de Oliveira C, Lodha R, Harmon L, Watson RS, Schlapbach LJ, Kissoon N, Argent AC, Society of Critical Care Medicine's Pediatric Sepsis Definition Taskforce. Operationalizing appropriate sepsis definitions in children worldwide: considerations for the pediatric sepsis definition taskforce. Pediatr Crit Care Med. 2023;24(6):e263–71. https://doi.org/10.1097/PCC.0000000000003263. Epub 2023 Apr 25. PMID: 37097029; PMCID: PMC10226471.
5. Evans L, Rhodes A, Alhazzani W, Antonelli M, Coopersmith CM, French C, Machado FR, Mcintyre L, Ostermann M, Prescott HC, Schorr C, Simpson S, Wiersinga WJ, Alshamsi F, Angus DC, Arabi Y, Azevedo L, Beale R, Beilman G, Belley-Cote E, Burry L, Cecconi M, Centofanti J, Coz Yataco A, De Waele J, Dellinger RP, Doi K, Du B, Estenssoro E, Ferrer R, Gomersall C, Hodgson C, Møller MH, Iwashyna T, Jacob S, Kleinpell R, Klompas M, Koh Y, Kumar A, Kwizera A, Lobo S, Masur H, McGloughlin S, Mehta S, Mehta Y, Mer M, Nunnally M, Oczkowski S, Osborn T, Papathanassoglou E, Perner A, Puskarich M, Roberts J, Schweickert W, Seckel M, Sevransky J, Sprung CL, Welte T, Zimmerman J, Levy M. Surviving sepsis campaign: international guidelines for management of sepsis and septic shock 2021.

Intensive Care Med. 2021;47(11):1181–247. https://doi.org/10.1007/s00134-021-06506-y. Epub 2021 Oct 2. PMID: 34599691; PMCID: PMC8486643.

6. Tuchschmidt J, Fried J, Astiz M, Rackow E. Elevation of cardiac output and oxygen delivery improves outcome in septic shock. Chest. 1992;102(1):216–20. https://doi.org/10.1378/chest.102.1.216. PMID: 1623756.
7. Shankar-Hari M, Phillips GS, Levy ML, Seymour CW, Liu VX, Deutschman CS, Angus DC, Rubenfeld GD, Singer M, Sepsis Definitions Task Force. Developing a new definition and assessing new clinical criteria for septic shock: for the third international consensus definitions for sepsis and septic shock (Sepsis-3). JAMA. 2016;315(8):775–87. https://doi.org/10.1001/jama.2016.0289. PMID: 26903336; PMCID: PMC4910392.
8. Lief L, Arbo J, Berlin DA. The physiology of early goal-directed therapy for sepsis. J Intensive Care Med. 2017;32(10):567–73. https://doi.org/10.1177/0885066616671705. Epub 2016 Oct 5. PMID: 27708007.
9. Seymour CW, Gesten F, Prescott HC, Friedrich ME, Iwashyna TJ, Phillips GS, Lemeshow S, Osborn T, Terry KM, Levy MM. Time to treatment and mortality during mandated emergency care for sepsis. N Engl J Med. 2017;376(23):2235–44. https://doi.org/10.1056/NEJMoa1703058. Epub 2017 May 21. PMID: 28528569; PMCID: PMC5538258.
10. Rackow EC, Astiz ME, Weil MH. Cellular oxygen metabolism during sepsis and shock. The relationship of oxygen consumption to oxygen delivery. JAMA. 1988;259(13):1989–93. PMID: 3279236.
11. Tuchschmidt J, Oblitas D, Fried JC. Oxygen consumption in sepsis and septic shock. Crit Care Med. 1991;19(5):664–71. https://doi.org/10.1097/00003246-199105000-00013. PMID: 2026029.
12. Gattinoni L, Brazzi L, Pelosi P, Latini R, Tognoni G, Pesenti A, Fumagalli R. A trial of goal-oriented hemodynamic therapy in critically ill patients. SvO2 Collaborative Group. N Engl J Med. 1995;333(16):1025–32. https://doi.org/10.1056/NEJM199510193331601. PMID: 7675044.
13. Tuchschmidt J, Fried J, Astiz M, Rackow E. Elevation of cardiac output and oxygen delivery improves outcome in septic shock. Chest. 1992;102:216–20.
14. Hayes MA, Timmins AC, Yau EH, Palazzo M, Hinds CJ, Watson D. Elevation of systemic oxygen delivery in the treatment of critically ill patients. N Engl J Med. 1994;330(24):1717–22. https://doi.org/10.1056/NEJM199406163302404. PMID: 7993413.
15. Friedman G, Silva E, Vincent JL. Has the mortality of septic shock changed with time. Crit Care Med. 1998;26(12):2078–86. https://doi.org/10.1097/00003246-199812000-00045. PMID: 9875924.
16. Haupt MT. Goal-oriented hemodynamic therapy. N Engl J Med. 1996;334(12):799; author reply 800. PMID: 8592561. https://doi.org/10.1056/NEJM199603213341213.
17. Sands KE, Bates DW, Lanken PN, Graman PS, Hibberd PL, Kahn KL, Parsonnet J, Panzer R, Orav EJ, Snydman DR, Black E, Schwartz JS, Moore R, Johnson BL Jr, Platt R. Academic Medical Center Consortium Sepsis Project Working Group. Epidemiology of sepsis syndrome in 8 academic medical centers. JAMA. 1997;278(3):234–40. PMID: 9218672.
18. Nugent KL, Coopersmith CM. Fluid management in Sepsis-Is There a Golden Hour (or Two)? Crit Care Med. 2017;45(10):1773–5. https://doi.org/10.1097/CCM.0000000000002612. PMID: 28915168.
19. Rivers E, Nguyen B, Havstad S, Ressler J, Muzzin A, Knoblich B, Peterson E, Tomlanovich M, Early Goal-Directed Therapy Collaborative Group. Early goal-directed therapy in the treatment of severe sepsis and septic shock. N Engl J Med. 2001;345(19):1368–77. https://doi.org/10.1056/NEJMoa010307. PMID: 11794169.
20. Kumar R, Kattimani B, Ojha PR, Khasage UJ. Quick sequential organ failure assessment score, lactate, and neutrophil-lymphocyte ratio help in diagnosis and mortality prediction during golden hour of sepsis in emergency department. J Emerg Trauma Shock. 2023;16(4):161–6. https://doi.org/10.4103/jets.jets_37_23. Epub 2023 Oct 24. PMID: 38292274; PMCID: PMC10824218.

21. Nguyen HB, Jaehne AK, Jayaprakash N, Semler MW, Hegab S, Yataco AC, Tatem G, Salem D, Moore S, Boka K, Gill JK, Gardner-Gray J, Pflaum J, Domecq JP, Hurst G, Belsky JB, Fowkes R, Elkin RB, Simpson SQ, Falk JL, Singer DJ, Rivers EP. Early goal-directed therapy in severe sepsis and septic shock: insights and comparisons to ProCESS, ProMISe, and ARISE. Crit Care. 2016;20(1):160. https://doi.org/10.1186/s13054-016-1288-3. PMID: 27364620; PMCID: PMC4929762.
22. Dellinger RP, Levy MM, Rhodes A, Annane D, Gerlach H, Opal SM, et al. Surviving sepsis campaign: international guidelines for management of severe sepsis and septic shock: 2012. Crit Care Med. 2013;41:580–637.
23. Osborn TM. Severe Sepsis and Septic Shock Trials (ProCESS, ARISE, ProMISe): what is optimal resuscitation? Crit Care Clin. 2017;33(2):323–44. https://doi.org/10.1016/j.ccc.2016.12.004. PMID: 28284298.
24. Gupta RG, Hartigan SM, Kashiouris MG, Sessler CN, Bearman GM. Early goal-directed resuscitation of patients with septic shock: current evidence and future directions. Crit Care. 2015;19(1):286. https://doi.org/10.1186/s13054-015-1011-9. PMID: 26316210; PMCID: PMC4552276.
25. ProCESS Investigators, Yealy DM, Kellum JA, Huang DT, Barnato AE, Weissfeld LA, Pike F, Terndrup T, Wang HE, Hou PC, LoVecchio F, Filbin MR, Shapiro NI, Angus DC. A randomized trial of protocol-based care for early septic shock. N Engl J Med. 2014;370(18):1683–93. https://doi.org/10.1056/NEJMoa1401602. Epub 2014 Mar 18. PMID: 24635773; PMCID: PMC4101700.
26. ARISE Investigators, ANZICS Clinical Trials Group, Peake SL, Delaney A, Bailey M, Bellomo R, Cameron PA, Cooper DJ, Higgins AM, Holdgate A, Howe BD, Webb SA, Williams P. Goal-directed resuscitation for patients with early septic shock. N Engl J Med. 2014;371(16):1496–506. https://doi.org/10.1056/NEJMoa1404380. Epub 2014 Oct 1. PMID: 25272316.
27. Mouncey PR, Osborn TM, Power GS, Harrison DA, Sadique MZ, Grieve RD, Jahan R, Tan JC, Harvey SE, Bell D, Bion JF, Coats TJ, Singer M, Young JD, Rowan KM. Protocolised Management In Sepsis (ProMISe): a multicentre randomised controlled trial of the clinical effectiveness and cost-effectiveness of early, goal-directed, protocolised resuscitation for emerging septic shock. Health Technol Assess. 2015;19(97):1–150. https://doi.org/10.3310/hta19970. PMID: 26597979; PMCID: PMC4781482
28. Bone RC, Balk RA, Cerra FB, Dellinger RP, Fein AM, Knaus WA, Schein RM, Sibbald WJ. Definitions for sepsis and organ failure and guidelines for the use of innovative therapies in sepsis. The ACCP/SCCM Consensus Conference Committee. American College of Chest Physicians/Society of Critical Care Medicine. Chest. 1992;101(6):1644–55. https://doi.org/10.1378/chest.101.6.1644. PMID: 1303622.
29. Knaus WA, Wagner DP, Draper EA, Zimmerman JE, Bergner M, Bastos PG, Sirio CA, Murphy DJ, Lotring T, Damiano A, et al. The APACHE III prognostic system. Risk prediction of hospital mortality for critically ill hospitalized adults. Chest. 1991;100(6):1619–36. https://doi.org/10.1378/chest.100.6.1619. PMID: 1959406.
30. PRISM Investigators, Rowan KM, Angus DC, Bailey M, Barnato AE, Bellomo R, Canter RR, Coats TJ, Delaney A, Gimbel E, Grieve RD, Harrison DA, Higgins AM, Howe B, Huang DT, Kellum JA, Mouncey PR, Music E, Peake SL, Pike F, Reade MC, Sadique MZ, Singer M, Yealy DM. Early, goal-directed therapy for septic shock - a patient-level meta-analysis. N Engl J Med. 2017;376(23):2223–34. https://doi.org/10.1056/NEJMoa1701380. Epub 2017 Mar 21. PMID: 28320242.
31. Angus DC, Barnato AE, Bell D, Bellomo R, Chong CR, Coats TJ, Davies A, Delaney A, Harrison DA, Holdgate A, Howe B, Huang DT, Iwashyna T, Kellum JA, Peake SL, Pike F, Reade MC, Rowan KM, Singer M, Webb SA, Weissfeld LA, Yealy DM, Young JD. A systematic review and meta-analysis of early goal-directed therapy for septic shock: the ARISE, ProCESS and ProMISe Investigators. Intensive Care Med. 2015;41(9):1549–60. https://doi.org/10.1007/s00134-015-3822-1. Epub 2015 May 8. PMID: 25952825.

32. Rhodes A, Evans LE, Alhazzani W, Levy MM, Antonelli M, Ferrer R, Kumar A, Sevransky JE, Sprung CL, Nunnally ME, Rochwerg B, Rubenfeld GD, Angus DC, Annane D, Beale RJ, Bellinghan GJ, Bernard GR, Chiche JD, Coopersmith C, De Backer DP, French CJ, Fujishima S, Gerlach H, Hidalgo JL, Hollenberg SM, Jones AE, Karnad DR, Kleinpell RM, Koh Y, Lisboa TC, Machado FR, Marini JJ, Marshall JC, Mazuski JE, McIntyre LA, McLean AS, Mehta S, Moreno RP, Myburgh J, Navalesi P, Nishida O, Osborn TM, Perner A, Plunkett CM, Ranieri M, Schorr CA, Seckel MA, Seymour CW, Shieh L, Shukri KA, Simpson SQ, Singer M, Thompson BT, Townsend SR, Van der Poll T, Vincent JL, Wiersinga WJ, Zimmerman JL, Dellinger RP. Surviving Sepsis Campaign: International Guidelines for Management of Sepsis and Septic Shock: 2016. Intensive Care Med. 2017;43(3):304–77. https://doi.org/10.1007/s00134-017-4683-6. Epub 2017 Jan 18. PMID: 28101605.
33. Sharif S, Owen JJ, Upadhye S. The end of early-goal directed therapy? Am J Emerg Med. 2016;34(2):292–4. https://doi.org/10.1016/j.ajem.2015.10.039. Epub 2015 Oct 24. PMID: 26612702.
34. Cecconi M, Corredor C, Arulkumaran N, Abuella G, Ball J, Grounds RM, Hamilton M, Rhodes A. Clinical review: goal-directed therapy-what is the evidence in surgical patients? The effect on different risk groups. Crit Care. 2013;17(2):209. https://doi.org/10.1186/cc11823. PMID: 23672779; PMCID: PMC3679445.

54 Dopamine Versus Norepinephrine in the Treatment of Shock: The SOAP II Trial

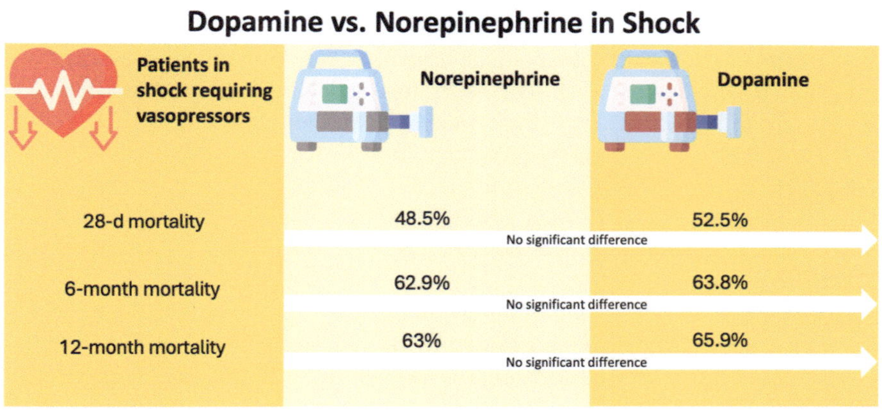

De Backer et al. (NEJM, 2010)

Quick Take
Which is the preferred vasopressor in shock—dopamine or norepinephrine?

The SOAP II trial compared the effects of dopamine and norepinephrine in patients with shock, evaluating their impact on mortality and adverse outcomes. This large, multicenter randomized controlled trial enrolled critically ill patients with shock and randomized them to receive either dopamine or norepinephrine as the primary vasopressor. The study revealed no improvement in survival with dopamine compared with norepinephrine in patients with shock. The most striking finding was the increase in the 28-day mortality with dopamine among patients with cardiogenic shock. Norepinephrine was associated fewer adverse events, including

---

De Backer D, Patrick B, Jacques D, Christian M, Didier C, Cesar A, et al. Comparison of Dopamine and Norepinephrine in the Treatment of Shock. N Engl J Med. 2010.

J. Chacko et al., *Landmark Studies in Critical Care*,
https://doi.org/10.1007/978-981-95-0673-6_54

arrhythmias, compared to dopamine. The findings suggest that norepinephrine should be preferred over dopamine as the first-line vasopressor in the treatment of shock, particularly due to its more favorable safety profile.

54.1 Introduction

Acute circulatory failure may be of varied etiology and carries a high mortality without expeditious evaluation and timely management. One of the basic tenets of circulatory support is the administration of catecholamines. They act on specific receptors to sustain the circulation, mainly as a temporizing measure, until specific therapeutic measures can take effect. Historically, norepinephrine and dopamine have been widely used as catecholamine support in acute circulatory failure.

Dopamine is a precursor of norepinephrine. Traditionally, several dose-specific effects have been attributed to dopamine, including the so-called "dopaminergic" effect at low doses, believed to increase renal blood flow and urine output. However, these potentially favorable observations have been largely confined to animals and healthy human volunteers [1]. The Australian and New Zealand Intensive Care Society group (ANZICS), in a large randomized controlled trial (RCT), demonstrated that dopamine in a "renal-protective" dose did not lower the peak creatinine levels, nor reduce the requirement for renal replacement therapy compared with placebo among patients with the systemic inflammatory response syndrome and early renal dysfunction. Besides, the ICU survival was not different compared with placebo [2].

The SOAP observational study, published in 2006, included 198 ICUs in Europe. This study included 3147 patients of whom 1058 developed shock. Among patients in shock, those who received dopamine had higher ICU and hospital mortality compared with those who did not (49.9% vs. 41.7%, $p = 0.01$). Furthermore, on multivariate analysis, dopamine was one of the independent predictors of ICU mortality in patients with shock [3]. However, despite a paucity of supporting evidence, consensus guidelines and expert recommendations continued to recommend dopamine as an initial vasopressor in patients with shock [4, 5].

Considering the lack of evidence to support a specific renal-protective effect of dopamine and observational data that supported the use of norepinephrine, the SOAP II investigators compared the two agents as first-line vasopressors in patients with shock [6].

54.2 Population and Design

The SOAP II trial was conducted between December 2003 and October 2007 across eight ICUs in Belgium, Austria, and Spain. The investigators randomly assigned patients with shock to receive dopamine or norepinephrine as the initial vasopressor. Clinicians and nursing staff who administered the drugs were unaware of the treatment assignment.

Adult patients >18 years who required vasopressors for shock were included.

Patients were considered to be in shock if the mean arterial pressure was <70 mm Hg or systolic BP <100 mm Hg after adequate fluid resuscitation with at least 1000 ml crystalloids or 500 ml colloids. Besides, signs of hypoperfusion were present, characterized by altered sensorium, skin mottling, urine output <0.5 ml/kg for 1 h, or a lactate level of >2 mmol/l.

54.2.1 Exclusions

Patients who had already received a vasopressor for >4 h, had a severe arrhythmia, and those who had been declared brain dead were excluded.

54.2.2 Dopamine Group

The dopamine dose was titrated by 2 mcg/kg/min at a time to a target blood pressure based on clinician judgment. Open-label norepinephrine was administered if the dose exceeded 20 mcg/kg/min.

54.2.3 Norepinephrine Group

The dose was titrated by 0.02 mcg/kg/min to attain the target blood pressure. Open-label norepinephrine was administered if a maximal dose of 0.19 mcg/kg/min was reached.

54.2.4 Common Management

Open-label dopamine was not allowed. Any vasopressor that was already being infused before study entry was replaced with the trial drug. Epinephrine or vasopressin could be used as rescue therapy based on the clinician's judgment. Inotropic agents could be administered specifically to improve the cardiac output at clinician discretion. Once hemodynamic stability was achieved, any open-label norepinephrine was weaned down first, followed by the study drug. If hypotension recurred after initial cessation of vasopressors, the study drug was reintroduced as the first option; open-label norepinephrine was added if required. The study protocol was followed for a maximum duration of 28 days. If an adverse event occurred, the patient could be withdrawn from the study and administered an open-label vasopressor based on the clinician's discretion. All other aspects of care were left to clinician judgment.

54.2.5 Sample Size

In the earlier SOAP observational trial, the mortality rate in the dopamine group was 43% compared with 36% in the norepinephrine group. Based on this finding, the authors calculated a sample size of 765 patients in each arm, assuming a 15% relative difference in the 28-day mortality. This sample size provided 80% power at a two-sided alpha level of 0.05.

54.3 Results

The study enrolled 1679 of the 2011 patients (83.5%) who were screened. In the dopamine group, 858 patients were included, compared with 821 patients in the norepinephrine group. All patients were followed up for 28 days. The baseline characteristics were similar. The median APACHE score was 20 and the median SOFA score, 9 in both groups. The most common cause of shock was septic (dopamine vs. norepinephrine: 63.2% vs. 61.1%), followed by cardiogenic shock (15.7% vs. 17.6%). In the dopamine group, 71.7% of patients were mechanically ventilated compared with 70.6% in the norepinephrine group. The mean arterial pressure was similar at baseline in both groups. Open-label norepinephrine was more often required in the dopamine group. The mean time taken to attain the target MAP was similar in both groups. The volume of fluid administered was similar in both groups. The urine output was higher in the dopamine group only in the first 24 h; the fluid balance was similar in both groups. Dopamine-treated patients experienced more tachycardia for up to 36 h after randomization. Similar changes were observed in the cardiac index, central venous pressure, venous oxygen saturation, and lactate levels in both groups.

Corticosteroids were administered to a similar number of patients in both groups. Recombinant activated protein C (drotrecogin alpha), considered to improve outcomes in sepsis based on the PROWESS trial, was in use during the study period; however, its use was similar in both groups of patients.

54.3.1 The Primary Outcome: 28-Day Mortality

There was no significant difference in the 28-day mortality between the dopamine and norepinephrine groups (52.5% vs. 48.5%, $p = 0.10$). On subgroup analysis, dopamine use was associated with a significantly higher 28-day mortality in patients with cardiogenic shock. There was no difference in mortality among patients with hypovolemic or septic shock.

54.3.2 Secondary Outcomes

Among the secondary outcomes, the 6- and 12-month mortality were also similar in both groups. The ICU mortality, hospital mortality, and the length of stay in the ICU and hospital were also similar. The number of ICU-free and organ support-free days was not significantly different. Death from refractory shock was more common among dopamine-treated patients.

54.3.3 Adverse Events

Arrhythmias occurred in 18.4% of patients, the most common being atrial fibrillation (86%). Patients in the dopamine group revealed a higher incidence of arrhythmia, particularly atrial fibrillation. Dopamine was discontinued in 6.1% of patients due to the onset of severe arrhythmias, while norepinephrine was discontinued in 1.6% of patients. Other adverse events, including myocardial infarction, new-onset infections, arterial occlusion, and ischemic events, were similar in both groups. The main study outcomes are summarized in Table 54.1.

54.4 Strengths

The SOAP II trial was adequately powered to evaluate the primary outcome of 28-day mortality. Of the 2011 patients screened, 1679 were randomized (83.5%); this constitutes a fairly high recruitment rate for a large RCT. Patients were well-matched at baseline, with a fairly high severity of illness, typical of a high acuity ICU. All patients were followed up until 28 days; hospital outcomes were available in 98.6% patients, adding to the strength of the study. The multicentric design also provides a high level of external validity.

The trial was conducted during the period when the American College of Cardiology—American Heart Association guidelines used to recommend dopamine as the preferred drug to increase arterial blood pressure in patients who were hypotensive following acute myocardial infarction [7]. In a multicentric, adequately powered RCT, the SOAP II trial vehemently challenged this recommendation—in fact, the 28-day mortality was higher among patients with cardiogenic shock who received dopamine compared with norepinephrine support. Currently, the Surviving Sepsis Guidelines recommend norepinephrine as the first-line vasopressor in patients with septic shock [8]. The American Heart Association also supports norepinephrine in cardiogenic shock, with dopamine as a second-line agent [9].

Table 54.1 Main study outcomes

Outcomes	Dopamine	Norepinephrine	Significance
ICU mortality	50.2%	45.9%	$P = 0.07$
Hospital mortality	59.4%	56.6%	$P = 0.24$
28-d mortality	52.5%	48.5%	$P = 0.10$
6-month mortality	63.8%	62.9%	$P = 0.71$
12-month mortality	65.9%	63.0%	$P = 0.34$
Median ICU LOS	5 days	5 days	$P = 0.12$
Median hospital LOS	11 days	12 days	$P = 0.22$

Abbreviation: *LOS* length of stay

54.5 Limitations

Initial fluid resuscitation with 1.0 l of crystalloid or 500 ml of colloid was considered adequate. A fixed volume of fluid resuscitation is debatable considering the heterogeneity associated with diverse types of shock. Clearly, hypovolemic or septic patients require a larger, often variable resuscitation volume; in contrast, volume resuscitation would be restricted in cardiogenic shock. However, the authors did not suggest any methodology to specifically evaluate volume responsiveness.

The target mean arterial pressure was based on clinician judgment, and may have cofounded the study findings.

A dose of 20 mcg/kg/min of dopamine was considered equipotent to 0.19 mcg/kg/min of norepinephrine. The authors offered no evidence to support the presumed equivalence of these doses.

Specific criteria, including an altered mental state, mottled skin, oliguria, and high serum lactate levels, were employed to define shock. However, the assessment of shock resolution appears to have been more subjective and perhaps prone to bias.

Details of specific interventions—including supportive measures like use of the intra-aortic balloon pump or coronary revascularization in cardiogenic shock—were not available. This may be relevant as 9.6% of patients had acute myocardial infarction. In patients with septic shock, the authors did not provide details on the source control interventions or the appropriateness of antibiotic therapy.

54.6 Subsequent Studies

In a retrospective cohort study, Fawzy et al. sought to evaluate factors associated with choice and outcomes with dopamine compared with norepinephrine as initial vasopressor in septic shock. Most clinicians preferred norepinephrine as the first-line vasopressor (77%). Dopamine seemed to be more in favor with cardiologists and more often used in non-teaching hospitals and in older patients with higher baseline comorbidities. On propensity-matched analysis, dopamine use was associated with increased hospital mortality [10].

A Cochrane review analyzed 28 studies comparing vasopressors in hypotensive shock. Only four RCTs fulfilled the quality criteria. No difference in mortality was observed when vasopressor regimens were compared. However, arrhythmias were more commonly observed with dopamine compared with norepinephrine.

54.7 Summary

Dopamine, an endogenous catecholamine, has been in use for decades for its presumed protective effect on the kidneys. This presumption was based on its potential to induce renal vasodilatation and improve renal blood flow at low doses. However, these favorable findings were largely confined to experimental studies involving animals and human volunteers. A dose-specific effect could not be discerned in critically ill patients. An increase in the urine output was observed in some studies, but has not been consistently evident. The ANZICS dopamine trial could identify no kidney-specific effect, with similar peak creatinine levels and no difference in the requirement for renal replacement therapy in dopamine-treated patients compared with placebo-treated patients. In the SOAP observational trial that followed, dopamine was found to be an independent predictor of mortality. Despite the dubious rationale, many guidelines continued to recommend dopamine as the preferred vasopressor in shock.

The SOAP II study, in a large, multicentric RCT, demonstrated no improvement in survival with dopamine compared with norepinephrine in patients with shock. The most striking finding was the increase in the 28-day mortality with dopamine among patients with cardiogenic shock. The SOAP II trial led to revised guidelines, with many recommending norepinephrine in preference to dopamine, triggering the decline of an all-pervasive, albeit irrational practice.

References

1. Dasta JF, Kirby MG. Pharmacology and therapeutic use of low-dose dopamine. Pharmacotherapy. 1986;6(6):304–10.
2. Bellomo R, Chapman M, Finfer S, Hickling K, Myburgh J. Low-dose dopamine in patients with early renal dysfunction: a placebo-controlled randomised trial. Australian and New Zealand Intensive Care Society (ANZICS) Clinical Trials Group. Lancet Lond Engl. 2000;356(9248):2139–43.
3. Sakr Y, Reinhart K, Vincent JL, Sprung CL, Moreno R, Ranieri VM, et al. Does dopamine administration in shock influence outcome? Results of the Sepsis Occurrence in Acutely Ill Patients (SOAP) Study. Crit Care Med. 2006;34(3):589–97.
4. Antman EM, Anbe DT, Armstrong PW, Bates ER, Green LA, Hand M, et al. ACC/AHA guidelines for the management of patients with ST-elevation myocardial infarction; a report of the American College of Cardiology/American Heart Association Task Force on Practice Guidelines (Committee to Revise the 1999 Guidelines for the Management of patients with acute myocardial infarction). J Am Coll Cardiol. 2004;44(3):E1–211.

5. Dellinger RP, Levy MM, Carlet JM, Bion J, Parker MM, Jaeschke R, et al. Surviving Sepsis Campaign: international guidelines for management of severe sepsis and septic shock: 2008. Intensive Care Med. 2008;34(1):17–60.
6. De Backer D, Patrick B, Jacques D, Christian M, Didier C, Cesar A, et al. Comparison of dopamine and norepinephrine in the treatment of shock. N Engl J Med. 2010;362:779.
7. Antman EM, Anbe DT, Armstrong PW, Bates ER, Green LA, Hand M, et al. ACC/AHA guidelines for the management of patients with ST-elevation myocardial infarction--executive summary: a report of the American College of Cardiology/American Heart Association Task Force on Practice Guidelines (Writing Committee to Revise the 1999 Guidelines for the Management of Patients With Acute Myocardial Infarction). Circulation. 2004;110(5):588–636.
8. Evans L, Rhodes A, Alhazzani W, Antonelli M, Coopersmith CM, French C, et al. Surviving Sepsis Campaign: International Guidelines for Management of Sepsis and Septic Shock 2021. Crit Care Med. 2021;49(11):e1063.
9. Vahdatpour C, Collins D, Goldberg S. Cardiogenic shock. J Am Heart Assoc. 2019;8(8):e011991.
10. Fawzy A, Evans SR, Walkey AJ. Practice patterns and outcomes associated with choice of initial vasopressor therapy for septic shock. Crit Care Med. 2015;43(10):2141–6.

55 Vasopressin Versus Norepinephrine in Septic Shock: The VASST Trial

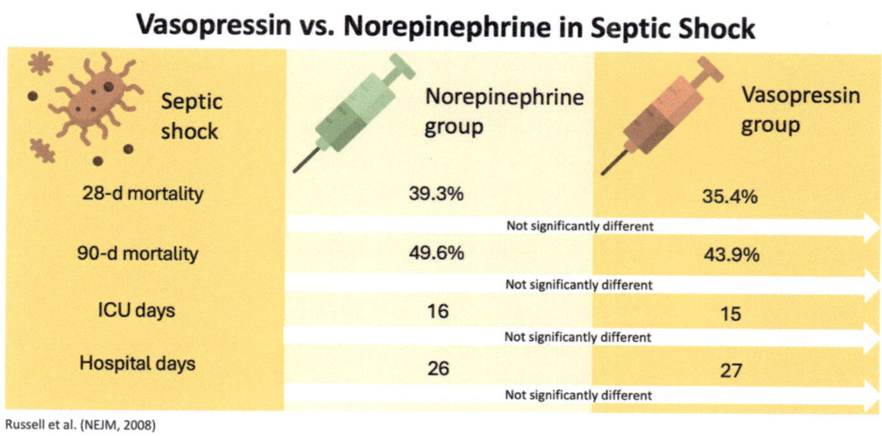

Quick Take

In patients with septic shock, does vasopressin, compared to norepinephrine, improve clinical outcomes when used as an adjunctive vasopressor therapy?

The Vasopressin and Septic Shock Trial (VASST) investigated whether low-dose vasopressin, compared to norepinephrine, improves outcomes in patients with septic shock requiring vasopressor support to maintain mean arterial pressure (MAP). This multicenter, randomized controlled trial enrolled 778 patients and randomized them to receive blinded infusions of either vasopressin (0.01–0.03 U/min) or norepinephrine (5–15 µg/min) in addition to standard care, titrated to a target MAP of 65–75 mm Hg. If infusion with the study drug was unable to sustain the target MAP,

---

Russell JA, Walley KR, Singer J, Gordon AC, Hébert PC, Cooper DJ, et al. Vasopressin versus *norepinephrine infusion in patients with septic shock. N Engl J Med. 2008 Feb 28;358(9):877–87.*

J. Chacko et al., *Landmark Studies in Critical Care*,
https://doi.org/10.1007/978-981-95-0673-6_55

open-label vasopressors were allowed. The primary outcome, 28-day mortality, showed no significant difference between the two groups overall. However, a subgroup analysis suggested a potential mortality benefit with vasopressin in patients with less severe septic shock (baseline norepinephrine requirement <15 μg/min), while no benefit was observed in patients with more severe shock. Secondary outcomes, including organ dysfunction scores, vasopressor-free days, and rates of adverse events such as arrhythmias, were similar between groups. The trial concluded that vasopressin is a safe adjunct to norepinephrine but does not improve overall mortality in septic shock, though it may offer benefits in less severe cases.

55.1 Introduction

The initial management of septic shock centers around intravenous fluid resuscitation and the infusion of catecholamines to support the circulation. Norepinephrine, the generally preferred vasopressor agent, may maintain perfusion pressure, albeit at the expense of reduced cardiac output, oxygen delivery, and compromised flow to vulnerable organs [1]. A relative deficiency of vasopressin may occur in septic shock, leading to a loss of vascular tone and reduced blood pressure. In this situation, exogenous vasopressin administration may revive vascular tone, and augment perfusion pressure to vital organs. Besides, it may also reduce the need for infusion of catecholamine vasopressors, including norepinephrine [2, 3]. At infusion rates <0.1 units/min, vasopressin has been demonstrated to improve blood pressure in patients with vasodilatory shock [2–4]. However, it may potentially lead to compromised blood flow to the heart, kidneys, and the gut.

Evidence from controlled clinical trials was confined to just two small randomized controlled trials (RCTs) before the conduct of the Vasopressin and Septic Shock Trial (VASST).

In a 1999 study, patients admitted to a trauma ICU with vasodilatory septic shock were randomized to vasopressin, 0.04 units/min or placebo in a randomized controlled trial (RCT). The systolic pressure increased in the vasopressin group, with a rise in the systemic vascular resistance; these parameters remained unchanged in the placebo group [5].

In a subsequent study, patients with septic shock, on high-dose vasopressor support, were randomized to receive a 4-h infusion of norepinephrine or vasopressin. Open-label vasopressors were titrated to target blood pressure. Vasopressin infusion resulted in a norepinephrine-sparing effect. Besides, an increase in the urine output was observed in the vasopressin group, compared with norepinephrine [4].

55.2 Population and Design

The VASST study was conducted across 27 centers in Canada, Australia, and the USA between July 2001 and April 2006 [6].

Adult patients with septic shock, who did not respond to fluid resuscitation and low-dose norepinephrine, were considered for inclusion. Septic shock was defined as proven or suspected infection, the presence of ≥ two systemic inflammatory response syndrome (SIRS) criteria, new-onset organ dysfunction, and persisting hypotension despite fluid resuscitation and the requirement for norepinephrine ≥5 μg/min for 6 h.

55.3 Exclusion

The study excluded patients who were on open-label vasopressin, those with severe traumatic brain injury with a GCS of <8, unstable coronary syndrome, suspected acute mesenteric ischemia, and Raynaud's phenomenon.

Patients were randomized to receive norepinephrine or vasopressin. The clinician was blinded to the vasopressor infused—the drugs were mixed in similar volumes of 5% dextrose (250 ml); infusions were commenced and titrated in a similar manner. The infusion of the study drug was commenced at 5 ml/h and increased by 2.5 ml/h over the first hour to a constant rate of 15 ml/h.

55.3.1 Vasopressin Group

The blinded vasopressin infusion commenced at 0.01 U/min, titrated to a maximum dose of 0.03 U/min.

55.3.2 Norepinephrine Group

The blinded norepinephrine infusion began at 5 μg/min, titrated to a maximum dose of 15 μg/min.

55.4 Common Management

The target mean arterial pressure (MAP) was set at 65–75 mm Hg; however, the clinician could choose a different target based on their judgment. If infusion with the study drug was unable to sustain the target MAP, open-label vasopressors were allowed. Open-label vasopressors were tapered down once the target MAP was achieved. However, the study drug infusion was tapered down only once the target MAP was sustained for 8 h after cessation of open-label vasopressors. The study drug was infused at 15 ml/h until open-label vasopressors were not required, a serious adverse event occurred, or until the patient died. Crossover to the other arm and open-label vasopressin were not allowed.

55.5 Sample Size

The authors assumed a mortality rate of 60% in the norepinephrine group. A sample size of 776 patients allowed the detection of an absolute difference in mortality of 10% between groups with a two-sided alpha error of 0.05, and 80% power.

55.6 Results

Among the 6229 patients screened, 802 were randomized. The final analysis included 778 patients—386 in the vasopressin and 382 in the norepinephrine group. The blood pressure in both groups was similar throughout the study; however, the heart rate was significantly lower in the vasopressin group during the initial 4 days of treatment. The infusion rate was significantly lower with vasopressin compared with norepinephrine in the first 4 days of treatment.

55.6.1 The Primary Outcome: All-Cause Mortality at 28 Days

The 28-day all-cause mortality was similar in the vasopressin and norepinephrine groups (35.4% vs. 39.3%, P = 0.26). The results remained similar on multivariate logistic regression analysis.

55.6.2 Secondary Outcomes

Among the secondary outcomes, the 90-day mortality was also similar in both groups (43.9% vs. 49.6%, $P = 0.11$). Multivariate logistic regression analysis also revealed no significant difference between the two groups.

In patients with less severe septic shock (norepinephrine dose 5–14 μg at baseline), a trend towards lower 28- and 90-days mortality was observed in the vasopressin group. However, the mortality was not different among patients with more severe septic shock (norepinephrine dose ≥15 μg at baseline).

Post hoc analysis based on baseline lactate levels and the number of vasopressors being infused revealed possible benefits in vasopressin-treated patients among those with less severe septic shock.

The number of days alive and free of organ dysfunction was similar in both groups. The ICU (16 vs. 15 days, $P = 0.14$) and hospital stay (26 vs. 27 days, $P = 0.23$) were also similar.

55.6.3 Adverse Events

The incidence of serious adverse events was similar in the vasopressin and the norepinephrine groups (10.3% vs. 10.5%, $P = 1.0$). The incidence of cardiac arrest was

Table 55.1 Main study outcomes

Outcomes	Vasopressin group	Norepinephrine group	Significance
28-d mortality	35.4%	39.3%	$P = 0.26$
90-d mortality	43.9%	49.6%	$P = 0.11$
Median ICU LOS	15 (7–29) days	16 (8–32) days	$P = 0.14$
Median hospital LOS	27 (13–52) days	26 (15–53) days	$P = 0.23$

Abbreviation: *LOS* length of stay

higher in the norepinephrine group, while digital ischemia occurred more often with vasopressin. The main study outcomes are summarized in Table 55.1.

55.7 Conclusion

The authors concluded that low-dose vasopressin, at 0.03 U/min, did not reduce mortality in combination with catecholamine vasopressors in patients with septic shock. They observed a trend towards reduced mortality in patients with less severe septic shock with the use of vasopressin.

55.8 Strengths

The VASST trial was multicentric, of robust design, and hence, lends external validity. The investigators assessed multiple clinically relevant endpoints, including the 28-day mortality, organ dysfunction, and safety profile, offering insights into the safety and efficacy of vasopressin in septic shock.

55.9 Weaknesses

A post hoc analysis suggested mortality benefit among patients with less severe septic shock with vasopressin compared with norepinephrine; however, this finding needs confirmation in future trials. The study did not explore the use of a variable dose protocol, which may be more in line with individual patient requirements. The exclusion of some categories of patients, including those with coronary artery disease, may limit its generalizability. The study included patients with a reasonably stable MAP—hence, the study may not apply to patients who experience refractory hypotension. The mortality observed in the study was lower than assumed for power calculation (60 vs. 40%); this may have led to an underpowered sample (Type II error).

55.10 Subsequent Evidence

The VANISH trial, a factorial double-blind RCT, enrolled patients with septic shock requiring vasopressors within 6 h of the onset of shock [7]. Patients were allocated to one of four groups—vasopressin titrated up to 0.06 U/min combined with hydrocortisone, vasopressin and placebo, norepinephrine combined with hydrocortisone, and norepinephrine with placebo.

The median kidney failure-free days among non-survivors, or those who developed kidney failure, or both, was 9 days in the vasopressin group and 13 days in the norepinephrine group; the difference was not statistically significant. Renal replacement therapy was used less often in the vasopressin group (25.4% vs. 35.3%). Although a lower mortality was observed with vasopressin, the difference did not reach statistical significance. The time to shock resolution also did not significantly differ between groups.

Thus, the VANISH trial left room for debate on whether vasopressin in preference to norepinephrine would exert a renal protective effect.

The VALOR observational trial evaluated the safety and efficacy of a loading dose of 1 U of vasopressin, followed by an infusion of 1 U/h among patients with septic shock who were on norepinephrine ≥0.2 μg/kg/min [8]. The authors sought to predict the response to vasopressin infusion using hemodynamic evaluation and catecholamine-sparing effect. Patients were categorized as responders or non-responders based on a MAP increase of more than 22 mmHg after the vasopressin bolus. They observed that the change in MAP following bolus vasopressin effectively predicted the catecholamine index during subsequent continuous infusion. A loading dose of vasopressin may thus enable the prediction of response to continuous infusion and choose an appropriate vasopressor strategy in septic shock.

55.11 Summary

Patients with septic shock often experience refractory hypotension despite adequate fluid resuscitation combined with the use of catecholamine vasopressors. Vasopressin levels were observed to be low in septic shock—could this lead to a loss of vascular tone and vasodilatory shock? Observational studies seemed to suggest that vasopressin infusion may exert a catecholamine-sparing effect. However, there was scant data to suggest any outcome benefit with vasopressin infusion in septic shock. Against this background, the VASST investigators conducted an RCT that compared the use of a combination of norepinephrine with vasopressin with norepinephrine infusion alone.

They did not observe a significant difference in hard-core clinical outcomes between norepinephrine and vasopressin infusion. There was no mortality benefit with the addition of vasopressin to conventional vasopressors. Besides, the incidence of organ dysfunction, the need for renal replacement therapy, and the length of stay in ICU and hospital were also similar in both groups. The incidence of adverse events was also similar. The authors observed a lower mortality among vasopressin-treated patients among those with less severe septic shock. However, these findings need corroboration in future trials.

References

1. Bomzon L, Rosendorff C. Renovascular resistance and noradrenaline. Am J Phys. 1975;229(6):1649–53.
2. Landry DW, Oliver JA. The pathogenesis of vasodilatory shock. N Engl J Med. 2001;345(8):588–95.
3. Holmes CL, Patel BM, Russell JA, Walley KR. Physiology of vasopressin relevant to management of septic shock. Chest. 2001;120(3):989–1002.
4. Patel BM, Chittock DR, Russell JA, Walley KR. Beneficial effects of short-term vasopressin infusion during severe septic shock. Anesthesiology. 2002;96(3):576–82.
5. Malay MB, Ashton RC, Landry DW, Townsend RN. Low-dose vasopressin in the treatment of vasodilatory septic shock. J Trauma. 1999;47(4):699–703; discussion 703–705.
6. Russell JA, Walley KR, Singer J, Gordon AC, Hébert PC, Cooper DJ, et al. Vasopressin versus norepinephrine infusion in patients with septic shock. N Engl J Med. 2008;358(9):877–87.
7. Gordon AC, Mason AJ, Thirunavukkarasu N, Perkins GD, Cecconi M, Cepkova M, et al. Effect of early vasopressin vs norepinephrine on kidney failure in patients with septic shock: the VANISH randomized clinical trial. JAMA. 2016;316(5):509–18.
8. Nakamura K, Nakano H, Ikechi D, Mochizuki M, Takahashi Y, Koyama Y, et al. The Vasopressin Loading for Refractory septic shock (VALOR) study: a prospective observational study. Crit Care. 2023;27(1):294.

Part XIII

Nutrition

Early Versus Late Parenteral Nutrition in the Critically Ill: The EPANIC Trial

56

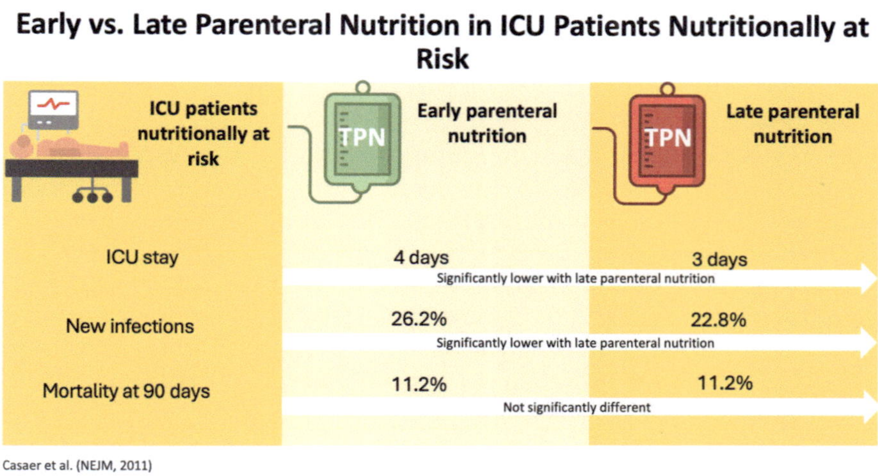

Quick Take

Is earlier the better with parenteral nutrition among critically ill patients in whom caloric targets cannot be met by enteral nutrition alone?

The EPANIC trial compared early versus late initiation of parenteral nutrition in critically ill adults who could not meet their nutritional needs with enteral feeding alone. In this multicenter, randomized controlled trial (RCT), patients were assigned to receive PN either within 24 h of ICU admission (early group) or after 7 days (late group). The study found no significant difference in the primary outcome of 90-day mortality between the two groups. Additionally, the early PN group had more

---

Casaer MP, Mesotten D, Hermans G, Wouters PJ, Schetz M, Meyfroidt G, et al. Early versus Late Parenteral Nutrition in Critically Ill Adults. N Engl J Med. 2011 Aug 11;365(6):506–17.

J. Chacko et al., *Landmark Studies in Critical Care*,
https://doi.org/10.1007/978-981-95-0673-6_56

infections and complications associated with nutrition delivery. The trial suggests that delaying PN for up to 7 days in critically ill patients does not compromise survival and may reduce complications associated with early parenteral feeding.

56.1 Introduction

The concept of intravenous nutrition arose during World War I with the introduction of sterile glucose solutions in water [1]. A decade later, intravenous protein hydrolysates were investigated, followed by the use of supplemental fat emulsions. Stanley Dudrick, during his surgical residency at the University of Pennsylvania, observed that malnutrition in the postoperative period led to poor outcomes among patients who were unable to absorb nutrients from the gut. In 1967, he tested the feasibility of parenteral nutrition in laboratory animals [2], followed by its initial use in malnourished infants [3]. The use of parenteral nutrition became more widespread with the safe and easy administration through central venous catheters. Initially, venous access was by cut-down; the advent of percutaneously inserted subclavian venous catheters facilitated long-term nutritional support through the parenteral route [4].

Considering the lower risk of complications and being less expensive, enteral nutrition is the preferred route in critically ill patients. However, enteral feeding alone often fails to achieve nutritional targets. Underfeeding has been shown to be associated with adverse clinical outcomes in critically ill patients, including a higher incidence of bloodstream infections [5], a longer duration of mechanical ventilation [6], and increased mortality [7]. Considering the failure to achieve nutritional targets through the enteral route alone among critically ill patients, parenteral nutrition may be combined with enteral nutrition to prevent nutritional deficit. However, the parenteral route may be associated with complications, including overfeeding, preponderance to nosocomial infections, and hyperglycemia [8, 9]. Clinical guidelines also differed; while the European Society of Parenteral and Enteral Nutrition (E.S.P.E.N.) recommended consideration of parenteral nutrition within 2 days of ICU admission if enteral nutrition was inadequate [10], the American and Canadian guidelines suggested nutritional support through the enteral route during the first week of ICU stay [11].

The Early Parenteral Nutrition Completing Enteral Nutrition in Adult Critically Ill Patients (EPaNIC) study included adult, critically ill patients who were at risk of undernutrition, but not chronically malnourished. The study question was whether early supplemental parenteral nutrition aimed to achieve caloric targets would reduce the risk of complications compared with delayed initiation of parenteral nutrition after a week [12].

56.2 Population and Design

The EPaNIC randomized controlled trial (RCT) was conducted between August 2007 and November 2010 in seven ICUs in Belgium. Eligible patients included those with a score ≥ 3 on nutritional risk screening (NRS), indicative of patients who were nutritionally at risk. The study excluded patients with ketoacidosis or hyperosmolar coma, a body mass index of <17, short bowel syndrome, and those who did not have a central venous catheter. Pregnant patients and those who were moribund and coded not for resuscitation were also excluded.

56.2.1 Early Initiation Group

Patients randomized to the early parenteral nutrition group received 20% glucose intravenously for a total energy intake of 400 kcal on day 1 and 800 kcal on day 2. On day 3, parenteral nutrition was commenced, combined with enteral nutrition as tolerated, aiming to achieve 100% of the caloric target. The caloric target was based on the corrected ideal body weight, age, and gender, with a maximum of 2880 kcal/day. Enteral nutrition was stepped up gradually; when the proportion of enteral nutrition had risen to 80% of the caloric target, parenteral nutrition was weaned off and ceased. If enteral nutrition dropped to below 50% of the caloric target at any stage, parenteral nutrition was recommenced.

56.2.2 Late Initiation Group

Patients assigned to the late initiation group were administered 5% glucose solution in similar volumes as the early initiation group to ensure adequate hydration. If oral intake was not feasible by day 2, enteral nutrition was commenced. After 7 days of ICU stay, if enteral nutrition was still insufficient, parenteral nutrition was initiated on day 8 to meet caloric targets.

56.2.3 Common Management

Patients in whom oral intake was not feasible by day 2 received enteral feeding. The rate of enteral feeding was stepped up twice a day; prokinetic drugs and post-pyloric feeding tubes were employed as appropriate. Trace elements, minerals, and vitamins were routinely administered. The blood glucose level was maintained between 80 and 110 mg/dl using insulin infusions as required. Weaning from mechanical ventilation was carried out based on local guidelines. If continued ICU care was considered futile, decisions on end-of-life care were made by consensus.

56.3 Sample Size Calculation

The sample size was calculated to detect a 1-day difference in the duration of ICU stay with 80% power, and concurrently, a 3% difference in the ICU mortality with 70% power.

56.4 Results

The EPaNIC study assessed 8703 patients for eligibility. After the exclusion of 4063 patients, 2312 patients were assigned to receive early parenteral nutrition and 2328 to late parenteral nutrition and were included in the final analysis. Baseline characteristics were similar in both groups of patients. As envisaged in the study protocol, the caloric target of 25–30 ml/kg was achieved by day 3 in the early initiation group, and by day 8 in the late initiation group. The higher caloric target in the first 7 days resulted in a greater requirement for insulin to maintain blood glucose levels within the target range in the early initiation group. Patients in the early initiation group received a significantly higher dose of insulin—a median of 31 units (interquartile range, 19–48) per day in the early initiation group compared with 58 units (interquartile range, 40–85) in the late initiation group. The levels of potassium, magnesium, and phosphorus were similar in both groups. The main clinical outcomes are summarized in Table 56.1.

56.4.1 The Primary Outcome

The duration of ICU stay was shorter by 1 day in the late initiation group [median: 3 days (interquartile range 2–7 days) vs. [median: 4 days (interquartile range 2–9 days), $P = 0.02$]. There were significantly more patients who stayed in the ICU for longer than 3 days in the early initiation group (51.3% vs. 48%, $P = 0.02$). Overall, patients in the late initiation group were more likely to be discharged alive from the ICU.

Table 56.1 Main clinical outcomes

Outcome	Late initiation (2328 patients)	Early initiation (2312 patients)	P-value
ICU stay (median, IQR)	3 (2–7) days	4 (2–9) days	0.02
ICU mortality	141 (6.1%)	146 (6.3%)	0.76
Hospital mortality	242 (10.4%)	251 (10.9))	0.63
90-d mortality	257 (11.2%)	255 (11.2%)	1.0
Mechanical ventilation >2 d	846 (36.3%)	930 (40.2%)	0.006
Hospital stay (median, IQR)	14 (9–27) days	16 (9–29) days	0.004
New infections	531 (22.8%)	605 (26.2%)	0.008
AKI	104 (4.6%)	131 (5.8)	0.06
Duration of RRT (median, IQR)	7 (3–16) days	10 (5–23)	0.008

Abbreviations: *IQR* interquartile range; *AKI* acute kidney injury; *RRT* renal replacement therapy

56.4.2 Safety Outcomes

In the late initiation group, more patients were discharged alive from the ICU within 8 days (75.2% vs. 71.7%, $P = 0.007$). There were no significant differences in the ICU or hospital mortality; mortality within 90 days after enrollment was also similar. Nutrition-related complications were similar in both groups; however, hypoglycemic episodes occurred more often in the late nutrition group (3.5% vs. 1.9%).

56.4.3 Secondary Outcomes

The overall incidence of new infections was higher in the early initiation group (26.2% vs. 22.8%, $P = 0.008$). Infections involving the airway or lungs, bloodstream, and wound infections were also more common in the early initiation group. There were significantly more patients in the early initiation group who required mechanical ventilation for more than 2 days (40.2% vs. 36.3%). The time to weaning from ventilator support was also longer with early initiation. The duration of hospital stay was longer in the early initiation group; furthermore, patients who required hospital admission for more than 15 days were also significantly higher with early initiation. The incidence of acute kidney injury based on the RIFLE criteria was significantly higher, and the duration of renal replacement therapy was longer in the early initiation group. Besides, early initiation of parenteral nutrition led to higher healthcare costs. The functional status at hospital discharge, assessed using the 6-min walk test, was similar in both groups.

56.4.4 Subgroup Analysis

The authors performed a predefined subgroup analysis of high-risk patients, including those with a body mass index <25 or > 40 and NRS score ≥ 5, post-cardiac surgical patients, and those presenting with sepsis. They found no difference in the duration of ICU stay or ICU mortality among these subgroups of patients.

On post hoc analysis, early vs. late initiation of parenteral nutrition was compared among patients in whom early enteral nutrition was contraindicated. Patients in this subgroup received a median of 0 calories (interquartile range, 0–163) per day until day 7. The incidence of infective complications was lower in the late initiation group; furthermore, they were more likely to be discharged alive from the ICU.

56.5 Study Conclusions

The EPaNIC study did not find a significant difference in mortality between early (within 48 h) and late initiation of parenteral nutrition (after 7 days) in ICU patients at high risk of malnutrition. Delaying parenteral nutrition for a week was associated with a lower incidence of infective complications. Late initiation of parenteral nutrition was associated with fewer days on mechanical ventilation, shorter ICU and hospital stay, lower duration of renal replacement therapy, and reduced healthcare costs. Late initiation of parenteral nutrition was associated with a higher incidence of hypoglycemia; however, the functional status at hospital discharge was comparable with early initiation.

56.6 Strengths

The EPaNIC trial was the first large RCT that compared clinical outcomes with early versus late initiation of parenteral nutrition in critically ill patients. Analysis was by intention to treat, and allocation concealment was maintained, adding to the robustness of the trial. The findings of the study strongly supported delaying parenteral nutrition by a week; late initiation resulted in improved clinical outcomes, although mortality remained similar.

56.7 Limitations

The study was unblinded owing to its design, and hence, may have been subject to bias. The dose of amino acids administered was less than recommended in clinical guidelines. The calorie requirement was calculated based on the corrected body weight, in contrast to the generally accepted method, based on indirect calorimetry.

The difference in clinical outcomes between the two groups was minimal, although statistically significant; besides, mortality rates were similar. The large majority of participants were not severely malnourished, with a nutrition score of ≤4. Sixty percent were postoperative cardiac surgical patients; hence, the results may not be extrapolatable to a general ICU setting. The study employed intensive insulin therapy aiming to maintain blood glucose levels below 110 mg/dl, in contrast to the generally accepted target of 140–180 mg/dl following the NICE-SUGAR study [13]. However, the blood glucose levels in both groups were similar and may not have influenced the difference in clinical outcomes. Overall, the median duration of ICU stay was short (3 days), suggesting a low severity of illness. The study protocol was not followed after discharge from the ICU.

56.8 Subsequent Analyses of EPaNIC Data

De Vlieger et al. evaluated the impact of the timing of supplemental parenteral nutrition on the incidence of invasive fungal infections by univariable and multivariable analysis of data from the EPaNIC trial. They observed that delaying parenteral nutrition until day 7 reduced the incidence of invasive fungal infections [14].

In another prospectively planned sub-analysis, intensive care-acquired muscular weakness was evaluated in 600 patients; skeletal muscle biopsy was performed in

122 patients and compared with 20 matched controls. Macronutrient deficiency during the early phase of critical illness did not affect muscle wasting; furthermore, recovery of muscle weakness was more rapid with late compared with early parenteral nutrition [15].

A cost analysis of the EPaNIC trial revealed that pharmacy-related expenditure was higher with the early use of parenteral nutrition. The increased costs were related to parenteral nutrition solutions and anti-infective agents [16].

56.9 Summary

The EPaNIC investigators conducted a large, multicentric RCT to address the uncertainty regarding when parenteral nutrition should be commenced in patients who were nutritionally at risk. How does early supplemental parenteral nutrition aimed to achieve 100% of the caloric target by day 3 compare with delayed initiation of parenteral nutrition after a week of ICU stay? The study found that later initiation of parenteral nutrition led to a more rapid recovery, a shorter ICU and hospital stay, and fewer infective complications. The likely beneficial effect of late parenteral nutrition was particularly evident among patients who underwent complicated pulmonary, esophageal, and abdominal surgery in whom early enteral nutrition was contraindicated. What are the putative mechanisms behind the apparent clinical benefits associated with a strategy of late initiation of parenteral nutrition? The authors hypothesized that parenteral nutrition may inhibit autophagy, leading to inadequate clearance of damaged cells and microorganisms. The more prolonged duration of ICU and hospital stay observed among recipients of early parenteral nutrition may be related to a higher incidence of infective complications and organ dysfunction. Based on the findings of the EPaNIC trial, the Society of Critical Care Medicine (SCCM) and the American Society for Parenteral and Enteral Nutrition (ASPEN) currently recommend that parenteral nutrition be withheld for the first 7 days following ICU admission among patients who cannot tolerate oral intake and in whom enteral nutrition is not feasible [17].

References

1. Moore FD, Brennan MF. Intravenous feeding. N Engl J Med. 1972;287(17):862–4.
2. Dudrick SJ. Early developments and clinical applications of total parenteral nutrition. JPEN J Parenter Enteral Nutr. 2003;27(4):291–9.
3. Wilmore DW, Dudrick SJ. Growth and development of an infant receiving all nutrients exclusively by vein. JAMA. 1968;203(10):860–4.
4. Dudrick SJ, Wilmore DW, Vars HM, Rhoads JE. Can intravenous feeding as the sole means of nutrition support growth in the child and restore weight loss in an adult? An affirmative answer. Ann Surg. 1969;169(6):974–84.
5. Rubinson L, Diette GB, Song X, Brower RG, Krishnan JA. Low caloric intake is associated with nosocomial bloodstream infections in patients in the medical intensive care unit. Crit Care Med. 2004;32(2):350–7.

6. Villet S, Chiolero RL, Bollmann MD, Revelly JP, Cayeux RNMC, Delarue J, et al. Negative impact of hypocaloric feeding and energy balance on clinical outcome in ICU patients. Clin Nutr Edinb Scotl. 2005;24(4):502–9.
7. Alberda C, Gramlich L, Jones N, Jeejeebhoy K, Day AG, Dhaliwal R, et al. The relationship between nutritional intake and clinical outcomes in critically ill patients: results of an international multicenter observational study. Intensive Care Med. 2009;35(10):1728–37.
8. Reid C. Frequency of under- and overfeeding in mechanically ventilated ICU patients: causes and possible consequences. J Hum Nutr Diet. 2006;19(1):13–22.
9. Dhaliwal R, Jurewitsch B, Harrietha D, Heyland DK. Combination enteral and parenteral nutrition in critically ill patients: harmful or beneficial? A systematic review of the evidence. Intensive Care Med. 2004;30(8):1666–71.
10. Singer P, Berger MM, Van den Berghe G, Biolo G, Calder P, Forbes A, et al. ESPEN Guidelines on Parenteral Nutrition: intensive care. Clin Nutr Edinb Scotl. 2009;28(4):387–400.
11. Heyland DK, Dhaliwal R, Drover JW, Gramlich L, Dodek P. Canadian Critical Care Clinical Practice Guidelines Committee. Canadian clinical practice guidelines for nutrition support in mechanically ventilated, critically ill adult patients. JPEN J Parenter Enteral Nutr. 2003;27(5):355–73.
12. Casaer MP, Mesotten D, Hermans G, Wouters PJ, Schetz M, Meyfroidt G, et al. Early versus late parenteral nutrition in critically ill adults. N Engl J Med. 2011;365(6):506–17.
13. NICE-SUGAR Study Investigators, Finfer S, Chittock DR, Su SYS, Blair D, Foster D, et al. Intensive versus conventional glucose control in critically ill patients. N Engl J Med. 2009;360(13):1283–97.
14. De Vlieger G, Ingels C, Wouters PJ, Debaveye Y, Vanhorebeek I, Wauters J, et al. Impact of supplemental parenteral nutrition early during critical illness on invasive fungal infections: a secondary analysis of the EPaNIC randomized controlled trial. Clin Microbiol Infect. 2019;25(3):359–64.
15. Hermans G, Casaer MP, Clerckx B, Güiza F, Vanhullebusch T, Derde S, et al. Effect of tolerating macronutrient deficit on the development of intensive-care unit acquired weakness: a subanalysis of the EPaNIC trial. Lancet Respir Med. 2013;1(8):621–9.
16. Vanderheyden S, Casaer MP, Kesteloot K, Simoens S, De Rijdt T, Peers G, et al. Early versus late parenteral nutrition in ICU patients: cost analysis of the EPaNIC trial. Crit Care Lond Engl. 2012;16(3):R96.
17. McClave SA, Taylor BE, Martindale RG, Warren MM, Johnson DR, Braunschweig C, et al. Guidelines for the provision and assessment of nutrition support therapy in the adult critically ill patient: Society of Critical Care Medicine (SCCM) and American Society for Parenteral and Enteral Nutrition (ASPEN). JPEN J Parenter Enteral Nutr. 2016;40(2):159–211.

Initial Trophic Versus Full Enteral Feeding in Acute Lung Injury: The EDEN Trial

57

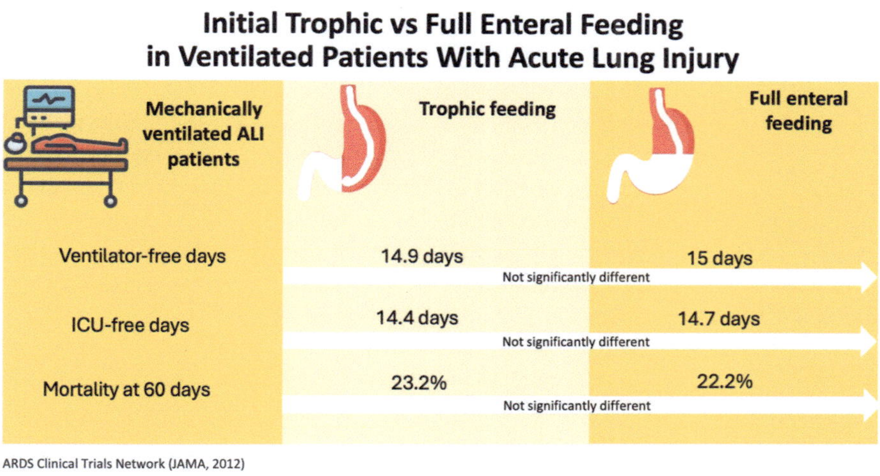

Quick Take

Is initial lower-volume enteral feeding safer in acute lung injury (ALI)?

The EDEN trial compared initial trophic feeding (low-calorie feeding) with full enteral feeding in patients with ALI to determine the optimal nutritional strategy in the early phase of critical illness. This randomized controlled trial showed no significant difference in 60-day mortality or ventilator-free days between the two groups. Patients receiving trophic feeding experienced fewer gastrointestinal complications, such as vomiting and elevated gastric residual

---

The National Heart, Lung, and Blood Institute Acute Respiratory Distress Syndrome (ARDS) Clinical Trials Network. Initial Trophic vs *Full Enteral Feeding in Patients with Acute Lung Injury: The EDEN Randomized Trial. JAMA J Am Med Assoc. 2012 Feb 22;307(8):795–803.*

J. Chacko et al., *Landmark Studies in Critical Care*,
https://doi.org/10.1007/978-981-95-0673-6_57

volumes. The study concluded that trophic feeding is a safe alternative to full enteral feeding in the first 6 days of ALI, potentially simplifying early nutritional management in the ICU.

57.1 Introduction

Patients on invasive mechanical ventilation routinely receive enteral nutrition. However, intolerance to enteral feeding is often encountered and may disrupt the delivery of nutritional targets. A lower incidence of infective complications, earlier liberation from mechanical ventilation, and reduced mortality have been noted when the actual delivery of nutrition is closer to the caloric requirement [1]. However, the optimal timing, formulation, and quantum of enteral nutrition remain unclear. In contrast, minimal enteral feeding, well below the target levels, may offer several putative benefits. Trophic feeding with low volumes of enteral feeds may preserve the integrity of the epithelial tight junctions in the intestines, thereby acting as a barrier to the translocation of bacteria from the lumen [2].

A nested cohort study evaluated the impact of the quantum of caloric intake over the initial week of ICU stay on clinical outcomes. A higher caloric intake, close to the target (>64.6%), was associated with increased hospital mortality, a more prolonged ICU and hospital stay, a higher incidence of ICU-acquired infections, and a longer duration of mechanical ventilation [3]. A retrospective observational study suggested that in obese, critically ill patients, hypocaloric enteral nutrition may be associated with more favorable clinical outcomes compared with eucaloric feeding. Patients who received hypocaloric enteral nutrition experienced a shorter duration of antibiotic therapy, mechanical ventilation, and ICU stay [4].

The EDEN investigators sought to investigate the clinical impact of initial trophic feeding compared with full feeding on clinical outcomes in light of observational studies that suggested benefit with trophic feeding. They hypothesized that initial trophic feeding would reduce the duration of mechanical ventilation by reducing the incidence of gastrointestinal intolerance.

57.2 Population and Design

The EDEN randomized controlled trial (RCT) was conducted between January 2008 and April 2011 across 44 hospitals in the National Heart, Lung, and Blood Institute ARDS Clinical Trials Network in the USA [5]. Adult patients, within 48 h of the onset of ALI and on invasive mechanical ventilation for <72 h, were eligible. ALI was defined by bilateral infiltrates on the chest radiograph, with no clinical evidence of left atrial hypertension, and a PaO_2/FiO_2 ratio of <300 mm Hg. Among those excluded were patients with neuromuscular disease requiring ventilatory assistance, burns involving >40% of body surface area, underlying disease with an expected 6-month mortality of >50%, severe chronic liver disease, intracranial hemorrhage, likely mortality within 24 h, refractory shock, mechanical bowel obstruction, current TPN use or intent to commence TPN within a week, and the presence of a high-output enterocutaneous fistula.

Patients were randomly assigned to receive either trophic or full enteral feeding during the initial 6 days of mechanical ventilation. The first 272 patients were also randomized, in a 2 by 2 factorial design, to another RCT that compared supplemental nutrition with omega-3 fatty acids and antioxidants with an isovolemic, isocaloric nutritional formula (the OMEGA study).

The assigned feeding strategy was commenced within 6 h of randomization; it was continued for 6 days, or until extubation or death, whichever occurred first.

57.2.1 Full Feeding

Enteral nutrition was commenced at 25 ml/h and stepped up to the target rate of 25–30 kcal/kg/day of non-protein calories and 1.2–1.6 g/kg/day of protein. The feeding rate was increased to reach target levels as rapidly as feasible, based on a protocol. Gastric residual volumes (GRVs) were checked 6 hourly as the feeding rate was being increased.

57.2.2 Trophic Feeding

Enteral nutrition was initiated at 10 ml/h (10–20 kcal/h) in the first 272 patients, who received nutritional supplements as part of a separate RCT, the OMEGA trial. After discontinuation of the OMEGA trial, the feeding rate was increased to 20 kcal/h to match the calories delivered during that trial. GRV was checked 12 hourly. If patients were still on mechanical ventilation at 6 days, enteral nutrition was stepped up to full energy feeding rates as in the full-feeding group.

57.2.3 Common Management in Both Groups

Enteral nutrition was withheld based on a protocol if the GRVs were > 400 ml, or if there was evidence of gastrointestinal intolerance. Patients were maintained in the semi-recumbent position if feasible. Lung-protective ventilation was carried out based on the ARDS-Network guidelines. Hemodynamic management was based on a fluid-conservative strategy. The blood glucose level was maintained between 80–150 mg/dl based on the local insulin protocol.

57.3 Sample Size

The authors assumed a mean of 14 ± 10.5 ventilator-free days at day 28. Enrollment of 1000 patients provided the study with 91% power to detect a difference of 2.25 days in the ventilator-free days between groups.

57.4 Results

The investigators screened nearly 8000 patients; after exclusions, 1000 were randomized. The primary analysis included 508 patients in the tropic feeding group and 492 patients in the full feeding group. Patients in both groups were well-matched regarding age, gender, severity of illness, underlying cause of ALI, ventilation parameters, and vasopressor use.

There was a clear separation between groups in the calories delivered—approximately 400 kcal/day in the trophic feeding group compared to 1300 kcal/day in the full feeding group; the difference persisted for the first 6 days. Post-pyloric feeding tubes were employed in less than 20% of the study population.

57.4.1 The Primary Endpoint: Ventilator-Free Days at Day 28

Patients who died before day 28 were considered to have 0 ventilator-free days. The number of ventilator-free days until day 28 was not significantly different between groups (trophic feeding vs. full feeding: 14.9 days vs. 15.0 days, $P = 0.89$).

57.4.2 Secondary Endpoints

The 60-day mortality was similar in both groups of patients (trophic feeding vs. full feeding: 23.2% vs. 22.2%, $P = 0.77$). The ICU-free and organ failure-free days were also similar. New-onset infections, including ventilator-associated pneumonia, Clostridium difficile colitis, and bacteremia, occurred at similar rates.

57.4.3 Other Outcomes

Gastrointestinal intolerance occurred less often in the trophic feeding group, with a lower incidence of regurgitation, vomiting, and high GRVs. Aspiration, diarrhea, abdominal distension, and cramping were equally common in both groups. Blood glucose levels and insulin requirements were higher in the full feeding group over the first 6 days. The full feeding group showed a higher net positive balance by day 7 (2.1 vs. 0.4 liters). However, the positive fluid balance did not seem to affect the hemodynamic or ventilatory parameters. The main study outcomes are summarized in Table 57.1.

Table 57.1 Main study outcomes

Outcome	Trophic feeding	Full feeding	P value (significance)
Ventilator-free days (mean, 95% CI)	14.9 (13.9–15.8)	15.0 (14.1–15.9)	0.89 (NS)
60-d mortality (%, 95% CI)	23.2 (19.6–26.9)	22.2 (18.5–25.8)	0.77 (NS)
ICU-free days (mean, 95% CI)	14.4 (13.5–15.3)	14.7 (13.8–15.6)	0.67 (NS)
VAP (%, 95% CI)	7.3 (5.0–9.5)	6.7 (4.5–8.9)	0.72 (NS)
C. Difficile infection (%, 95% CI)	3.0 (1.5–4.4)	2.6 (1.2–4.1)	0.77 (NS)
Bacteremia (%, 95% CI)	11.6 (8.8–14.4)	9.3 (6.8–11.9)	0.24 (NS)

Abbreviations: *CI* confidence interval; *NS* not significant

57.5 Study Conclusions

The authors concluded that in patients with ALI on invasive mechanical ventilation, low-calorie trophic feeding in the first 6 days did not result in improved clinical outcomes compared to a strategy of full feeding. The number of ventilator-free days, mortality at 60 days, and the incidence of infective complications were similar in both groups. Trophic feeding was associated with reduced gastrointestinal intolerance.

57.6 Strengths

The EDEN trial was a large, multicentric RCT that was adequately powered to address the question regarding the impact of a trophic feeding compared with a full feeding strategy in ventilated patients with ALI. There was a clear separation between groups in the caloric intake during the first 6 days. The overall mortality in the trial was as predicted in previous RCTs of patients with ALI. As planned, the caloric intake after the first 6 days was similar in both groups. The definition and management of gastrointestinal intolerance were standardized. Ventilation strategy, fluid management, and glucose control were also protocolized.

57.7 Weaknesses

About 87% of screened patients were excluded for various reasons, limiting generalizability. Owing to the unblinded design, caregivers were aware of the assigned group; this may have led to bias in the reporting of gastrointestinal intolerance. The full feeding group experienced a more positive fluid balance by day 7, which could have impacted outcomes. Most patients had an underlying medical illness; hence, the applicability of the study results to surgical patients remains unclear. The study did not use parenteral nutrition—which may have an influence on clinical outcomes. Malnourished and underweight patients were excluded; the results may not be extrapolatable to these subgroups. Patients who were off ventilator support and discharged before day 60 were assumed to be alive at 60 days. This may have led to an underestimation of the 60-day mortality.

57.8 Subsequent Evidence

Two follow-up studies were carried out on survivors of the EDEN trial. In one study, a substantial impairment of physical, cognitive, and psychological function was noted at 6 and 12 months in both study groups. Survivors experienced a reduced quality of life with the inability to return to work; these outcomes did not differ between the initial trophic and full feeding groups [6].

Another follow-up study observed physical and cognitive performance at 6 and 12 months among survivors. The investigators assessed the 6-minute walk distance, cognitive ability, and other secondary outcomes. They observed that performance levels were lower than predicted values at 6 and 12 months, with slow improvement over time. The initial feeding strategy—trophic vs. full feeding—did not appear to influence outcomes [7].

57.9 Summary

The EDEN trial aimed to evaluate the potential advantages of initial trophic feeding compared with full feeding among mechanically ventilated patients with ALI for the first 6 days. Patients in the trophic feeding group were randomized to receive 10–20 kcal/h, while the full feeding group received 25–30 kcal/kg/day. The authors observed no difference in the main study outcomes, including ventilator-free days, the 60-day mortality, and infectious complications. Gastrointestinal intolerance was lower in the trophic feeding group. The study was not designed to demonstrate the equivalence of both strategies. However, it suggested that aggressive ramping up of enteral feeding in the first few days of mechanical ventilation to reach calculated nutritional targets may not make a difference in clinical outcomes; a strategy of low-calorie, trophic feeding may be adequate in the first few days in mechanically ventilated patients with ALI.

References

1. Rubinson L, Diette GB, Song X, Brower RG, Krishnan JA. Low caloric intake is associated with nosocomial bloodstream infections in patients in the medical intensive care unit. Crit Care Med. 2004;32(2):350–7.
2. Kotani J, Usami M, Nomura H, Iso A, Kasahara H, Kuroda Y, et al. Enteral nutrition prevents bacterial translocation but does not improve survival during acute pancreatitis. Arch Surg Chic Ill 1960. 1999;134(3):287–92.

3. Arabi YM, Haddad SH, Tamim HM, Rishu AH, Sakkijha MH, Kahoul SH, et al. Near-target caloric intake in critically ill medical-surgical patients is associated with adverse outcomes. JPEN J Parenter Enteral Nutr. 2010;34(3):280–8.
4. Dickerson RN, Boschert KJ, Kudsk KA, Brown RO. Hypocaloric enteral tube feeding in critically ill obese patients. Nutrition. 2002;18(3):241–6.
5. The National Heart, Lung, and Blood Institute Acute Respiratory Distress Syndrome (ARDS) Clinical Trials Network, Rice TW, Wheeler AP, Thompson BT, Steingrub J, Hite RD, et al. Initial trophic vs full enteral feeding in patients with acute lung injury: the EDEN randomized trial. JAMA. 2012;307(8):795–803.
6. Needham DM, Dinglas VD, Morris PE, Jackson JC, Hough CL, Mendez-Tellez PA, et al. Physical and cognitive performance of patients with acute lung injury 1 year after initial trophic versus full enteral feeding. EDEN trial follow-up. Am J Respir Crit Care Med. 2013;188(5):567–76.
7. Needham DM, Dinglas VD, Bienvenu OJ, Colantuoni E, Wozniak AW, Rice TW, et al. One year outcomes in patients with acute lung injury randomised to initial trophic or full enteral feeding: prospective follow-up of EDEN randomised trial. BMJ. 2013;346:f1532.

Part XIV

Therapeutic Hypothermia

58 Therapeutic Hypothermia After Out-of-Hospital Cardiac Arrest: The HACA Trial

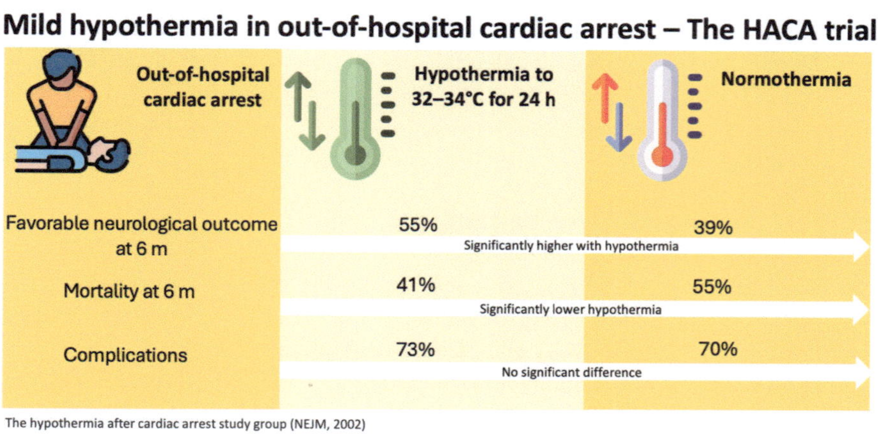

Quick Take

Does cooling after out-of-hospital cardiac arrest save lives?

The HACA trial was a multicenter, randomized controlled trial (RCT) that aimed to evaluate the effectiveness of therapeutic hypothermia in patients who had suffered a cardiac arrest and remained comatose. The study compared the outcomes of patients who were treated with therapeutic hypothermia (cooling to 32–34 °C for 24 h) versus those who were treated with normothermia (maintaining normal body temperature). The results showed that therapeutic hypothermia significantly improved neurologic outcomes and survival at 6 months compared to the

---

Hypothermia after Cardiac Arrest Study Group. Mild therapeutic hypothermia to improve the neurologic outcome after cardiac arrest. N Engl J Med. 2002 Feb 21;346 (8):549–56.

J. Chacko et al., *Landmark Studies in Critical Care*,
https://doi.org/10.1007/978-981-95-0673-6_58

normothermic group. The trial concluded that therapeutic hypothermia was a safe and effective intervention for improving outcomes in patients who had survived a cardiac arrest but remained comatose.

58.1 Introduction

Cooling down the body as a therapeutic modality has been prevalent since ancient times. The Edwin Smith Papyrus, an Egyptian medical treatise dating back to 3500 B.C.E, describes the use of hypothermia as a treatment for various ailments [1]. Temple Fay reinvigorated interest in hypothermia in modern-day practice in the 1930s with his experiments on whole-body refrigeration and localized cryotherapy for brain lesions. He invented the cooling blanket, circulating cold fluids through a rubber tube [2]. During the Second World War, hypothermia fell into disrepute following Nazi experiments on prisoners at the Dachau concentration camp, in gross violation of basic human rights [3]. There was a resurgence of interest in the 1950s with the intraoperative use of hypothermia as a brain-protective strategy [4].

58.2 Early Reports

58.2.1 Case Reports from Baltimore

In 1958, Williams Jr. et al. reported four patients who underwent hypothermia following in-hospital cardiac arrest at the Johns Hopkins University School of Medicine and Hospital, Baltimore, Maryland. Chest compression was performed within 4–6 min, followed by induced hypothermia to 30–34 °C and maintained for 72 h. All the patients had evidence of severe neurological injury. Three of these patients made a complete neurological recovery. The authors observed that patients with similar neurological injury following cardiac arrest had rarely survived previously [5]. They attributed the apparent neuroprotective effect of hypothermia to the alleviation of brain swelling following cardiac arrest.

58.2.2 The Boy Who Rose From the Dead After Being Struck by Lightning

On the afternoon of July 24, 1958, a 10-year-old boy was brought to the Baltimore City Hospital following a lightning strike. A Boy Scout had found the victim slumped over his bike at the scene. He thought that he could feel a pulse and performed artificial respiration on the victim using the back thrust-arm lift technique in vogue during those days. There was no sign of life when the boy was seen in the accident room 22 minutes after the event. He lay pulseless, with no respiratory efforts, looking pale, his lips cyanotic, and pupils widely dilated. Those were the days of open-chest cardiac massage, three years before external chest compression was first proposed by Kouwenhoven and Knickerbocker [6]. The boy's chest was opened rapidly; the heart was found to be motionless. Following the administration of epinephrine into the heart and massage, spontaneous cardiac activity returned. He was ventilated initially through an oropharyngeal airway and thereafter through an endotracheal tube. He was packed in crushed ice to induce hypothermia down to a temperature of 31.5 °C. Over the next few days, he developed status epilepticus and hemiparesis. He began showing signs of neurological improvement after remaining in a coma for six days. After nearly a month of hospitalization, he was discharged home with no significant neurological deficits. The authors concluded that the timely performance of artificial respiration, open cardiac massage, and expeditious induction of hypothermia likely contributed to his miraculous recovery [7].

58.2.3 Case Series

In 1961, Benson et al. reported 27 patients who suffered in-hospital cardiac arrest. Among them, there were 19 patients with neurological injury, of whom 12 had undergone induced hypothermia to 31–32 °C using a cooling blanket. There were six survivors in the hypothermia group, compared to just a lone survivor among seven patients who did not undergo induced hypothermia. The authors concluded that induced hypothermia in patients with a demonstrable neurological injury following cardiac arrest conferred a significant survival advantage [8].

58.2.4 Peter Safar: The Concept of Cardiopulmonary-Cerebral Resuscitation

Peter Safar pioneered the use of therapeutic hypothermia in patients who remained comatose after resuscitation from cardiac arrest. In his 1964 publication on the "ABCs" of resuscitation, he recommended initiation of hypothermia within 30 min of resuscitation if there were no signs of neurological recovery [9]. He espoused the concept of cardiopulmonary-cerebral resuscitation, advocating hypothermia as a brain-protective strategy. Widely regarded as the father of cardiopulmonary resuscitation, Safar was thrice nominated for the Nobel Prize.

58.3 The Dandenong Hospital Studies

The first prospective clinical trial using hypothermia in survivors of out-of-hospital cardiac arrest was conducted at the Dandenong Hospital in Australia. Twenty-two patients, who remained unconscious after return of spontaneous circulation (ROSC), underwent therapeutic hypothermia to 33 °C. Hypothermia was maintained for 12 h, followed by rewarming. These patients were compared with a historical control group of 22 patients. Hypothermia was associated with significantly more patients with a favorable neurological recovery compared to the control group. No incidence of clinically significant complications was noted with hypothermia [10]. The same group carried out a later RCT of 77 patients comparing hypothermia to 33 °C with normothermia. In this RCT, significantly more patients randomized to hypothermia were discharged home or to a rehabilitation facility compared to the normothermia group. This RCT [11] and the landmark HACA trial [12], were published in the February 21, 2002, edition of The New England Journal of Medicine. These epoch-making trials marked an important breakthrough in the history of cardiopulmonary resuscitation, providing strong evidence that hypothermia may improve outcomes in out-of-hospital survivors of cardiac arrest.

58.4 The Landmark HACA Trial

58.4.1 Population and Design

The HACA trial enrolled patients from nine centers in Europe over a 4-year period between March 1996 and July 2000. It compared the impact of mild hypothermia with normothermia in patients between 18 and 75 years who had sustained out-of-hospital cardiac arrest. The cardiac arrest was witnessed, with ventricular fibrillation or pulseless ventricular tachycardia as the presenting rhythm. The underlying etiology was presumed to be of cardiac origin. The time to commencement of resuscitation attempts by emergency personnel was 5–15 min. The time to ROSC was no more than 60 min. Patients who responded to commands after ROSC were excluded.

Patients who were randomized to receive induced hypothermia were cooled to 32–34 °C using an external cooling device, within 4 h of ROSC. The temperature was maintained in the target range for 24 h, followed by passive rewarming. Normothermia was targeted in the control group. In both groups of patients, sedation was maintained with intravenous infusions of fentanyl and midazolam. In case of shivering, muscle relaxants were administered as appropriate.

A total of 275 patients were enrolled; 137 were randomized to undergo induced hypothermia while 138 were assigned to receive standard care. There were marginal differences in patient characteristics between the two groups at baseline. In the normothermia group, more patients had diabetes mellitus and coronary artery disease. Bystander-administered cardiopulmonary resuscitation was performed more often in the normothermia group.

58.4.2 Outcomes

The primary outcome was based on the neurologic status at six months, evaluated using the Pittsburgh cerebral-performance scale. A score of 1 or 2 represented a favorable neurological outcome. Significantly more patients in the hypothermia group experienced a favorable neurological outcome, 75/136 (55%), compared with patients in the normothermia group, 54/137 (39%). The risk ratio was 1.4, with a 95

Table 58.1 Main study outcomes

Outcomes	Hypothermia (43 patients)	Normothermia (34 patients)	Significance
Good neurological outcome	21 (49%)	9 (26%)	$P = 0.14$
Hospital mortality	22 (51.2%)	23 (67.6%)	Not significantly different
6-month mortality	41%	55%	$P = 0.02$
Complications	93/132	98/135	Not significantly different

percent confidence interval of 1.08 to 1.81, in favor of induced hypothermia. Six patients treated with induced hypothermia were estimated to prevent one unfavorable neurologic outcome.

Among the secondary outcomes, the 6-month mortality was also significantly lower in the hypothermia group (41% vs. 55%, $p = 0.02$). Seven patients treated with induced hypothermia were estimated to prevent one death at 6 months.

Overall, the incidence of complications was not significantly different between the two groups (93/132 vs. 98/135, $p = 0.70$). However, septic complications occurred more commonly with hypothermia (13% vs. 7%), although the difference was not statistically significant. The incidence of arrhythmias, a known complication of hypothermia, was similar in both groups. The main study outcomes are summarized in Table 58.1.

58.5 Study Conclusions

The HACA trial found that in patients who suffered out-of-hospital cardiac arrest due to ventricular fibrillation, cooling down to a temperature of 32–24 °C led to improved neurological outcomes and reduced mortality.

58.5.1 Criticisms

The study was unblinded, which may have resulted in bias. Of the 3551 patients screened, only 275 (7.7%) were enrolled, raising the possibility of selection bias and limited generalizability. The neurological status prior to cooling was not evaluated in detail; hence, it is questionable whether the two groups of patients had suffered similar neurological injury at baseline. Diabetes mellitus and coronary artery disease were more common in the normothermia group; however, the difference in the primary outcome remained significant on multivariate regression analysis. The target temperature was attained at a median of 8 h after ROSC, although the study aimed to attain the target temperature at 4 h after ROSC. Many patients in the control group developed fever that could have potentially caused harm and confounded the results. The trial did not calculate a prospective sample size based on the expected difference in the primary outcome, nor did it report any interim analysis or stopping rules.

58.6 The Post-HACA Era

Following the HACA and the Australian trial, observational studies and a meta-analysis [13] also echoed similar findings, with favorable neurological outcomes among patients treated with hypothermia following cardiac arrest. This prompted the International Liaison Committee on Resuscitation (ILCOR) recommendation for therapeutic hypothermia to 32–34 °C in survivors of out-of-hospital cardiac arrest [14]. Although the strategy of cooling gained widespread acceptance, several questions remained unanswered, opening the door for further studies across larger, more generalizable populations and using different target temperatures.

58.6.1 The Targeted Temperature Management-1 (TTM-1) Trial

Conducted across 36 centers in Europe and Australia, the TTM-1 trial included out-of-hospital cardiac arrest survivors [15]. Patients remained unconscious with a GCS of <8 on arrival at hospital. In contrast to the HACA and the Australian trial, which only included patients with ventricular fibrillation as the presenting rhythm, this study included patients with any arrest rhythm. In the intervention arm, the target temperature of 36 °C, compared to 33 °C in the control group. The target temperature was maintained for 28 h in both groups, followed by rewarming. Following the intervention period, the temperature was maintained below 37.5 °C among patients who remained unconscious in both groups.

Clinical outcomes in the TTM-1 trial contrasted with the findings of the HACA and Australian trials. The all-cause mortality during the study period was similar between the two groups. Among patients in the 33 °C group, the mortality was 50% compared with 48% in the 36 °C group (hazard ratio: 1.06; 95% confidence interval, 0.89 to 1.28; $P = 0.51$). At 180 days, 54% of patients randomized to 33 °C had died or experienced poor neurological outcomes assessed using the cerebral performance category scale, compared with 52% of patients in the 36 °C group; the difference was not statistically significant.

58.6.2 The TTM-2 Trial

In light of the TTM-1 results, the question remained whether fever control alone would provide equivalent clinical outcomes compared to active reduction of temperature below the normal range. The TTM-2 trial included 2000 patients, randomized to hypothermia to 33 °C or fever control alone [16]. In the latter group, if the temperature reached 37.8 °C, a temperature control device was used to maintain the temperature at 37.5 °C. The target temperatures were maintained for a 40-h period in both groups, followed by maintenance of normothermia (36.5–37.7 °C) from 40 to 72 h. No difference in mortality was observed between the two groups at 6 months. Besides, the functional outcomes based on the modified Rankin scale and the health-related quality of life at 6 months were also similar. This well-conducted study strongly suggested that, in contrast to previous studies, maintenance of normal temperature alone would result in similar outcomes compared to therapeutic hypothermia.

58.6.3 The HYPERION Trial

The effect of moderate hypothermia in out-of-hospital cardiac arrest with non-shockable rhythms was evaluated in the HYPERION trial [17]. Patients were randomized to moderate hypothermia of 33 °C in the first 24 h compared with targeted temperature management of 37 °C. At 90 days, a significantly larger number of patients randomized to moderate hypothermia survived with a favorable neurological outcome (CPC score of 1or 2) compared with patients who underwent targeted normothermia (10.2% vs. 5.7%, $p = 0.04$). The 90-day mortality was similar between the two groups.

58.7 Summary

During the period that the HACA trial was conducted, clinical outcomes from out-of-hospital cardiac arrest had remained dismal, despite advances in the field of resuscitation. Induced hypothermia was presumed to affect the brain through reduced metabolism and oxygen consumption at lower temperatures. Although intraoperative cooling was employed from the 1950s, reports of hypothermia following cardiac arrest were few and far between and remained dormant for several decades. The HACA trial represented a landmark and triggered a radical change in the management of survivors of out-of-hospital cardiac arrest. The study held the promise of improving the dismal outcomes following out-of-hospital cardiac arrest, despite several limitations. More recent trials, including the TTM 1 and 2 trials, have not corroborated the beneficial effects observed in the HACA trial; they suggest that control of fever alone may lead to improved clinical outcomes. However, questions regarding the optimal timing and duration of cooling, and specifically, the possible beneficial effects in more severe cardiac arrest syndromes, especially following non-shockable rhythms, remain unanswered.

References

1. Wang H, Olivero W, Wang D, Lanzino G. Cold as a therapeutic agent. Acta Neurochir. 2006;148(5):565–70; discussion 569–570.
2. Alzaga AG, Salazar GA, Varon J, Resuscitation great. Breaking the thermal barrier: Dr. temple fay. Resuscitation. 2006;69(3):359–64.

3. Berger RL. Nazi science — the Dachau hypothermia experiments. N Engl J Med. 1990;322(20):1435–40.
4. Lazorthes G, Campan L. Hypothermia in the treatment of craniocerebral traumatism. J Neurosurg. 1958;15(2):162–7.
5. Williams GR, Spencer FC. The clinical use of hypothermia following cardiac arrest. Ann Surg. 1958;148(3):462–6.
6. Kouwenhoven WB, Jude JR, Knickerbocker GG. Closed-chest cardiac massage. JAMA. 1960;173:1064–7.
7. Ravitch MM, Lane R, Safar P, Steichen FM, Knowles P. Lightning stroke. Report of a case with recovery after cardiac massage and prolonged artificial respiration. N Engl J Med. 1961;264:36–8.
8. Benson DW, Williams GR, Spencer FC, Yates AJ. The use of hypothermia after cardiac arrest. Anesth Analg. 1959;38:423–8.
9. Safar P. Community-wide cardiopulmonary resuscitation. J Iowa Med Soc. 1964;54:629–35.
10. Bernard SA, Jones BM, Horne MK. Clinical trial of induced hypothermia in comatose survivors of out-of-hospital cardiac arrest. Ann Emerg Med. 1997;30(2):146–53.
11. Bernard SA, Gray TW, Buist MD, Jones BM, Silvester W, Gutteridge G, et al. Treatment of comatose survivors of out-of-hospital cardiac arrest with induced hypothermia. N Engl J Med. 2002;346(8):557–63.
12. Hypothermia after Cardiac Arrest Study Group. Mild therapeutic hypothermia to improve the neurologic outcome after cardiac arrest. N Engl J Med. 2002;346(8):549–56.
13. Holzer M, Bernard SA, Hachimi-Idrissi S, Roine RO, Sterz F, Müllner M, et al. Hypothermia for neuroprotection after cardiac arrest: systematic review and individual patient data meta-analysis. Crit Care Med. 2005;33(2):414–8.
14. Nolan JP, Morley PT, Vanden Hoek TL, Hickey RW, Kloeck WGJ, Billi J, et al. Therapeutic hypothermia after cardiac arrest: an advisory statement by the advanced life support task force of the international liaison committee on Resuscitation. Circulation. 2003;108(1):118–21.
15. Nielsen N, Wetterslev J, Cronberg T, Erlinge D, Gasche Y, Hassager C, et al. Targeted temperature management at 33°C versus 36°C after cardiac arrest. N Engl J Med. 2013;369(23):2197–206.
16. Dankiewicz J, Cronberg T, Lilja G, Jakobsen JC, Levin H, Ullén S, et al. Hypothermia versus normothermia after out-of-hospital cardiac arrest. N Engl J Med. 2021;384(24):2283–94.
17. Lascarrou JB, Merdji H, Le Gouge A, Colin G, Grillet G, Girardie P, et al. Targeted temperature Management for Cardiac Arrest with nonshockable rhythm. N Engl J Med. 2019;381(24):2327–37.

59 Targeted Temperature Management After Cardiac Arrest: 33 °C Versus 36 °C: The TTM Trial

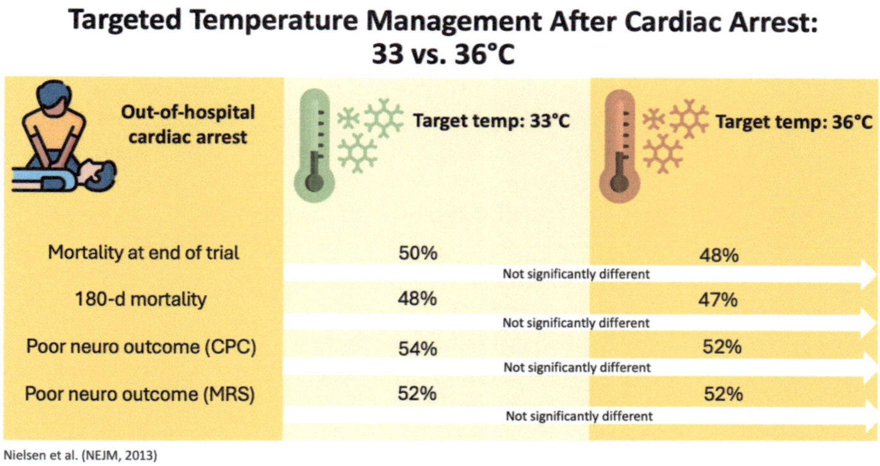

Quick Take

What is the optimal temperature target for patients who remain unconscious after resuscitation from out-of-hospital cardiac arrest?

The TTM trial sought to answer this question by comparing two temperature targets—33 °C and 36 °C—for targeted temperature management (TTM) in patients who remained unconscious following out-of-hospital cardiac arrest. This large, multicenter, randomized controlled trial (RCT) included 939 adult patients who were resuscitated after a presumed cardiac cause of arrest. Participants were randomly assigned to receive hypothermia at either 33 °C or 36 °C for 24 h, followed

Nielsen N, Wetterslev J, Cronberg T, Erlinge D, Gasche Y, Hassager C, et al. Targeted temperature management at 33 °C versus 36 °C after cardiac arrest. N Engl J Med. 2013 Dec 5;369(23):2197–206.

J. Chacko et al., *Landmark Studies in Critical Care*,
https://doi.org/10.1007/978-981-95-0673-6_59

by slow rewarming. The study revealed no significant difference in mortality at 180 days or in neurological recovery between the groups. Adverse events, including arrhythmias and infections, were also similar. The TTM trial concluded that targeted temperature management at 33 °C did not provide a clear advantage over 36 °C, challenging previous practices and reinforcing the importance of avoiding fever in post-cardiac arrest care.

59.1 Background

Out-of-hospital cardiac arrest carries high mortality; besides, survivors are often left with severe neurological disability [1]. Two landmark studies from 2002 revealed improved survival and neurological function among patients who received therapeutic hypothermia to 32–34 °C compared with standard care following out-of-hospital cardiac arrest [2, 3].

Bernard et al. randomly assigned 77 out-of-hospital cardiac arrest patients to hypothermia targeted to 33 °C or normothermia [3]. Targeted hypothermia resulted in improved outcomes, with significantly more patients being discharged home or to a rehabilitation facility (49% vs. 26%). The HACA (Hypothermia After Cardiac Arrest) trial compared a target temperature of 32 °C to 34 °C with standard care, aiming for normothermia. The neurologic outcome was more favorable in the hypothermia group (55% vs. 39%); besides, the 6-month mortality was also lower (41% vs. 55%) [2].

Based on these findings, therapeutic hypothermia was recommended by international guidelines following resuscitation from cardiac arrest [4]. Furthermore, the application of therapeutic hypothermia became more widespread, including in the in-hospital setting [4]. However, the question remained whether prevention of fever alone would be equally efficacious, considering that many patients in the standard care group developed fever in the control group in the HACA trial [2]. The Target Temperature Management (TTM) trial investigators aimed to evaluate clinical outcomes with two temperature targets—33 °C compared with 36 °C—among out-of-hospital cardiac arrest patients. Both strategies were intended to prevent fever in a broader patient population compared to previous studies [5].

59.2 Population and Design

The TTM trial was conducted between November 2010 and January 2013 across 36 centers in Australia and Europe. The study included adult patients who were admitted to the hospital following out-of-hospital cardiac arrest and remained unconscious with a score of <8 on the Glasgow Coma Scale. The underlying cause was presumed to be of cardiac origin; patients were eligible regardless of the initial rhythm. A minimum duration of 20 consecutive minutes of spontaneous circulation was required for study inclusion.

59.2.1 Excluded

Patients who suffered an unwitnessed arrest with asystole as the initially identified rhythm and those who experienced more than 240 min of spontaneous circulation at the time of screening were excluded. Other exclusion criteria were suspected or known intracranial bleed or stroke, and a body temperature of <30 °C. Trauma-related cardiac arrests and those with a known terminal illness were also excluded.

59.3 Study Groups: Temperate Maintained at 33 °C Versus 36 °C

Eligible patients were randomly assigned to targeted temperature management to a body temperature of 33 °C or 36 °C. Randomization was carried out in permuted blocks and stratified by site. Cooling was carried out expeditiously using ice-cold intravenous fluids, ice packs, and intravascular or surface cooling devices based on feasibility at the study site. The target temperature was maintained for a 36-h period, beginning at the time of randomization. Patients were sedated, and neuromuscular blockade was administered.

At 28 h post-randomization, slow rewarming was commenced in both groups at 0.5 °C per hour. Sedation was stopped or weaned down at the end of the 36-h study period. The aim was to maintain the body temperature <37.5 °C for a 72-h period post-cardiac arrest. Fever control was carried out at the clinician's discretion.

59.4 Sample Size

The authors calculated a sample size of 900 patients that provided the study with 90% power to identify a 20% reduction in the hazard ratio for mortality in the 33 °C group. Additionally, they assumed a mortality of 44% in the 33 °C group compared to 55% in the 36 °C group—a relative risk reduction of 20% in the 33 °C group. Based on these assumptions, a sample size of 950 patients was arrived at, allowing a loss to follow-up of 50 patients.

59.5 Results

As planned, the study enrolled 950 patients—476 were assigned to the 33 °C and 474 to the 36 °C group. Baseline characteristics were similar in both groups. There was a clear difference between temperatures between the two groups, beginning at 2–3 h after randomization, and maintained for 36 h ($P < 0.001$ for separation of the temperature curves).

Life-support measures were withdrawn using a protocolized approach in 247 patients (132 in the 33 °C group, 115 in the 36 °C group) during the first week of hospitalization.

59.5.1 The Primary Outcome: Mortality at the End of the Trial Period

At the end of the trial period, the all-cause mortality was similar in both groups. In the 33 °C group, 235/473 (50%) of patients had died by the time the trial ended, compared with 225/466 (48%) in the 36 °C group (hazard ratio: 1.06 (0.89–1.28), $P = 0.51$).

59.5.2 Secondary Outcomes

The main secondary outcome was a composite of death or a poor neurological outcome at 180 days, assessed using the Cerebral Performance Category (CPC) score and the modified Rankin score. The composite outcome was considered poor if the CPC score was 3–5 (3 = severe disability, 4 = coma or vegetative state, 5 = brain death), and the modified Rankin score was 4–6 (4 = moderately severe disability, 5 = severe disability, 6 = death).

There was no significant difference in the composite outcome of death or poor neurological outcome between the 33 °C group and the 36 °C group at 180 days—either by assessment using the CPC or the modified Rankin scale. The authors analyzed the individual components of the composite outcome separately; the 180-day mortality, a CPC score of 3–5, and a modified Rankin score of 4–6 occurred at similar rates in both groups. Analysis by intention-to-treat or per-protocol yielded similar results.

Subgroup analysis based on age (65 years vs. higher), gender, time to return of spontaneous circulation (25 min or less vs. more), initial rhythm (shockable vs. not shockable), presence of shock at admission, and study site (large vs. small) did not reveal a significant difference between groups.

59.6 Adverse Events

Serious adverse events occurred in 93% of patients in the 33 °C group and 90% of patients in the 36 °C group. The common adverse events related to infections, arrhythmias, and electrolyte abnormalities. The main study outcomes are summarized in Table 59.1.

Table 59.1 Main study outcomes

Outcome	33 °C group	36 °C group	P value
Mortality at end of trial period	235/473 (50%)	225/466 (48%)	0.51
180-d mortality	226/473 (48%)	220/466 (47%)	0.92
CPC 3–5 (poor neurological outcome)	251/469 (54%)	242/464 (52%)	0.78
MRS 4–6 (poor neurological outcome	245/469 (52%)	239/464 (52%)	0.87
Serious adverse events	439/472 (92%)	417/464 (90%)	0.09

Abbreviations: *CPC* cerebral performance category scale; *MRS* modified Rankin scale

59.7 Study Conclusion

The authors concluded that among survivors of out-of-hospital cardiac arrest who remained unconscious, therapeutic hypothermia targeting a temperature of 33 °C did not lead to improvement in clinical outcomes compared with a targeted temperature of 36 °C.

59.8 Strengths

The TTM investigators addressed an important clinical question—does targeted hypothermia to 33 °C confer important clinical outcome benefits compared with a near-normal target of 36 °C. This question remained pertinent against the background of two previous RCTs that had shown improved clinical outcomes with a temperature target of 32–34 °C compared with standard care. The multicentric design involving 36 centers across Europe and Australia lent external validity to the study. The TTM trial was more than twice the limited sample size of the 2002 trials and was conducted with meticulous attention to detail. Follow-up was carried out by face-to-face interview in 86% of patients. The study enrolled 950/1242 (76.5%) of eligible patients. The investigators evaluated meaningful clinical outcomes, including mortality and long-term neurological status. Analysis was performed by intention-to-treat and per-protocol. The investigators who assessed outcomes were blinded to the study assignment. Loss to follow-up was minimal. A protocolized approach was employed for neurologic prognostication and withdrawal of life-sustaining interventions.

59.9 Limitations

The study is not generalizable to cardiac arrests with long or unclear downtime; patients who suffered unwitnessed arrest and those with asystole as the initial rhythm were excluded. The median time to initiation of basic (≈ 1 min) and advanced life support (≈ 10 min) was relatively short and may not be reproducible in other healthcare settings. Patients were randomized within 4 h of return of spontaneous circulation. Would earlier commencement of cooling (during or immediately after the arrest) make a difference? Seven patients did not receive the assigned intervention—three in the 33 °C group and four in the 36 °C group. Besides, rewarming was performed before the intended 28-h duration among 16 patients assigned to the 33 °C, which could have impacted outcomes. Details of the type of sedation were not available and could have influenced neurological prognostication. Understandably, the treating team was not blinded to the study assignment.

59.10 Subsequent Evidence: The TTM2 Trial

How does therapeutic hypothermia targeted to 33 °C compare with the maintenance of normothermia, with early treatment of fever if the temperature rose above 37.8 °C following out-of-hospital cardiac arrest? The TTM2 trial compared these two strategies of temperature control. In the intervention group, patients were cooled with surface or intravascular devices to a target temperature of 33 °C [6]. In the control group, the temperature was maintained at ≤37.5 °C with conservative and pharmacological measures alone. If the body temperature rose to 37.8 °C, device cooling was performed, aiming for a target temperature of 37.5 °C. The study evaluated 1850 patients for 6-month mortality, the primary outcome. At the end of 6 months, the mortality was similar in the hypothermia and normothermia groups (50% vs. 48%, $P = 0.37$). Among the secondary outcomes, the proportion of patients with poor functional outcome (modified Rankin scale score: 4–6) was 55% in both groups (relative risk for hypothermia, 1.00; 95% CI, 0.92 to 1.09). The health-related quality of life was also similar in both groups. Among the adverse events, the incidence of arrhythmias causing hemodynamic instability was significantly higher in the hypothermia group. Thus, the TTM2 trial suggested that induced hypothermia to 33 °C does not improve clinical outcomes compared with maintenance of normothermia and treatment of fever when the body temperature rose to >37.8 °C among patients who suffer out-of-hospital cardiac arrest.

59.11 Summary

Two RCTs from 2002 had revealed improved survival and neurological outcomes among survivors of out-of-hospital cardiac arrest who underwent therapeutic hypothermia to 32–34 °C. The TTM investigators addressed the question of whether prevention of fever alone would be equally efficacious. They randomly assigned patients who remained unconscious following out-of-hospital cardiac arrest to a temperature target of 33 °C compared with 36 °C. The study enrolled 950 patients, including 476 assigned to the 33 °C, and 474 to the 36 °C group. The primary outcome, the all-cause-mortality at the end of the trial period, was similar in both groups. The composite of death or a poor neurological outcome at 180 days was also similar. Therapeutic hypothermia targeting a temperature of 33 °C did not lead to improved clinical outcomes in subgroups of patients based on age, gender, time to return of spontaneous circulation, initial rhythm, the presence of shock at admission, and study site. The incidence of serious adverse events was similar in both groups.

The TTM trial clearly demonstrated that hypothermia targeted to 33 °C did not confer a meaningful clinical outcome benefit compared with maintenance of a near-normal body temperature of 36 °C.

References

1. Moulaert VRMP, Verbunt JA, van Heugten CM, Wade DT. Cognitive impairments in survivors of out-of-hospital cardiac arrest: a systematic review. Resuscitation. 2009;80(3):297–305.
2. Hypothermia after Cardiac Arrest Study Group. Mild therapeutic hypothermia to improve the neurologic outcome after cardiac arrest. N Engl J Med. 2002;346(8):549–56.
3. Bernard SA, Gray TW, Buist MD, Jones BM, Silvester W, Gutteridge G, et al. Treatment of comatose survivors of out-of-hospital cardiac arrest with induced hypothermia. N Engl J Med. 2002;346(8):557–63.
4. Peberdy MA, Callaway CW, Neumar RW, Geocadin RG, Zimmerman JL, Donnino M, et al. Part 9: post-cardiac arrest care: 2010 American Heart Association Guidelines for Cardiopulmonary Resuscitation and Emergency Cardiovascular Care. Circulation. 2010;122(18 Suppl 3):S768–86.
5. Nielsen N, Wetterslev J, Cronberg T, Erlinge D, Gasche Y, Hassager C, et al. Targeted temperature management at 33°C versus 36°C after cardiac arrest. N Engl J Med. 2013;369(23):2197–206.
6. Dankiewicz J, Cronberg T, Lilja G, Jakobsen JC, Levin H, Ullén S, et al. Hypothermia versus normothermia after out-of-hospital cardiac arrest. N Engl J Med. 2021;384(24):2283–94.

60 Hypothermia or Normothermia After Out-of-Hospital Cardiac Arrest? The TTM 2 Trial

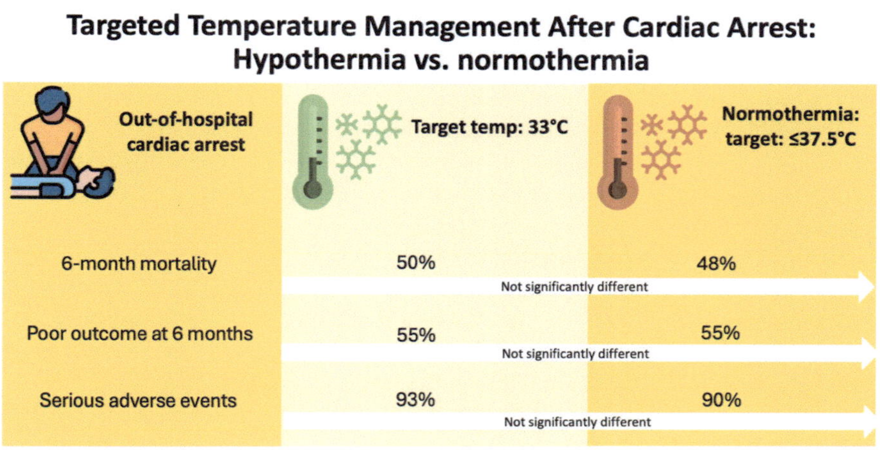

Dankiewicz et al. (NEJM, 2021)

Quick Take

What is the effect of hypothermia versus normothermia on outcomes in patients after out-of-hospital cardiac arrest (OHCA)?

The TTM 2 trial aimed to address this question by comparing the efficacy of therapeutic hypothermia and normothermia in improving survival and neurological outcomes in patients who survived OHCA. In this large, multicenter, randomized controlled trial, 1848 patients who had been resuscitated after OHCA with an initial rhythm of either shockable or non-shockable were randomly assigned to either a hypothermia group (target temperature 33 °C) or a normothermia group (target

---

Dankiewicz J, Cronberg T, Lilja G, Jakobsen JC, Levin H, Ullén S, et al. Hypothermia versus *Normothermia after Out-of-Hospital Cardiac Arrest. N Engl J Med. 2021 Jun 17;384(24):2283–94.*

J. Chacko et al., *Landmark Studies in Critical Care*,
https://doi.org/10.1007/978-981-95-0673-6_60

temperature ≤ 37.5 °C), with temperature control for 24 h followed by gradual rewarming. There was no significant difference between the groups in 6-month survival. Furthermore, there was no difference in neurological outcomes, with similar proportions of patients achieving a favorable neurological recovery. The TTM 2 trial concluded that, in patients with OHCA, targeted temperature management at 33 °C did not provide a survival or neurological benefit over normothermia. These findings further reinforced the importance of normothermic management post-cardiac arrest, shifting the paradigm toward less aggressive cooling strategies in clinical practice.

60.1 Introduction and Background

Two landmark randomized controlled trials (RCTs) of 2002 revealed improved survival and neurological outcomes with therapeutic hypothermia at 32–34 °C compared to standard care in comatose survivors of out-of-hospital cardiac arrest [1, 2]. Following the publication of these trials, international guidelines recommended targeted temperature management following cardiac arrest [3, 4].

The TTM trial of 2013 compared targeted temperature management of 33 °C vs. 36 °C in out-of-hospital cardiac arrest, irrespective of the initial rhythm. In this study, the all-cause mortality and the neurological outcome were similar in both groups [5].

The HYPERION trial compared targeted hypothermia to 33 °C with normothermia (37 °C) in post-cardiac arrest patients with an initial nonshockable rhythm who remained in coma. At 90 days, survival to a favorable neurological outcome was significantly higher in the hypothermia group (10.2% vs. 5.7%). Besides, the incidence of adverse events was similar in both groups [6].

A 2011 meta-analysis, including 478 patients from five randomized controlled trials (RCTs) indicated a lack of robust evidence of benefit with hypothermia on trial sequential analysis. Besides, the included trials had a high risk of bias and random error [7].

Although fever was considered a risk factor for unfavorable outcomes from cardiac arrest, a cause-and-effect relationship had not been established. There was a lack of firm evidence regarding the beneficial effect of hypothermia compared to maintenance of normal body temperature. The TTM2 investigators aimed to evaluate the impact of hypothermia compared to normothermia with early treatment of fever in comatose survivors of out-of-hospital cardiac arrest [8].

60.2 Population and Design

The TTM2 trial was conducted between November 2017 and January 2020 across 61 centers in 14 countries. The study included patients admitted after out-of-hospital cardiac arrest of presumed cardiac or unknown etiology, regardless of the initial rhythm. Patients remained unconscious and unable to obey commands, corresponding to a score of <4 on the Full Outline of Unresponsiveness (FOUR) scale, with no verbal response to pain. Twenty consecutive minutes should have elapsed since the return of spontaneous circulation for eligibility.

60.2.1 Excluded

Patients were excluded if more than 180 min had elapsed since the return of spontaneous circulation. Patients who suffered unwitnessed arrest with asystole as the initial rhythm, and those with limitation of care orders were also excluded.

Eligible patients were randomly assigned to undergo hypothermia or normothermia in a 1:1 ratio. Randomization was in permuted blocks and stratified based on the trial center. The intervention period was 40 h and commenced at the time of randomization.

60.3 The Hypothermia Group

Hypothermia was induced by surface cooling or with an intravascular temperature-management device to a target temperature of 33 °C. The target temperature was maintained for 28 h post-randomization, followed by rewarming. During rewarming, the temperature was increased by one-third of a degree per hour.

60.4 Normothermia Group

In the normothermia group, the temperature was maintained at ≤37.5 °C. If the temperature rose to ≥37.8 °C despite conservative and pharmacological measures, surface or intravascular cooling was performed to maintain the temperature at 37.5 °C. If the temperature remained <37.8 °C, no active cooling was applied.

60.5 Both Groups

There was no standardized sedation protocol; however, short-acting agents or volatile anesthetics were recommended. Sedation was titrated, targeting a Richmond Agitation-Sedation Scale (RASS) of minus 4 (No response to voice, but presence of any movement to physical stimulation). Sedation was maintained until the completion of the 40-h intervention period. Following this, normothermia (36.5 °C to 37.7 °C) was targeted for 72 h post-randomization in patients who were sedated or remained comatose.

Neurologic assessment was carried out by a physician who was blinded to the study arm at 96 h post-randomization or later. Decisions on withdrawal of life-support measures were guided by protocol, but the final decision was at the discretion of the clinician.

60.6 Sample Size

The authors estimated a relative risk reduction in mortality by 15% in the hypothermia group based on earlier trials of therapeutic hypothermia following cardiac arrest [9]. They calculated a sample size of 1862 patients, providing the study with 90% power at a two-sided alpha level of 0.05 to detect a relative risk reduction of 15% and an absolute risk reduction of 7.5%. The final sample size of 1900 allowed for loss to follow-up and withdrawal of consent.

60.7 Results

The intention-to-treat analysis included 1861 patients—930 in the hypothermia group and 931 in the normothermia group. Patients were well-matched at baseline. A shockable rhythm was present in 72% of patients in the hypothermia group and 75% of patients in the normothermia group. The most common rhythm was ventricular fibrillation. Most cardiac arrests were witnessed (91% vs. 92%), with a high rate of bystander-initiated cardiopulmonary resuscitation (82% vs. 78%). The median time from cardiac arrest to the return of spontaneous circulation was 25 min in both groups. The median time from cardiac arrest to randomization was 136 min in the hypothermia group compared with 133 min in the normothermia group.

There was a clear difference in temperatures between the two groups until the end of the 40-h intervention period. The median time to attain a temperature of 34 °C was 3 h in the hypothermia group.

60.7.1 The Primary Outcome: All-Cause Mortality at 6 Months

The all-cause mortality at 6 months was similar in the hypothermia and the normothermia groups (50% vs. 48%; relative risk in the hypothermia group, 1.04; 95% confidence interval, 0.94–1.14; $P = 0.37$). On pre-specified subgroup analysis, there was no difference in mortality based on gender, age (65 years or more vs. less), time to return of spontaneous circulation (25 min or more vs. less), the initial rhythm (shockable vs. non-shockable), or the presence of shock on admission.

60.7.2 Secondary Outcomes

The main secondary endpoint was the functional outcome at 6 months. A poor functional outcome was defined as a score of 4–6 on the modified Rankin scale (4 = moderately severe disability, 5 = severe disability, 6 = dead). If a structured assessment was not feasible, a binary assessment was performed based on available data—as good or poor (a score on the modified Rankin scale of 0–3 was classified as a good outcome and 4–6 as a poor outcome.

At 6 months, there was no significant difference in the number of patients with a poor functional outcome, based on a modified Rankin scale score of 4–6 (55% in both groups; relative risk in the hypothermia group, 1.00; 95% CI, 0.92–1.09). A poor functional outcome based on binary assessment was also similar in both groups (54% in both groups, relative risk in the hypothermia group, 1.00; 95% CI, 0.91–1.08).

The health-related quality of life among survivors was also similar in both groups. The number of days alive and out of the hospital did not differ significantly between the two groups.

60.8 Adverse Events

Among the serious adverse events, arrhythmias leading to hemodynamic instability was significantly higher in the hypothermia group (24% vs. 16%. $P < 0.001$). The incidence of other adverse events, including pneumonia, sepsis, and bleeding, was similar in both groups. The main study outcomes are summarized in Table 60.1.

Table 60.1 Main study outcomes

Outcome	Hypothermia	Normothermia	RR (95% CI)
6 month all-cause mortality	465/925 (50%)	446/925 (48%)	1.04 (0.94–1.14)
Poor outcome at 6 months (mRS 4–6)	488/881 (55%)	479/866 (55%)	1.00 (0.92–1.09)
Poor outcome at 6 months (binary assessment)	495/918 (54%)	493/911 (54%)	1.00 (0.91–1.08)
Serious adverse events (overall)	439 (93%)	417 (90%)	Not significant
Serious adverse events—arrhythmias with hemodynamic instability	222/927 (24%)	152/921 (16%)	1.45 (1.21–1.75)

Abbreviations: *RR* relative risk; *CI* confidence interval; *mRS* modified Rankin scale

60.9 Study Conclusions

The TTM2 trial found that targeted hypothermia (33 °C) did not improve survival or neurological outcomes compared to maintaining normothermia (≤37.8 °C) in patients resuscitated from out-of-hospital cardiac arrest. Both groups had similar mortality rates (50% vs. 48%) and neurological outcomes at 6 months. The study suggests that avoiding fever, rather than inducing hypothermia, should be the focus of temperature management during post-cardiac arrest care.

60.10 Strengths

The TTM2 trial was by far the largest RCT that evaluated temperature management on outcomes following out-of-hospital cardiac arrest. The multicentric design offered external validity. The actual mortality was similar to the presumed mortality employed for sample size calculation. The outcome assessment was performed by investigators who were blinded to the assignment arm. Analysis was by intention-to-treat, adding to the strength of the study. There was a clear separation of temperatures between the study groups with near complete follow-up. The important facets of care, including neurological prognostication, were protocolized.

60.11 Limitations

The caregivers were aware of the assignment arm, with the likelihood of bias. The trial protocol, including mechanical ventilation, sedation, and neuromuscular blockade, may not represent real-world practice. Withdrawal of life support was also based on a conservative protocol that may differ in other centers and may have impacted outcomes. The study did not evaluate the effect of no specific temperature management; in fact, 46% of patients in the normothermia group underwent device cooling to control fever, which may not reflect usual care. Apart from sedation and assessment of prognosis, other aspects of care were left to the clinician's discretion. The trial included patients who had suffered out-of-hospital cardiac arrest of presumed cardiac or unknown cause; the results may not be extrapolatable to other clinical scenarios. The median time to reach 34 °C was 3 h in the hypothermia group. Would earlier initiation of cooling make a difference in outcomes? One-fifth of patients were also enrolled in another trial, although the investigators did not expect any interaction.

60.12 Summary

Although international guidelines recommend targeted temperature management following cardiac arrest, there was no robust evidence to support therapeutic hypothermia. The multicentric TTM2 trial compared two strategies of temperature management in out-of-hospital cardiac arrest of presumed cardiac or unknown cause—induced hypothermia to 33 °C compared with maintenance of normothermia with early treatment of fever (≥37.8 °C). The large, adequately powered RCT included 1850 patients in the assessment of the primary outcome—the all-cause mortality at 6 months. The 6-month mortality was similar in the hypothermia and normothermia groups (50% vs. 48%). Besides, the occurrence of moderately severe disability or worse, based on a modified Rankin scale score of ≥4, was also similar (55% in both groups). Among other outcomes, the health-related quality of life among survivors and the number of days alive and out of the hospital were also similar. Among important adverse events, the incidence of arrhythmia leading to hemodynamic instability was more common in the hypothermia group.

In the largest RCT of targeted temperature management following out-of-hospital cardiac arrest, the TTM2 trial failed to reveal improvement in clinical outcomes with hypothermia at 33 °C compared to normothermia between 36 °C to 37.5 C and prevention of fever. The study highlights to continued need to refine protocols and identify subgroups of patients who might benefit from targeted hypothermia.

References

1. Hypothermia after Cardiac Arrest Study Group. Mild therapeutic hypothermia to improve the neurologic outcome after cardiac arrest. N Engl J Med. 2002;346(8):549–56.
2. Bernard SA, Gray TW, Buist MD, Jones BM, Silvester W, Gutteridge G, et al. Treatment of comatose survivors of out-of-hospital cardiac arrest with induced hypothermia. N Engl J Med. 2002;346(8):557–63.
3. Nolan JP, Soar J, Cariou A, Cronberg T, Moulaert VRM, Deakin CD, et al. European resuscitation council and European society of intensive care medicine guidelines for post-resuscitation care 2015: section 5 of the European resuscitation council guidelines for resuscitation 2015. Resuscitation. 2015;95:202–22.
4. Panchal AR, Bartos JA, Cabañas JG, Donnino MW, Drennan IR, Hirsch KG, et al. Part 3: adult basic and advanced life support: 2020 American Heart Association guidelines for cardiopulmonary resuscitation and emergency cardiovascular care. Circulation. 2020;142(16_suppl_2):S366–468.
5. Nielsen N, Wetterslev J, Cronberg T, Erlinge D, Gasche Y, Hassager C, et al. Targeted temperature management at 33°C versus 36°C after cardiac arrest. N Engl J Med. 2013;369(23):2197–206.
6. Lascarrou JB, Merdji H, Le Gouge A, Colin G, Grillet G, Girardie P, et al. Targeted temperature management for cardiac arrest with nonshockable rhythm. N Engl J Med. 2019;381(24):2327–37.
7. Nielsen N, Friberg H, Gluud C, Herlitz J, Wetterslev J. Hypothermia after cardiac arrest should be further evaluated--a systematic review of randomised trials with meta-analysis and trial sequential analysis. Int J Cardiol. 2011;151(3):333–41.
8. Dankiewicz J, Cronberg T, Lilja G, Jakobsen JC, Levin H, Ullén S, et al. Hypothermia versus normothermia after out-of-hospital cardiac arrest. N Engl J Med. 2021;384(24):2283–94.
9. Dankiewicz J, Cronberg T, Lilja G, Jakobsen JC, Bělohlávek J, Callaway C, et al. Targeted hypothermia versus targeted Normothermia after out-of-hospital cardiac arrest (TTM2): a randomized clinical trial-rationale and design. Am Heart J. 2019;217:23–31.

Part XV

Sedation in the ICU

61 Daily Interruption of Sedation in Mechanically Ventilated Patients: Kress et al.

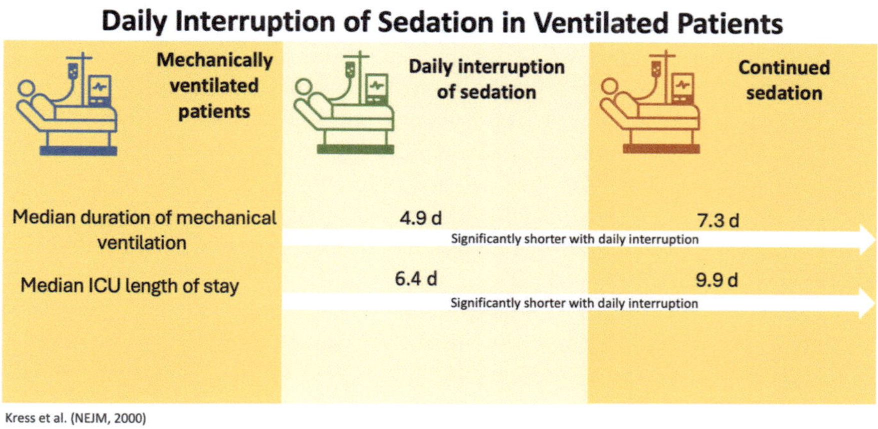

Quick Take

Could a simple change in sedation management lead to better outcomes for ICU patients?

The Kress et al. study was a randomized controlled trial (RCT) designed to evaluate the effects of daily interruption of sedative infusions on the duration of mechanical ventilation and the length of stay in the ICU. The trial involved critically ill patients who were mechanically ventilated and found that daily interruptions of sedation resulted in improved patient outcomes, including a shorter duration of

---

Kress JP, Pohlman AS, O'Connor MF, Hall JB. Daily interruption of sedative infusions in critically ill patients undergoing mechanical ventilation. N Engl J Med. 2000 May 18;342(20):1471–7.

J. Chacko et al., *Landmark Studies in Critical Care*,
https://doi.org/10.1007/978-981-95-0673-6_61

mechanical ventilation, and reduced ICU length of stay without compromising patient comfort or safety. This practice was shown to be an effective and safe strategy for managing sedation in critically ill patients.

61.1 Introduction

Dating back to the 1980s, sedative agents were increasingly used to improve patient comfort during mechanical ventilation. The practice evolved over time with the nearly routine use of a cocktail of narcotics, benzodiazepines, propofol, and major tranquilizers. These drugs provide analgesia, a sense of comfort during stressful, often painful interventions, enable synchronization with mechanical ventilation, and offer a margin of safety with invasive lines and devices in patients who may become restless or agitated [1]. Unfortunately, in many situations, sedation use may go overboard to the point of drug-induced "suspended animation." According to John Kress, the lead author of this landmark paper, by the 1990s, it was fairly common to administer deep sedation, often in combination with neuromuscular blockers, to mechanically ventilated patients in the ICU—a practice that took roots from the operating room [2]. The late Thomas Petty poignantly wrote in 1998, "What I see these days are paralyzed, sedated patients, lying without motion, appearing to be dead, except for the monitors that tell me otherwise" [3]. At the University of Chicago, where the study was conducted, patients would take several days to wake up after ceasing sedative agents. Although there was a policy of daily cessation of sedation, it was rarely followed [2].

Sedative medications are usually administered as intravenous infusions. Compared to intermittent bolus administration, continuous infusions maintain a constant level of sedation and presumably, an increased level of comfort [4]. Clearly, excessive sedation carries the risk of adverse outcomes. Too much sedation may prolong the duration of mechanical ventilation and ICU stay, and may lead to an increase in the incidence of ventilator-associated pneumonia [5]. Besides, neurological assessment may be rendered difficult, often leading to needless, often misguided imaging or other modalities of investigation. Interruption of sedation on a daily basis may offer a window allowing patients to awaken without compromising comfort. Against this background, the authors hypothesized that a policy of daily interruption of sedation might reduce the duration of mechanical ventilation, ICU, and hospital stay.

61.2 Population and Design

The study was conducted in the medical intensive care unit of the University of Chicago [6]. Patients were intubated and mechanically ventilated and required continuous infusion of sedatives according to the clinician judgment. Those who were transferred from elsewhere and already on sedation, and those who were resuscitated after cardiac arrest, were excluded. Patients were randomly assigned to daily interruption or continued sedation.

61.3 Intervention

Sedatives were interrupted daily, beginning 48 h after study enrollment. The sedative (midazolam or propofol) and morphine (as an analgesic) infusions were interrupted until patients were awake and able to follow commands or if they became uncomfortable, restless, or agitated. The sedative and morphine infusions were resumed as deemed appropriate. If patients were on neuromuscular blockade, it was ceased before stopping the sedative infusion.

61.4 Control

Sedatives were continued; cessation was at the discretion of the ICU team.

Within each group, patients were randomized to receive either midazolam or propofol as the sedative infusion, thus creating four groups of patients. Midazolam was administered as an initial bolus of 0.5–5 mg every 1–5 min, followed by a continuous infusion of 1–2 mg/h. The infusion rate was increased by 1–2 mg/h for the desired level of sedation. Propofol was commenced at 5 mcg/kg/min; the infusion rate was increased by 5–10 mcg/kg/min every 2 min until the desired level of sedation was attained.

61.5 Common Management

Bedside nurses titrated the dose of the sedative infusion to a score of 3–4 on the Ramsay sedation scale. All four groups of patients received morphine as an analgesic. Morphine was administered as an initial bolus of 2–10 mg and followed up with a continuous infusion of 1–5 mg/h. The overall care was left to the discretion of the ICU team. Patients were considered awake if they were able to perform three of the following four actions: (1) open eyes to call, (2) follow the investigator with their eyes, (3) squeeze hand on command, and (4) protrude tongue on command.

61.6 Results

61.6.1 Patient Characteristics

A total of 150 patients were randomized, 75 to each group. After excluding patients who were extubated early or died, 68 patients in the intervention group and 60 in the control group were included in the final analyses. In the interruption group, 37 patients received midazolam while 31 received propofol as the sedative agent. In the control group, 29 received midazolam, while 31 received propofol infusion. Baseline characteristics, including demographic characteristics, the baseline APACHE II scores, and the underlying diagnosis, were similar between the two groups.

Table 61.1 Main study outcomes

Outcomes	Daily interruption	Control	Significance
Median ventilation days	4.9	7.3	$P = 0.004$
Median ICU length of stay	6.4	9.9	$P = 0.02$
Median hospital length of stay	13.3	16.9	$P = 0.19$
Hospital mortality	36.0%	46.7%	$P = 0.25$

61.6.2 Outcomes

The median duration of mechanical ventilation was significantly shorter in the daily interruption group compared to the control group [4.9 (2.5–8.6) vs. 7.3 (3.4–16.1) days, $p = 0.004$]. Patients in the daily interruption group were extubated earlier compared to the control group. The median ICU length of stay was also significantly shorter with daily interruption of sedation [6.4 (3.9–12.0) vs. 9.9 (4.7–17.9) days, $p = 0.02$]. The duration of hospital stay was longer in the control group; however, the difference was not statistically significant. Failed extubation requiring reintubation was similar between the two groups. The hospital mortality was also similar in both groups; 36% of patients died in the daily interruption group compared with 47.6% in the control group. Significantly more patients in the daily interruption group were discharged home compared to the control group. The choice of the sedative agent, midazolam vs. propofol, did not affect the duration of mechanical ventilation, ICU stay, and hospital stay.

Diagnostic imaging to assess the neurological status was performed less often in the daily interruption group. In the control group, 13 CT scans, two MRI scans, and one lumbar puncture and cerebrospinal fluid examination were carried out, compared to six CT scans in the daily interruption group. In the control group, 15 patients (13 died in a coma) never awakened during the ICU stay, compared with seven patients (six died in a coma) in the daily interruption group.

Adverse events were similar in both groups; two accidental extubations and one accidental removal of a central venous catheter occurred in the daily interruption group; none of these events occurred during the period of interruption of sedation. Four accidental extubations occurred in the control group. Main study outcomes are summarized in Table 61.1.

61.7 Study Conclusions

The Kress et al. trial found that daily interruption of sedative infusions in mechanically ventilated ICU patients reduced the duration of mechanical ventilation (median 4.9 vs. 7.3 days) and ICU stay (median 6.4 vs. 9.9 days) without increasing adverse events. The study suggests that routine sedation breaks improve outcomes and should be part of the ICU sedation protocol.

61.8 Relevance of the Study

This landmark study by Kress et al. revealed that daily interruption of sedative agents is safe, practicable, and helps reduce the duration of mechanical ventilation and ICU stay. Besides, this strategy enables a more precise clinical evaluation of the neurological status and results in fewer investigations being performed. This landmark trial turned out to be a wake-up call for ICU physicians and reaffirmed the "less is more" principle regarding the depth of sedation in the critically ill. The study triggered a departure from the widespread use of sedatives as a continuous infusion in mechanically ventilated patients during the 1980s and 90 s. When sedative agents are used indiscriminately, without titration to objective endpoints, patients may remain obtunded for a prolonged duration, leading to adverse clinical outcomes. The long-term impact of sedative agents may be more profound in the critically ill, with alterations in the volume of distribution and elimination due to impaired hepatic and renal function. Heavy-handed use of sedative agents may also be more prevalent in units that may have less than optimal skilled nursing available by the bedside.

61.9 Weaknesses

Although the study did not reveal any evidence of compromised safety with a policy of daily interruption of sedation, the number of events was too few to come to a definite conclusion. The psychological impact emanating from the daily cessation of sedation was not assessed, particularly regarding the perception of pain and discomfort. Cardiovascular compromise arising from the sympathetic surge that may accompany the interruption of sedation could conceivably lead to harm, particularly in patients with coronary artery disease. The study was unblinded, which may have led to bias. In the control group, some patients had cessation of sedation in between, which could have impacted outcomes. The findings of the study, conducted in a medical ICU, may not be directly extrapolatable to surgical ICUs.

61.10 Later Studies

Many RCTs followed in light of the findings of this landmark trial on "sedation vacation," as it came to be popularly known in intensive care circles.

Girard et al. compared daily awakening combined with a spontaneous breathing trial with a usual sedation practice combined with daily awakening. The strategy of a spontaneous breathing trial combined with daily awakening led to more ventilator-free days, ICU, and hospital stay compared with daily awakening alone [7]. Another study by Mehta et al. demonstrated that a protocolized sedation strategy is as effective as daily interruption combined with protocolized sedation [8]. The NONSEDA trial compared a strategy of no sedation with light sedation to an arousable level. The authors did not find a significant difference in the mortality, ventilation-free days, and duration of ICU stay between the two groups. However, the intended difference in the level of sedation between the two groups was not attained [9].

61.11 Summary

More than three decades ago, it was customary to maintain mechanically ventilated patients under deep sedation, often combined with neuromuscular blockade. This practice percolated through contemporary anesthetic practice and was based on the presumption that a deep level of sedation improved patient comfort. Besides, a deeper level of sedation facilitated nursing care, especially in understaffed units. The question of patient safety was also a consideration with the likely potential for accidental removal of care-related devices and the possibility of adverse outcomes from such incidents. The authors of this landmark trial embarked upon a policy of daily interruption, with the resumption of sedative medication as appropriate. This strategy was compared to a conventional approach with continued sedation and cessation based on the judgment of the ICU team. They found that daily interruption of sedation among mechanically ventilated patients led to earlier extubation and resulted in a shorter duration of ventilator support overall. The length of stay in the ICU was also shorter with the daily interruption strategy.

Although there have been conflicting results from subsequent RCTs, the Kress et al. study marked a paradigm shift from the traditional practice of deep sedation in mechanically ventilated patients. This study is particularly relevant considering the relatively unpredictable effect of sedative agents among critically ill patients with altered pharmacokinetic profiles, especially in the presence of multiorgan dysfunction.

References

1. Jacobs JR, Reves JG, Glass PS. Rationale and technique for continuous infusions in anesthesia. Int Anesthesiol Clin. 1991;29(4):23–38.
2. Balzer F, Weiß B, Kumpf O, Treskatsch S, Spies C, Wernecke KD, et al. Early deep sedation is associated with decreased in-hospital and two-year follow-up survival. Crit Care Lond Engl. 2015;19:197.
3. Petty TL. Suspended life or extending death? Chest. 1998 Aug;114(2):360–1.
4. Shafer A. Complications of sedation with midazolam in the intensive care unit and a comparison with other sedative regimens. Crit Care Med. 1998;26(5):947–56.
5. Klompas M. Prevention of intensive care unit-acquired pneumonia. Semin Respir Crit Care Med. 2019;40(4):548–57.
6. Kress JP, Pohlman AS, O'Connor MF, Hall JB. Daily interruption of sedative infusions in critically ill patients undergoing mechanical ventilation. N Engl J Med. 2000;342(20):1471–7.
7. Girard TD, Kress JP, Fuchs BD, Thomason JWW, Schweickert WD, Pun BT, et al. Efficacy and safety of a paired sedation and ventilator weaning protocol for mechanically ventilated patients in intensive care (Awakening and Breathing Controlled trial): a randomised controlled trial. 2008;371:9.
8. Mehta S. Daily sedation interruption in mechanically ventilated critically ill patients cared for with a sedation protocol: a randomized controlled trial. JAMA. 2012;308(19):1985.
9. Olsen HT, Nedergaard HK, Strøm T, Oxlund J, Wian KA, Ytrebø LM, et al. Nonsedation or light sedation in critically ill, mechanically ventilated patients. N Engl J Med. 2020;382(12):1103–11.

62 A Combined Sedation and Ventilator Weaning Protocol for Mechanically Ventilated Patients: The ABC Trial

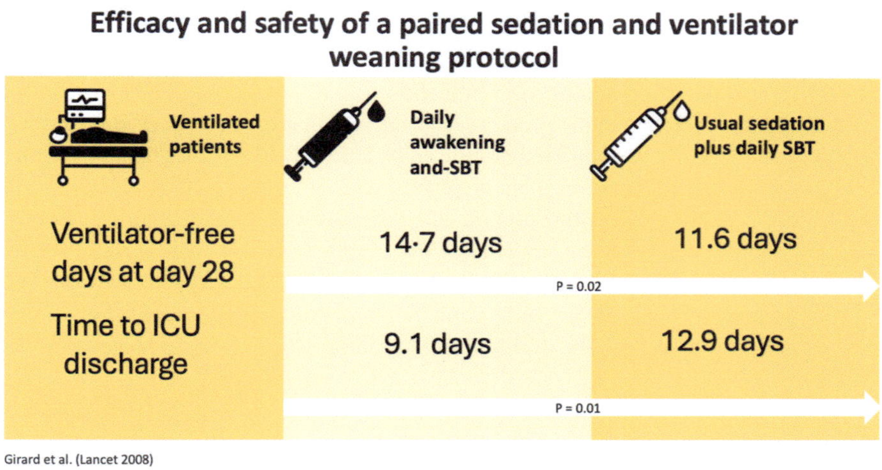

Quick Take

In mechanically ventilated patients, does a paired strategy of daily interruption of sedation and spontaneous breathing trials reduce the duration of mechanical ventilation?

This pivotal randomized controlled trial (RCT) evaluated the impact of pairing daily sedation interruptions with spontaneous breathing trials in mechanically ventilated ICU patients. The patient group that received the paired protocol experienced

---

Girard TD, Kress JP, Fuchs BD, Thomason JWW, Schweickert WD, Pun BT, et al. Efficacy and safety of a paired sedation and ventilator weaning protocol for mechanically ventilated patients in intensive care (Awakening and Breathing Controlled trial): a randomised controlled trial. 2008;371.

J. Chacko et al., *Landmark Studies in Critical Care*,
https://doi.org/10.1007/978-981-95-0673-6_62

significantly shorter durations of mechanical ventilation and ICU stay compared to the control group, which followed standard care. Importantly, the trial demonstrated no increase in serious adverse events in the paired protocol group. The findings underscored the importance of minimizing sedation and promoting early liberation from mechanical ventilation to improve patient outcomes.

62.1 Introduction

Analgesic and sedative agents are administered to patients on mechanical ventilation to provide pain relief and alleviate anxiety [1]. Besides, they enhance patient safety and facilitate nursing care [1]. However, they may also be associated with undesirable effects, including excessive sedation, delirium [2], and prolonged mechanical ventilation [3]. Although scoring systems are employed to titrate sedation [4], observational studies suggest that ICU patients are often sedated to inordinate levels [5].

Kress et al. compared daily interruption with continued sedation, ceased only at the clinician's discretion, among mechanically ventilated patients [6]. They observed a significantly shorter duration of mechanical ventilation and ICU stay among patients who underwent daily interruption of sedation. Besides, diagnostic imaging to assess neurological function was employed less often with a daily interruption strategy. A policy of daily interruption did not lead to an increase in the rate of adverse events.

Protocolized weaning from mechanical ventilation has been extensively studied [7]. These protocols center around spontaneous breathing trials (SBT), and have been established to reduce the duration of ventilatory support across heterogenous patient populations [7].

A cohesive approach of titrated sedation combined with ventilator weaning protocols carries the potential to improve clinical outcomes. However, in many parts of the world, ventilator weaning and titration of sedation are compartmentalized and handled by separate care teams. The ABC investigators hypothesized that daily interruption of sedation represented by spontaneous awakening trials (SAT), combined with SBT, may be superior to a strategy of continued protocolized sedation with standard SBTs.

The Awakening and Breathing Controlled (ABC) trial was conducted between October, 2003 and March 2006 in four large medical centers in the US [8]. Adult patients receiving mechanical ventilation for ≥12 h were screened. Patients who were on full ventilator support and those being weaned were eligible.

62.1.1 Excluded

Patients who were admitted following cardiopulmonary arrest, and those on mechanical ventilation for ≥2 weeks, were excluded. The study also excluded patients who were at imminent risk of dying, those in whom life support measures were being withdrawn, and those with severe neurological impairment.

62.2 Management of Sedation: All Patients

Patients were managed with a patient-targeted sedation strategy, titrated to maintain a level of arousal and comfort as deemed appropriate, using a validated scale. Patients were randomly allocated to a paired SAT and SBT strategy (intervention) or usual care (control). Patient management was protocolized according to the group assigned.

Patients were randomized in a 1:1 ratio to SBT (control) or SAT plus SBT (intervention).

62.3 Usual Care (Control Group): SBT

Sedatives and analgesics were continued based on the patient-targeted strategy.

Patients were screened for SBT safety. SBT was considered safe if: oxygenation was adequate, spontaneous respiratory efforts were present, there was no agitation, arrhythmias, significant vasoactive drug infusions, and no evidence of raised ICP.

If SBT screening was successful, spontaneous breathing was allowed through a T-tube or supported with a continuous positive airway pressure of 5 cm H_2O or pressure support of <7 cm H_2O. The FiO_2 and PEEP levels were maintained at the same level. SBT was considered to have failed if any of the following occurred: respiratory rate >35 or <8/min for 5 min or longer, hypoxemia, new onset change in mental status, arrhythmias, and respiratory distress. SBT was deemed successful if none of the failure criteria occurred during the 120-minute trial period, and patients were considered for extubation based on clinician judgment.

Those who failed SBT were recommenced on the pre-SBT ventilator settings.

62.4 Intervention: SAT Plus SBT

Patients were screened every morning for the safety of SAT. SAT was withheld in the presence of active seizures, alcohol withdrawal, agitation, neuromuscular blockade, active myocardial ischemia, or raised intracranial pressure. If they passed the safety screen, SAT was performed.

SAT involved cessation of all sedatives and analgesics except those considered essential for pain relief. Following cessation of sedatives and analgesics, patients were monitored for up to 4 h.

SAT was considered to have failed if patients experienced anxiety, agitation, or pain; a respiratory rate >35/min, desaturation to 88% or less, occurrence of cardiac arrhythmia, or any signs of respiratory distress. If the SAT failed, sedatives were recommenced at half the previous dose and titrated to an adequate level.

Those who passed the SAT underwent an SBT, as in the control group.

62.5 Sample Size Calculation

The authors assumed a mean of 12.9 (±10.4) ventilator-free days in the control group. They calculated a sample size of 334 patients that would enable the detection of a 25% increase in the ventilator-free days in the intervention group. This sample size provided the study with 80% power at a two-sided significance level of 0.05.

62.6 Results

Among 1658 patients considered eligible, 336 were enrolled—168 to each group. The baseline characteristics were similar in both groups, including age, gender, and severity of illness. Opiate and benzodiazepine use was similar in both groups before enrollment; propofol use was higher in the intervention group.

62.7 The Primary Outcome: Ventilator-Free Days from Day 1 to 28

Death during the study period was counted as 0 ventilator-free days. The number of ventilator-free days at day 28 was significantly higher in the intervention group (14.7 ± 0.9 vs. 11.6 ± 0.9 days, $P = 0.02$). No significant interaction was observed between the study center and ventilator-free days.

62.8 Secondary Outcomes

The time to discharge from ICU (9.1 vs. 12.9 days) and the time to discharge from hospital (14·9 vs. 19·2 days) were significantly lower in the intervention group. The 28-day all-cause mortality was similar in both groups (28% vs. 35%).

The 1-year mortality was lower in the intervention group (44% vs. 58%, $P = 0.01$). One life was saved for every 7 patients managed with the SAT-SBT strategy (number needed to treat = 7.4).

Patients in the SAT-SBT group were more awake and alert compared to control patients on the day of SBT safety evaluation. There was no significant difference in the incidence of delirium between the two groups.

Fewer tracheostomies were performed in the SAT-SBT group (13% vs. 20%); the median time to placement of tracheostomy was similar in both groups.

The overall rate of reintubation was similar in both groups. Self-extubations occurred more often in the SAT-SBT group (10% vs. 4%). However, among those who experienced self-extubation, only a few patients required reintubation in either group; the between-group difference was not significant. The main findings of the study are summarized in Table 62.1.

Table 62.1 Main Study Outcomes

Outcome	SAT plus SBT (167 patients)	Usual care plus SBT (168 patients)	Significance
Mean ventilator-free days	14·7	11·6	$P = 0.02$
Median time to ICU discharge (days)	9·1	12·9	$P = 0.01$
Median time to hospital discharge (days)	14·9	19·2	$P = 0.04$
28-d mortality	28%	35%	$P = 0.21$
1-y mortality	44%	58%	$P = 0.01$
Self extubation	10%	4%	$P = 0.03$
Self extubation, reintubated	3%	2%	$P = 0.47$

Abbreviations: *SAT* spontaneous awakening trial, *SBT* spontaneous breathing trial

62.9 Study Conclusions

The ABC trial found that daily sedation interruption combined with spontaneous breathing trials significantly reduced time on mechanical ventilation (median 9 vs. 12 days) and 1-year mortality (44% vs. 58%) compared to usual care. The study supports integrating both sedation breaks and breathing trials to improve ICU outcomes.

62.10 Strengths

The ABC trial was an adequately powered RCT that compared the efficacy and safety of the combination of daily sedation interruption and SBTs with a control group that received continued titrated sedation and SBTs. The investigators followed a pragmatic, easy-to-follow protocol. Patients in both intervention and control groups were well matched at baseline, and follow-up was nearly complete. The trial demonstrated the favorable impact of a combined sedation and weaning protocol, instead of dealing separately with these important facets of care.

62.11 Limitations

A sizeable proportion (79.7%) of eligible patients were not enrolled, many due to physician's refusal to participate. The study was unblinded owing to its design; extubation was entirely based on clinician judgment and may have led to bias. The study did not include surgical patients; extrapolation may not be appropriate among this subgroup. The participating ICUs were part of large academic medical centers, with ready availability of skilled staff, including respiratory therapists. It remains to be seen if the results may be replicable at lower-level centers. A combined SAT plus SBT protocol may also be time-consuming, labor-intensive, and not feasible at smaller centers.

The 1-year mortality was significantly lower in the SAT-SBT group; however, mortality at 28 days was similar in both groups. It is difficult to explain how longer-term survival may be more favorable based on a strategy involving sedation and weaning. The control group did not require cessation of sedation, which may have led to spontaneous breathing trials being carried out in patients who were not awake enough. This may explain the relatively higher number of failures of spontaneous breathing trials in the control group (456 vs. 284 failures). Functional and psychological outcomes were not evaluated; daily awakening may have impacted these outcomes.

62.12 Subsequent Evidence

The NONSEDA trial randomized mechanically ventilated ICU patients to a strategy of no sedation or light sedation—to a level at which the patient is arousable. The 90-day mortality, the primary outcome, was similar in both groups of patients. Secondary outcomes, including ICU- and ventilator-free days, and the incidence of delirium, were also similar [9].

The 2018 PADIS guidelines of the Society of Critical Care Medicine recommend a multifaceted approach towards improving the care of critically ill patients. SAT and SBT, as suggested by the ABC investigators, are key components of this bundled approach. The full ABDCEF bundle includes the following: A: assessment, prevention, and management of pain, B: both SAT and SBT, C: choice of analgesics and sedatives, D: delirium—assessment, prevention, and management, E: early mobilization and exercise, and F: family engagement and empowerment [10].

62.13 Summary

Daily sedation hold had been previously demonstrated to reduce the duration of mechanical ventilation and ICU stay among critically ill patients. Similar favorable outcomes were also observed with a strategy of SBTs. The ABC trial evaluated a combination of both approaches—titrated sedation with daily interruption combined with SBTs (SAT plus SBT). They compared this approach with SBT alone, with continued, titrated sedation. Patients who underwent a paired approach of SAT combined with SBT experienced more favorable clinical outcomes—they spent more days breathing without assistance during the 28-day study period. Besides, they were discharged from the ICU and hospital earlier than their counterparts in the control group. The 1-year mortality was also lower in the SAT plus SBT group. The ABC trial led to the incorporation of spontaneous awakening and spontaneous breathing trials into guidelines aimed at improving outcomes of mechanically ventilated patients.

References

1. Jacobi J, Fraser GL, Coursin DB, Riker RR, Fontaine D, Wittbrodt ET, et al. Clinical practice guidelines for the sustained use of sedatives and analgesics in the critically ill adult. Crit Care Med. 2002;30(1):119–41.
2. Pandharipande P, Shintani A, Peterson J, Pun BT, Wilkinson GR, Dittus RS, et al. Lorazepam is an independent risk factor for transitioning to delirium in intensive care unit patients. Anesthesiology. 2006;104(1):21–6.
3. Kollef MH, Levy NT, Ahrens TS, Schaiff R, Prentice D, Sherman G. The use of continuous i.v. sedation is associated with prolongation of mechanical ventilation. Chest. 1998;114(2):541–8.
4. Ely EW, Truman B, Shintani A, Thomason JWW, Wheeler AP, Gordon S, et al. Monitoring sedation status over time in ICU patients: reliability and validity of the Richmond agitation-sedation scale (RASS). JAMA. 2003;289(22):2983–91.
5. Weinert CR, Calvin AD. Epidemiology of sedation and sedation adequacy for mechanically ventilated patients in a medical and surgical intensive care unit. Crit Care Med. 2007;35(2):393–401.
6. Kress JP, Pohlman AS, O'Connor MF, Hall JB. Daily interruption of sedative infusions in critically ill patients undergoing mechanical ventilation. N Engl J Med. 2000;342(20):1471–7.
7. Blackwood B, Burns KEA, Cardwell CR, O'Halloran P. Protocolized versus non-protocolized weaning for reducing the duration of mechanical ventilation in critically ill adult patients. Cochrane Database Syst Rev. 2014;2014(11):CD006904.
8. Girard TD, Kress JP, Fuchs BD, Thomason JWW, Schweickert WD, Pun BT, et al. Efficacy and safety of a paired sedation and ventilator weaning protocol for mechanically ventilated patients in intensive care (Awakening and Breathing Controlled trial): a randomised controlled trial. 2008;371.
9. Olsen HT, Nedergaard HK, Strøm T, Oxlund J, Wian KA, Ytrebø LM, et al. Nonsedation or light sedation in critically ill, mechanically ventilated patients. N Engl J Med. 2020;382(12):1103–11.
10. Marra A, Ely EW, Pandharipande PP, Patel MB. The ABCDEF bundle in critical care. Crit Care Clin. 2017;33(2):225–43.

63 No Sedation Vs. Light Sedation in Mechanically Ventilated Patients: The NONSEDA Trial

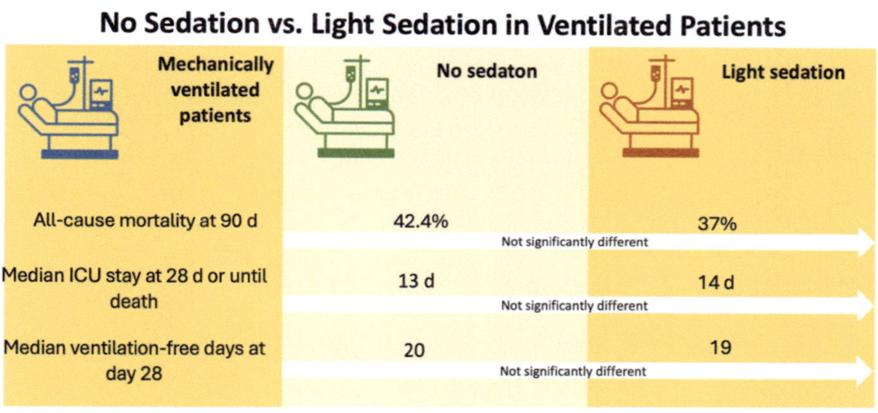

Olsen et al. (NEJM, 2020)

Quick Take

Could a no-sedation policy improve outcomes in ventilated ICU patients?

The NONSEDA trial investigated whether a strategy of no sedation compared with light sedation would result in improved outcomes in mechanically ventilated patients. This multicenter randomized trial enrolled critically ill patients requiring mechanical ventilation and assigned them to either nonsedation or light sedation with daily interruption. The study found no significant difference in mortality between the groups; besides, the duration of mechanical ventilation, ICU, and hospital stay were also similar.

Olsen HT, Nedergaard HK, Strøm T, Oxlund J, Wian KA, Ytrebø LM, et al. Nonsedation or Light Sedation in Critically Ill, Mechanically Ventilated Patients. N Engl J Med. 2020 Mar 19;382(12):1103–11.

J. Chacko et al., *Landmark Studies in Critical Care*,
https://doi.org/10.1007/978-981-95-0673-6_63

63.1 Introduction

Although present-day ventilators are more tuned to patient needs, mechanically ventilated patients in the ICU are usually administered continuous sedative infusions to ensure comfort and compliance with care. The practice of continued sedation, as opposed to analgesia alone, has been questioned, with some studies demonstrating worse outcomes. In a randomized controlled trial (RCT) published in 2000, daily interruption of sedative infusions resulted in lower mortality and shorter hospital stay compared with patients who received uninterrupted sedation [1]. Eight years later, yet another RCT demonstrated the advantages of a daily interruption policy, with patients experiencing a shorter duration of mechanical ventilation and ICU stay [2].

In their earlier single-center RCT, the investigators of the present study had compared a policy of no sedation with daily interruption among mechanically ventilated patients in the ICU [3]. A no-sedation strategy was associated with a shorter ICU and hospital stay; besides, patients who received no sedation experienced significantly more ventilation-free days. Among other findings of this study, acute renal failure was lower with a no-sedation policy. However, the study was not powered to evaluate a difference in survival rates between the two groups. Hence, they designed a multicentric study to investigate whether a no-sedation strategy would lead to improved survival compared with light sedation and daily interruption.

63.1.1 Population and Design

The NONSEDA trial was conducted between January 2014 and November 2017 across eight centers in Denmark, Norway, and Sweden [4]. Adult patients who had been commenced on invasive mechanical ventilation within 24 h of screening and expected to remain ventilated for >24 h were eligible.

63.1.2 Excluded

Patients who were being ventilated for severe traumatic brain injury, status epilepticus, and those undergoing therapeutic hypothermia were excluded. Patients who were treated in another ICU for >48 h, those who were comatose, brain dead, severely hypoxic with a PaO_2/FiO_2 ratio ≤9 kPa (67.5 mm Hg), those who required sedative agents for maintaining oxygenation, and those who were ventilated in the prone position were also excluded.

Eligible patients were randomly assigned in a 1:1 ratio to a strategy of no sedation or light sedation with daily interruption. Randomization was stratified based on study center, age, and presence of shock.

63.2 No Sedation Group

Patients in the no sedation group received bolus doses of morphine for pain relief, based on clinical judgment. They were awake and able to communicate, with the goal to maintain a natural sleep rhythm. If reassurance and analgesia were inadequate, sedative agents could be used as in the light sedation group; however, crossover was not allowed.

63.3 Light Sedation Group

Patients received a continuous infusion of sedative agents; however, they remained arousable, corresponding to a score of −2 to −3 on the Richmond Agitation and Sedation Scale (RASS). During the first 48 h, propofol was preferentially used for sedation, and midazolam thereafter. The sedative infusion was ceased every morning, aiming for full wakefulness and the ability to obey simple commands. Weaning off ventilator support was attempted during the period of wakefulness. Sedation was resumed at half the original dose. If the PEEP level could be weaned down to 5 cm H_2O and the FiO_2 below 0.4, sedation was withheld; however, it could be resumed in case of patient discomfort. Bolus doses of clonidine could be administered for anxiety or mild agitation.

63.4 Common Management

Both groups of patients received analgesics including paracetamol, opioid boluses, and epidural analgesia as appropriate. The study protocol discouraged the use of dexmedetomidine.

Delirium was assessed twice daily, at 08:00 and 20:00 h, using the Confusion Assessment Method for the ICU (CAM-ICU). Patients were categorized based on the assessment to have delirium, no delirium, or comatose, and hence unable to evaluate. If delirium was diagnosed, the first step was to resort to non-pharmacological methods, including reassurance and mobilization. If delirium persisted, haloperidol or olanzapine was administered according to protocol. Following extubation, patients were transferred out of the ICU based on local policies and clinician discretion.

63.5 Sample Size Calculation

Based on previous studies, the authors assumed a 25% reduction in the relative risk of hospital mortality with a strategy of no sedation. Considering a maximum risk of 5% type 1 error and 20% type 2 error, they calculated a sample size of 350 patients in each group, providing the study with 80% power.

63.6 Results

The study enrolled 710 of 2300 patients who were screened; after the exclusion of 10 patients (five in each group), 700 were included in the modified intention-to-treat analysis. Overall, 38.4% of patients in the no sedation group received sedative medication at some point, the main reason being delirium. The mean RASS score was significantly higher in the no sedation group from days 1–7, indicating a more alert state.

63.7 The Primary Outcome: 90-Day Mortality

On modified intention-to-treat analysis, the 90-day mortality was similar in both groups (no sedation vs. sedation: 42.4% vs. 37.0%, $P = 0.65$).

63.8 Secondary Outcomes

The median time until death up to 90 days post-randomization was similar in the no sedation and sedation groups (13 [1–27] vs. 12 [5–28]). Major thromboembolic events occurred in 10 (2.8%) patients in the sedation group compared with just one patient (0.3%) in the no sedation group. The median number of coma- or delirium-free days was similar (27 [21–28] vs. 26 [22–28]). The renal function, assessed using the highest RIFLE score within 28 days of randomization, was identical in both groups. Mechanical ventilation-free days up to 28 days were not significantly different between groups (20 [0–26] vs. 19 [0–25]).

63.9 Adverse Events

Accidental extubation requiring reintubation within an hour occurred at similar rates in both groups (1.1% vs. 0.3%, $P = 0.2$). However, accidental extubation that required reintubation within 24 h occurred significantly more often in the no sedation group (8.9% vs. 4%, $P = 0.01$). Accidental removal of central venous catheters and peripheral IV lines was similar in both groups. The main study results are summarized in Table 63.1.

Table 63.1 Main study outcomes

Outcome	No sedation group	Sedation group	Significance
90-d all-cause mortality	42.4%	37%	Not significant
Median coma or delirium-free days at 28 days	27	26	Not significant
Median ICU days until death or at 28 days	13	14	Not significant
Median ventilation-free days at day 28	20	19	Not significant
Highest RIFLE score at day 28	2	2	Not significant

Abbreviation: *RIFLE* Classification of acute kidney injury by Risk, Injury, Failure, Loss of function, and End-stage kidney disease

63.10 Study Conclusions

The NONSEDA trial found that a policy of no sedation compared with light sedation did not improve the 90-day mortality among mechanically ventilated patients in the ICU. The duration of ICU and hospital stay also did not differ significantly between the two groups. Patients in the nonsedation group were coma- and delirium-free for a day more compared to the light sedation group; besides, they experienced fewer thromboembolic events.

63.11 Strengths

The multicentric randomized controlled design enhances the generalizability of the NONSEDA trial. The study groups were clearly defined and divided into the no sedation and light sedation groups, based on the RASS score. A broad ICU patient population was included, reflecting real-world practice. The primary outcome, the 90-day mortality, was a clinically meaningful endpoint. Outcome assessors were blinded to the study arm, reducing the likelihood of bias. The study evaluated extensive and meaningful data, including ventilation-free days, ICU length of stay, and incidence of adverse events, including delirium. There was no loss to follow-up, adding to the robustness of the trial.

63.12 Weaknesses

The findings of the study may not apply to ICUs of healthcare systems with a lower nurse-to-patient ratio. A no-sedation protocol requires additional staffing, diligent bedside monitoring, and focused care, which may be difficult to reproduce in other settings. Lack of blinding of clinicians may have led to bias. The incidence of delirium and accidental extubation was higher in the no-sedation group, raising concerns about the safety of this practice. The difference in the level of sedation was marginal; besides, there was a substantial number of patients in the no-sedation group who required some form of sedation, which could have impacted clinical outcomes. About 14% of patients refused to participate in the study, raising the possibility of selection bias. The study did not assess longer-term outcomes, including quality of life and cognitive outcomes.

63.13 Post-hoc Analysis

In a subsequent study, Nedergaard et al. performed a retrospective post-hoc analysis of the NONSEDA trial [5]. Patients who were randomized to the no-sedation arm in their original trial were classified into those who did not require sedation—the "non-sedation success" group and those who ended up requiring sedation at least on one occasion—the "non-sedation failure" group.

Among 348 patients who were randomized to the no sedation group, 199 were classified as "success" and 149 as "failure".

Failure of the no-sedation strategy was associated with adverse outcomes, including fewer days alive without mechanical ventilation and organ support. Besides, patients who failed the no-sedation strategy and required sedation also experienced a longer duration of mechanical ventilation, ICU, and hospital stay. However, there was no difference in mortality and long-term outcomes between the two groups.

63.14 Summary

Evidence from previously published studies had revealed improved outcomes, including a shorter duration of mechanical ventilation and a shorter duration of stay in the ICU and in hospital with a policy of daily sedation interruption or no sedation. In their previous single-center trial, the same investigators had observed significantly more ventilator-free days and a shorter stay in the ICU and hospital among mechanically ventilated patients who did not receive sedation. Considering this background, the multicentric NONSEDA trial was designed with a larger sample size that would allow a more robust evaluation of outcomes, including mortality.

The eight-center RCT allocated patients to a strategy of no sedation or light sedation, titrated to a RASS score of −2 to −3.

The 90-day mortality, the primary outcome, was similar in both groups. Among the secondary outcomes, both groups of patients experienced similar ICU- and ventilator-free days. Major thromboembolic events occurred more often in the sedation group. The authors reasoned that, in contrast to their hypothesis, clinical outcomes were not superior in the no-sedation group, probably because the level of sedation was not substantially different between groups, especially during the early phase of mechanical ventilation.

The NONSEDA trial is a significant contribution to the debate on how much sedation may be appropriate in critically ill patients who are mechanically ventilated. Considering the findings of this study, a deep level of sedation is probably not appropriate in most ICU patients. It is important to highlight that a strategy of low or no sedation calls for an adequate level of staff and diligent bedside monitoring.

References

1. Kress JP, Pohlman AS, O'Connor MF, Hall JB. Daily interruption of sedative infusions in critically ill patients undergoing mechanical ventilation. N Engl J Med. 2000;342(20):1471–7.
2. Girard TD, Kress JP, Fuchs BD, Thomason JWW, Schweickert WD, Pun BT, et al. Efficacy and safety of a paired sedation and ventilator weaning protocol for mechanically ventilated patients in intensive care (awakening and breathing controlled trial): a randomised controlled trial. Lancet. 2008;371(9607):126–34.
3. Strøm T, Martinussen T, Toft P. A protocol of no sedation for critically ill patients receiving mechanical ventilation: a randomised trial. Lancet. 2010;375(9713):475–80.
4. Olsen HT, Nedergaard HK, Strøm T, Oxlund J, Wian KA, Ytrebø LM, et al. Nonsedation or light sedation in critically ill, mechanically ventilated patients. N Engl J Med. 2020;382(12):1103–11.
5. Nedergaard HK, Korkmaz S, Olsen HT, Jensen HI, Strøm T, Toft P. Failure of non-sedation strategy in critically ill, mechanically ventilated patients—a retrospective, post-hoc analysis of the NONSEDA trial. J Crit Care. 2022;68:66–71.

Part XVI

Pulmonary Embolism

64 Thrombolysis for Moderate Pulmonary Embolism: The MOPPET Trial

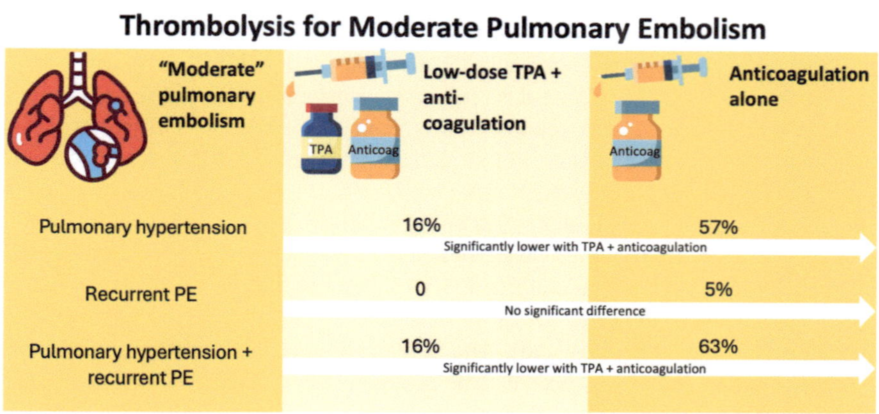

Sharifi et al. (J Cardiol, 2013)

Quick Take

Could low-dose thrombolysis impact outcomes in moderate pulmonary embolism (PE)?

The MOPETT trial by Sharifi et al. investigated whether reduced-dose thrombolysis improves outcomes in patients with PE. Moderate PE was defined as embolism with right ventricular dysfunction but without systemic hypotension. Patients receiving low-dose thrombolysis (50 mg tissue plasminogen activator) in addition to anticoagulation were compared to those treated with anticoagulation alone. The results showed a significant reduction in pulmonary hypertension and recurrent PE in the thrombolysis group, without an increase in major bleeding. These findings

---

Sharifi M, Bay C, Skrocki L, Rahimi F, Mehdipour M. Moderate Pulmonary Embolism Treated with Thrombolysis (from the "MOPETT" Trial). Am J Cardiol. 2013 Jan;111(2):273–7.

J. Chacko et al., *Landmark Studies in Critical Care*,
https://doi.org/10.1007/978-981-95-0673-6_64

suggest that reduced-dose thrombolysis offers a safer, effective strategy for improving long-term outcomes in moderate PE, challenging the traditional reliance on anticoagulation alone.

64.1 Introduction

Thrombolysis is well established as an effective therapeutic strategy in acute massive pulmonary embolism [1, 2]. Besides, it is also recommended in patients who are hemodynamically stable following submassive pulmonary embolism, characterized by right ventricular dilatation or hypokinesia, or increased level of biomarkers [3]. Thrombolytic treatment carries with it an increased risk of bleeding; particularly, intracerebral hemorrhage is a dreaded complication that occurs in 0.7–6.4% of patients and often leads to poor clinical outcomes [4, 5]. Considering the risk, clinicians are often reluctant to resort to thrombolysis among patients who remain hemodynamically stable following symptomatic acute pulmonary embolism.

Thrombi in the pulmonary circulation may be remarkably responsive to low-dose as opposed to conventional-dose intravenous thrombolysis, given that the lung is the final destination of the venous return. Nearly the entire dose of the thrombolytic agent traverses the lungs through a "first pass" effect. Considering that the brain receives 15% of the cardiac output, and the heart, 5%, the thrombolytic dose required for pulmonary embolism may be substantially lower than the dose conventionally used for acute stroke and myocardial infarction. A previous study by the same authors appeared to be congruent with this theory; they had observed a profound pulmonary response to low-dose thrombolysis during endovenous intervention for deep vein thrombosis [6]. The authors of the MOPETT trial raised the question—is it necessary to use the same dose of thrombolysis designed for organs that receive a fraction of the cardiac output, compared to the lungs that receive almost the entire cardiac output? They hypothesized that a lower than conventional thrombolytic dose may be just as effective in acute pulmonary embolism while substantially reducing the risk of hemorrhagic complications.

Against this background, the MOPETT randomized controlled trial (RCT) was designed to evaluate the efficacy of low-dose tissue plasminogen activator (tPA) in reducing the development of pulmonary artery hypertension among patients with "moderate" pulmonary embolism [7].

64.2 Population and Design

The MOPETT (Moderate Pulmonary Embolism Treated with Thrombolysis) trial was a single-center, open label, RCT that enrolled adult patients with "moderate" acute pulmonary embolism during a 22-month period beginning May 2008. Patients who presented with clinical features of acute pulmonary embolism, confirmed on imaging by CT angiography or ventilation-perfusion scan, were eligible. At least two of the following signs and symptoms had to be present for eligibility—chest pain, respiratory rate >22/min, heart rate >90/min, dyspnea, cough, drop in oxygen saturation to <95%, or raised jugular venous pressure >12 cm H_2O. Moderate pulmonary embolism was defined by the presence of two or more of the above clinical criteria with >70% involvement of thrombus by CT angiography in two lobar or the left or right main pulmonary arteries or by a high probability ventilation/perfusion scan demonstrating mismatch in 2 lobes.

64.3 Excluded

- Symptom onset of >10 days
- More than 8 h since the commencement of parenteral anticoagulation
- Eligible for full-dose thrombolysis
- Systolic BP of <95 or >200/100 mm Hg
- Severe thrombocytopenia with a platelet count of <50,000/mm^3
- Major hemorrhage within the previous 2 months that needed transfusion
- Surgery or major trauma within 2 weeks
- Mass lesion in the brain or neurosurgery
- Intracerebral hemorrhage
- Subdural hemorrhage within the previous year
- Contraindication for unfractionated or low-molecular-weight heparin
- Echocardiography not feasible due to technical reasons

Patients were randomized in a 1:1 ratio to the thrombolysis group or the control group.

64.3.1 Thrombolysis Group

In the thrombolysis group, 50% of the standard thrombolytic dose was administered. Patients with a body weight ≥50 kg received a total dose of 50 mg of tPA; 10 mg was administered over 1 min, followed by infusion of the remaining 40 mg over 2 h. Those weighing <50 mg received 0.5 mg/kg of tPA; 10 mg was administered over 1 min, followed by the remaining dose over 2 h.

Enoxaparin, or unfractionated heparin, was administered as anticoagulant. Enoxaparin was administered subcutaneously in a dose of 1 mg/kg twice a day, with the initial dose not exceeding 80 mg. If unfractionated heparin was used, the initial dose was 70 units/kg to a maximum limit of 6000 units intravenously. The maintenance dose of unfractionated heparin was 10 units/kg/hour while tPA was being infused; the dose was increased to 18 units/kg/hour after cessation of the tPA dose. The rate of infusion of unfractionated heparin was titrated, aiming for an activated partial thromboplastin time of 1.5–2 times the baseline value.

64.3.2 Control Group

Patients in the control group received anticoagulation alone—enoxaparin, 1 mg/kg subcutaneously, twice daily, or unfractionated heparin 80 units/kg/hour intravenously as a bolus followed by 18 units/kg/hour, aiming for an activated partial thromboplastin time of 1.5–2 times the baseline value.

In both groups, enoxaparin was the preferred anticoagulant. Unfractionated heparin was considered in the presence of impaired renal function or according to patient preference. Warfarin was commenced at admission in all patients. Pulmonary artery systolic pressure was estimated from the velocity of the tricuspid regurgitant jet by continuous-wave Doppler, using the modified Bernoulli equation.

$$\text{Pulmonary artery systolic pressure} = 4V^2 + \text{right atrial pressure}$$

(V = velocity of the tricuspid regurgitant jet by continuous-wave Doppler)

The right atrial pressure was estimated based on the size of the right atrium—10 mm Hg for mild, 12 for moderate, and 18 for severe right atrial enlargement.

64.4 Sample Size

Based on previous studies that evaluated long-term changes in pulmonary artery pressures in patients with acute pulmonary embolism who underwent thrombolysis, the authors assumed a 10% reduction of pulmonary artery pressures in the thrombolysis group. A sample size of 55 patients per group provided 90% power at a two-sided alpha level of 0.05 to detect this difference. Allowing for a 10% drop-out, the study planned to enroll 60 patients in each group.

64.5 Results

Among 121 patients who were randomized, 61 were assigned to the thrombolysis group and 60 to the control group. Patients were well-matched at baseline. The study population was predominantly female; the mean age was 58 ± 9 years in the thrombolysis group and 59 ± 10 in the control group. Co-morbidities, including hypertension, diabetes mellitus, cardiovascular disease, hypercholesterolemia, and pulmonary and renal disease, were similar in both groups. Concomitant deep vein thrombosis was noted in 57% of patients in the thrombolysis group and 55% in the control group. The baseline pulmonary artery pressures were similar in both groups: 50 ± 6 mm Hg in the thrombolysis group and 51 ± 7 in the control group.

Follow-up was carried out for a mean duration of 28 ± 5 months in 58 patients in the thrombolysis group and 56 patients in the control group.

64.6 Primary Endpoints

The development of pulmonary hypertension at 28 ± 5 months of follow-up, defined as a pulmonary artery pressure of >40 mm Hg by echocardiography, was significantly lower in the thrombolysis group compared to the control group [9/58 (16%) vs. 32/56 (57%), $P < 0.001$]. The composite primary endpoint of pulmonary hypertension and recurrent pulmonary embolism was significantly lower with thrombolysis [9/58 (16%) vs. 35/56 (63%), $P < 0.001$].

The pulmonary artery pressure was also significantly lower in the thrombolysis group at 48 h and 6 months of follow-up.

64.7 Secondary Endpoints

At 28 months of follow-up, recurrent pulmonary embolism had not occurred in any patient in the thrombolysis group compared to three patients who experienced recurrence in the control group. One patient died in the thrombolysis group, compared to three in the control group. The composite of mortality and recurrent pulmonary embolism occurred in one (1.6%) patient in the thrombolysis group compared with 6 patients in the control group (10%) ($P = 0.049$). No bleeding occurred in either group during the index hospitalization. The duration of stay in hospital was significantly lower in the thrombolysis group (2.2 ± 0.5 days) compared to the control group (4.9 ± 0.8 days) ($P < 0.001$). The main findings are summarized in Table 64.1.

Table 64.1 Main findings on follow-up at 28 ± 5 months

Outcome	Thrombolysis group	Control group	*P* value
Pulmonary hypertension	9/58 (16%)	32/56 (57%)	<0.001
Recurrent pulmonary embolism	0/61	3/60 (5%)	0.08
Composite of pulmonary hypertension and recurrent pulmonary embolism	9/58 (16%)	35/56 (63%)	<0.001
Mortality	1/61 (1.6%)	3/60 (5%)	0.30
Hospital days	2.2 ± 0.5	4.9 ± 0.8	<0.001

64.8 Study Conclusion

The authors concluded that low-dose thrombolysis with tPA is safe and effective in moderate pulmonary embolism, with an early reduction of pulmonary artery pressures that was maintained at 28 months of follow-up.

64.9 Strengths

The RCT design was appropriate to address the clinical question—in moderate pulmonary embolism, does a lower dose of thrombolysis combined with anticoagulation lead to improved outcomes compared with anticoagulation alone? All except seven of 121 patients were followed up for a period of 28 months. The pulmonary artery pressure was assessed using the standard, commonly employed method by measuring the velocity of the tricuspid regurgitant jet by continuous wave Doppler. The investigators who performed echocardiography were blinded to the study allocation arm, thus eliminating bias in the assessment of pulmonary artery pressures. The authors triggered interest in low-dose intravenous thrombolysis for acute pulmonary embolism and suggested that this strategy may be comparable to catheter-directed thrombolysis.

64.10 Limitations

The MOPETT trial was a single-center, open-label study with a propensity to bias. The main primary outcome, the reduction in pulmonary artery pressure over time, was not patient-centric. The study was not powered to evaluate clinical outcomes. The incidence of recurrent pulmonary embolism, one of the components of the composite primary outcome, was low and not significantly different between groups (none in the thrombolysis group vs. three in the control group). The sample size was calculated based only on the reduction in pulmonary artery pressure in the thrombolysis group; no calculation was carried out for the second, composite primary outcome of pulmonary hypertension and recurrent pulmonary embolism. The authors did not report the hazard ratio or risk ratio with confidence intervals—a lacuna in the statistical analysis.

Submassive pulmonary embolism has been conventionally defined on the basis of right ventricular dilatation and hypokinesia [8]. However, the MOPETT trial employed anatomical criteria based on the extent of clot involvement by CT angiography or ventilation/perfusion scan to define "moderate" pulmonary embolism. The incidence of right ventricular dilatation (21%) and dysfunction (6%) was low, suggesting a cohort of patients who were less severely ill at baseline.

64.11 Subsequent Studies

Several investigators have subsequently evaluated the option of low-dose thrombolysis in acute pulmonary embolism, especially in patients with a high risk of hemorrhagic complications. Based on the promising results of the MOPETT trial, a low-dose strategy was more commonly employed by clinicians as a therapeutic approach in intermediate-risk pulmonary embolism. Although the literature is replete with case reports, observational studies, and RCTs of small sample size [9, 10], there is a paucity of firm evidence to support low-dose thrombolysis.

A retrospective cohort study compared outcomes among 3768 patients who received 50 mg (half-dose) with those who received 100 mg (full dose) of alteplase in acute pulmonary embolism. On propensity matching with 548 patients in each group, half-dose alteplase was associated with a higher rate of escalation of treatment—mainly driven by additional thrombolysis and catheter-directed therapy. The mortality rate was similar in both groups; the incidence of major bleeding was also similar [11].

An open-label, non-randomized, single-center trial compared low molecular weight heparin and low-dose rt-PA 50 mg with low molecular weight heparin alone. The study subjects, 38 in each group, had echocardiographic or CT evidence of pulmonary hypertension or right ventricular dilatation. Hemodynamic decompensation and mortality were lower in the rt-PA compared to the low molecular weight heparin group at 7 and 30 days. The incidence of recurrent pulmonary embolism and pulmonary hypertension at 6 months was similar in both groups. No intracranial hemorrhage occurred in either group. Minor and major bleeding complications were also similar in both groups [12].

64.12 Summary

Thrombolysis is established therapy for acute massive pulmonary embolism. Besides, it may be the preferred strategy in submassive pulmonary embolism, characterized by right ventricular dilatation or hypokinesia, or increased levels of biomarkers. Would a lower than conventional dose of thrombolysis be effective and potentially safer in pulmonary embolism? The concept of a low, "safe" dose arose from a physiological standpoint—unlike the brain or the heart, the entire dose of intravenously administered thrombolytic agent passes through the lungs. The MOPETT trial investigators embarked upon an RCT that compared low-dose tPA with anticoagulation alone among patients with "moderate" pulmonary embolism. They observed that low-dose thrombolysis is safe and effective; at 28 months of follow-up, the incidence of pulmonary hypertension was lower with thrombolysis. Recurrent pulmonary embolism occurred in only three patients, all in the control group. No bleeding complications were observed in the entire study cohort. The MOPETT trial stimulated interest in an important clinical question—is a lower dose of thrombolysis safer and equally effective in acute pulmonary embolism, and hence, enable use among patients who are less severely ill? The authors hypothesized that low-dose intravenous thrombolysis may be safe, effective, and comparable to more invasive techniques, including catheter-directed interventions.

References

1. Kearon C, Akl EA, Comerota AJ, Prandoni P, Bounameaux H, Goldhaber SZ, et al. Antithrombotic therapy for VTE disease: antithrombotic therapy and prevention of thrombosis, 9th ed: American College of Chest Physicians Evidence-Based Clinical Practice Guidelines. Chest. 2012;141(2 Suppl):e419S–96S.
2. Wan S, Quinlan DJ, Agnelli G, Eikelboom JW. Thrombolysis compared with heparin for the initial treatment of pulmonary embolism: a meta-analysis of the randomized controlled trials. Circulation. 2004;110(6):744–9.
3. Meyer G, Vicaut E, Danays T, Agnelli G, Becattini C, Beyer-Westendorf J, et al. Fibrinolysis for patients with intermediate-risk pulmonary embolism. N Engl J Med. 2014;370(15):1402–11.
4. Berkowitz SD, Granger CB, Pieper KS, Lee KL, Gore JM, Simoons M, et al. Incidence and predictors of bleeding after contemporary thrombolytic therapy for myocardial infarction. The Global Utilization of Streptokinase and Tissue Plasminogen activator for Occluded coronary arteries (GUSTO) I Investigators. Circulation. 1997;95(11):2508–16.
5. National Institute of Neurological Disorders and Stroke rt-PA Stroke Study Group. Tissue plasminogen activator for acute ischemic stroke. N Engl J Med. 1995;333(24):1581–7.
6. Sharifi M, Bay C, Mehdipour M, Sharifi J, TORPEDO Investigators. Thrombus Obliteration by Rapid Percutaneous Endovenous Intervention in Deep Venous Occlusion (TORPEDO) trial: midterm results. J Endovasc Ther Off J Int Soc Endovasc Spec. 2012;19(2):273–80.
7. Sharifi M, Bay C, Skrocki L, Rahimi F, Mehdipour M. Moderate pulmonary embolism treated with thrombolysis (from the "MOPETT" trial). Am J Cardiol. 2013;111(2):273–7.
8. Konstantinides S, Geibel A, Heusel G, Heinrich F, Kasper W. Heparin plus Alteplase compared with heparin alone in patients with submassive pulmonary embolism. N Engl J Med. 2002;347(15):1143–50.
9. Wang C, Zhai Z, Yang Y, Wu Q, Cheng Z, Liang L, et al. Efficacy and safety of low dose recombinant tissue-type plasminogen activator for the treatment of acute pulmonary thromboembolism: a randomized, multicenter, controlled trial. Chest. 2010;137(2):254–62.
10. Mi YH, Liang Y, Lu YH, Li YM, Liu WX, Qian W. Recombinant tissue plasminogen activator plus heparin compared with heparin alone for patients with acute submassive pulmonary embolism: one-year outcome. J Geriatr Cardiol JGC. 2013;10(4):323–9.
11. Kiser TH, Burnham EL, Clark B, Ho PM, Allen RR, Moss M, et al. Half-dose versus full-dose Alteplase for treatment of pulmonary embolism. Crit Care Med. 2018;46(10):1617–25.
12. Yilmaz ES, Uzun O. Low-dose thrombolysis for submassive pulmonary embolism. J Investig Med Off Publ Am Fed Clin Res. 2021;69(8):1439–46.

65 Fibrinolysis in Intermediate-Risk Pulmonary Embolism: The PEITHO Trial

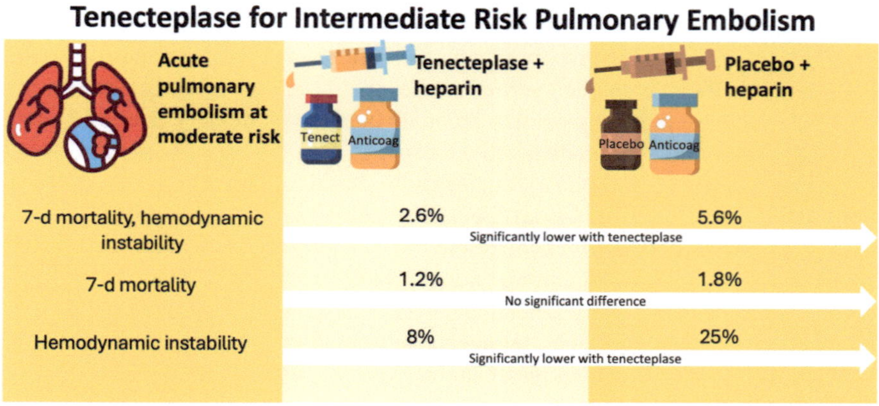

Meyer et al. (J Cardiol, 2014)

Quick Take

Can fibrinolysis improve outcomes in patients with intermediate-risk pulmonary embolism (PE)?

The PEITHO trial investigated whether fibrinolysis could reduce mortality and complications in patients with intermediate-risk PE. This multicenter randomized controlled trial enrolled patients with intermediate-risk PE, characterized by right ventricular dysfunction and elevated biomarkers but without systemic hypotension. The study found that fibrinolysis significantly reduced the incidence of hemodynamic collapse and in-hospital mortality, but it also led to a higher rate of major

---

Meyer G, Vicaut E, Danays T, Agnelli G, Becattini C, Beyer-Westendorf J, et al. Fibrinolysis for Patients with Intermediate-Risk Pulmonary Embolism. N Engl J Med. 2014 Apr 10;370(15):1402–11.

J. Chacko et al., *Landmark Studies in Critical Care*,
https://doi.org/10.1007/978-981-95-0673-6_65

bleeding. Despite the risks, the trial suggested that fibrinolysis may be beneficial in select intermediate-risk PE patients, prompting further debate about the optimal management of this patient group.

65.1 Introduction and Background

The history of thrombolytic therapy dates back to 1933 when William Smith Tillet, an Associate Professor of Medicine at the Johns Hopkins University, serendipitously observed that Lancefield Group A beta-hemolytic streptococci produced a fibrinolytic substance. Tillet called this substance "streptococcal fibrinolysin" [1]. Years of research, along with his student Sol Sherry, fuelled an increasing interest in its potential application in acute myocardial infarction. It was finally left to Fletcher et al. to embark upon a pivotal clinical trial with streptokinase [2]. They infused massive doses of streptokinase over prolonged periods in patients with acute myocardial infarction. Although a bleeding diathesis occurred in a few patients, mortality was lower in those who received streptokinase compared to other therapies. The 1960s witnessed animal studies that tested the efficacy of streptokinase and urokinase in lysing massive blood clots in the pulmonary arteries. One of the early pioneering studies involved 21 patients with massive pulmonary embolism, demonstrated by pulmonary angiography. In this 1968 study from Australia, 18 patients were treated with intravenous streptokinase, with clear improvement on pulmonary angiography and a perceptible increase in peripheral pulmonary perfusion 24 h later. In contrast, pulmonary angiography on three patients who received heparin alone demonstrated little change, with persistent, high-grade obstruction of the main pulmonary arteries [3]. Intravenous thrombolytic therapy was found to be clinically feasible, easy to administer, and relatively safe in acute pulmonary embolism, leading to the first multinational randomized controlled trial (RCT). The Urokinase in Pulmonary Embolism (UPETP) trial of 1970 compared urokinase combined with heparin to heparin alone in acute pulmonary embolism [4]. The study revealed significantly greater clot resolution at 24 h evidenced by pulmonary angiography, lung scans, and right heart pressure measurements. The only complication observed was a relatively higher incidence of bleeding with urokinase. Thrombolytic therapy for acute pulmonary embolism gained widespread acceptance in the 1980s, with focused research in specific clinical settings.

While acute pulmonary embolism with hypotension is a clear indication for fibrinolytic therapy, standard anticoagulation alone was considered adequate in hemodynamically stable patients [5]. However, the presence of acute right ventricular pressure overload may also be an important determinant of the severity and impact on outcomes from acute pulmonary embolism [6]. Such patients may have acute right ventricular dysfunction and myocardial injury without overt hemodynamic instability. This group of patients may represent an "intermediate-risk" group and may benefit from early fibrinolytic therapy.

Although fibrinolytic therapy had been in use for acute pulmonary embolism for more than four decades, there were few RCTs that compared fibrinolysis with anticoagulation. Particularly, the potential efficacy of fibrinolytic therapy in improving clinical outcomes among patients who remained hemodynamically stable was not adequately investigated.

The Pulmonary Embolism Thrombolysis (PEITHO) was an RCT that evaluated patients who carried an intermediate risk of adverse outcomes following acute pulmonary embolism [7]. The study aimed to assess the safety and efficacy of fibrinolytic therapy with a single dose of tenecteplase combined with standard anticoagulation therapy compared with anticoagulation alone in this setting.

65.2 Population and Design

The PEITHO trial was conducted between November 2007—and July 2012 in 76 centers across 13 countries. Adult patients (>18 years old) who were diagnosed to have acute pulmonary embolism by V/Q scan, CT, or pulmonary angiogram within 15 days of symptom onset were eligible. Right ventricular dysfunction was confirmed by echocardiography or spiral CT scan of the chest; myocardial injury was confirmed by a positive test for troponin I or T.

65.2.1 Excluded

Patients with a contraindication to fibrinolytic therapy were excluded. Those with hemodynamic decompensation evidenced by the requirement for cardiopulmonary resuscitation, a systolic BP of <90 mm Hg for >15 min, a drop in systolic BP by >40 mm Hg for >15 min with features of end-organ hypoperfusion, and the requirement for catecholamine support were excluded. Block randomization, stratified by center, was carried out to ensure a balanced distribution of treatment groups. Randomization was aimed to be performed within 2 h of identification of right ventricular dysfunction and myocardial injury.

65.3 Fibrinolysis Group (Tenecteplase)

Patients randomized to receive fibrinolysis were administered an intravenous bolus of 30–50 mg of tenecteplase, based on body weight.

65.4 Control Group (Placebo)

In the control group, a single bolus dose of placebo of the same volume and appearance was administered.

65.5 Common Management

Unfractionated heparin was administered as an intravenous bolus immediately after randomization in both groups, except among those who had already received a bolus dose or infusion of heparin. The bolus dose of unfractionated heparin was withheld among patients who had received a therapeutic dose of low-molecular-weight heparin or fondaparinux; the infusion of unfractionated heparin was commenced after 12 h of the last dose of low-molecular-weight heparin and 24 h after the last dose of fondaparinux. Heparin infusion was titrated to an activated partial thromboplastin time of 2.0–2.5 times the upper limit of normal. Anticoagulant drugs other than unfractionated heparin were not allowed until 48 h post-randomization.

65.6 Sample Size

The authors calculated the sample size based on a meta-analysis of trials on thrombolysis [8] and the MAPPETT 3 trial [9], the largest RCT on pulmonary embolism until the study date. The primary endpoint of death or hemodynamic collapse within 7 days was presumed to be approximately 7%. The study was planned to include 1000 patients, providing 80% power to detect a difference between the two groups.

65.7 Results

The study enrolled 1006 patients—506 were assigned to receive tenecteplase combined with unfractionated heparin, and 500 to receive placebo combined with unfractionated heparin. Excluding the lone patient with missing informed consent, 1005 patients were included in the intention-to-treat analysis. The overall median age was 70 years; patients were normotensive at randomization. The diagnosis of pulmonary embolism was confirmed by CT in nearly 95% of patients. Right ventricular dysfunction was confirmed by either echocardiography or CT in all patients; myocardial injury was diagnosed based on Troponin T or I testing in all except nine patients.

65.8 Efficacy Outcomes

65.8.1 The Primary Outcome

The primary composite endpoint of death or hemodynamic collapse within 7 days of randomization was significantly lower in patients assigned to receive tenecteplase (2.6% vs. 5.6%; odds ratio, 0.44, 95% CI, 0.23–0.87; $P = 0.02$). Among the individual components of the primary outcome, mortality at 7 days was not significantly different between the tenecteplase and the placebo groups (1.2% vs. 1.8%, $P = 0.42$). Hemodynamic collapse occurred more often in the placebo group (5% vs. 1.6%, $P = 0.002$). More patients in the placebo group received catecholamine support; cardiopulmonary resuscitation was required for five patients in the placebo group compared with one patient in the tenecteplase group.

On prespecified subgroup analysis, the primary outcome was more favorable in patients 75 years of age or younger, compared to older patients. Tenecteplase was equally efficacious in men and women.

65.8.2 Other Outcomes

Twenty-three patients (4.6%) received open-label, rescue fibrinolysis; however, crossover occurred after the onset of hemodynamic instability in all except nine patients. The 30-day mortality was similar in both groups (tenecteplase: 2.4% vs. placebo: 3.2%, $P = 0.42$). In the tenecteplase group, eight patients (1.6%) underwent mechanical ventilation compared to 15 patients (3.0%) in the placebo group.

65.8.3 Safety

Major bleeding within 7 days was more common among patients who received tenecteplase (11.5% vs. 2.4%). Major extracranial bleeding was more common among those >75 years old compared to younger subjects. The incidence of stroke was also more common in the tenecteplase group. Ten patients suffered hemorrhagic stroke and two, ischemic stroke in the tenecteplase group compared with a lone patient who suffered a hemorrhagic stroke in the placebo group. The main study outcomes are summarized in Table 65.1.

Table 65.1 Main study outcomes

Outcome	Tenecteplase (506 patients)	Placebo (499 patients)	OR (95% CI)	*P* value
7-day mortality, hemodynamic instability	13 (2.6%)	28 (5.6%)	0.44 (0.23–0.87)	0.02
7-day mortality	6 (1.2%)	9 (1.8%)	0.65 (0.23–1.85)	0.42
Hemodynamic instability	8 (1.6%)	25 (5.0%)	0.30 (0.14–0.68)	0.002
Major extracranial bleeding	32 (6.3%)	6 (1.2%)	5.55 (2.3–13.39)	<0.001
Stroke by day 7	12 (2.4%)	1 (0.2%)	12.10 (1.57–93.39)	0.003

Abbreviations: *OR* odds ratio, *CI* confidence interval

65.9 Study Conclusion

The findings of the study suggested that fibrinolytic therapy may reduce the likelihood of hemodynamic decompensation or death in intermediate-risk patients with acute pulmonary embolism. Patients who are hemodynamically stable with right ventricular dysfunction on echocardiography or CT and myocardial injury evidenced by positive troponin levels may represent patients with intermediate risk.

65.10 Strengths

The PEITHO trial evaluated a key clinical question—is timely fibrinolytic therapy efficacious among intermediate-risk patients with acute pulmonary embolism and stable blood pressure? In a double-blinded, randomized controlled design with an adequate sample size, the authors convincingly demonstrated that fibrinolytic therapy reduces hemodynamic instability, although the mortality was similar in both groups. Being multi-centered, the study provided external validity.

65.11 Limitations

The primary outcome was a composite of death or hemodynamic instability at 7 days; the beneficial effect was driven almost entirely by the latter outcome. Evaluation of longer-term mortality may have been a more appropriate clinical endpoint. Rescue fibrinolysis was administered in 23 (4.6%) patients in the control group, mostly after the onset of hemodynamic instability. The question arises whether it may be more appropriate to consider fibrinolysis expeditiously once hemodynamic instability is evident. The overall mortality was low, and the study was not powered to detect a mortality difference, a more relevant clinical outcome.

65.12 Long-Term Follow-Up Study

The long-term survival was evaluated in 28 study sites comprising a total of 709 patients who participated in the long-term follow-up (median of 37.8 months; interquartile range: 24.6 to 54.8 months) [10]. Mortality was assessed in 353 of 359 (98.3%) of patients who received tenecteplase and 343 of 350 (98.0%) of patients in the placebo group. The overall mortality was 19.2%, with no difference between groups (tenecteplase vs. placebo, 2.2% vs. 2.9%). Mortality between 30 days and longer-term occurred due to cancer, acute or chronic respiratory failure, acute infections, or chronic systemic inflammatory disease.

65.13 Summary

Fibrinolytic therapy had previously been shown to be effective among high-risk patients with acute pulmonary embolism who were hemodynamically unstable. The PEITHO trial suggested that fibrinolytic therapy may be associated with improved hemodynamic stability among intermediate-risk patients with acute pulmonary embolism. As expected, fibrinolytic therapy was associated with a higher risk of major bleeding, including intracranial hemorrhage. The risk of hemorrhagic complications may be especially higher among the elderly population. Hence, the cornerstone of management lies in the assessment of the balance between risk and benefit and individualization of care. The trial underlined the impending need for robust risk stratification among patients who are at intermediate risk of death.

References

1. Tillett WS, Garner RL. The fibrinolytic activity of hemolytic streptococci. J Exp Med. 1933;58(4):485–502.
2. Fletcher AP, Alkjaersig N, Smyrniotis FE, Sherry S. The treatment of patients suffering from early myocardial infarction with massive and prolonged streptokinase therapy. Trans Assoc Am Phys. 1958;71:287–96.
3. Hirsh J, Hale GS, McDonald IG, McCarthy RA, Pitt A. Streptokinase therapy in acute major pulmonary embolism: effectiveness and problems. Br Med J. 1968;4(5633):729–34.
4. Urokinase pulmonary embolism trial. Phase 1 results: a cooperative study. JAMA. 1970;214(12):2163–72.
5. Kearon C, Akl EA, Comerota AJ, Prandoni P, Bounameaux H, Goldhaber SZ, et al. Antithrombotic therapy for VTE disease: antithrombotic therapy and prevention of thrombosis, 9th ed: American College of Chest Physicians Evidence-Based Clinical Practice Guidelines. Chest. 2012;141(2 Suppl):e419S–96S.
6. Konstantinides S. Clinical practice. Acute pulmonary embolism. N Engl J Med. 2008;359(26):2804–13.
7. Meyer G, Vicaut E, Danays T, Agnelli G, Becattini C, Beyer-Westendorf J, et al. Fibrinolysis for patients with intermediate-risk pulmonary embolism. N Engl J Med. 2014;370(15):1402–11.
8. Wan S, Quinlan DJ, Agnelli G, Eikelboom JW. Thrombolysis compared with heparin for the initial treatment of pulmonary embolism: a meta-analysis of the randomized controlled trials. Circulation. 2004;110(6):744–9.
9. Konstantinides S, Geibel A, Heusel G, Heinrich F, Kasper W. Heparin plus Alteplase compared with heparin alone in patients with submassive pulmonary embolism. N Engl J Med. 2002;347(15):1143–50.
10. Konstantinides SV, Vicaut E, Danays T, Becattini C, Bertoletti L, Beyer-Westendorf J, et al. Impact of thrombolytic therapy on the long-term outcome of intermediate-risk pulmonary embolism. J Am Coll Cardiol. 2017;69(12):1536–44.

66 Retrievable Inferior Vena Cava Filter Plus Anticoagulation Vs. Anticoagulation Alone and Recurrent Pulmonary Embolism: The PREPIC2 Trial

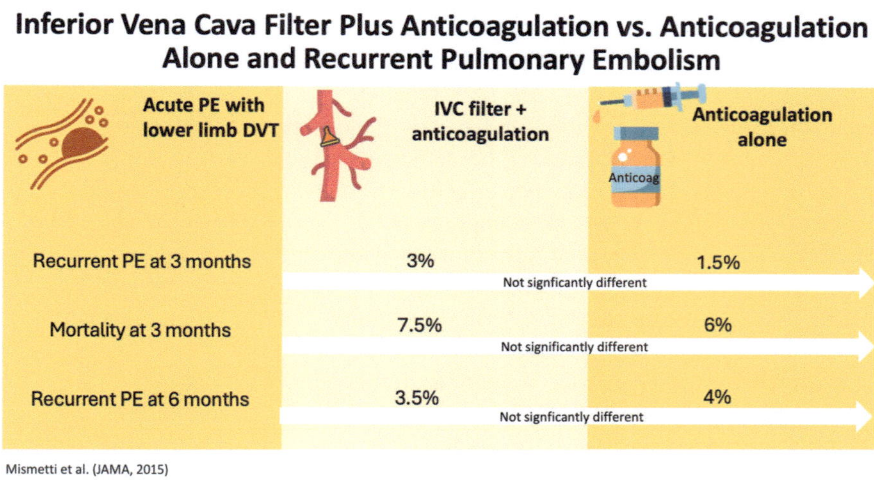

Quick Take

Does placement of a retrievable inferior vena cava (IVC) filter reduce the risk of recurrent pulmonary embolism?

The PREPIC2 trial investigated whether combining a retrievable IVC filter with anticoagulation therapy reduces the risk of recurrent pulmonary embolism (PE) in high-risk patients. This multicenter, randomized clinical trial enrolled patients following a first episode of PE and contraindications to long-term anticoagulation. The study found no significant difference in the incidence of recurrent PE between the

---

Mismetti P, Laporte S, Pellerin O, Ennezat PV, Couturaud F, Elias A, et al. Effect of a Retrievable Inferior Vena Cava Filter Plus Anticoagulation vs Anticoagulation Alone on Risk of Recurrent Pulmonary Embolism: A Randomized Clinical Trial. JAMA. 2015 Apr 28;313(16):1627.

J. Chacko et al., *Landmark Studies in Critical Care*,
https://doi.org/10.1007/978-981-95-0673-6_66

two groups, despite the ability of the filter to trap emboli. However, patients with the IVC filter experienced more complications related to the device. The findings suggest that IVC filters, when combined with anticoagulation, do not significantly improve outcomes in preventing recurrent PE and highlight the need for careful consideration of the risks and benefits of filter placement.

66.1 Introduction

More than half a century ago, Kazi Mobin-Uddin et al. reported the use of an intracaval prosthetic device for the prevention of pulmonary embolism in 15 patients [1]. A graduate of King Edward Medical College, Lahore, Mobin-Uddin underwent training in thoracic and vascular surgery at the Jackson Memorial Hospital, Miami. During his tenure as assistant professor, he conceptualized the passage of a filter into the inferior vena cava through the internal jugular vein that would impede the passage of clots. The umbrella device consisted of stainless-steel spokes arising from a central hub, enmeshed with a thin sheet of silicon rubber. In a later study, the umbrella filter was placed in a series of 100 patients [2]. The device appeared effective, with recurrent embolism occurring in only two patients. There were no deaths directly related to the procedure. The authors concluded that the umbrella filter placement appeared to be a safe and effective technique to prevent recurrent pulmonary embolism. Refinements in technology led to the introduction of the Kimray-Greenfield filter, which carried a lower incidence of inferior vena caval occlusion compared to the groundbreaking Mobin–Uddin umbrella filter. In 1984, Tadavarthy et al. described the percutaneous insertion technique of the Kimray–Greenfield filter through the internal jugular or femoral approach [3].

The inferior vena cava filter is often used in conjunction with full-dose anticoagulant therapy in patients with acute pulmonary embolism with a large clot burden, compromised cardio-pulmonary function, or when the risk of recurrence is deemed to be high. Clinicians generally resorted to filter placement based on their judgment, considering the lack of prospective controlled studies that evaluated clinical outcomes. Despite the absence of robust evidence regarding clinical benefit, a sharp increase in filter placement was observed over the years; besides, guideline recommendations also remained variable [4, 5]. Inferior vena cava filters are associated with complications, including device migration, fracture, and embolization, vena caval occlusion, and perforation.

The PREPIC 1 randomized controlled trial (RCT) had previously evaluated the placement of permanent inferior vena cava filters compared with anticoagulation alone in patients with proximal deep vein thrombosis who were considered to be at high risk for pulmonary embolism. At 12 days, pulmonary embolism, symptomatic or otherwise, was less common among patients who received filters compared to those who did not. However, at the 2-year follow-up, there was a significantly higher incidence of recurrent deep vein thrombosis in the filter group [6]. A further follow-up study was carried out at 8 years to evaluate long-term outcomes. Symptomatic pulmonary embolism remained significantly lower in the filter group compared with the no-filter group. However, the incidence of deep vein thrombosis continued to remain higher in the filter group. There was no difference in all-cause mortality between the two groups [7].

The advent of retrievable filters held the potential to reduce the incidence of long-term, device-related complications. Temporary filter placement to cover the period of risk with subsequent removal, in combination with anticoagulation, could potentially prevent early, recurrent pulmonary embolism, while minimizing filter-related complications.

The PREPIC 2 trial evaluated the potential benefit of placement of a retrievable inferior vena cava filter combined with anticoagulation compared with anticoagulation alone in patients with acute pulmonary embolism with a high risk of recurrence [8]. Filter retrieval was mandatory after 3 months; anticoagulation was continued for a minimum duration of 6 months.

66.2 Population and Design

The PREPIC 2 (Prevention du Risque d'Embolie Pulmonaire par Interruption Cave) multicenter trial was conducted between August 2006 and July 2012 across 17 centers in France. Adult patients, 18 years or older, with symptomatic acute pulmonary embolism and venous thrombosis of the lower limb were eligible. Pulmonary embolism was confirmed by standard testing, including spiral CT, ventilation-perfusion scan, or pulmonary angiography; lower limb venous thrombosis was diagnosed by compression ultrasonography and or venography. One of the following additional severity criteria had to be met for study inclusion.

- Age >75 years
- Chronic cardiac or respiratory insufficiency
- Ischemic stroke with paralysis of the lower limb in the preceding 6 months
- Deep vein thrombosis involving the ilio-caval segment or bilateral, or at least one sign of right ventricular dysfunction or myocardial injury, as evident on echocardiography, or by an increase in the level of biomarkers

Excluded

- Insertion of vena cava filter was otherwise indicated
- Thrombosis of the vena cava that precluded insertion
- Full anticoagulation was administered for >72 h before randomization.
- Non-cancer surgery in the preceding 3 months or cancer surgery within 10 days
- Allergy to contrast media
- Raised serum creatinine level of >2.04 mg/dl
- Life expectancy <6 months
- Pregnancy

Patients were randomized to the filter group or the control group. Randomization was carried out in permuted blocks of 4 or 6, stratified by center and creatinine clearance.

66.3 Intervention (the Filter Group)

A retrievable vena cava filter was inserted within 72 h of randomization; among those who underwent thrombolysis, insertion was performed after 36 h of therapy. Adequately experienced vascular or interventional radiologists carried out the procedure according to standardized guidelines. Filter retrieval was planned 3 months after insertion.

66.4 Anticoagulation Alone (the Control Group)

In both groups, anticoagulation therapy was continued for a minimum duration of 6 months; continued treatment was individualized and left to the clinician's discretion. Although the choice of anticoagulant medication was based on clinician choice, unfractionated heparin was recommended in the presence of renal dysfunction. Long-term anticoagulant therapy was continued with vitamin K antagonists. In patients with cancer, low-molecular-weight heparin was preferred over vitamin K antagonists.

66.5 Sample Size

The primary outcome was recurrent pulmonary embolism at 3 months; recurrence could be fatal, or symptomatic, but non-fatal. The authors hypothesized a 75% reduction in the primary outcome in the filter group. A sample size of 400 patients provided the study with 80% power to detect a significant difference between groups.

66.6 Results

During the 6-year study period, the PREPIC 2 trial randomized a total of 399 patients—200 to the filter group and 199 to the control group. In the filter group, device insertion was successful in 193 of 195 patients (99%) on whom it was attempted. Filter removal was attempted in 164 patients and was successful in 153 patients. In the control group, six patients underwent filter insertion; these patients could not be anticoagulated—an invasive procedure or surgery was required in four patients, while bleeding complications occurred in the other two. Patients were well-matched at baseline. In the filter group, 55% of patients were aged >75 years, compared to 49.7% in the control group. Active cancer was present in 16.6% and 14.6% of patients, respectively. Bilateral deep vein thrombosis was identified in nearly 13% of patients in both groups. There was evidence of right ventricular dysfunction or myocardial injury in 66.7% patients in the filter group and 65.2% of patients in the control group. In most cases (74% in the filter group and 79.4% in the control group), pulmonary embolism was unprovoked.

66.7 Outcomes

66.7.1 Recurrent Pulmonary Embolism—The Primary Outcome

Recurrent pulmonary embolism at 3 months of follow-up occurred in six (3%) of patients in the filter group and three (1.5%) of patients in the control group. The absolute difference was +1.5% in the filter group. The relative risk (RR) with filter insertion was not significantly different compared with the control group (RR, 2.00 [95% CI, 0.51 to 7.89]; $P = 0.50$). Among the nine patients who developed recurrent pulmonary embolism, there was a lone survivor in the control group. Between 3 and 6 months, one patient developed pulmonary embolism in each group.

66.7.2 Other 3-Month Outcomes

The mortality at 3 months was not significantly different between the two groups (7.5% vs. 6.0%). Recurrent deep vein thrombosis, venous thromboembolism, and major bleeding also occurred with similar frequency in both groups.

66.7.3 Six-Month Outcomes

Clinical outcomes at 6 months were similar in both groups. By then, recurrent pulmonary embolism had occurred in 7 patients (3.5%) in the filter group and 4 (2.0%) in the control group. Among these 11 patients, there was just the lone survivor in the control group among those who developed recurrent pulmonary embolism. Recurrent deep vein thrombosis was uncommon (one patient in the filter group and 2 in the control group). Major bleeding occurred in 13 patients (6.5%) in the filter group and 15 (7.5%) in the control group. By 6 months, 21 patients (10.6%) had died in the filter group compared with 15 (7.5%) in the control group.

66.8 Adverse Events Related to Filter Insertion

Among 193 patients who underwent filter insertion, hematoma at the site of insertion occurred in 5 patients (2.6%), and filter thrombosis, in 3 (1.6%) patients. Cardiac arrest occurred in one patient during insertion. Retrieval was unsuccessful in 11 patients (5.7%) due to mechanical problems. The main study outcomes are summarized in Table 66.1.

Table 66.1 Main study outcomes

Outcomes	Retrievable IVC filter	Anticoagulation alone	Significance
Recurrent pulmonary embolism at 3 months	3.0%	1.5%	$P = 0.50$
Recurrent pulmonary embolism at 6 months	3.5%	2.0%	$P = 0.54$
Recurrent DVT at 3 months	0.5%	0.5%	$P > 0.99$
Major bleeding at 3 months	4%	5%	$P = 0.63$
Major bleeding at 6 months	6.5%	7.5%	$P = 0.69$
Mortality at 3 months	7.5%	6.0%	$P = 0.55$
Mortality at 6 months	10.6%	7.5%	$P = 0.29$

Abbreviations: *IVC* inferior vena cava, *DVT* deep vein thrombosis

66.9 Study Conclusions

Among hospitalized patients with severe acute PE, the placement of a retrievable IVC filter combined with anticoagulation does not reduce the risk of recurrent PE or mortality at 3 months.

66.10 Strengths

Although the use of inferior vena cava filters had increased over the years, there was no firm evidence regarding its efficacy in the prevention of recurrent pulmonary embolism. Besides, the use of permanent filters carries their own share of complications. The introduction of retrievable filters in the early 2000s was a step forward in reducing filter-related complications. The PREPIC 2 trial addressed an important clinical question—does the use of retrievable filters combined with anticoagulation reduce the incidence of recurrent pulmonary embolism among patients at high risk? The trial was multicentric, including 17 centers in France. Analysis was by intention-to-treat, and follow-up was nearly complete at 6 months. The study came up with robust findings regarding the lack of efficacy of the inferior vena cava filter in reducing the incidence of recurrent pulmonary embolism among patients who were appropriately anticoagulated.

66.11 Limitations

The trial was unblinded; however, a concealed randomization system and a central adjudication committee who were blinded to treatment assignment mitigated the risk of bias. The incidence of recurrent pulmonary embolism was only 1.5% in the control arm—well below the expected incidence of 8%, which may have led to an inadequate sample size. The filter retrieval rate was high (153/193 patients), which may be generally hard to achieve in the real world.

The PREPIC 2 trial studied a cohort of patients in whom full anticoagulant therapy was feasible. Filter placement may, however, be an alternative treatment option among patients in whom anticoagulation is contraindicated or ineffective. Furthermore, in patients with a large, mobile, lower limb thrombus, filter placement could potentially prevent massive pulmonary embolism.

66.12 Summary

The PREPIC 2 demonstrated that the use of a retrievable inferior vena cava filter in combination with anticoagulation, compared with anticoagulation alone, does not reduce the incidence of symptomatic recurrent pulmonary embolism associated with deep vein thrombosis among patients at high risk of recurrence. The findings of the study fail to substantiate the placement of retrievable filters in patients who can be safely treated with anticoagulation. Based on the findings of this trial, inferior vena cava filter placement should probably be confined to patients with contraindications to anticoagulation or those who have recurrent pulmonary embolism despite adequate anticoagulation. The PREPIC 2 trial enabled increased clarity regarding the appropriate use of inferior cava filters in patients who are at high risk of recurrent pulmonary embolism.

References

1. Mobin-Uddin K, McLean R, Bolooki H, Jude JR. Caval interruption for prevention of pulmonary embolism: long-term results of a new method. Arch Surg. 1969;99(6):711–5.
2. Mobin-Uddin K, Callard GM, Bolooki H, Rubinson R, Michie D, Jude JR. Transvenous Caval interruption with umbrella filter. N Engl J Med. 1972;286(2):55–8.
3. Tadavarthy SM, Castaneda-Zuniga W, Salomonowitz E, Lund G, Cragg A, Hunter D, et al. Kimray-greenfield vena cava filter: percutaneous introduction. Radiology. 1984;151(2):525–6.
4. Torbicki A, Perrier A, Konstantinides S, Agnelli G, Galiè N, Pruszczyk P, et al. Guidelines on the diagnosis and management of acute pulmonary embolism: the task force for the diagnosis and management of acute pulmonary embolism of the European Society of Cardiology (ESC). Eur Heart J. 2008;29(18):2276–315.
5. Caplin DM, Nikolic B, Kalva SP, Ganguli S, Saad WEA, Zuckerman DA, et al. Quality improvement guidelines for the performance of inferior vena cava filter placement for the prevention of pulmonary embolism. J Vasc Interv Radiol JVIR. 2011;22(11):1499–506.
6. Decousus H, Leizorovicz A, Parent F, Page Y, Tardy B, Girard P, et al. A clinical trial of vena caval filters in the prevention of pulmonary embolism in patients with proximal deep-vein thrombosis. Prévention du Risque d'Embolie Pulmonaire par Interruption Cave Study Group. N Engl J Med. 1998;338(7):409–15.
7. PREPIC Study Group. Eight-year follow-up of patients with permanent vena cava filters in the prevention of pulmonary embolism: the PREPIC (Prevention du Risque d'Embolie Pulmonaire par Interruption Cave) randomized study. Circulation. 2005;112(3):416–22.
8. Mismetti P, Laporte S, Pellerin O, Ennezat PV, Couturaud F, Elias A, et al. Effect of a retrievable inferior vena cava filter plus anticoagulation vs anticoagulation alone on risk of recurrent pulmonary embolism: a randomized clinical trial. JAMA. 2015;313(16):1627.

Part XVII

Glucose Control

Intensive vs. Conventional Glucose Control in the ICU: The NICE-SUGAR Trial

67

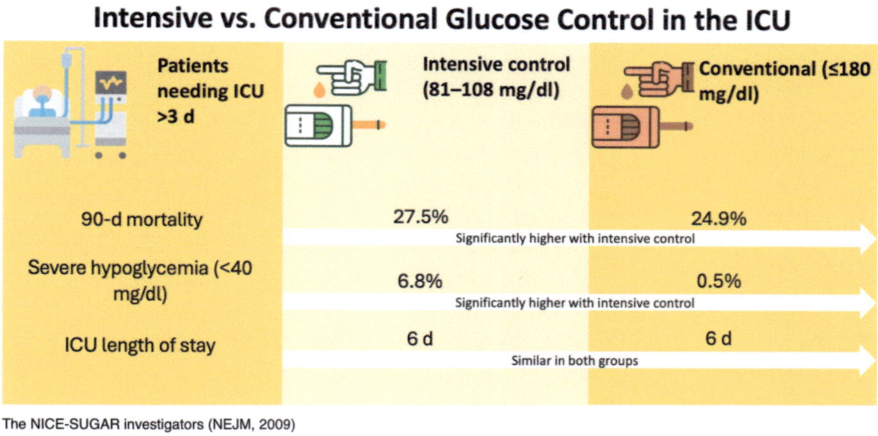

Quick Take

Does intensive glucose control save lives in critically ill patients—or put them at risk?

The NICE-SUGAR trial compared intensive glucose control (targeting blood glucose levels of 81–108 mg/dL) with conventional control (≤180 mg/dL) in critically ill patients to evaluate the impact on mortality. This large, multicenter randomized controlled trial enrolled over 6000 patients in both medical and surgical ICUs. The findings revealed higher 90-day mortality in the intensive glucose control group, driven by an increased incidence of severe hypoglycemia. Conventional glucose control was associated with better survival and fewer adverse events, reshaping

The NICE-SUGAR Study Investigators. Intensive versus conventional glucose control in critically ill patients. N Engl J Med. 2009 Mar 26;360(13):1283–97.

J. Chacko et al., *Landmark Studies in Critical Care*,
https://doi.org/10.1007/978-981-95-0673-6_67

the management of glycemic targets in critically ill patients. The NICE-SUGAR trial established that overly aggressive glucose control may do more harm than good, advocating for a more balanced approach to glycemic management in the ICU.

67.1 Introduction

Uncontrolled blood glucose levels have been associated with poor clinical outcomes among critically ill patients. Stress-related release of counterregulatory hormones, including catecholamines, corticosteroids, and glucagon, tends to increase blood glucose levels in critical illness [1]. Hyperglycemia may lead to harm through cytokine release and generation of reactive oxygen species [2]. Furthermore, it may impair the bactericidal and chemotactic effects of neutrophils. High blood glucose levels may also lead to a procoagulant state [3]. These putative mechanisms behind adverse clinical outcomes led to an increasing focus on the management of hyperglycemia in hospitalized, particularly ICU patients. It remains unclear whether adverse outcomes are directly related to hyperglycemia or if it is just a marker of such outcomes.

The Leuven trials were landmark studies that targeted control of blood glucose within a narrow range in critically ill patients. The Leuven 1 (2001) trial revealed a significantly reduced mortality among surgical patients when the blood glucose levels were maintained between 80 and 110 mg/dl [4]. The authors could not reproduce the results in their second trial (Leuven 2, 2006) on medical ICU patients. However, they observed reduced mortality in a subgroup of patients who stayed in the ICU for longer than 3 days [5]. Based on the findings of these two trials, many healthcare systems across the globe began adopting tight control of blood glucose levels as a key facet in the care of critically ill patients. However, it became abundantly clear that maintenance of blood glucose levels within a narrow, lower range may be difficult to achieve among the sickest of patients. Furthermore, aiming for tight control may also increase the likelihood of hypoglycemia and adverse outcomes.

In the meantime, the Glucontrol trial compared a target of 140–180 with 80–110 mg/dl in 21 medico-surgical ICUs. Protocol violations occurred frequently; hence, the study was stopped early. The investigators observed no clinical benefit with a lower blood glucose target. Furthermore, episodes of hypoglycemia were more common in the 80–110 mg/dl group [6]. In another RCT, Brunkhorst et al. also observed a significantly higher incidence of hypoglycemia with intensive compared to conventional insulin therapy [7].

Two meta-analyses were performed in the wake of the clinical conundrum related to glycemic control. Pittas et al. analyzed 35 RCTs to evaluate the effect of insulin therapy in critically ill patients [8]. They observed a 15% reduction in mortality with insulin therapy compared with controls. The effect was particularly prominent when insulin therapy was titrated to pre-set glucose levels. However, a later meta-analysis by Wiener et al., including 8432 patients from 29 RCTs, came up with contrasting results. Tight control of glucose levels did not reduce mortality, regardless of target glucose levels of <110 mg/dl or < 150 mg/dl. The mortality was also similar on subgroup analysis of medical, surgical, and mixed ICU patients [9].

In light of contrasting evidence, it remained unclear whether aiming for a narrow range of blood glucose levels with intensive insulin therapy would lead to improved outcomes. The two Leuven trials that appeared to support intensive control were single-center trials that called for external validation in a larger RCT. The Normoglycemia in Intensive Care Evaluation–Survival Using Glucose Algorithm Regulation (NICE-SUGAR) was a randomized controlled trial (RCT) designed to test the hypothesis that intensive glucose control reduces the 90-day mortality in critically ill patients.

67.2 Population and Design

The NICE-SUGAR trial was conducted between December 2004 to November 2008. The study involved 42 hospitals in Australia, New Zealand, and North America [10]. The study population consisted of patients who were within 24 h of ICU admission. Patients were expected to require continued care in the ICU for 3 or more consecutive days. Using a parallel group, randomized, controlled design, patients were allocated to intensive or conventional glucose control. A stratified randomization was followed based on admission type (medical or surgical) and the study region (Australia and New Zealand or North America).

67.2.1 Excluded

Patients who were admitted with diabetic ketoacidosis or hyperosmolar state were excluded. Also excluded were patients expected to have oral nutrition by day 3, those with a high risk of hypoglycemia, or had fulminant hepatic failure.

67.3 Intensive Glucose Control

In the intensive control group, intravenous insulin infusion was titrated to a target blood glucose level of 81–108 mg/dl (multiply by 0.0555 for conversion to mmol/l).

67.4 Conventional Group

Insulin was administered when the blood glucose level was >180 mg/dl. The dose was titrated to maintain a blood glucose level of ≤180 mg/dl. If the blood glucose level was <144 mg/dl, the insulin dose was weaned down and stopped.

67.5 Management Common to both Groups

Management of blood glucose level was guided by an online treatment algorithm. Control of blood glucose levels was part of the routine duties of the staff at the participating center. The intervention was discontinued at the time of ICU discharge; however, if readmission to the ICU occurred, the assigned treatment was continued. The maximum duration of the intervention was up to 90 days or until death. Samples from the arterial line were used for blood glucose measurement if possible. Capillary samples were discouraged. All other care, including management of nutrition, was left to the clinician's judgment.

67.6 Sample Size

The original sample size was 4000 patients; it was later increased to 6100 based on the results of the second Leuven 2 trial of medical ICU patients [5]. The study provided 90% power to detect an absolute mortality difference of 3.8% between groups at a baseline mortality of 30% and a two-sided alpha level of <0.05. All data were analyzed on an intention-to-treat basis.

67.7 Results

The investigators screened 40,171 patients; 6104 underwent randomization—3054 were assigned to the intensive glucose control group and 3500 to the conventional glucose control group. Among these, 6030 patients were included in the final analysis. Most were nonoperative admissions (intensive control vs. conventional: 63.1% vs. 62.8%). The mean APACHE II score was 21.1 ± 7.91 in the intensive control group and 21.1 ± 8.3 in the conventional group. The baseline blood glucose levels were also similar between the two groups. Patients in the intensive control group received insulin more often, and in significantly higher doses compared to the conventional group. The mean, time-weighted blood glucose level was significantly lower in the intensive control group (115 ± 18 vs. 144 ± 23 mg/dl). Patients in the intensive control group received corticosteroids more often compared to the conventional group—the most common indication was septic shock.

67.8 The Primary Outcome: 90-Day Mortality

Mortality at 90 days after randomization was significantly higher in the intensive control group compared with the conventional group (27.5% vs. 24.9%; odds ratio: 1.14, 95% CI, 1.02–1.28; $p = 0.02$). The difference in mortality remained significant on adjusted analysis based on predefined risk factors. The proximate cause of death was similarly distributed in both groups; however, cardiovascular deaths were more common in the intensive control group. On subgroup analysis, there was no significant difference in the 90-day mortality between treatment groups among operative vs. nonoperative patients, those with diabetes, severe sepsis, and patients with APACHE II scores ≥25.

67.9 Secondary Outcomes

In contrast to the 90-day mortality, the mortality at 28 days was not significantly different between the intensive control and the conventional groups (22.3% vs. 20.8%). The median length of stay in the ICU was 6 days, and the median length of stay in hospital was 17 days in both groups. The median duration of mechanical ventilation was 6.6 days in both groups. The use and duration of renal replacement therapy were similar. Packed red cells were transfused in a similar number of patients in both groups; the volume of transfusion was also similar. Positive blood cultures and new-onset single or multiorgan failure occurred at similar frequencies in both groups.

67.10 Hypoglycemia

The incidence of hypoglycemia was markedly different between groups.

Severe hypoglycemia with blood glucose levels ≤40 mg/dl occurred much more often in the intensive control group (6.8% vs. 0.5%, $p = 0.001$). There were 272 episodes of hypoglycemia in the intensive control group compared with 16 in the conventional group. No long-term sequelae directly related to hypoglycemia were reported. The main findings of the study are summarized in Table 67.1.

Table 67.1 Main findings of the study

Outcome	Intensive control (81–108 mg/dl)	Conventional (≤180 mg/dl)	OR (95% CI)	*P*-value
Primary outcome, 90-day mortality	27.5%	24.9%	1.14 (1.02–1.28)	0.02
28-d mortality	22.3%	20.8%	1.09 (0.96–1.23)	0.17
Severe hypoglycemia (<40 mg/dl)	6.8%	0.5%	14.7 (9.0–25.9)	<0.001
Median ICU LOS	6 (2–11)	6 (2–11)	0	0.84
Mean ventilation days	6.6 ± 6.6	6.6 ± 6.5	0	0.56
Median hospital LOS	17 (8–35)	17 (8–35)	0	0.86
New-onset organ failure	41.4%	42.7%		
RRT	15.4%	14.5%	0.9 (−0.9–2.7)	0.34

67.11 Study Conclusions

The NICE-SUGAR trial revealed increased 90-day mortality with the intensive control strategy of blood glucose management (81–108 mg/dl) mg/dl compared with conventional control (equal to or less than 180 mg/dl). The increase in the absolute risk of death was 2.6 percentage points. The number needed to cause harm was 38—one additional death when 38 patients are treated with an intensive control strategy. Besides, severe hypoglycemia with a blood glucose level of ≤40 mg/dl was more common when the intensive control strategy was employed.

67.12 Strengths

The NICE-SUGAR trial was a large, pragmatic RCT that evaluated clinical outcomes in a heterogenous group of ICU patients with intensive glucose control compared with a conventional strategy. A uniform protocol of insulin dosing was applied across centers. The multicentric design offered generalizability of the results. The study explored the most relevant clinical outcomes in critically ill patients. There was robust adherence to the treatment algorithm and minimal loss to follow-up. The mean blood glucose levels differed substantially between groups during the 90-day study period, as envisaged by the investigators. The incidence of hypoglycemia was low compared with that reported in contemporaneous studies.

67.13 Limitations

The mean, time-weighted blood glucose level was slightly higher (115 ± 18 mg/dl) than the target range of 81–108 mg/dl in the intensive control group. This finding exemplifies the practical difficulty in maintaining the blood glucose level within a narrow range for extended periods. Blinding was not feasible and could have led to bias. It is unclear if the higher use of corticosteroids in the intensive control group may have influenced the outcomes. Most patients received early enteral feeds; the outcomes may be different among patients who receive early or supplemental parenteral nutrition in the first few days of ICU admission. In the intensive control group, the treatment protocol was discontinued prematurely, based on clinician judgment or a switch to palliative care. These patients were analyzed on an intention-to-treat basis, as belonging to the intensive control group. It is unclear whether this aspect of the study would have impacted outcomes. The 90-day mortality was significantly lower with conventional glucose control. Yet, the absence of a significant difference in the 28-day mortality and the similar incidence of new-onset organ dysfunction between the two groups was difficult to explain.

67.14 Post-hoc Analysis

The NICE-SUGAR investigators evaluated the association between the degree of hypoglycemia and the risk of death in a subsequent post-hoc analysis [11]. A blood glucose level between 41 and 70 mg/dl was considered to represent moderate hypoglycemia, and a level < 40 mg/dl, severe hypoglycemia. Intensive glucose control resulted in a higher incidence of moderate and severe hypoglycemia compared to conventional control; both were associated with a higher risk of death. There was a dose-response relationship; an increase in mortality was related to the severity of hypoglycemia. However, the study does not establish a cause and effect relationship between hypoglycemia and the risk of death.

67.15 Summary

In one of the largest RCTs in the history of critical care, the NICE-SUGAR trial demonstrated increased mortality with an intensive glucose control strategy with target levels between 81 to 108 mg/dl compared with conventional control between 144 and 180 mg/dl. Severe hypoglycemia was more common in the intensive control group. There was a strong association between hypoglycemia and mortality, with lower glucose levels resulting in a higher risk of death. The NICE-SUGAR trial provided robust evidence that lowering the blood glucose level below a threshold level of 144 mg/dl does not offer any additional benefit; on the contrary, it carries a higher risk of poor outcomes related to hypoglycemia. This well-conducted, multicentric trial, with robust statistical analysis, dampened the unfettered enthusiasm aroused by earlier RCTs with a tight glucose control strategy.

References

1. McCowen KC, Malhotra A, Bistrian BR. Stress-induced hyperglycemia. Crit Care Clin. 2001;17(1):107–24.
2. Stentz FB, Umpierrez GE, Cuervo R, Kitabchi AE. Proinflammatory cytokines, markers of cardiovascular risks, oxidative stress, and lipid peroxidation in patients with hyperglycemic crises. Diabetes. 2004;53(8):2079–86.
3. Boden G, Rao AK. Effects of hyperglycemia and hyperinsulinemia on the tissue factor pathway of blood coagulation. Curr Diab Rep. 2007;7(3):223–7.
4. van den Berghe G, Wouters P, Weekers F, Verwaest C, Bruyninckx F, Schetz M, et al. Intensive insulin therapy in critically ill patients. N Engl J Med. 2001;345(19):1359–67.
5. Van den Berghe G, Wilmer A, Hermans G, Meersseman W, Wouters PJ, Milants I, et al. Intensive insulin therapy in the medical ICU. N Engl J Med. 2006;354(5):449–61.
6. Preiser JC, Devos P, Ruiz-Santana S, Mélot C, Annane D, Groeneveld J, et al. A prospective randomised multi-centre controlled trial on tight glucose control by intensive insulin therapy in adult intensive care units: the Glucontrol study. Intensive Care Med. 2009;35(10):1738–48.
7. Brunkhorst FM, Engel C, Bloos F, Meier-Hellmann A, Ragaller M, Weiler N, et al. Intensive insulin therapy and pentastarch resuscitation in severe sepsis. N Engl J Med. 2008;358(2):125–39.

8. Pittas AG, Siegel RD, Lau J. Insulin therapy for critically ill hospitalized patients: a meta-analysis of randomized controlled trials. Arch Intern Med. 2004;164(18):2005–11.
9. Wiener RS, Wiener DC, Larson RJ. Benefits and risks of tight glucose control in critically ill adults: a meta-analysis. JAMA. 2008;300(8):933–44.
10. NICE-SUGAR Study Investigators. Intensive versus conventional glucose control in critically ill patients. N Engl J Med. 2009;360(13):1283–97.
11. NICE-SUGAR Study Investigators, Finfer S, Liu B, Chittock DR, Norton R, Myburgh JA, et al. Hypoglycemia and risk of death in critically ill patients. N Engl J Med. 2012;367(12):1108–18.

68 Intensive Insulin Therapy in the Surgical ICU: The Leuven 1 Trial

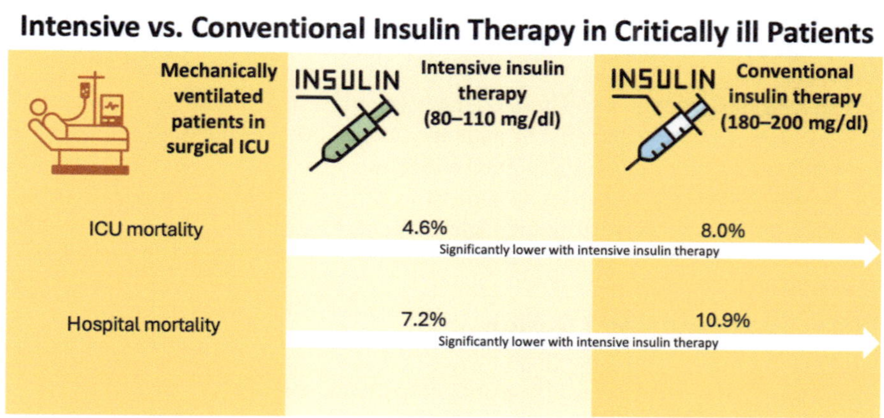

Van Den Berghe et al. (NEJM, 2001)

Quick Take

Does intensive glucose control lead to improved outcomes in the surgical ICU?

The study by Van den Berghe et al. investigated the effects of intensive insulin therapy in surgical ICU patients. The trial showed that maintaining strict blood glucose control (targeting a glucose level of 80–110 mg/dL) led to improved outcomes, including reduced mortality, fewer infections, and less organ dysfunction compared to conventional insulin therapy. However, the study also raised concerns about the risk of hypoglycemia, which can have serious consequences. Despite these concerns, the overall findings supported the benefits of tight glycemic control in ICU settings.

Van den Berghe G, Wouters P, Weekers F, Verwaest C, Bruyninckx F, Schetz M, et al. Intensive insulin therapy in critically ill patients. N Engl J Med. 2001 Nov 8;345(19):1359–67.

J. Chacko et al., *Landmark Studies in Critical Care*,
https://doi.org/10.1007/978-981-95-0673-6_68

68.1 Introduction and Background

Insulin resistance and hyperglycemia commonly occur in critically ill patients, regardless of their pre-existing diabetic status [1]. Hyperglycemia predisposes to a high rate of infection and poor wound healing [2]. Uncontrolled blood glucose levels have been shown to worsen outcomes following stroke [3]. Diabetic patients with high blood glucose levels are more prone to complications following coronary artery surgery, including postoperative arrhythmias, respiratory complications, and wound infections [4].

In the DIGAMI study, diabetic patients with acute myocardial infarction were assigned to a ≥ 24-hour insulin-glucose infusion followed by subcutaneous insulin. In the control group, patients received standard antidiabetic therapy. At 3.4 years of follow-up, the mortality was lower in the intensive insulin group [5]. The authors proposed a blood glucose target <215 mg/dl in patients who sustain acute myocardial infarction [5]. Among non-diabetic patients with prolonged critical illness, hepatocyte response to insulin may be impaired, leading to a higher risk of mortality [6].

Van Den Berghe et al. hypothesized that hyperglycemia or relative insulin insufficiency may occur in critically ill patients, leading to an increased likelihood of morbidity and mortality. They designed a randomized controlled trial (RCT) to test the hypothesis whether tight blood glucose control with intensive insulin therapy would confer clinical benefits among such patients [7].

68.2 Population and Design

The study enrolled mechanically ventilated patients admitted to the surgical ICU over a 1-year period between February 2000 and January 2001. Patients were randomized to receive intensive or conventional insulin therapy for control of blood glucose levels. Randomization was stratified based on the type of illness requiring ICU admission. Patients who were enrolled in other trials and those who were terminally ill with do-not-resuscitate orders were excluded.

68.3 Conventional Insulin Therapy

In the conventional group, patients received a continuous infusion of insulin (50 IU/50 ml), titrated to maintain the blood glucose levels between 180 and 200 mg/dl.

68.4 Intensive Insulin Therapy

In this group, insulin infusion was commenced if the blood glucose level rose above 110 mg/dl; the rate of infusion was titrated to maintain blood glucose levels between 80 and 110 mg/dl.

68.5 Common Management

Glucose levels were measured 1–4 hourly on whole-blood samples of arterial blood. Adjustment of the insulin dose was based on a strict algorithm, with the maximum dose set at 50 IU/hour. On the first day of ICU admission, 200–300 mg of intravenous glucose was administered intravenously. From the next day onwards, regular feeding was commenced—either enteral, parenteral, or a combination of both, based on a standard schedule. Total enteral nutrition was instituted as early as feasible. Following discharge from the ICU, a conventional approach of blood glucose control was adopted in both groups. Patients were considered ready for discharge to the ward when life support interventions were not required and two-thirds of caloric intake was through the enteral route.

The outcome assessors were blinded to the allocation arm; the clinical team was not.

68.6 Sample Size

The sample size was calculated based on a 5% difference in mortality among patients with ICU stay of >5 days and 2% difference among all patients admitted to the ICU. The study was planned to enrol 2500 patients to identify a difference between groups at a two-sided alpha level of <0.05.

68.7 Results

The study was terminated after enrollment of 1548 patients when the fourth scheduled interim analysis suggested inferiority of conventional glucose control. Demographic and clinical characteristics of patients were similar at baseline. Surgical patients represented >90% of the study population. Most patients were postoperative cardiac surgical—63% in the conventional treatment group and 62% in the intensive treatment group. The median APACHE II score was identical in both groups (median: 9, interquartile range: 7–13). The incidence of pre-existing diabetes and renal failure was similar in both groups.

There was a clear separation between groups in the blood glucose levels measured at 6 AM every morning—103 ± 19 mg/dl in the intensive insulin therapy group and 153 ± 33 mg/dl in the conventional insulin therapy group. Hypoglycemia occurred in more patients who received intensive therapy group (39 vs. 6).

68.7.1 The Primary Outcome—ICU Mortality

Among all study patients, the ICU mortality was significantly lower with intensive compared with conventional therapy (4.6% vs. 8%, $P < 0.04$), representing a relative risk reduction of 42%. Mortality during the first 5 days of ICU stay was similar in both groups (1.7% vs. 1.8%). The observed mortality difference was confined to patients who stayed longer. Among those with an ICU stay >5 days, the mortality was significantly reduced with intensive therapy (10.6% vs. 20.2%, $P = 0.005$).

On multivariate analysis, independent predictors of mortality included APACHE II score of ≥9 in the first 24 h, older age, admission for reasons other than cardiac surgery, tertiary referral, and conventional insulin therapy. History of diabetes or hyperglycemia at admission did not influence mortality.

68.7.2 Secondary Outcomes

The overall hospital mortality was lower in the intensive therapy group (7.2 vs. 10.9, $P = 0.01$); besides, hospital mortality was also lower among those with ICU stay of >5 days (16.8% vs. 26.3%, $P = 0.01$).

The duration of stay in the ICU did not differ significantly between groups. However, among those who stayed longer than 5 days in the ICU, the duration of stay was shorter in the intensive therapy group.

The duration of mechanical ventilation was shorter in the intensive therapy group among patients who stayed in the ICU for >5 days (median: 12 vs. 10 days). Fewer patients in the intensive therapy group required ventilator support for >14 days (7.5% vs. 11.9%).

Vasopressor and inotrope use were similar in both groups. The incidence of renal impairment and the use of renal replacement therapy was more common in the conventional therapy group. Septicemia occurred more often with conventional therapy. Electromyographic evidence of critical illness-related polyneuropathy was more common in the conventional therapy group. Patients who underwent conventional therapy received more blood transfusions compared with those who received intensive therapy. Markers of inflammation were lower in the intensive therapy group. The main study outcomes are summarized in Table 68.1.

Table 68.1 Main study outcomes

Outcome	Intensive insulin therapy	Conventional therapy	Significance
ICU mortality	4.6%	8.0%	$P < 0.04$
Hospital mortality	7.2%	10.9%	$P = 0.01$
Median ICU days	3	3	$P = 0.2$
Median ventilation days	2	2	$P = 0.06$
Septicemia	4.8%	7.2%	$P = 0.003$
Critical illness-related polyneuropathy	28.7%	51.9%	$P < 0.001$
Median units of RBC transfusions	1	1	$P < 0.001$

68.8 Study Conclusions

Among surgical patients, intensive insulin therapy led to a significant reduction in ICU mortality. Besides, it resulted in reduced bloodstream infections, a lower incidence of AKI requiring renal replacement therapy, fewer red cell transfusions, and a reduced number of patients with critical illness-related polyneuropathy. Patients who received intensive insulin therapy were less likely to require prolonged mechanical ventilation and ICU care.

68.9 Strengths

The randomized controlled design and the target blood glucose levels were appropriate to evaluate the clinical equipoise that existed relating to the glucose control in critically ill patients. The study excluded only 14 patients, allowing broad applicability. The assessors were blinded to group allocation, reducing the risk of bias that may have occurred to the clinical team being unblinded to the study arm. Besides, glycemic control was based on a strict protocol based on regular monitoring of blood glucose levels.

68.10 Limitations

The study was confined to the surgical ICU of a single center. Blinding of the clinical team to the allocation arm was not feasible, considering the requirement for monitoring of blood glucose levels and titration of the insulin dose. Lack of blinding may have led to bias. The study population was >90% surgical; most patients had undergone cardiac surgery, with a low baseline severity of illness (median APACHE II score = 9). Hence, the results may not be extrapolatable to more severely ill patients in a general ICU. The study was stopped early based on more favorable outcomes in the intensive therapy group on interim analysis, and hence did not attain the calculated sample size. Details of adverse events related to the allocated modality of treatment were not available.

68.11 Subsequent Evidence

68.11.1 The Leuven II Trial

In contrast to their surgical trial, the investigators could not reproduce the favorable outcomes in the study of patients admitted to a medical ICU, using the same blood sugar targets [8]. The Leuven II trial included 1200 patients admitted to a medical ICU. Intensive insulin therapy did not significantly reduce the hospital mortality (intensive therapy: 37.3% vs. conventional therapy: 40%). The authors observed a higher mortality with intensive therapy among patients who had an ICU stay of <3 days; conversely, a lower mortality was observed among patients who had an extended ICU stay of ≥3 days (43.0% vs. 52.5%, $P = 0.009$). Improvement in some secondary outcomes was noted, including a lower incidence of new-onset AKI and earlier weaning from mechanical ventilation.

68.11.2 The NICE-SUGAR Trial

Considering the lack of certainty regarding appropriate blood glucose targets in critically ill patients, the The NICE-SUGAR Study Investigators conducted a large, multicentric RCT comparing intensive vs. conventional glucose control [9]. The study randomized 6104 patients—3054 to the intensive control and 3050 to the conventional control group. The target blood glucose level was aimed between 81–108 mg/dl and ≤180 mg/dl, respectively. The 90-day all-cause mortality, the primary outcome, was significantly higher with intensive compared with conventional control (27.5% vs. 24.9%, $P = 0.02$). The effect on mortality did not differ between medical compared with surgical patients. Severe hypoglycemia, defined as a blood glucose level of ≤40 mg/dl, was significantly more common with the intensive approach (6.8% vs. 0.5%). The ICU and hospital stay, the duration of mechanical ventilation, and initiation of renal replacement therapy did not differ significantly between the two groups. The findings of the NICE-SUGAR trial suggested that aiming for normoglycemia in critically ill patients may not lead to improved outcomes; indeed, it may be harmful.

68.12 Summary

Critically ill patients have a predilection to insulin resistance and high blood glucose levels, regardless of their diabetic state. Tight control of blood glucose levels was shown to be associated with improved outcomes in patients with stroke, acute myocardial infarction, and post-coronary artery bypass surgery. It was unclear at the time of conduct of the Leuven trial whether normalization of blood glucose levels with an intensive approach would lead to improved outcomes in critically ill patients. The Leuven investigators randomized patients in a surgical ICU to undergo intensive insulin therapy aiming to maintain a blood glucose level of 80–110 mg/dl compared with a conventional line of management, with target blood glucose levels less than 215 mg/dl.

Intensive insulin therapy resulted in a significantly lower ICU mortality compared with conventional therapy. The mortality benefit was mainly evident among patients who experienced a prolonged ICU stay of more than 5 days. The hospital mortality was lower in the intensive therapy group; the duration of mechanical ventilation was lower among patients who had an ICU stay of >5 days. Septicemia was more common in the conventional therapy group. Besides, the incidence of renal impairment and use of renal replacement therapy was lower, and critical illness-related neuromuscular weakness was less common with intensive insulin therapy.

The favorable clinical outcomes observed in the Leuven trial were not corroborated by the findings of the NICE-SUGAR trial, which revealed higher 90-day all-cause mortality with intensive insulin therapy. However, it highlighted the importance of blood glucose control among critically ill patients and the need for further investigation. Strict control of blood glucose levels carries the risk of hypoglycemia, which may offset any benefit, as observed in the NICE-SUGAR trial. As technology evolves, the use of more robust devices to monitor blood glucose levels with algorithms supported by artificial intelligence may enable tighter control while reducing the risk of hypoglycemia.

References

1. Shangraw RE, Jahoor F, Miyoshi H, Neff WA, Stuart CA, Herndon DN, Wolfe RR, et al. Differentiation between septic and postburn insulin resistance. Metab Clin Exp [Internet]. 1989[cited 2024 Apr 19];38(10). Available from: https://pubmed.ncbi.nlm.nih.gov/2677612/.
2. McCowen KC, Malhotra A, Bistrian BR. Stress-induced hyperglycemia. Crit Care Clin. 2001;17(1):107–24.
3. O'Neill PA, Davies I, Fullerton KJ, Bennett D. Stress hormone and blood glucose response following acute stroke in the elderly. Stroke [Internet]. 1991 [cited 2024 Apr 19];22(7). Available from: https://pubmed.ncbi.nlm.nih.gov/1853403/.
4. Fietsam R, Bassett J, Glover JL. Complications of coronary artery surgery in diabetic patients. Am Surg. 1991 Sep;57(9):551–7.
5. Malmberg K, Norhammar A, Wedel H, Rydén L. Glycometabolic state at admission: important risk marker of mortality in conventionally treated patients with diabetes mellitus and acute myocardial infarction: long-term results from the Diabetes and Insulin-Glucose Infusion in Acute Myocardial Infarction (DIGAMI) study. Circulation [Internet]. 1999 [cited 2024 Apr 19];99(20). Available from: https://pubmed.ncbi.nlm.nih.gov/10338454/.
6. Van den Berghe G, Wouters P, Weekers F, Mohan S, Baxter RC, Veldhuis JD, et al. Reactivation of pituitary hormone release and metabolic improvement by infusion of growth hormone-releasing peptide and thyrotropin-releasing hormone in patients with protracted critical illness. J Clin Endocrinol Metab. 1999;84(4):1311–23.

7. Van den Berghe G, Wouters P, Weekers F, Verwaest C, Bruyninckx F, Schetz M, et al. Intensive insulin therapy in critically ill patients. N Engl J Med. 2001;345(19):1359–67.
8. Van den Berghe G, Wilmer A, Hermans G, Meersseman W, Wouters PJ, Milants I, et al. Intensive insulin therapy in the medical ICU. N Engl J Med. 2006;354(5):449–61.
9. NICE-SUGAR Study Investigators, Finfer S, Chittock DR, Su SYS, Blair D, Foster D, et al. Intensive versus conventional glucose control in critically ill patients. N Engl J Med. 2009;360(13):1283–97.

Intensive Insulin Therapy in the Medical ICU: The Leuven 2 Trial

69

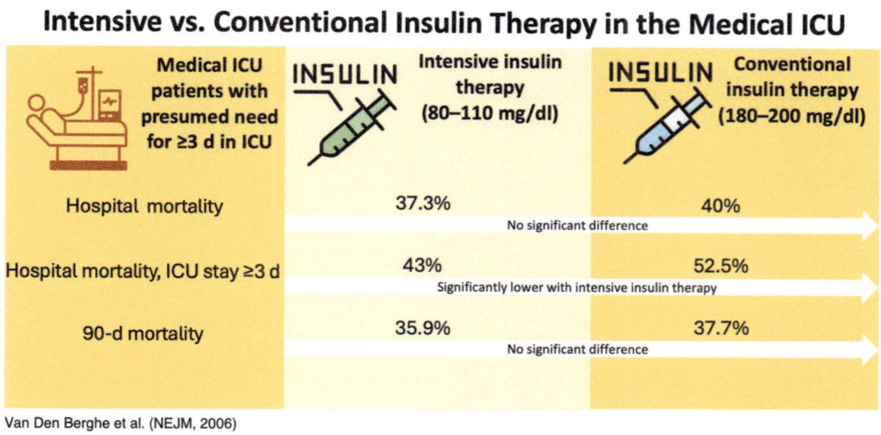

Quick Take

Does intensive insulin therapy improve outcomes compared to conventional insulin therapy in critically ill medical ICU patients?

The Leuven 2 trial, a single-center randomized controlled study, investigated this question among 1200 adult patients admitted to the medical ICU at the University Hospital in Leuven, Belgium. Patients were randomized to receive either intensive insulin therapy (targeting blood glucose 80–110 mg/dL) or conventional insulin therapy (targeting <220 mg/dL). The primary outcome was all-cause hospital mortality. Overall mortality was not significantly different between groups. However, among the 767 patients who remained in ICU for ≥3 days, hospital mortality was

---

Van den Berghe G, Wilmer A, Hermans G, Meersseman W, Wouters PJ, Milants I, et al. Intensive insulin therapy in the medical ICU. N Engl J Med. 2006 Feb 2;354(5):449–61.

J. Chacko et al., *Landmark Studies in Critical Care*,
https://doi.org/10.1007/978-981-95-0673-6_69

significantly lower with intensive therapy. Intensive therapy also led to earlier weaning from mechanical ventilation, shorter ICU and hospital stays, and a lower incidence of new-onset acute kidney injury. Hypoglycemia occurred more frequently with intensive treatment and was associated with higher ICU mortality. The study concluded that while intensive insulin therapy did not reduce overall mortality, it may benefit long-staying ICU patients—though these patients cannot be identified at admission.

69.1 Introduction and Background

Uncontrolled blood glucose levels may lead to adverse clinical outcomes among critically ill patients [1]. In their previous study on surgical patients, Van den Berghe et al. had observed improved outcomes, including reduced mortality in patients admitted to a surgical intensive care unit [2]. The impact of strict glucose control was most pronounced in patients who experienced an ICU stay of 3 or more days [2]. However, it remained unclear whether the favorable outcomes would be reproducible in patients admitted to medical ICUs, who are likely to be more severely ill and carry a higher risk of mortality.

The authors designed a randomized controlled trial (RCT) among patients admitted to their medical ICU to evaluate the impact of intensive glucose control with a special focus on patients who required intensive care for at least 3 days [3].

69.2 Population and Design

The Leuven 2 trial was conducted over a 3-year period between March 2002 and May 2005 among patients admitted to the medical ICU of the University Hospital in Leuven, Belgium. Eligible patients included those who were judged to require at least a third day of intensive care.

69.2.1 Exclusion

The study excluded patients who could be fed orally and those with do-not-resuscitate orders on admission.

Patients were randomly assigned to receive intensive insulin treatment or conventional insulin treatment.

69.3 Intensive Treatment Group

A continuous infusion of insulin, containing 50 IU in 50 ml of normal saline, was commenced when the blood glucose level rose above 110 mg/dL (6.1 mmol/L). The dose was titrated targeting a blood glucose level between 80 and 110 mg/dL

(4.4–6.1 mmol/L). On discharge from the ICU, a conventional approach was followed, targeting blood glucose levels of 200 mg/dL.

69.4 Conventional Treatment Group

In this group, insulin infusion was commenced when the blood glucose was >215 mg/dL; the rate of infusion was adjusted to maintain glucose levels between 180 and 220 mg/dL (10–11 mmol/L). The infusion was tapered and ceased when the blood glucose level dropped below 180 mg/dL.

69.5 Common Management

Blood glucose levels were measured based on whole-blood glucose levels from an arterial line. In the absence of an arterial line, capillary glucose levels were measured using a point-of-care glucometer. Titration of the insulin dose was performed by bedside nursing staff, using predefined guidelines. Enteral feeding was commenced as early as feasible, once hemodynamic stability was attained. Blood glucose levels were measured at admission to the ICU, followed by 4-hourly, or more often, as deemed appropriate by the bedside nurse.

69.6 Sample Size

The authors hypothesized an absolute reduction in mortality by 7% based on their study on surgical ICU patients. They calculated a sample size of 1200 patients for a two-sided alpha level <0.05 and beta level <0.2.

69.7 Results

The study enrolled 1200 patients—595 in the intensive treatment group and 605 in the conventional treatment group. Of these, 767 patients experienced an ICU stay of at least until the third day.

69.7.1 The Primary Outcome: All-Cause Hospital Mortality

The overall hospital mortality was not significantly different between the intensive and conventional treatment groups—222/595 (37.3%) patients died in the intensive treatment group compared with 242/605 (40%) in the conventional treatment group (P = 0.33). However, among patients who experienced an ICU stay of 3 or more days, the hospital mortality was lower in the intensive treatment group [166/386 (43%) vs. 200/381 (52.5%), $P = 0.009$]. Furthermore, among patients who stayed in ICU for >5 days, the mortality was lower in the intensive treatment group (54.9% vs. 45.9%, $P = 0.03$)

69.7.2 Secondary Outcomes

The 28- (29.9% vs. 30%, $P = 0.95$) and 90-day mortality (35.9% vs. 37.7%, $P = 0.53$) were similar in both the intensive and conventional treatment groups. The difference between groups remained non-significant regardless of the duration of stay in the ICU ≥3 days or less.

Among patients who stayed in the ICU for ≥3 days, intensive insulin therapy led to more rapid weaning from mechanical ventilation ($P = 0.03$), earlier discharge from ICU ($P = 0.04$), and hospital ($P = 0.05$).

New-onset acute kidney injury was lower in the intensive treatment group (8.9% vs. 5.9%, $P = 0.04$). However, a similar number of patients underwent renal replacement therapy in both groups. There was no significant difference between groups in the incidence of bacteremia or the requirement for prolonged antibiotic therapy.

Hypoglycemia was observed more often with intensive insulin treatment, although the severity of hypoglycemia was similar in both groups. On logistical regression analysis, the ICU mortality was higher among patients who experienced hypoglycemia. The main findings of the study are summarized in Table 69.1A, B.

Table 69.1 Main study findings

(A) Mortality outcomes

Outcome	Overall, intensive treatment	Overall, conventional treatment	*P* value	≥3 days in ICU, intensive treatment	≥3 days in ICU, conventional treatment	*P* value
Hospital mortality	37.3%	40%	0.33	43%	52.5%	0.009
28-day mortality	29.9%	30%	0.95	34.5%	39.1%	0.18
90-day mortality	35.9%	37.7%	0.53	42.2%	49.1%	0.06

(B) Other outcomes

Outcome	Intensive treatment	Conventional treatment	Significance
ICU stay	Shorter stay	Longer stay	$P = 0.04$
Weaning from mechanical ventilation	Earlier weaning	More prolonged	$P = 0.03$
Hospital stay	Shorter stay	Longer stay	$P = 0.05$
Acute kidney Injury	Lower incidence	Higher incidence	$P = 0.04$

69.8 Study Conclusions

Overall, intensive insulin treatment had no impact on hospital mortality compared with conventional treatment. A significant reduction in mortality was observed in patients who experienced an ICU stay of ≥3 days, although this subgroup of patients could not be identified beforehand. The authors observed reduced morbidity with intensive insulin therapy among patients who stayed in the ICU for ≥3 days, including quicker weaning from mechanical ventilation, and earlier ICU and hospital discharge.

69.9 Strengths

The study employed a robust methodology and protocolized management of blood glucose levels. Besides, previous experience from their study in the surgical ICU ensured consistent implementation of the insulin protocol. The large sample size of 1200 medical patients added to the validity of the study. The authors evaluated clinically meaningful outcomes, including mortality, weaning from mechanical ventilation, and duration of ICU and hospital stay. They analyzed outcomes specifically related to the duration of ICU stay—those who stayed ≥3 days vs. less.

69.10 Limitations

Strict blinding to the allocated treatment group was not feasible as patient safety dictated frequent monitoring of blood glucose levels. Intensive insulin treatment heightened the risk of hypoglycemia, with a potential for complications, including mortality. In contrast to their earlier trial in the surgical ICU, the strategy of intensive insulin therapy did not result in improved hospital mortality among critically ill medical patients, although long stayers revealed a possible benefit. However, the identification of patients who require longer ICU stay is often fraught with uncertainty; hence, a much larger sample size would be required to address this issue. Although the single-center design facilitated protocolized care, it limits generalizability to other settings. Particularly, the requirement for nursing expertise and heavier workload may impact feasibility in broader clinical practice. The study did not evaluate the potential impact of nutritional management and comorbidities on the final outcomes.

69.11 Subsequent Evidence—The NICE-SUGAR Trial

In a large, multicentric RCT of 6104 patients, the NICE-SUGAR trial sought to provide robust evidence on glucose control among critically ill patients [4]. The study, conducted between 2004 and 2008, included patients from Australia, New Zealand, Canada, and the US. The authors compared intensive glucose control

(81–108 mg/dL) with a conventional strategy (<180 mg/dL). This large RCT revealed that intensive glucose control may be potentially harmful—the 90-day mortality was significantly higher compared with conventional glucose control (27.5% vs. 24.9%, $P = 0.02$). The increased mortality may have arisen from a higher incidence of hypoglycemia (≤40 mg/dL) in the intensive glucose control group (6.8% vs. 0.5%), highlighting the risks associated with intensive glucose control. Besides, there was no favorable impact of intensive control on the ICU length of stay, requirement for renal replacement therapy, or the incidence of infections. The NICE-SUGAR trial led to a change of paradigm, targeting a more conventional glucose target of <180 mg/dL.

69.12 Summary

The Leuven 2 trial of intensive insulin treatment in the medical ICU followed up on the earlier trial among surgical ICU patients. However, the authors could not replicate the benefits of intensive treatment that they had previously demonstrated in the surgical ICU. Conducted in 1200 medical ICU patients, intensive insulin treatment did not reduce hospital mortality overall compared with a conventional strategy. Patients who stayed in ICU for a longer duration (revealed improved survival ≥3 days), although they could not be identified at the outset. Hypoglycemia was a potential hazard and could lead to increased mortality.

The Leuven 2 trial dispelled the presumed benefits of intensive insulin therapy in general critically ill patients. This pivotal study, along with the NICE-SUGAR trial that followed, led to a shift away from aggressive control of glucose levels in ICU patients.

References

1. Capes SE, Hunt D, Malmberg K, Gerstein HC. Stress hyperglycaemia and increased risk of death after myocardial infarction in patients with and without diabetes: a systematic overview. Lancet. 2000;355(9206):773–8.
2. Van den Berghe G, Wouters P, Weekers F, Verwaest C, Bruyninckx F, Schetz M, et al. Intensive insulin therapy in critically ill patients. N Engl J Med. 2001;345(19):1359–67.
3. Van den Berghe G, Wilmer A, Hermans G, Meersseman W, Wouters PJ, Milants I, et al. Intensive insulin therapy in the medical ICU. N Engl J Med. 2006;354(5):449–61.
4. NICE-SUGAR Study Investigators, Finfer S, Chittock DR, Su SYS, Blair D, Foster D, et al. Intensive versus conventional glucose control in critically ill patients. N Engl J Med. 2009;360(13):1283–97.

Part XVIII

Transfusion Thresholds

70 Transfusion Thresholds in the Critically Ill: The TRICC Trial

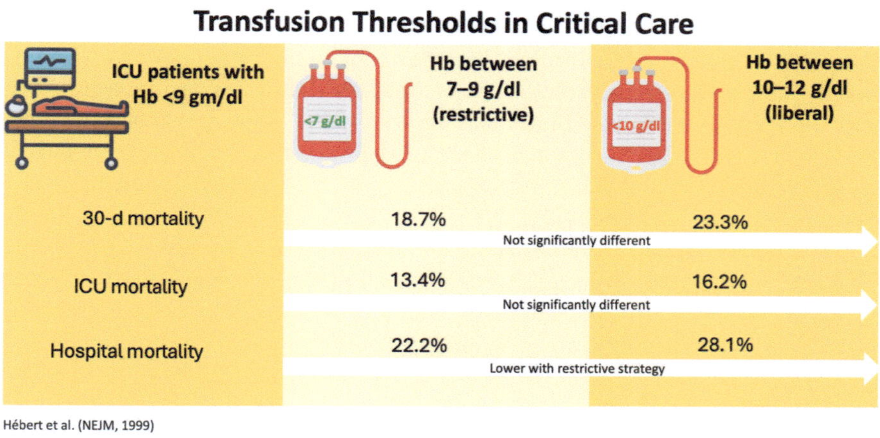

Quick Take

Does a restrictive transfusion strategy improve outcomes for critically ill patients?

The TRICC trial was a landmark randomized controlled trial (RCT) that compared restrictive versus liberal red blood cell transfusion strategies in critically ill patients. The trial enrolled over 800 patients who were admitted to intensive care units with acute illness and randomized them to receive either a restrictive transfusion strategy (transfusions only when hemoglobin levels fell below 7 g/dL) or a liberal strategy (transfusions when hemoglobin levels fell below 10 g/dL). The results of the study demonstrated that the restrictive transfusion strategy was non-inferior to the liberal strategy in terms of 30-day mortality, and was associated with

---

Hébert PC, Martin C, Yetisir E. A Multicenter, Randomized, Controlled Clinical Trial of Transfusion Requirements in Critical Care. N Engl J Med. 1999.

J. Chacko et al., *Landmark Studies in Critical Care*,
https://doi.org/10.1007/978-981-95-0673-6_70

fewer complications and a lower incidence of transfusion-related side effects. This study provided robust evidence that, in critically ill patients, a restrictive approach to red blood cell transfusion—aimed at maintaining hemoglobin levels above 7 g/dL—can safely improve patient outcomes and reduce the risks associated with transfusion. The TRICC trial helped establish restrictive transfusion protocols as the standard of care in critically ill patients, highlighting the importance of avoiding unnecessary transfusions in the ICU.

70.1 Introduction

Transfusion of blood was first reported in the early nineteenth century. In the early days of transfusion history, direct donor-to-recipient transfusion was commonly practiced. By 1914, the addition of citrate was found to prevent clotting, thus opening the door to the storage of collected blood. As World War I broke out in Europe, there was an increasing transfusion requirement for soldiers wounded in battle. Similar to other medical innovations that took root on the battlefield, type O blood mixed with citrate-glucose solution was stored for emergency use in army units. With the entry of the United States into the war in 1917, physicians became more familiar with transfusion practices. During the war, blood was collected from healthy soldiers, citrated and refrigerated, followed by transportation to the battlefront in sterilized milk bottles [1].

It took several years before Bernard Fantus established the first blood bank at the Cook County Hospital in Chicago in March 1937. In the following year, the number of transfusions saw a phenomenal rise, with a considerable decrease in the incidence of adverse reactions from 33% to 8% [1].

70.2 Early Transfusion Practices

Red cell transfusions were often administered based on clinician judgment, leading to wide variability in transfusion thresholds. In their treatise of 1942, titled "Anesthesia in Cases of Poor Surgical Risk: Some Suggestions for Decreasing the Risk," Adam and Lundy [2] proposed that "When the concentration of hemoglobin is less than 8 to 10 grams per 100 cubic centimeters of whole blood, it is wise to give a blood transfusion before operation." This suggestion appears to have been rapidly indoctrinated into anesthetic practice in that era. The widespread adoption of the 10/30 rule followed, with transfusion of red cells below a threshold hemoglobin level of 10 g/dl or a hematocrit of less than 30%. This approach was based on the physiological rationale that the hemoglobin level is the key determinant of oxygen delivery. However, it failed to take into account compensatory mechanisms that are activated, including a rise in the cardiac output and an increase in the oxygen extraction at the tissue level.

70.3 Rising Concerns with Transfusion-Transmitted Infection

Transfusion practices became the subject of intense scrutiny from the 1980s with increasing concern regarding the transmission of infection, particularly with the human immunodeficiency virus (HIV) [3]. It was soon realized that blood transfusions, once considered relatively safe, carry risks and may be potentially dangerous. In the meantime, the National Institutes of Health Consensus Conference in the United States of 1988 reported that there was no evidence to support a rigid threshold for transfusion of red cells [4]. The term "transfusion trigger" was coined by Friedman et al. in 1981, comparing transfusion practices among 535,031 male and female surgical patients [5].

70.4 Background to the Transfusion Requirements in Critical Care (TRICC) Trial

Besides the transmission of infection, the potential immunosuppressive [6] and microcirculatory complications of blood transfusion [7] were realized by the early 1990s. However, there was no credible evidence to support transfusion thresholds in critically ill patients, balancing the risks compared to possible benefits. Against this background, the Canadian Critical Care Trials Group planned an RCT to identify optimal transfusion thresholds among critically ill patients. They aimed to compare a liberal with a more restrictive transfusion strategy among normovolemic critically ill patients with anemia [8].

70.5 The Study Population and Design

The TRICC trial enrolled patients from 22 tertiary and 3 community-level ICUs across Canada during a 3-year period between 1994 and 1997. The study patients had a hemoglobin level of 9.0 g/dl or less within 72 h of ICU admission, and were expected to stay in the ICU for more than 24 h. Patients with ongoing bleeding, chronic anemia, following elective cardiac surgery, and those in whom death seemed imminent were excluded. Patients were randomly assigned to a liberal or restrictive transfusion strategy, stratified by center and disease severity. Stratification by disease severity was based on an APACHE II score of ≤ 15 or >15.

70.6 The Restrictive vs. Liberal Strategies

The hemoglobin level in the restrictive group was maintained between 7.0 and 9.0 g/dl; red cell transfusion was carried out if the hemoglobin level dropped below 7.0 g/dl. In the liberal group, the aim was to maintain a hemoglobin level of 10–12 g/dl, with transfusion of red cells if the level dropped below 10 g/dl. One unit of blood, between 240 and 340 ml, was transfused at a time, with hemoglobin levels measured after each unit. The overall care was left to the clinician's judgment.

A total of 6451 patients were screened, 418 patients were randomized to receive a restrictive transfusion strategy, and 420 to a liberal strategy. Baseline characteristics were well matched between the two groups. Respiratory and cardiac disease were the most common underlying causes for ICU admission. More than 80% of patients received mechanical ventilation. Vasoactive drugs were administered in 37% and the baseline hemoglobin level was 8.2 ± 0.7 g/dl in both groups.

70.7 Hemoglobin Levels and the Number of Units Transfused

The mean daily hemoglobin levels through the study period were significantly different between the two groups (restrictive vs. liberal: 8.5 ± 0.7 vs. 10.7 ± 0.7 g/dl). The liberal strategy led to significantly more units of red cell transfusion compared with the restrictive strategy (5.6 ± 5.3 vs. 2.6 ± 4.1 units), equating to a 54% reduction in transfusions with the restrictive strategy.

70.8 Outcomes

The all-cause mortality at 30 days post ICU admission, the primary outcome, was similar among both groups of patients. The mortality was 18.7% in the restrictive group compared with 23.3% in the liberal group ($p = 0.11$). The hospital mortality was significantly lower in the restrictive group (22.2% vs. 28.1%, $P = 0.05$). The 60-day and ICU mortality were comparable between the two groups. The number of patients with multiorgan failure was also similar between the two groups.

70.9 Subgroup Analysis

The authors analyzed subgroups of patients who were less than 55 years old and APACHE II score ≤20. In both these subgroups, the mortality at 30 days post ICU admission was significantly lower with a restrictive compared with a liberal strategy on Kaplan-Meier analysis ($p = 0.02$ for both subgroups). No difference in the primary outcome was observed between the two groups among patients with trauma, primary or secondary cardiac disease, severe infections, and septic shock.

70.10 Adverse Events

Cardiac adverse events, mainly acute pulmonary edema and acute myocardial infarction, were more common in the liberal group. The main study outcomes are summarized in Table 70.1.

Table 70.1 Main study outcomes

Outcomes	Restrictive transfusion	Liberal transfusion	Significance
ICU mortality	13.4%	16.2%	0.29
Hospital mortality	22.2	28.1	0.05
30-day mortality	18.7%	23.3%	0.11
60-day mortality	22.7%	26.5%	0.23
Mean ICU LOS	11.0 ± 10.7 days	11.5 ± 11.3 days	0.53
Mean hospital LOS	34.8 ± 19.5 days	35.5 ± 19.4 days	0.58

Abbreviation: *LOS* length of stay

70.11 Conclusions

The authors concluded that among normovolemic critically ill patients, a restrictive strategy with a transfusion threshold of 7.0 g/dl is at least as effective as a liberal strategy using a transfusion threshold of 10.0 gm/dl. A target hemoglobin level of 7–9 g/dl was comparable or even superior to a higher target level of 10.0–12.0 g/dl. In contrast to previous studies, a low transfusion trigger of 7 g/dl did not lead to adverse outcomes in patients with cardiac disease. The authors suggested that a transfusion threshold of 7.0 g/dl may be generalizable to most critically ill patients, except those with acute coronary syndrome.

70.12 Comments

The TRICC trial challenged the use of tradition-borne, arbitrary transfusion thresholds and provided strong evidence that injudicious administration of red cells might lead to adverse outcomes. It questioned the purported benefits of targeting oxygen delivery by raising hemoglobin levels in critically ill patients. The trial addressed appropriate clinical outcomes, with analysis by intention to treat. The mean APACHE II score was 21, with 80% patients on mechanical ventilation, and nearly 37% on vasoactive medication, all suggesting a fairly high severity of illness at baseline. Thus, the study is applicable to most real-world ICUs. There was a substantial difference in the number of units transfused between the restrictive and liberal groups, with 33% patients in the restrictive group not receiving any transfusion.

70.13 Criticisms

The study excluded a large number of patients. Nearly 87% of patients who were initially screened were excluded for various reasons; of the 3206 eligible subjects, only 838 were randomized (26.1%). A substantial number of patients were excluded either because the clinician did not agree to participate (598 patients) or the family refused consent (603 patients). Randomization was stratified according to an

APACHE II score of ≤15 or >15; however, inexplicably, subgroup analysis was based on an APACHE II score of ≤20 compared with >20. The study included only 838 patients, against the calculated sample size of 1620 patients. Patients with traumatic brain injury were considered to be a population vulnerable to the harmful effects of anemia; perhaps a subgroup analysis may have been relevant. The study excluded elective cardiac surgical patients, leading to many cardiac surgical units holding on tenaciously to the time-honored hemoglobin threshold of 10 g/dl. The study was performed during a period when leucodepletion was not in common practice. The question remained whether transfusion of leucodepleted blood would make a difference in clinical outcomes.

70.14 The Aftermath and Relevance in Today's World

Historically, transfusion practices were largely based on tradition. Critically ill patients were considered to be especially prone to adverse outcomes related to anemia. A hemoglobin level of 10, corresponding to a hematocrit of 30% was considered to optimize oxygen delivery in critical illness. This dogmatic approach may have led to overzealous transfusion practices and resulted in innumerable adverse clinical outcomes.

The TRICC trial triggered a wind of change among clinicians, supporting lower hemoglobin levels under most clinical circumstances. The findings of this landmark study were bolstered by many clinical trials that were published later. The TRISS trial, using leucodepleted blood, compared transfusion thresholds of 7.0 vs. 9.0 g/dl in patients with septic shock and found no difference in the 90-day mortality [9]. The TRACS trial evaluated patients who underwent cardiac surgery under cardiopulmonary bypass. A target hematocrit of ≥24% was compared with ≥30% in the liberal group [10]. The composite primary outcome, including the 30-day all-cause mortality, cardiogenic shock, acute respiratory distress syndrome, and acute kidney injury requiring renal replacement therapy, was similar between the two groups. The TRICS III RCT further strengthened the evidence for a restrictive strategy among cardiac surgical patients using a transfusion trigger of 7.5 g/dl [11].

The TRICC trial was carried out in an era when clinicians were sharply divided on red cell transfusion thresholds in critically ill patients. Although the study was planned to recruit 2300 patients over 5 years, with just a year remaining, physicians and patients were increasingly reluctant to participate. The study was closed after randomizing 838 patients, well short of the calculated sample size. Paul Hébert and his co-investigators were surprised when their analysis revealed that a restrictive transfusion strategy seemed to be no worse, and even superior compared with a liberal strategy [12]. Subsequent studies over the years largely corroborated their findings. This pioneering trial from more than two decades ago, comparing transfusion thresholds, remains a landmark in the field of critical care medicine.

70.15 Summary

The TRICC trial was a multicenter, randomized, controlled trial that investigated the impact of different red blood cell (RBC) transfusion strategies in critically ill patients. The study compared a restrictive transfusion strategy (maintaining hemoglobin levels between 7.0 and 9.0 g/dL) with a liberal transfusion strategy (maintaining hemoglobin levels between 10.0 and 12.0 g/dL). A total of 838 critically ill patients were enrolled and randomly assigned to one of the two strategies.

The primary outcome was 30-day mortality, with secondary outcomes including organ dysfunction and ICU length of stay. The results showed no significant difference in overall mortality between the two groups, but the restrictive strategy was associated with lower in-hospital mortality in less critically ill patients and those under 55 years of age. Additionally, the restrictive group required fewer transfusions and experienced fewer complications, such as infections and cardiac events.

The TRICC trial concluded that a restrictive transfusion strategy is at least as effective as a liberal one in most critically ill patients and may be beneficial in certain subgroups. This study has had a significant impact on transfusion practices, promoting a more conservative approach in ICU settings.

References

1. Meyer KA. The history of the Cook County Hospital blood bank. Q Bull Northwest Univ Evanst Ill Med Sch. 1949;23(3):318–20.
2. Adams RC, Lundy JS. Anesthesia in cases of poor surgical risk: some suggestions for decreasing the risk. Anesthesiology. 1942;3(5):603–7.
3. Welch HG. Prudent strategies for elective red blood cell transfusion. Ann Intern Med. 1992;116(5):393.
4. Perioperative red blood cell transfusion. JAMA. 1988;260(18):2700–3.
5. Friedman BA, Burns TL, Schork MA. An analysis of blood transfusion of surgical patients by sex: a question for the transfusion trigger. Transfusion (Paris). 1980;20(2):179–88.
6. Bordin JO, Heddle NM, Blajchman MA. Biologic effects of leukocytes present in transfused cellular blood products. Blood. 1994;84(6):1703–21.
7. Baker CH, Wilmoth FR, Sutton ET. Reduced RBC versus plasma microvascular flow due to endotoxin. Circ Shock. 1986;20(2):127–39.
8. Hébert PC, Martin C, Yetisir E. A multicenter, randomized, controlled clinical trial of transfusion requirements in critical care. N Engl J Med. 1999;340(6):409–17.
9. Holst LB, Haase N, Wetterslev J, Wernerman J, Guttormsen AB, Karlsson S, et al. Lower versus higher hemoglobin threshold for transfusion in septic shock. N Engl J Med. 2014;371(15):1381–91.
10. Hajjar LA, Vincent JL, Galas FRBG, Nakamura RE, Silva CMP, Santos MH, et al. Transfusion requirements after cardiac surgery: the TRACS randomized controlled trial. JAMA. 2010;304(14):1559.
11. Mazer CD, Whitlock RP, Fergusson DA, Hall J, Belley-Cote E, Connolly K, et al. Restrictive or liberal red-cell transfusion for cardiac surgery. N Engl J Med. 2017;377(22):2133–44.
12. Transfusion Trigger [Internet]. 50 Landmark Papers every Intensivist Should Know. CRC Press; 2021 [cited 2023 Jan 3]. Available from: https://www.taylorfrancis.com/chapters/edit/10.1201/9781003042136-39/transfusion-trigger-manish-patel-jeffrey-carson.

Transfusion Thresholds in Septic Shock: The TRISS Trial

71

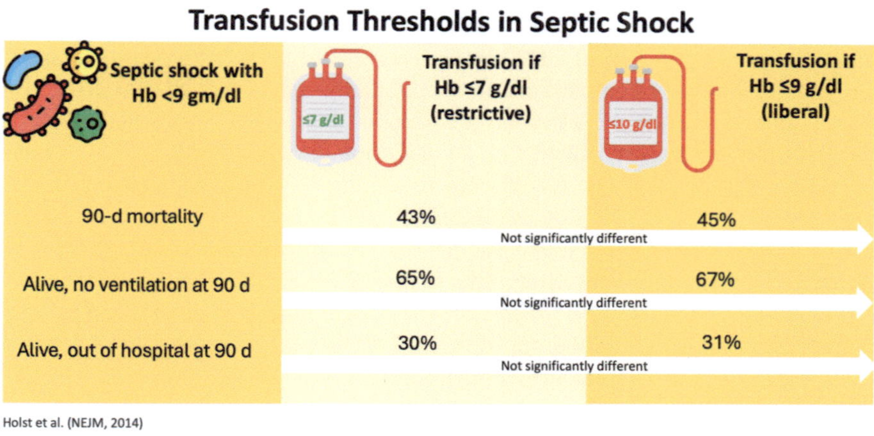

Quick Take

Does a lower hemoglobin threshold for transfusion improve outcomes in patients with septic shock?

The TRISS trial aimed to determine whether a lower hemoglobin threshold for red blood cell transfusion could improve outcomes in patients with septic shock. This multicenter, randomized controlled trial enrolled over 1000 critically ill patients with septic shock and randomized them to receive either a lower hemoglobin threshold for transfusion (7 g/dL) or a higher threshold (9 g/dL). The study demonstrated that a lower hemoglobin threshold (7 g/dL) did not result in higher

---

Holst LB, Haase N, Wetterslev J, Wernerman J, Guttormsen AB, Karlsson S, et al. Lower versus higher hemoglobin threshold for transfusion in septic shock. N Engl J Med. 2014 Oct 9;371(15):1381–91.

J. Chacko et al., *Landmark Studies in Critical Care*,
https://doi.org/10.1007/978-981-95-0673-6_71

mortality compared to the higher threshold (9 g/dL). Furthermore, the lower threshold group showed comparable or better outcomes in terms of organ failure and mechanical ventilation. These findings suggested that a restrictive transfusion strategy (7 g/dL threshold) is safe and may be preferable in septic shock patients.

71.1 Introduction

Patients with septic shock often require blood transfusion [1]. At the time of the conduct of the TRISS trial, the surviving sepsis guidelines recommended a hematocrit >30% during the initial phase of resuscitation among patients in septic shock with evidence of hypoperfusion. Following the initial phase, a hemoglobin level of 7–9 gm/dl was recommended, with a transfusion threshold of <7 gm/dl, in those with no evidence of myocardial ischemia, severe hypoxemia, or acute hemorrhage [2]. However, there was no firm evidence to support these guidelines. Besides, the PROCESS trial had already been published, in which patients randomized to the early goal-directed therapy (EGDT) group received red cell transfusions to maintain the hematocrit >30% [3]. In this three-armed randomized controlled trial (RCT), the 60-day mortality in the EGDT group was similar to those who received a protocol-based standard therapy managed with a transfusion threshold of 7.5 gm/dl, or usual care, thus casting doubts on the efficacy of aiming for a higher hemoglobin level during the resuscitation phase of septic shock.

The landmark TRICC trial had compared transfusion thresholds in critically ill patients who were euvolemic after initial treatment [4]. Patients were randomized to a restrictive or liberal arm. In the restrictive arm, patients received red cell transfusions if the hemoglobin level dropped below 7.0 gm/dl, to maintain a level between 7 and 9 gm/dl; in the liberal arm, a higher threshold of 10 gm/dl was followed, to maintain the hemoglobin level between 10 and 12 gm/dl. The 30-day mortality was similar overall in both groups; subgroup analysis did not reveal a difference in mortality and among patients ≥55 years or those with more severe disease at baseline [4].

Park et al. analyzed a prospective observational database aiming to evaluate the impact of blood transfusions on patients with severe sepsis or septic shock [5]. On propensity analysis of 152 matched pairs, they observed a lower risk of 7-day, 28-day, and in-hospital mortality in patients who were transfused compared with those who were not.

It remained unclear whether the transfusion strategy in patients with septic shock—liberal vs. restrictive—would have a significant impact on clinical outcomes. The TRISS trial was conceived considering the paucity of evidence regarding optimal transfusion thresholds, amid concerns of safety. The trial aimed to evaluate clinical outcomes associated with a lower compared with a higher transfusion threshold among patients with septic shock [6].

71.2 Population and Design

The TRISS trial was conducted during a 2-year period between December 2011 and December 2013 across 32 ICUs in Denmark, Sweden, Norway, and Finland. The study population included patients who fulfilled the criteria for septic shock with a hemoglobin concentration of ≤9 g/dl. Patients were randomly assigned in a 1:1 ratio to receive blood transfusion at a higher or a lower hemoglobin threshold [6].

71.2.1 Excluded

Patients who refused blood transfusion, those with serious adverse reactions to blood products, acute myocardial ischemia, and life-threatening bleeding were excluded. Patients who had already received red cell transfusion during the current ICU admission, acute burn injury, and those in whom active therapy had been discontinued were also excluded.

71.3 Lower Hemoglobin Threshold

Patients were transfused with single units of cross-matched, pre-storage leukoreduced red cells when the hemoglobin concentration dropped to ≤7 g/dl.

71.4 Higher Hemoglobin Threshold

Transfusion was carried out when the hemoglobin concentration was ≤9 g/dl

71.5 Both groups

Transfusion was carried out in single units; the hemoglobin level was re-estimated within 3 h of transfusion before carrying out another transfusion. The total duration of intervention was the entire ICU stay, or 90 days post-randomization. Transfusion was allowed in case of life-threatening bleeding or ischemia and during the use of extracorporeal membrane oxygenation based on a threshold determined by the clinician.

71.6 Sample Size

The sample size was calculated based on the 90-day mortality, the primary outcome. The authors assumed a mortality reduction of 9 percentage points in the lower-threshold group (from 45% in the higher-threshold group to 36% in the lower-threshold group). A sample size of 1000 patients provided the study with 80%

power at a two-sided alpha level of 5% to demonstrate this difference in the 90-day mortality.

71.7 Results

A total of 1005 patients underwent randomization; 998 were included in the analysis of the 90-day mortality—502 in the lower-threshold group and 496 in the higher-threshold group. Patients were well-matched at baseline, with a median age of 67 years. The lowest median hemoglobin level in the 24 h preceding randomization was 8.4 g/dl in both groups. The most common source of infection was the lung, followed by intra-abdominal and urinary tract infection. The severity of illness was similar at baseline, with a median SOFA score of 10 in both groups. In the lower-threshold group, 348/502 (68.7%) patients underwent mechanical ventilation compared with 350/496 (70.6%) in the higher-threshold group. Renal replacement therapy was performed at baseline among 13.5% of patients in the lower-threshold group and 10.7% of patients in the higher-threshold group. Protocol violations were significantly higher in the lower-threshold group.

During the trial period, the number of transfusions administered was much higher in the higher-threshold group (3088 vs. 1545, $P = 0.001$). The median cumulative transfusion was one unit in the lower-threshold group compared with four units in the higher-threshold group ($P < 0.001$). In the lower-threshold group, 36.1% of patients did not receive a transfusion compared with 1.2% in the higher-threshold group.

71.8 The Primary Outcome: 90-Day Mortality

At 90 days post-randomization, the mortality was similar in both groups. In the lower threshold group, 216/502 (43%) patients had died compared with 223/496 (45%) in the higher threshold group (relative risk, 0.94; 95% CI, 0.78–1.09; $P = 0.44$). The results were similar on per-protocol and risk-adjusted analysis. On pre-defined subgroup analysis, there was no difference in mortality between the two groups among patients who were 70 years or older, those with a SAPS II score of >53, or chronic cardiovascular disease.

71.9 Secondary Outcomes

The use of life support measures (vasopressor or inotropic support, mechanical ventilation, or renal replacement therapy) at days 5, 14, and 28 after randomization was similar in both groups. The incidence of ischemic events (myocardial, cerebral, intestinal, or limb ischemia) was similar. At 90 days of follow-up, the number of days alive without vasopressor or inotropic support, alive without mechanical ventilation, and alive without renal replacement therapy were not significantly different

Table 71.1 Main study outcomes

Outcome	Lower hemoglobin threshold	Higher hemoglobin threshold	Relative risk, *P* value
90-day mortality	216/502 (43.0%)	223/496 (45.0%)	0.94 (0.78–1.09) $P = 0.44$
Alive without vasopressor or inotropic therapy at 90 days (mean % of days)	73	75	$P = 0.93$
Alive without mechanical ventilation at 90 days (mean % of days)	65	67	$P = 0.49$
Alive without renal-replacement therapy at 90 days (mean % of days)	85	83	$P = 0.54$
Alive and out of the hospital at 90 days—mean % of days	30	31	$P = 0.89$
Ischemic events in the ICU (%)	7.2%	8.0%	0.90 (0.58–1.39) $P = 0.64$

between the two groups. Furthermore, the number of days alive and out of the hospital at 90 days was also similar. The main clinical outcomes are summarized in Table 71.1.

71.10 Study Conclusions

In septic shock, transfusion at a lower hemoglobin threshold of ≤7 g/dl resulted in similar rates of 90-d mortality, ischemic events, and the use of life support compared to a higher threshold of ≤9 g/dl. The findings were similar in patients with chronic cardiovascular disease, older age groups, and those with more severe illness. Those allocated to the lower threshold group received 50% less transfusions; 36% in this group did not receive transfusions compared with just 1% in the higher threshold group.

71.11 Strengths

The TRISS trial was an adequately powered, multicentric trial that evaluated hemoglobin thresholds for transfusion among patients with septic shock. The study followed a pragmatic protocol that adhered to standard practice in the management of patients with septic shock. There was a clear separation in median hemoglobin levels between the two groups of 1.5–2.0 gm/dl throughout the duration of the study. The study established the safety of the use of a lower transfusion threshold in septic shock—contrary to the approach followed in the Early Goal-Directed Therapy (EGDT) protocol proposed by Rivers et al. Investigators who assessed the primary outcome were blinded to group assignment, limiting the possibility of bias. The majority of patients who were screened were included in the study; furthermore, patients were recruited from hospitals that offered different levels of care—including university and non-university hospitals. Patient characteristics and outcomes were similar to observations from contemporaneous clinical trials of septic shock, enhancing generalizability [1, 2].

71.12 Weaknesses

The study was unblinded due to practical reasons—investigators and clinicians were aware of the study arm, which could have led to bias. Protocol violations occurred; however, per protocol analysis did not reveal a significant difference between groups in the 90-day mortality, the primary outcome. Sepsis-related interventions were not evaluated, although the large sample size and the multicentric design reduced the likelihood of imbalance between groups. The wide confidence interval suggested that a 9% relative increase or 22% decrease in the 90-day mortality could not be entirely ruled out. The study was not powered to assess secondary outcomes, including ischemic events and the impact of chronic cardiovascular disease.

71.13 Follow-Up Study

In a subsequent study, the TRISS investigators evaluated outcomes at 1-year follow-up, including mortality and health-related quality of life. The 1-year mortality was similar in both groups (lower-threshold vs. higher-threshold: 53.5% vs. 54.6%); the mortality rates remained similar at the longest median follow-up of 21 months. Data on health-related quality of life was available in 629 patients recruited from Denmark; there was no significant difference between the two groups [7].

71.14 Summary

The TRISS trial randomized patients with septic shock to a lower (7 gm/dl) compared with a higher (9 gm/dl) transfusion threshold during the ICU stay. Baseline characteristics were similar in both groups. The lower-threshold group received a median of 1 unit of blood during the ICU stay compared with 4 units in the higher-threshold group. The 90-day mortality, the primary outcome, was similar in both groups. Among the secondary outcomes, the use of life support measures was similar in both groups at days 5, 14, and 28 post-randomization. The restrictive strategy halved the transfusion rates, with no evidence of harm. Three large multicentric RCTs that compared EGDT with usual care [PROCESS [3], PROMISE [8], and

ARISE [9]] subsequently confirmed the lack of benefit of liberal transfusion strategy during the resuscitation phase of septic shock, thus echoing the findings of the TRISS trial.

References

1. Rosland RG, Hagen MU, Haase N, Holst LB, Plambech M, Madsen KR, et al. Red blood cell transfusion in septic shock – clinical characteristics and outcome of unselected patients in a prospective, multicentre cohort. Scand J Trauma Resusc Emerg Med. 2014;22:14.
2. Dellinger RP, Levy MM, Rhodes A, Annane D, Gerlach H, Opal SM, et al. Surviving Sepsis Campaign: international guidelines for management of severe sepsis and septic shock, 2012. Intensive Care Med. 2013;39(2):165–228.
3. PROCESS Investigators, Yealy DM, Kellum JA, Huang DT, Barnato AE, Weissfeld LA, et al. A randomized trial of protocolbased care for early septic shock. N Engl J Med. 2014;370(18):1683–93.
4. Hébert PC, Wells G, Blajchman MA, Marshall J, Martin C, Pagliarello G, et al. A multicenter, randomized, controlled clinical trial of transfusion requirements in critical care. N Engl J Med. 1999;340(6):409–17.
5. Park DW, Chun BC, Kwon SS, Yoon YK, Choi WS, Sohn JW, et al. Red blood cell transfusions are associated with lower mortality in patients with severe sepsis and septic shock: a propensity-matched analysis*. Crit Care Med. 2012;40(12):3140–5.
6. Holst LB, Haase N, Wetterslev J, Wernerman J, Guttormsen AB, Karlsson S, et al. Lower versus higher hemoglobin threshold for transfusion in septic shock. N Engl J Med. 2014;371(15):1381–91.
7. Rygård SL, Holst LB, Wetterslev J, Winkel P, Johansson PI, Wernerman J, et al. Long-term outcomes in patients with septic shock transfused at a lower versus a higher haemoglobin threshold: the TRISS randomised, multicentre clinical trial. Intensive Care Med. 2016;42(11):1685–94.
8. Mouncey PR, Osborn TM, Power GS, Harrison DA, Sadique MZ, Grieve RD, et al. Trial of early, goal-directed resuscitation for septic shock. N Engl J Med. 2015;372(14):1301–11.
9. ARISE Investigators, ANZICS Clinical Trials Group, Peake SL, Delaney A, Bailey M, Bellomo R, et al. Goal-directed resuscitation for patients with early septic shock. N Engl J Med. 2014;371(16):1496–506.

Part XIX

COVID-19 Pneumonia

Remdesivir for COVID-19 Pneumonia: The ACTT-1 Trial

72

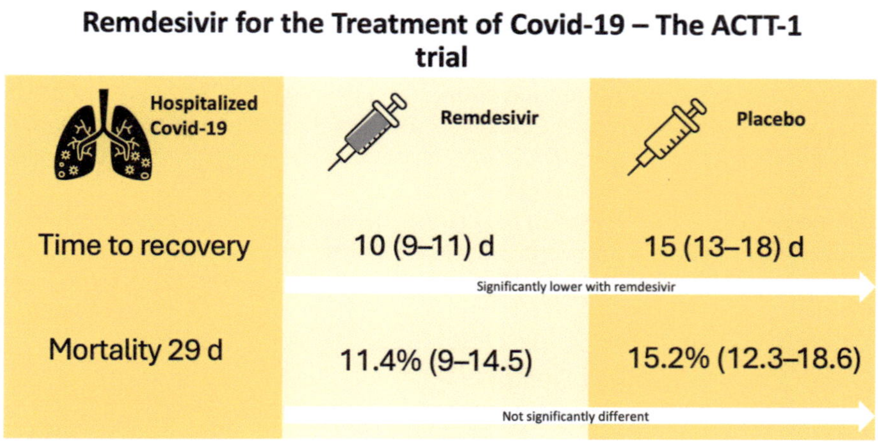

Beigel et al. (NEJM 2020)

Quick Take

Does the anti-viral agent, remdesivir, improve outcomes in hospitalized patients with COVID-19?

This multicenter, double-blind, randomized, placebo-controlled trial evaluated the efficacy of remdesivir in hospitalized patients with COVID-19. The study included 1062 patients and demonstrated that a 10-day course of remdesivir significantly reduced the median time to recovery (from 15 days to 10 days) compared to placebo. While there was a trend toward reduced mortality in the remdesivir group (11.4% vs. 15.2%), this finding did not reach statistical

---

Beigel JH, Tomashek KM, Dodd LE, Mehta AK, Zingman BS, Kalil AC, et al. Remdesivir for the Treatment of COVID-19 – Final Report. N Engl J Med. 2020 Nov 5;383(19):1813–26.

J. Chacko et al., *Landmark Studies in Critical Care*,
https://doi.org/10.1007/978-981-95-0673-6_72

significance. The trial established remdesivir as the first antiviral agent to show clinical benefit in COVID-19, particularly for patients requiring oxygen support but not yet on mechanical ventilation. The ACTT-1 trial reveals how remdesivir shortens recovery time for hospitalized COVID-19 patients, marking a milestone in antiviral therapy.

72.1 Introduction and Background

A severe type of acute respiratory syndrome was first reported from Wuhan, China, in December 2019. Within weeks, it spread across the globe, carrying with it a heavy toll of mortality and morbidity. The causative agent was identified as SARS-CoV-2, a novel coronavirus; the disease was designated as COVID-19 by the World Health Organization. Around the world, healthcare resources were rapidly overwhelmed, and the quest for effective therapy commenced with a sense of urgency.

The antiviral agent, remdesivir, an inhibitor of viral RNA synthesis, was previously shown to have in vitro activity against the SARS-CoV-1 and the MERS-CoV viruses. Considering its in vitro inhibitory effect on SARS-CoV-2, remdesivir held promise as an antiviral agent in COVID-19. Besides, studies of remdesivir in rhesus macaques inoculated with MERS-CoV revealed a reduction in viral levels and attenuation of lung involvement [1].

Considering the pressing need for therapeutic options in severe COVID-19, the ACTT-1 investigators designed an adaptive platform clinical trial to evaluate the safety and efficacy of remdesivir [2].

72.2 Population and Design

The ACTT-1 trial was conducted across 73 sites in the United States, Denmark, the United Kingdom, Greece, Germany, Korea, Mexico, Spain, Japan, and Singapore. The study population included adult patients admitted to the hospital with a laboratory-confirmed diagnosis of COVID-19. Patients were randomized to receive remdesivir or a placebo. Randomization was stratified by trial site and severity of the disease at baseline. The disease was considered severe if oxygen saturation was $\leq$94% on ambient air, the respiratory rate was $\geq$24/minute, and if supplemental oxygen or mechanical ventilation was required.

72.3 Remdesivir Group

Intravenous remdesivir was administered in a loading dose of 200 mg on day 1 of treatment, followed by 100 mg daily from day 2 to day 10 or until discharge from the hospital or death.

72.4 Placebo Group

Patients were allocated to receive a matching placebo of the same volume and according to the same schedule.

72.5 Common Management

Supportive care was based on the standard of care at the trial site. The study did not allow the use of other experimental or off-label treatment specific for COVID-19 from day 1 to day 29.

Patients were considered to have recovered based on an eight-category ordinal scale if: 1, if they were not hospitalized with no limitation of activity, 2, not hospitalized, but with limitation of activity, or requirement for home oxygen, or 3, hospitalized, but not requiring supplemental oxygen or continued medical care (hospitalized to prevent disease transmission or other non-medical reasons). The clinical status in categories 4–8 on the scale (considered not to have recovered) was as follows:

4. Hospitalized for continued medical care, but not requiring supplemental oxygen
5. Hospitalized and requiring supplemental oxygen
6. Hospitalized, on non-invasive ventilation or high-flow devices
7. Hospitalized, on invasive mechanical ventilation or extracorporeal respiratory support
8. Death

A comparison of the clinical status on day 15 on the eight-category ordinal scale was initially proposed as the primary outcome; however, it became apparent during the study that COVID-19 ran a more prolonged course. Hence, the primary outcome was revised to a comparison of the time to recovery by day 29.

72.6 Results

Over the approximately 2-month study period, 1062 COVID-19 patients were randomized—541 were assigned to the remdesivir arm, and 521 to the placebo group, representing the intention-to-treat population. The study population was predominantly male (64.4%) and the mean age was 58.9 years. The median duration of illness until randomization was 9 days (interquartile range, 6–12 days).

72.6.1 The Primary Outcome: Time to Recovery

Patients who received remdesivir recovered more rapidly compared with placebo. By day 29, the median time to recovery was 10 days in the remdesivir group compared with 15 days in the placebo group. The rate ratio for recovery was 1.29 (95% confidence interval: 1.12 to 1.49) in favor of remdesivir. Among patients with severe disease at baseline, the median time to recovery was 11 days in the remdesivir group, compared with 18 days in the placebo group (rate ratio for recovery, 1.31; 95% CI, 1.12 to 1.52, in favor of remdesivir). However, among patients on mechanical ventilation or ECMO, there was no significant difference in the time to recovery between the two groups.

The recovery rate was highest among patients with an ordinal score of 5 at baseline. Earlier treatment with remdesivir, within the first 10 days of illness, was associated with a higher rate of recovery compared to later treatment.

72.6.2 Secondary Outcomes

By day 15, mortality was lower in the remdesivir group (6.7% vs. 11.9%; hazard ratio, 0.55; 95% CI, 0.36–0.83). The mortality rate by day 29 was not significantly different between the two groups (11.4% vs. 15.2%). Akin to recovery rates, the highest impact of remdesivir on mortality was seen among patients with an ordinal score of 5 at baseline.

Improvement by one or two categories on the ordinal scale was higher among remdesivir-treated patients compared with placebo. Time to discharge or to attain a National Early Warning Score (NEWS) of 2 or less was shorter in the remdesivir group. Treatment with remdesivir resulted in a shorter initial duration of hospitalization; however, readmissions occurred slightly more often in the remdesivir group.

Among patients who were on supplemental oxygen at enrollment, the duration of oxygen therapy was lower with remdesivir compared to placebo. Among those who were not on oxygen at baseline, the use of supplemental oxygen was less in the remdesivir group. Commencement of non-invasive ventilation and high-flow oxygen therapy was lower in those who received remdesivir.

72.6.3 Safety Outcomes

The incidence of adverse events was similar in both groups. No deaths were attributed to either treatment arm. The main study outcomes are summarized in Table 72.1.

Table 72.1 Main study outcomes

Outcome	Remdesivir	Placebo	Significance
Time to recovery (median, 95% CI)	10 (9–11) days	15 (13–18) days	RR, 1.29; 95% CI, 1.12–1.49 $P < 0.001$
Time to recovery in severe disease (median, 95% CI)	11 (10–14) days	18 (15–20) days	RR, 1.31; 95% CI, 1.12–1.52
Mortality, day 15 (%, 95% CI)	6.7 (4.8–9.2)	11.9 (9.4–15)	HR, 0.55; 95% CI, 0.36–0.83
Mortality, day 29 (%, 95% CI)	11.4 (9–14.5)	15.2 (12.3 –18.6)	HR, 0.73; 95% CI, 0.52 –1.03
Time to discharge or MEWS ≤2 for 24 h (median, 95% CI)	8.0 (7.0–9.0) days	12.0 (10.0–15.0) days	HR, 1.27; 95% CI, 1.10–1.46

Abbreviations: *CI* confidence interval, *RR* rate ratio, *HR* hazard ratio, *MEWS* modified early warning score

72.7 Study Conclusions

The ACTT-1 trial found that remdesivir significantly shortened the recovery time in hospitalized COVID-19 patients, reducing the median recovery from 15 to 10 days compared to placebo. The greatest benefit was observed in patients requiring supplemental oxygen but not mechanical ventilation. However, remdesivir did not show a significant reduction in mortality.

72.8 Strengths

The ACTT-1 authors conducted the first large RCT to evaluate the efficacy of remdesivir in COVID-19 at an early stage of the pandemic in multiple centers across the globe. The investigators overcame arduous challenges against the background of travel restrictions, continued clinical responsibilities, and illness among staff members. The multicentric design offered generalizability. Randomization was stratified by center and disease severity, and analysis was based on intention-to-treat, adding to the robustness of the trial.

72.9 Limitations

The efficacy of remdesivir was largely confined to less requirement for respiratory support, especially among patients who required supplemental oxygen (category 5 on the ordinal scale). Concomitant therapies were not standardized and were based on local practice. The primary outcome was initially based on the clinical status on day 15 on the eight-category ordinal scale. However, as the pandemic progressed, it became apparent that COVID-19 ran a more prolonged course. Hence, after the enrolment of 72 patients, the primary outcome was revised to the time to recovery.

Recovery was defined as meeting categories 1, 2, or 3 on the eight-category ordinal scale in the first 28 days after study enrolment. Due to a shortage of matching placebo, normal saline was used at some sites, which may have affected blinding with the possibility of bias. Follow-up was limited to 29 days after enrolment; hence, longer-term outcomes remained unknown.

72.10 Subsequent Evidence

In a 2023 systematic review, Grundeis et al. assessed the impact of remdesivir on clinical outcomes compared with standard care among patients with COVID-19 infection [3]. They included nine RCTs with 11,218 patients, of whom 5932 were assigned to receive remdesivir. Most patients were on supplemental oxygen at baseline. Based on moderate-certainty evidence, the authors found no significant difference in the all-cause mortality for up to 28 or 60 days. Besides, there was no significant difference in hospital mortality for up to 150 days.

Clinical improvement at 28 days occurred more often, and the risk of clinical worsening was lower with remdesivir. The rate of hospitalization was lower with remdesivir in a single study including patients with mild to moderate disease [4].

The authors concluded that remdesivir does not impact all-cause or in-hospital mortality in patients with moderate to severe COVID-19. However, it may have a positive impact on disease progression with more rapid clinical improvement among hospitalized and non-hospitalized patients, although the certainty of evidence was limited.

72.11 Summary

The ACTT-1 RCT supported the efficacy of remdesivir as antiviral therapy in the treatment of COVID-19. Remdesivir treatment led to a more rapid recovery compared with placebo. Improvement by one or two categories on the ordinal scale occurred earlier, and the time to discharge from the hospital was shorter. However, the all-cause mortality did not differ significantly between the two groups. Progression to more severe disease appeared to be lower with remdesivir treatment. Patients with a baseline ordinal score of 5 (hospitalized, requiring supplemental oxygen) appeared to benefit the most with remdesivir. Based on the findings of the trial, the Food and Drug Administration in the US issued an Emergency Use Authorization for remdesivir use.

References

1. de Wit E, Feldmann F, Cronin J, Jordan R, Okumura A, Thomas T, et al. Prophylactic and therapeutic remdesivir (GS-5734) treatment in the rhesus macaque model of MERS-CoV infection. Proc Natl Acad Sci USA. 2020;117(12):6771–6.
2. Beigel JH, Tomashek KM, Dodd LE, Mehta AK, Zingman BS, Kalil AC, et al. Remdesivir for the treatment of COVID-19 – final report. N Engl J Med. 2020;383(19):1813–26.
3. Grundeis F, Ansems K, Dahms K, Thieme V, Metzendorf MI, Skoetz N, et al. Remdesivir for the treatment of COVID-19. Cochrane Database Syst Rev. 2023;1(1):CD014962.
4. Gottlieb RL, Vaca CE, Paredes R, Mera J, Webb BJ, Perez G, et al. Early remdesivir to prevent progression to severe COVID-19 in outpatients. N Engl J Med. 2022;386(4):305–15.

73 Dexamethasone in COVID-19 Infection: The RECOVERY Trial

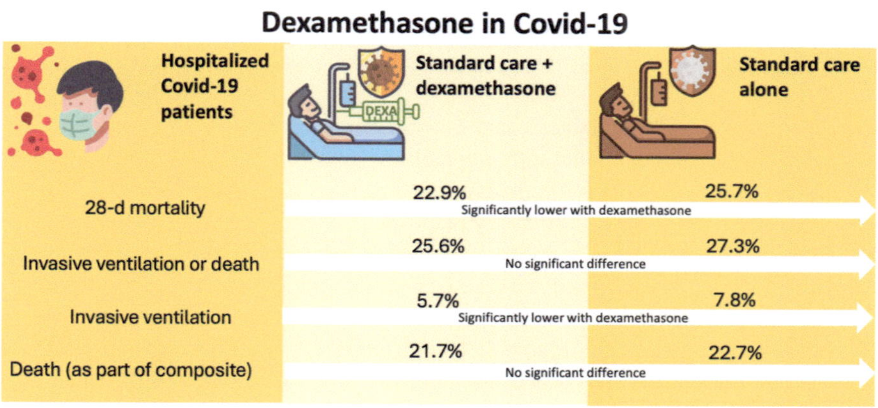

Quick Take

Does dexamethasone improve survival in hospitalized COVID-19 patients?

The RECOVERY trial investigated whether dexamethasone, a corticosteroid, could improve survival in patients hospitalized with COVID-19. This large, multicenter randomized controlled trial enrolled over 6000 patients and compared the effects of dexamethasone (6 mg daily for up to 10 days) with standard care. The study found that dexamethasone significantly reduced 28-day mortality in patients receiving invasive mechanical ventilation or oxygen, but it had no benefit in patients who did not require respiratory support. The trial provided strong evidence that

---

The RECOVERY Collaborative Group. Dexamethasone in Hospitalized Patients with COVID-19. N Engl J Med. 2021 Feb 25;384(8):693–704.

J. Chacko et al., *Landmark Studies in Critical Care*,
https://doi.org/10.1007/978-981-95-0673-6_73

low-dose dexamethasone improves survival in severe COVID-19, establishing it as a key treatment in managing the disease in hospitalized patients, especially those with respiratory distress.

73.1 Introduction

A novel coronavirus infection caused by the SARS-CoV-2 virus broke out in the Chinese city of Wuhan in late 2019 [1]. Although most infections were mild, the outbreak rapidly spread across Asia, Europe, and the rest of the world by early 2020, leading to substantial mortality and morbidity. Amid increasing concern following the affliction of large patient populations, the World Health Organization (WHO) declared COVID-19 a pandemic in March 2020 [2]. Severe hypoxemic respiratory failure requiring respiratory support led to the rapid overwhelming of healthcare systems across the globe. Several agents were employed by clinicians in the early phase of the pandemic; however, apart from the administration of the antiviral agent remdesivir [3], no therapeutic agent revealed a favorable impact on clinical outcomes.

Severe COVID-19 is characterized by widespread consolidation and extensive radiological involvement. The pathophysiology involves diffuse alveolar damage, inflammatory changes, and microvascular thrombosis [4]. Corticosteroids were employed to counter the inflammatory response in other types of viral pneumonia, including severe acute respiratory syndrome (SARS), avian influenza, and seasonal influenza; however, there was considerable debate regarding efficacy and impact on clinical outcomes [5].

In a previous randomized controlled trial (RCT), 64 patients with COVID-19 who were on supplemental oxygen, but not receiving ventilatory support, with evidence of systemic inflammatory response were evaluated to assess the efficacy of corticosteroids. Patients were assigned to receive methylprednisolone 40 mg twice daily, intravenously, for 3 days, followed by 20 mg twice daily for another 3 days, compared with standard care alone. The primary outcome, a composite of death, non-invasive ventilation, or ICU admission, did not significantly differ between the methylprednisolone and standard care groups. However, on per-protocol analysis, the composite endpoint was significantly lower in methylprednisolone-treated patients [6].

When the RECOVERY trial was designed, there was no evidence from large RCTs regarding the benefit of corticosteroid therapy in COVID-19. Guideline recommendations varied, but the general consensus seemed to suggest that corticosteroids may be harmful. Practices among clinicians across the globe were also variable; some case series reported corticosteroid use in up to 50% of cases [7]. Considering the lack of consistent evidence and diverse practice, the RECOVERY investigators designed a large RCT to evaluate the efficacy of dexamethasone among hospitalized patients with COVID-19 [8].

73.2 Study Design

The RECOVERY trial aimed to evaluate the impact of different treatment modalities among patients hospitalized with COVID-19 across 176 hospitals of the National Health Service in the United Kingdom. The trial was based on an adaptive platform design that tested multiple treatments simultaneously in different arms of the study. New treatment arms could be added as fresh evidence emerged.

Eligible patients included those hospitalized with a clinical or laboratory-confirmed diagnosis of COVID-19 infection. The initial multi-arm design randomized patients in a 2:1 ratio to receive usual care alone or usual care combined with dexamethasone, hydroxychloroquine, lopinavir-ritonavir, or azithromycin in a 2:1:1:1:1 ratio.

73.3 The Standard Care vs. Dexamethasone Arm

The standard care vs. standard care plus dexamethasone study was conducted between March and June 2020 and included 6425 patients with COVID-19 infection. The study initially included patients who were >18 years old but was later modified to include patients in all age groups. Pregnant and breastfeeding women could also be included.

73.3.1 Exclusion

Based on the clinician's judgement, those with a medical history likely to subject them to significant risk if they participated in the trial were excluded. Patients in whom dexamethasone was considered to be definitely indicated or contraindicated based on clinician judgment were also excluded. Patients were excluded from the dexamethasone arm of the trial if the drug was unavailable at the time of randomization.

73.4 Dexamethasone Group

Dexamethasone was administered in a dose of 6 mg per day, by the intravenous or oral route, for up to 10 days or until hospital discharge, whichever occurred earlier. Pregnant and breastfeeding women were administered prednisolone 40 mg orally or hydrocortisone 80 mg twice daily intravenously.

73.5 Usual Care Group

Standard care represented the usual care provided at the participating hospital.

73.6 Sample Size

The sample size was based on the 28-day mortality, the primary outcome. However, COVID-19-related mortality was unclear at the time of commencement of the trial. During the course of the trial, the steering committee estimated the mortality to be 20%. Assuming an absolute reduction in mortality of 4 percentage points with dexamethasone, the authors calculated a sample size of 6000 patients (2000 in the dexamethasone group and 4000 in the control group). This sample size provided the study with at least 90% power at a two-sided P value of 0.01.

73.7 Results

Recruitment was ceased on June 8, 2020, after reaching the target sample size. By this time, 6425 patients had been randomized—2104 to the dexamethasone group and 4321 to standard care.

The mean age of patients was 66.1 ± 15.7 years; the majority were male patients (64%). Major comorbidities were present in 56% of patients, including diabetes (24%), heart disease (27%), and chronic lung disease (21%). The median duration of dexamethasone treatment was 7 days; 95% of patients received at least one dose. Only five patients received remdesivir as it was not available during the early phase of the study.

At randomization, 60% of patients were receiving supplemental oxygen with or without non-invasive ventilation, while 16% were on invasive mechanical ventilation or extracorporeal support.

73.8 The Primary Outcome: 28-Day Mortality

The 28-day mortality was significantly lower with dexamethasone compared with standard care alone. At 28 days, 482/2104 (22.9%) of patients had died in the dexamethasone group compared with 1110/4321 (25.7%) in the standard care group ($P < 0.001$). The mortality benefit was most profound with dexamethasone treatment among patients on invasive mechanical ventilation (29.3% vs. 41.4%). Lower mortality was also observed among patients receiving supplemental oxygen with or without non-invasive ventilation (23.3% vs. 26.2%). There was an age-adjusted absolute mortality reduction of 12.3 percentage points among patients on invasive ventilation and 4.2 percentage points among those receiving supplemental oxygen alone.

The mortality was not significantly different among patients who were not on any respiratory support; in fact, there was a suggestion of possible harm in this subgroup of patients (28-day mortality: 17.8% vs. 14.0%).

Dexamethasone-related mortality reduction was greater among patients with a more prolonged illness at randomization. Patients with a duration of illness of <7 days did not appear to benefit from dexamethasone.

Table 73.1 Main study outcomes

Outcome	Dexamethasone	Standard care	Rate ratio or risk ratio (95% CI)
28-day mortality	482/2104 (22.9%)	1110/4321 (25.7%)	0.83 (0.75–0.93)
Discharged alive at 28 days	1413/2104 (67.2%)	2745/4321 (63.5%)	1.10 (1.03–1.17)
Composite of invasive ventilation or death (among those not on invasive ventilation at randomization)	25.6%	27.3%	0.92 (0.84–1.01)
Invasive ventilation (as part of the above composite outcome)	5.7%	7.8%	0.77 (0.62–0.95)
Death (as part of the above composite outcome)	21.7%	22.7%	0.93 (0.84–1.03)
Median duration of hospitalization	12 days	13 days	

73.9 Secondary Outcomes

The median duration of hospital stay was one day shorter in the dexamethasone group compared to the standard care group (12 vs. 13 days). Dexamethasone-treated patients were also more likely to be discharged alive at 28 days—this effect was most pronounced in patients who were on invasive mechanical ventilation at the time of randomization.

Among those who were not on invasive mechanical ventilation at randomization, the composite outcome of invasive mechanical ventilation or death was lower in the dexamethasone group—an effect more profound among those who were on supplemental oxygen at randomization. Overall, the likelihood of progression to invasive ventilation was lower in the dexamethasone group. The main study outcomes are summarized in Table 73.1.

73.10 Study Conclusions

In hospitalized patients with COVID-19, dexamethasone was associated with a lower 28-day mortality among those on invasive mechanical ventilation or receiving supplemental oxygen at randomization. There was no benefit observed in patients who did not require respiratory support at randomization; the findings suggested possible harm among these patients.

73.11 Strengths

The RECOVERY trial was a large RCT that adopted a simple approach and enrolled patients over a relatively brief period in the middle of the COVID-19 pandemic. The trial was an important milestone that clearly demonstrated the feasibility of conducting crucial clinical research in the setting of an outbreak. The adaptive platform allowed newer agents to be added to the trial as new data emerged; besides, agents that were proven to be ineffective could be removed from the investigative platform. Nearly 10% of patients hospitalized in the National Health Service in the United Kingdom were included in the trial, adding robustness and validity to the study. Approximately 95% of patients allocated to the dexamethasone arm received at least one dose of the drug. The study evaluated clinically important outcomes, including mortality; follow-up was nearly complete. Analysis was by intention to treat; besides, the authors also performed age-adjusted analysis. The study also included clinically relevant subgroup analysis.

The RECOVERY trial revealed that dexamethasone, a cheap, easily available agent, could save lives in patients with severe COVID-19. The efficacy appeared to be more profound in the most severely ill patients and the later phase of the disease.

73.12 Limitations

The trial was unblinded, raising the likelihood of bias. Due to the lack of availability of dexamethasone at some centers, a few patients were excluded. Follow-up was not carried out in 5% of the study population as they had not completed 28 days post-randomization at the time of publication. Standard care was not protocolized, considering the severe constraints on healthcare systems imposed by the pandemic, and the relative lack of evidence regarding the efficacy of therapeutic interventions in the initial phase of the outbreak. The sample size could not be calculated at the outset due to a lack of data regarding outcomes from COVID-19 and could have led to a false-positive result (type I error). Longer-term follow-up is likely to be important, especially considering the possibility of disease sequelae. Details regarding the baseline severity of illness were not available, particularly considering that the reported mortality appeared higher compared to contemporaneous data from other healthcare systems [9].

73.13 Other Evidence

Many investigators evaluated the efficacy of corticosteroids in COVID-19 around the same period that the RECOVERY trial was conducted. Most of these trials were terminated once the results of the RECOVERY trial became available.

The CoDEX RCT was conducted in 41 Brazilian ICUs and compared dexamethasone 20 mg, once daily for 5 days, intravenously, followed by 10 mg intravenously once daily for 5 more days or until ICU discharge with standard care alone among patients with COVID-19-related severe acute respiratory distress syndrome [10]. The study was terminated before reaching the calculated sample size as the results of the RECOVERY trial were published, and continuation of the trial was considered unethical in the face of strong evidence suggesting benefit with dexamethasone. The study had enrolled 299 patients at the time of cessation—151 in the dexamethasone group and 148 in the standard care group. The number of days alive and mechanical ventilation-free in the first 28 days was significantly higher in the dexamethasone group compared with the standard care group (mean: 6.6 days vs. 4.0 days). There was no significant difference between groups in the 28-day all-cause mortality, ICU-free days, and the duration of mechanical ventilation.

The multi-centric CAPE-COVID trial from France was conducted as an embedded trial as part of an ongoing RCT evaluating the efficacy of corticosteroids in treating community-acquired pneumonia [11]. This trial was also terminated when the RECOVERY trial results became available. In this RCT, hydrocortisone did not reduce mortality or persistent dependence on mechanical ventilation or high-flow oxygen at 21 days (defined as treatment failure) compared with placebo. Furthermore, there was no significant difference in the proportion of patients undergoing mechanical ventilation on day 21.

The REMAP-CAP trial was an adaptive platform trial that tested multiple therapeutic interventions in patients with severe COVID-19 [12]. In the corticosteroid domain of the study, patients were randomized to one of three arms—a 7-day treatment with hydrocortisone 50 or 100 mg intravenously every 6 h, or 50 mg every 6 h only when shock was clinically evident, or no hydrocortisone. This study revealed a potential benefit of hydrocortisone in reducing the requirement for organ support. The 7-day and the shock-dependent course revealed 93% and 80% probabilities of superiority compared with no hydrocortisone regarding higher organ support-free days at 21 days.

73.14 Summary

The RECOVERY trial was conducted during the peak of the COVID-19 pandemic when healthcare systems around the globe became severely overburdened. At that time, no specific or effective therapeutic interventions were on the horizon, although several were being evaluated, including hydroxychloroquine, azithromycin, convalescent plasma, ivermectin, and several antiviral agents. Against this background, the RECOVERY investigators embarked upon a clinical trial based on an adaptive platform that planned to evaluate multiple treatment modalities. In the dexamethasone arm of the study, hospitalized patients with clinically suspected or laboratory-confirmed disease were randomized to receive dexamethasone or standard care alone in a 1:2 ratio. Dexamethasone was administered in a dose of 6 mg per day, by the intravenous or oral route for up to 10 days or until hospital discharge, whichever occurred earlier. Overall, the 28-day mortality was significantly lower among dexamethasone-treated patients. Among patients who received dexamethasone, mortality was lowest among patients on invasive mechanical ventilation, followed by those on supplemental oxygen or non-invasive ventilatory support. No mortality difference was observed among patients who were not on respiratory support at randomization. The median duration of hospital stay was shorter among patients treated with dexamethasone. The likelihood of being discharged alive at 28 days was also higher in the dexamethasone arm—an effect that was most pronounced among patients on invasive mechanical ventilation at randomization. In the midst of a global pandemic, the RECOVERY trial offered robust evidence for a cheap and effective therapy in improving survival among patients with severe COVID-19 infection.

References

1. Zhu N, Zhang D, Wang W, et al. A novel coronavirus from patients with pneumonia in China, 2019. N Engl J Med [Internet]. 2020 [cited 2024 May 24];382(8).
2. Cucinotta D, Vanelli M. WHO declares COVID-19 a pandemic. Acta Biomed. 2020;91(1):157–60.
3. Beigel JH, Tomashek KM, Dodd LE, Mehta AK, Zingman BS, Kalil AC, et al. Remdesivir for the treatment of COVID-19 – final report. N Engl J Med. 2020;383(19):1813–26.
4. Carsana L, Sonzogni A, Nasr A, Rossi RS, Pellegrinelli A, Zerbi P, et al. Pulmonary postmortem findings in a series of COVID-19 cases from northern Italy: a two-centre descriptive study. Lancet Infect Dis. 2020;20(10):1135–40.
5. Shang L, Zhao J, Hu Y, Du R, Cao B. On the use of corticosteroids for 2019-nCoV pneumonia. The Lancet. 2020;395(10225):683–4.
6. Corral-Gudino L, Bahamonde A, Arnaiz-Revillas F, Gómez-Barquero J, Abadía-Otero J, García-Ibarbia C, et al. Methylprednisolone in adults hospitalized with COVID-19 pneumonia: an open-label randomized trial (GLUCOCOVID). Wien Klin Wochenschr. 2021;133(7–8):303–11.
7. Wang D, Hu B, Hu C, Zhu F, Liu X, Zhang J, et al. Clinical characteristics of 138 hospitalized patients with 2019 novel coronavirus-infected pneumonia in Wuhan, China. JAMA. 2020;323(11):1061–9.
8. RECOVERY Collaborative Group, Horby P, Lim WS, Emberson JR, Mafham M, Bell JL, et al. Dexamethasone in hospitalized patients with COVID-19. N Engl J Med. 2021;384(8):693–704.
9. Hodgson CL, Higgins AM, Bailey MJ, Mather AM, Beach L, Bellomo R, et al. Comparison of 6-month outcomes of survivors of COVID-19 versus non–COVID-19 critical illness. Am J Respir Crit Care Med. 2022;205(10):1159–68.
10. Tomazini BM, Maia IS, Cavalcanti AB, Berwanger O, Rosa RG, Veiga VC, et al. Effect of dexamethasone on days alive and ventilator-free in patients with moderate or severe acute respiratory distress syndrome and COVID-19: the CoDEX randomized clinical trial. JAMA. 2020;324(13):1307–16.
11. Dequin PF, Heming N, Meziani F, Plantefève G, Voiriot G, Badié J, et al. Effect of hydrocortisone on 21-day mortality or respiratory support among critically ill patients with COVID-19. JAMA. 2020;324(13):1–9.
12. Angus DC, Derde L, Al-Beidh F, Annane D, Arabi Y, Beane A, et al. Effect of hydrocortisone on mortality and organ support in patients with severe COVID-19: The REMAP-CAP COVID-19 corticosteroid domain randomized clinical trial. JAMA. 2020;324(13):1317–29.

Part XX

Miscellaneous

74 Acetaminophen for Fever in the Critically Ill: The HEAT Trial

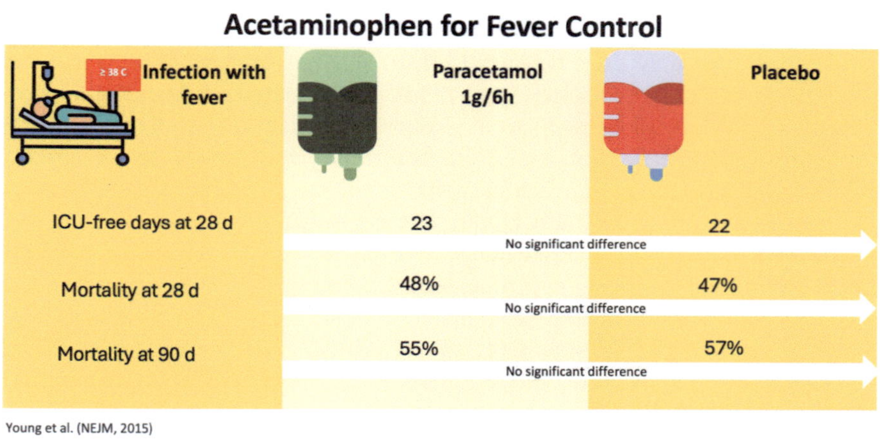

Quick Take

Does fever control matter in critically ill patients?

The HEAT randomized controlled trial (RCT) investigated the use of acetaminophen (paracetamol) to reduce fever in critically ill patients with suspected infection. The study compared the effects of acetaminophen administration to a placebo in these patients, specifically looking at outcomes including mortality, organ dysfunction, and temperature regulation. The results showed no significant difference in mortality or major clinical outcomes between the acetaminophen and placebo groups, despite a reduction in body temperature in the acetaminophen group. The

---

Young P, Saxena M, Bellomo R, Freebairn R, Hammond N, van Haren F, et al. Acetaminophen for Fever in Critically Ill Patients with Suspected Infection. N Engl J Med. 2015 Dec 3;373(23):2215–24.

J. Chacko et al., *Landmark Studies in Critical Care*,
https://doi.org/10.1007/978-981-95-0673-6_74

study concluded that fever reduction with acetaminophen in critically ill patients with suspected infection does not confer a survival benefit and is not associated with improvements in major clinical outcomes.

74.1 Introduction

Clinicians often resort to measures to control fever among critically ill patients based on the premise that elevation of body temperature places additional physiological stress and increases oxygen consumption [1]. The effect of external cooling to maintain normothermia in patients with septic shock was evaluated in an RCT [2]. The control group received no external cooling. After two hours of treatment, the body temperature was significantly lower in the external cooling group. A 50% reduction in the vasopressor dose and shock reversal were observed more often in patients who underwent external cooling. Furthermore, the 14-day mortality was also significantly lower in the external cooling group. On the other hand, a rise in body temperature may exert beneficial effects through augmentation of immune function [3], inhibition of bacterial growth [4], and increased efficacy of antimicrobial agents [5]. A previous retrospective cohort study had suggested that temperature control may be beneficial in traumatic brain injury and stroke. However, among patients with infections of the central nervous system, a rise in body temperature was not associated with mortality but, in turn, suggested benefit [6].

There was a paucity of robust evidence to evaluate the impact of acetaminophen administration in controlling fever of infective etiology among critically ill patients. The HEAT investigators hypothesized that fever control with acetaminophen would lead to an increase in ICU-free days among critically ill patients with probable infection and undertook an RCT to test their hypothesis [7].

74.2 Population and Design

The HEAT (Permissive Hyperthermia through Avoidance of Acetaminophen in Known or Suspected Infection in the Intensive Care Unit) trial was conducted between February 2013 and July 2014 in 23 medical-surgical ICUs in Australia and New Zealand. Adult patients with known or suspected infection and a temperature of ≥38 °C within 12 h prior to enrollment were eligible. Those with acute brain disorders, liver dysfunction, hyperthermia, and ongoing treatment with non-steroidal anti-inflammatory agents were excluded. Patients who were currently undergoing or likely to require therapeutic hypothermia and those who were moribund were also excluded. Eligible patients were randomly assigned in a 1:1 ratio to receive intravenous acetaminophen or a matching placebo. Randomization was carried out in blocks of six and stratified by center.

74.3 The Acetaminophen Group

Intravenous acetaminophen was administered in a dose of 1 g every 6 h as a 100 ml solution.

74.4 The Control Group

Patients in the control group received 5% dextrose in water every 6 h from an indistinguishable 100 ml container.

74.5 Both Groups

The study drug was continued until 28 days, discharge from the ICU, death, fever resolution, cessation of antimicrobial treatment, or emergence of a contraindication to acetaminophen. Fever resolution was determined using an algorithm and necessitated a temperature <38 °C for 48 h after withholding the study medication. Rescue physical cooling was allowed if the temperature rose to ≥39.5 °C. Following the course of the study agent, open-label acetaminophen was permitted.

74.6 Sample Size

The investigators assumed 16.0 ± 9.2 ICU-free days in the control group based on a previous prospective observational study [8]. The sample size was increased by 20%, allowing for loss to follow-up and to account for a rank-based test in statistical analysis. Thus, 700 patients provided the study with 80% power to detect a difference of 2.2 ICU-free days at 28 days, at an alpha level of 0.05.

74.7 Results

Among the 3601 patients who met the inclusion criteria, 700 were randomized; 346 patients in the paracetamol group and 344 patients in the placebo group were included in the final analysis.

Patients were well-matched at baseline. The mean APACHE II score was 19.1 ± 6.7 in the acetaminophen group and 18.7 ± 7.5 in the placebo group. More than 50% of patients in both groups were on invasive mechanical ventilation and vasopressor therapy. The lungs and the abdomen were the most common sites of infection. A causative pathogen was identified in a similar number of patients in both arms (acetaminophen vs. placebo: 62.5% vs. 62.2%). Open-label acetaminophen administration was similar in both groups (30% vs. 29.4%). Physical cooling and non-steroidal anti-inflammatory medications were used in a similar number of patients.

74.7.1 Fever Control

The peak (38.4 ± 1.0 °C vs. 38.6 ± 0.8 °C) and mean body temperatures (37.0 ± 0.6 °C vs. 37.3 ± 0.6 °C) were significantly lower in the acetaminophen group. Cessation of the study drug due to resolution of fever occurred more often in the acetaminophen group compared to the placebo group (22.8% vs. 16.9%).

74.7.2 The Primary Outcome: ICU-Free Days at Day 28

There was no significant difference between the acetaminophen and the placebo groups in the median number of ICU-free days until day 28 [23 days; IQR: 13–25 days vs. 22 days; IQR: 12–25 days; $P = 0.07$). The number of ICU-free days did not differ significantly among subgroups of patients with septic shock or temperature >39 °C; the primary outcome was also similar regardless of the location where the infection was acquired—community, hospital, or ICU.

74.7.3 Secondary Outcomes

The 28-day mortality (acetaminophen vs. placebo: 48% vs. 47%); and the 90-day mortality (55% vs. 57%) were not significantly different between groups. Other key secondary outcomes at 28 days were also similar in the acetaminophen and the control groups, including the median hospital-free days (12 vs. 10 days), mechanical ventilation-free days (27 vs. 26 days), inotrope and vasopressor-free days (27 days in both groups), renal replacement therapy-free days (28 days in both groups), and ICU support-free days (26 vs. 25 days).

Among 28-day survivors, the median length of stay in the ICU was significantly shorter with acetaminophen compared with placebo (3.5 vs. 4.3 days, $P = 0.1$). In contrast, among non-survivors, the median length of ICU stay was significantly longer among those who received acetaminophen (10.4 vs. 4.0 days, $P = <0.001$).

74.7.4 Adverse Events

The incidence of liver dysfunction was similar with acetaminophen and placebo (8.1% vs. 9.9%). A markedly elevated body temperature was observed in a patient who received a placebo; this patient did not survive. The main study findings are summarized in Table 74.1.

Table 74.1 Main study findings

Outcome	Acetaminophen (346 patients)	Placebo (344 patients)	Significance
ICU-free days at 28 days (median, IQR)	23 (13–25)	22 (12–25)	0.07
28-day mortality (number, %)	48 (13.9)	47 (13.7)	0.94
90-day mortality (number, %)	55 (15.9)	57 (16.6)	0.84
Ventilation-free days (median, IQR)	27 (19–28)	26 (17–28)	0.14
Vasoactive drug-free days (median, IQR)	27 (25–28)	27 (24–28)	0.36
RRT-free days (median, IQR)	28 (28–28)	28 (28–28)	0.53
ICU support-free days (median, IQR)	26 (16–27)	25 (15–27)	0.14

74.8 Study Conclusions

Acetaminophen administration for fever control in critically ill patients with suspected infection was associated with no significant impact on mortality or ICU-free days compared to placebo. Although acetaminophen use reduced fever more rapidly, there was no improvement in clinical outcomes, suggesting no clear benefit with routine use among critically ill patients.

74.9 Strengths

The HEAT trial sought answers to a hitherto unsettled clinical question—does acetaminophen administration among critically ill patients with fever impact important clinical outcomes? The multicentric study was conducted across 23 mixed ICUs in Australia and New Zealand, including a broad population of critically ill patients. The study was double-blinded; the placebo was dispensed in an indistinguishable 100 ml bottle. All analyses were carried out before unmasking the study groups, adding to the robustness of the trial. Follow-up was nearly complete, with data analyses of 98.6% of patients who were randomized.

74.10 Limitations

Data on patients who received acetaminophen before randomization were not available, which may have impacted outcomes. The duration of administration of acetaminophen was relatively short; it is unclear whether a longer duration of administration would improve outcomes. About one-third of patients in both groups received acetaminophen after completion of the course of the study drug. Hence, it may be argued that the study results apply only to the early administration of acetaminophen. Protocol violation and open-label administration of paracetamol occurred in nearly 30% of patients. The number of antibiotic days, a clinically meaningful outcome, was not reported. The ICU length of stay was shorter among 28-day survivors who received acetaminophen compared with placebo, and longer among non-survivors. The authors hypothesized that this paradox may arise due to earlier discharge from the ICU of patients in whom the fever had resolved; alternatively, clinicians may perceive fever control as a sign of clinical improvement and continue treatment for a longer duration in patients who are otherwise unlikely to survive. Finally, would the findings apply to enterally administered acetaminophen?

74.11 Subsequent Evidence

Holgersson et al. performed a systematic review with meta-analysis to evaluate the impact of fever therapy in a broad population. They included RCTs in patients with fever of varied etiology. The experimental group included patients who underwent any type of therapeutic intervention for fever; the control group received no fever therapy. The study included 42 trials of 5140 patients. Among the study subjects, 3007 were critically ill, while 1892 were not. Infectious fever occurred in 3277 compared with 1139 patients who had fever of non-infectious origin. The authors carried out meta-analysis and trial sequential analysis. Fever therapy was not found to reduce the risk of death (risk ratio 1.04, 95% confidence interval 0.90–1.19; $P = 0.62$) nor the risk of serious adverse events risk ratio 1.02, 95% confidence interval 0.89–1.17; $P = 0.78$).

74.12 Summary

In a binational, blinded RCT, the HEAT investigators evaluated the clinical effect of early administration of intravenous acetaminophen in ICU patients for the control of fever suspected to be of infective origin. Acetaminophen administration resulted in a modest, but statistically significant reduction in body temperature compared to patients who received a placebo (the peak temperature was 0.2 °C lower and the mean temperature 0.3 °C lower in the acetaminophen group). The median number of ICU-free days until day 28, the primary outcome, was not significantly different between the two groups. Among the important secondary outcomes, the mortality at 28 and 90 days, and the survival time until day 90 were also similar. The authors observed a shorter ICU stay among survivors and a longer stay among non-survivors in the acetaminophen group compared to the placebo group. They hypothesized that the difference in ICU stay may be related to the physiological effects of fever reduction or the clinician's perception of the severity of illness. The HEAT trial did not reveal improved clinical outcomes from acetaminophen use among critically ill patients with fever presumed to be of infective origin, a finding corroborated in a later meta-analysis of RCTs.

References

1. Manthous CA, Hall JB, Olson D, Singh M, Chatila W, Pohlman A, et al. Effect of cooling on oxygen consumption in febrile critically ill patients. Am J Respir Crit Care Med. 1995;151(1):10–4.
2. Schortgen F, Clabault K, Katsahian S, Devaquet J, Mercat A, Deye N, et al. Fever control using external cooling in septic shock: a randomized controlled trial. Am J Respir Crit Care Med. 2012;185(10):1088–95.
3. Berman JD, Neva FA. Effect of temperature on multiplication of Leishmania amastigotes within human monocyte-derived macrophages in vitro. Am J Trop Med Hyg. 1981;30(2):318–21.
4. Small PM, Täuber MG, Hackbarth CJ, Sande MA. Influence of body temperature on bacterial growth rates in experimental pneumococcal meningitis in rabbits. Infect Immun. 1986;52(2):484–7.
5. Mackowiak PA, Ruderman AE, Martin RM, Many WJ, Smith JW, Luby JP. Effects of physiologic variations in temperature on the rate of antibiotic-induced bacterial killing. Am J Clin Pathol. 1981;76(1):57–62.
6. Saxena M, Young P, Pilcher D, Bailey M, Harrison D, Bellomo R, et al. Early temperature and mortality in critically ill patients with acute neurological diseases: trauma and stroke differ from infection. Intensive Care Med. 2015;41(5):823–32.
7. Young P, Saxena M, Bellomo R, Freebairn R, Hammond N, van Haren F, et al. Acetaminophen for fever in critically ill patients with suspected infection. N Engl J Med. 2015;373(23):2215–24.
8. Young P, Saxena M, Eastwood GM, Bellomo R, Beasley R. Fever and fever management among intensive care patients with known or suspected infection: a multicentre prospective cohort study. Crit Care Resusc. 2011;13(2):97–102.

Step-Up Approach vs. Open Necrosectomy for Acute Necrotizing Pancreatitis: The PANTER Trial

75

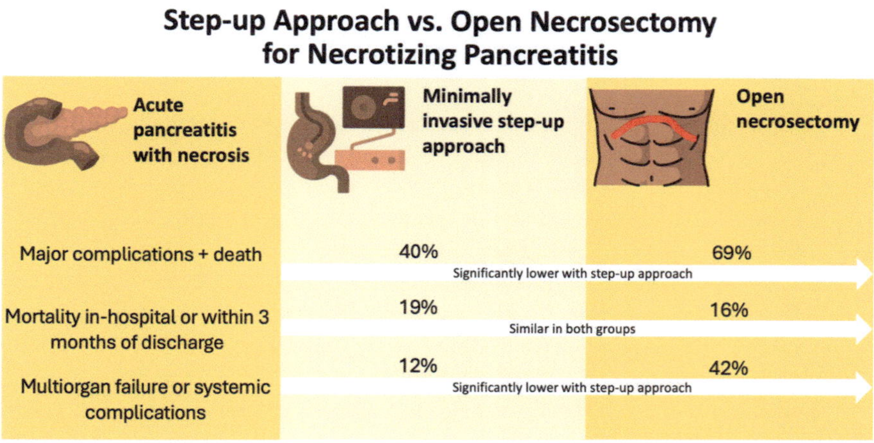

Van Santvoort et al. (NEJM, 2010)

Quick Take

Which strategy improves outcomes for patients with necrotizing pancreatitis—step-up or open necrosectomy?

The PANTER trial compared a step-up approach, involving minimally invasive techniques, with traditional open necrosectomy for the management of infected pancreatic necrosis in patients with severe acute pancreatitis. This randomized controlled trial enrolled over 200 patients and found that the step-up approach, which involved drainage followed by necrosectomy if necessary, resulted in fewer

---

Van Santvoort HC, Besselink MG, Bakker OJ, Hofker HS, Boermeester MA, Dejong CH, et al. A step-up approach or open necrosectomy for necrotizing pancreatitis. N Engl J Med. 2010 Apr 22;362(16):1491–502.

J. Chacko et al., *Landmark Studies in Critical Care*,
https://doi.org/10.1007/978-981-95-0673-6_75

complications, a shorter hospital stay, and similar or better survival rates compared to open surgery. The trial established that the step-up approach is a safer, more effective strategy for managing necrotizing pancreatitis, challenging the long-standing preference for open necrosectomy.

75.1 Introduction

Acute pancreatitis may be complicated by necrosis of the pancreatic or peripancreatic tissue, leading to sepsis and multiorgan failure, with a relatively high mortality [1]. Infected necrosis necessitates intervention as a source control measure [2, 3]. The conventional approach in this situation was open necrosectomy and complete removal of the infected, necrotic tissue [4]. However, an open approach may be associated with complications and high mortality, besides the risk of pancreatic insufficiency among survivors due to inadvertent excision of viable pancreatic tissue [5, 6]. Less invasive approaches include percutaneous [7] or endoscopic, transgastric drainage [8], and video-assisted necrosectomy through the retroperitoneal route [9].

Less invasive interventions may be performed in a stepwise manner, with percutaneous or endoscopic drainage initially, followed by retroperitoneal necrosectomy if the patient fails to improve. A step-up approach may ameliorate the impact of surgical trauma, the severe inflammatory reaction that often follows, and potentially reduce the incidence of complications [5].

Observational studies had previously suggested favorable outcomes with minimally invasive necrosectomy [5, 10] and endoscopic drainage [8, 11]. However, many of these studies did not have a control group; besides, less invasive procedures may have been preferred for patients with milder disease, leading to selection bias.

Considering the lack of robust evidence to support a minimally invasive strategy, the PANTER group of investigators conducted a randomized controlled trial (RCT) that compared a step-up approach with open necrosectomy among patients with necrotizing pancreatitis [12].

75.2 Population and Design

The Dutch Pancreatitis Study Group conducted the PANTER study between November 2005 and October 2008 across 19 centers in the Netherlands. The study enrolled adult patients with acute pancreatitis with signs of pancreatic or peripancreatic necrosis evident on a contrast-enhanced CT scan. Patients with suspected infected necrosis, in whom surgical intervention was planned, and those in whom drainage of the collection was considered feasible were also included. Suspected infected necrosis was defined as the persistence of sepsis or clinical worsening despite maximal supportive measures in the ICU, although infection of the necrotic tissue was not documented.

Patients were randomized to undergo primary open necrosectomy or a minimally invasive, step-up approach. Randomization was carried out in permuted blocks of four and stratified by center.

75.3 Open Necrosectomy

Laparotomy was performed through a bilateral subcostal incision. Necrotic tissue was excised by blunt dissection, followed by the insertion of two large-bore drains and abdominal closure.

75.4 Minimally Invasive Step-Up Approach

The first step of the minimally invasive approach was drainage of the collection percutaneously or by the endoscopic transgastric route. Lack of clinical improvement after 72 h was followed by a second drainage if the initial drain was inadequately positioned, or new drainable collections had formed in the meantime. If a second drainage was not feasible or if there were no signs of improvement after a further 72 h, the next step was followed. These patients, who failed to improve after the initial steps, underwent video-assisted retroperitoneal debridement guided by the retroperitoneal drain. Two large-bore drains were placed, and postoperative lavage was performed. If there was no retroperitoneal access and video-assisted drainage was not feasible, laparotomy and necrosectomy was carried out as in the control group.

75.5 Sample Size

The sample size was calculated based on the primary endpoint—a composite of major complications, and mortality in hospital or in the first 3 months after discharge. Major complications included new-onset multiorgan failure or systemic complications, perforation of a viscus requiring intervention, development of an enterocutaneous fistula, or intra-abdominal hemorrhage. The authors assumed a 64% relative reduction in the primary endpoint with the step-up approach (45% vs. 16%). A sample size of 88 patients was calculated, providing the study with 80% power at a two-sided alpha level of 0.05.

75.6 Results

A total of 88 patients were randomized during the 3-year trial period, including 45 patients in the primary open necrosectomy group and 43 in the minimally invasive step-up group.

75.6.1 The Primary Composite Endpoint: Major Complications or Death

The primary endpoint was significantly lower among patients who underwent the minimally invasive step-up approach [17/43 (40%) vs. 31/45 (69%), $P = 0.006$].

75.6.2 Components of the Primary Outcome

All the components of the primary outcome occurred more often in the open necrosectomy group; among these, the incidence of new-onset multiorgan failure and multiple systemic complications was significantly lower with the minimally invasive step-up approach.

Mortality in hospital or within 3 months of discharge was similar in both groups. Eight patients (19%) died in the minimally invasive step-up group compared with seven (16%) patients in the open necrosectomy group ($P = 0.70$).

Among the eight patients who died in the minimally invasive step-up group, seven died of multiorgan failure, and one due to hemorrhage. Among the seven who died in the open necrosectomy group, multiorgan failure was the cause of death in six; one patient died of pneumonia.

75.6.3 Other Outcomes

At 6 months of follow-up, incisional hernias (24% vs. 7%, $P = 0.03$) and new-onset diabetes (38% vs. 16%, $P = 0.02$) were more common in the open necrosectomy group. Healthcare resource utilization was lower in the minimally invasive step-up group. The minimally invasive step-up approach led to a reduction in the overall cost of care by 12%.

75.6.4 Subgroup Analysis

Treatment effect on the primary endpoint was similar across subgroups of patients based on the presence of organ failure at the time of randomization, and the timing of the intervention. The main study findings are summarized in Table 75.1.

Table 75.1 Main study outcomes

Outcome	Step-up approach (43 patients)	Open necrosectomy (45 patients)	P value
Mortality or major complications at 3 months (n, %)	17 (40)	31 (69)	0.006
Multiorgan failure or systemic complications	5 (12)	19 (42)	0.001
Intra-abdominal bleed requiring intervention	7 (16)	10 (22)	0.48
Enterocutaneous fistula or perforation of viscus requiring intervention	6 (14)	10 (22)	0.32

75.7 Study Conclusions

In patients with acute necrotizing pancreatitis with infection, a minimally invasive step-up approach compared with open necrosectomy reduced mortality and major complications, including new-onset multiorgan failure or systemic complications, perforation of a viscus requiring intervention, development of an enterocutaneous fistula, and intra-abdominal hemorrhage.

75.8 Strengths

The PANTER trial established the feasibility and efficacy of a minimally invasive approach in acute necrotizing pancreatitis, compared to the traditional open approach. Although minimally invasive interventions were already in vogue at the time of the conduct of the study, they had not been systematically evaluated in a controlled clinical trial.

75.9 Limitations

The study had a relatively small sample size, which could have resulted in a Type I error.

Repeated interventions were required in approximately one-third of patients in both groups, which was higher than the rate of reinterventions in contemporaneous studies [13]. The duration of hospitalization and overall mortality were also longer than previously reported [13–15]. Patients who underwent video-assisted retroperitoneal drainage required a protracted period of post-procedure lavage and drainage, which could have likely extended the duration of hospital stay and added to the cost of care.

The study did not address the question of whether video-assisted retroperitoneal debridement may be superior to the open technique when necrosectomy is necessary; the comparison was only between percutaneous drainage followed by video-assisted retroperitoneal drainage vs. open necrosectomy. The efficacy of treatment may vary depending on the consistency of the necrotic tissue—liquified necrosis may be more amenable to drainage, while solid tissue may still require open debridement. A minimally invasive approach is generally aimed at reducing the infective load by removing as much of the infected tissue as feasible, implying a higher number of interventions compared to open necrosectomy.

75.10 Follow-Up Study

In 2019, the Dutch Pancreatitis Study Group published results from long-term follow-up of patients who participated in the PANTER trial. Among the 88 patients who were originally randomized, all 73 survivors were followed up for a median duration of 86 months. The primary endpoint of death or major complications was significantly lower in the step-up group (44% vs. 73%). The incidence of incisional hernias (23% vs. 53%), and pancreatic exocrine (29% vs. 56%) or endocrine insufficiency (40% vs. 64%) was lower with the step-up strategy. The requirement for repeated interventions or pancreatic surgery was not significantly higher in the step-up group (11% vs. 13%). The incidence of chronic or recurrent acute pancreatitis was also similar in both groups. The overall quality of life increased in both groups. The authors concluded that a step-up approach for necrotizing pancreatitis is superior to open necrosectomy, with no increase in the requirement for repeated interventions.

75.11 Summary

In a multicentric RCT, the PANTER trial randomized patients with infected, acute necrotizing pancreatitis to undergo a minimally invasive step-up approach or open necrosectomy. The primary composite endpoint of mortality or the incidence of major complications was significantly lower with a minimally invasive strategy. Among the individual components of the primary outcome, new onset multiorgan failure was significantly lower with a minimally invasive approach; however, there was no difference in mortality between the two groups. Among other complications, the incidence of incisional hernias and new-onset diabetes was lower in the minimally invasive group.

The PANTER trial offered robust evidence that a minimally invasive step-up approach may be preferable compared to open necrosectomy in patients with infected, necrotizing pancreatitis. The step-up approach represented a paradigm shift, with open debridement considered only as a last step if minimally invasive interventions do not lead to clinical improvement. Following this ground-breaking trial, a minimally invasive step-up approach became more widespread and largely replaced open necrosectomy as the initial strategy in infected, necrotizing pancreatitis.

References

1. Whitcomb DC. Clinical practice. Acute pancreatitis. N Engl J Med. 2006;354(20):2142–50.
2. Nathens AB, Curtis JR, Beale RJ, Cook DJ, Moreno RP, Romand JA, et al. Management of the critically ill patient with severe acute pancreatitis. Crit Care Med. 2004;32(12):2524–36.
3. Uhl W, Warshaw A, Imrie C, Bassi C, McKay CJ, Lankisch PG, et al. IAP guidelines for the surgical management of acute pancreatitis. Pancreatology. 2002;2(6):565–73.
4. Traverso LW, Kozarek RA. Pancreatic necrosectomy: definitions and technique. J Gastrointest Surg. 2005;9(3):436–9.
5. Connor S, Alexakis N, Raraty MGT, Ghaneh P, Evans J, Hughes M, et al. Early and late complications after pancreatic necrosectomy. Surgery. 2005;137(5):499–505.
6. Tsiotos GG, Luque-de León E, Sarr MG. Long-term outcome of necrotizing pancreatitis treated by necrosectomy. Br J Surg. 1998;85(12):1650–3.
7. Freeny PC, Hauptmann E, Althaus SJ, Traverso LW, Sinanan M. Percutaneous CT-guided catheter drainage of infected acute necrotizing pancreatitis: techniques and results. AJR Am J Roentgenol. 1998;170(4):969–75.
8. Papachristou GI, Takahashi N, Chahal P, Sarr MG, Baron TH. Peroral endoscopic drainage/debridement of walled-off pancreatic necrosis. Ann Surg. 2007;245(6):943–51.
9. van Santvoort HC, Besselink MGH, Horvath KD, Sinanan MN, Bollen TL, van Ramshorst B, et al. Videoscopic assisted retroperitoneal debridement in infected necrotizing pancreatitis. HPB (Oxford). 2007;9(2):156–9.
10. Carter CR, McKay CJ, Imrie CW. Percutaneous necrosectomy and sinus tract endoscopy in the management of infected pancreatic necrosis: an initial experience. Ann Surg. 2000;232(2):175–80.
11. Gardner TB, Chahal P, Papachristou GI, Vege SS, Petersen BT, Gostout CJ, et al. A comparison of direct endoscopic necrosectomy with transmural endoscopic drainage for the treatment of walled-off pancreatic necrosis. Gastrointest Endosc. 2009;69(6):1085–94.
12. Van Santvoort HC, Besselink MG, Bakker OJ, Hofker HS, Boermeester MA, Dejong CH, et al. A step-up approach or open necrosectomy for necrotizing pancreatitis. N Engl J Med. 2010;362(16):1491–502.
13. Rodriguez JR, Razo AO, Targarona J, Thayer SP, Rattner DW, Warshaw AL, et al. Debridement and closed packing for sterile or infected necrotizing pancreatitis: insights into indications and outcomes in 167 patients. Ann Surg. 2008;247(2):294–9.
14. Howard TJ, Patel JB, Zyromski N, Sandrasegaran K, Yu J, Nakeeb A, et al. Declining morbidity and mortality rates in the surgical management of pancreatic necrosis. J Gastrointest Surg. 2007;11(1):43–9.
15. Parikh PY, Pitt HA, Kilbane M, Howard TJ, Nakeeb A, Schmidt MC, et al. Pancreatic necrosectomy: North American mortality is much lower than expected. J Am College Surg. 2009;209(6):712.

76 Intra-aortic Balloon Counterpulsation in Cardiogenic Shock Following Acute Myocardial Infarction: The IABP-SHOCK II Trial

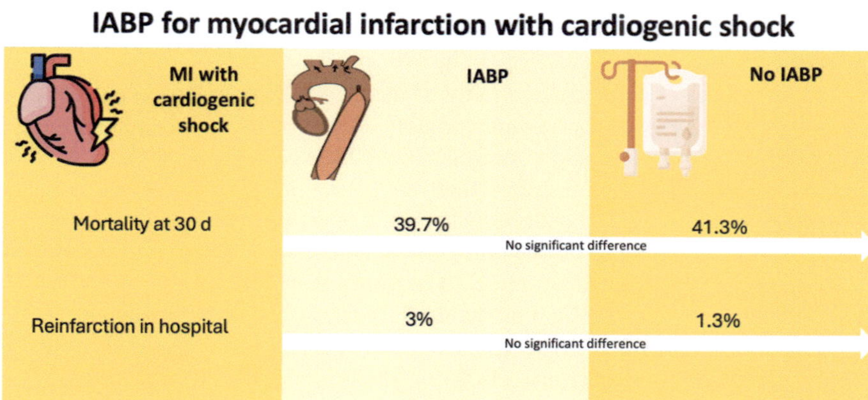

Thiele et al. (NEJM, 2012)

Quick Take

Does the intra-aortic balloon pump (IABP) save lives in cardiogenic shock following acute myocardial infarction?

The IABP-SHOCK II trial was a multicenter, randomized controlled trial that aimed to evaluate the effectiveness of IABP therapy in patients with acute myocardial infarction (MI) complicated by cardiogenic shock. The study compared the outcomes of patients treated with IABP and those who received standard medical therapy without IABP. The trial found no significant difference in 30-day mortality between the two groups, suggesting that IABP did not provide a mortality benefit in

---

Thiele H, Zeymer U, Neumann FJ, Ferenc M, Olbrich HG, Hausleiter J, et al. Intraaortic Balloon Support for Myocardial Infarction with Cardiogenic Shock. N Engl J Med. 2012 Oct 4;367(14):1287–96.

J. Chacko et al., *Landmark Studies in Critical Care*,
https://doi.org/10.1007/978-981-95-0673-6_76

this cohort. Despite prior suggestions of the benefit of IABP for improving survival in cardiogenic shock, the findings of the IABP-SHOCK II trial led to a reassessment of its routine use in these patients.

76.1 Introduction

The concept of diastolic augmentation of coronary blood flow in patients with left ventricular failure arose in the 1950s. Animal experimenters attempted wrapping of the hemidiaphragm around the distal thoracic aorta with stimulation in diastole to provide counterpulsation [1]. Following laboratory studies, early investigations employed a latex balloon at the tip of a small plastic catheter using carbon dioxide as the driving gas [2]. The balloon inflated in diastole to augment coronary blood flow and deflated in systole, thereby reducing left ventricular afterload. Early attempts at balloon augmentation were unsuccessful, probably because the relatively high viscosity of carbon dioxide resulted in slow transit through the tubing and delayed balloon filling.

Cardiogenic shock carried a mortality of more than 85% in those days, despite pharmacological support. The administration of vasopressors, including norepinephrine by continuous infusion, seemed to have little effect on mortality. In 1968, Kantrovitz and colleagues described their early experience with the "intra-aortic cardiac assistance" device in patients with cardiogenic shock following acute myocardial infarction [3]. Their device consisted of a 60 cm long polytetrafluoroethylene tubing with a 14.8 cm long pumping chamber at the distal end. In contrast to earlier studies, they used helium as the driving gas; its low density enabled rapid transit through the tubing. The device was timed to inflate in systole and deflate in diastole by synchronizing with the ECG or the arterial pressure transducer. After many years of animal experimentation, the device was ready for clinical use.

On the early morning of June 29, 1967, a 45-year-old woman presented with acute myocardial infarction to the Maimonides Medical Center in Brooklyn, New York. She was clearly in distress, cold and blue, and had no palpable pulses. She was treated with digitalis and infusions of norepinephrine and isoprenaline; however, after nearly 5 h, she was in unrelenting shock. As her condition appeared hopeless, they commenced balloon pumping as a last resort. Within the first few hours, her blood pressure rose, the central venous pressure dropped, and urine started flowing. By 7 h of pumping, she had turned the corner—the cyanosis had disappeared, and her extremities felt warm. She was off pharmacological support throughout the duration of pumping and remained stable after the removal of the device. Following this, her hospital stay was relatively uneventful, and she was discharged home. Similar encouraging results were observed in a 58-year-old man with acute myocardial infarction and cardiogenic shock. However, during a brief interruption of pumping to reposition the balloon, he developed refractory ventricular fibrillation that rendered the balloon ineffective [3].

Although initial results were encouraging, long years of disappointment followed; there were few survivors in these early case series. The intra-aortic balloon pump (IABP) seemed to be on the verge of quietly fading away into history. However, considering the apparent hemodynamic effects, sporadic use continued among patients with acute low-output syndromes.

More than five decades have passed since the first report of IABP. The management of acute myocardial infarction has witnessed a sea change in the meantime, with several watershed moments, including early revascularization by percutaneous coronary intervention (PCI), the introduction of novel therapeutic agents, and advancements in intensive care support. However, the mortality from cardiogenic shock continued to be high [4]. Although the hunt for the holy grail of mechanical support continues, the IABP remains the most sought-after device in cardiogenic shock following acute myocardial infarction.

76.2 Background to the Study

The earlier IABP-SHOCK trial had evaluated the efficacy of IABP combined with PCI in reducing the onset of multiorgan dysfunction syndrome in patients with cardiogenic shock following acute myocardial infarction. In a randomized controlled trial (RCT) conducted between 2003 and 2004, 45 consecutive patients were assigned to standard care combined with IABP or standard care alone. IABP support did not lead to a significant improvement in the multiorgan dysfunction syndrome over 4 days, based on the APACHE II scores. IABP use did not have any significant impact on the cardiac index or activation of systemic inflammation, based on plasma IL-6 levels [5]. However, the study was limited by a small sample size and its single-center design. The question of any beneficial effect on mortality also remained unanswered. The recommendations for IABP use by the American and European guidelines were largely based on limited evidence from registry data. IABP use had also remained highly variable, ranging between 25% and 40% [6]. Against this background, the IABP-SHOCK II Trial investigators proposed testing their hypothesis that the additional use of this support modality may reduce mortality among patients with acute myocardial infarction and cardiogenic shock compared with medical therapy alone [7].

76.3 Population and Design

The IABP-SHOCK II trial was conducted between June 2009 to March 2012 across 37 centers in Germany. Patients who presented with acute myocardial infarction and cardiogenic shock and planned for early revascularization were eligible. Cardiogenic shock was defined as a systolic BP of <90 mm Hg for >30 min, or the requirement for catecholamines, with pulmonary congestion and impaired organ perfusion. The diagnosis of organ perfusion was based on one of the following features: altered sensorium, cold and clammy extremities, urine output of <30 ml/h, or serum lactate levels >2 mmol/l. Patients were randomly assigned to receive IABP or standard care alone (control group).

76.3.1 Excluded

They study excluded patients older than 90 years, those who had undergone resuscitation for >30 min, had fixed dilated pupils, or developed a mechanical complication leading to shock, including ventricular septal defect or ruptured papillary muscle. Patients who were in shock for >12 h, had severe peripheral vascular disease that prevented device insertion, severe aortic regurgitation, or were not expected to survive for >6 months were also excluded.

76.4 IABP Group

Device insertion was carried out before or immediately after PCI based on the clinician's judgment. Support was commenced with 1:1 triggering and weaned down once the systolic BP remained >90 mm Hg for 30 min without catecholamine support.

76.5 Common Management

Early revascularization was planned along with the most optimal medical management based on guidelines. The mode of revascularization—target lesion alone, or correction of other lesions, either at the same time or at a later stage, was at clinician's discretion. The option for coronary artery bypass grafting was also left to the clinician's judgment.

76.6 Sample Size

The study was powered to detect a difference of 12 percentage points in the 30-day survival, the primary endpoint, assuming 56% mortality in the control group. The type I error level was set at 0.05. The authors calculated a sample size of 282 patients in each group with two planned interim analyses after enrollment of 33% and 66% of the original sample size.

76.7 Results

Seven hundred and ninety patients were screened over a 3-year period; 600 were included—301 in the IABP group and 299 in the control group. Patients were well-matched at baseline. A similar number of patients in both groups underwent resuscitation and fibrinolysis before randomization. The baseline systolic BP and lactate levels were also similar. ST-elevation myocardial infarction occurred in 66.7% of patients in the IABP group compared with 71.1% in the control group. IABP was inserted in 30 patients who were randomized to the control group; 26 of these crossovers were protocol violations. Thirteen patients randomized to undergo IABP did not receive the intervention; most had died before the procedure could be carried out. Revascularization was by PCI in most patients (95.8%), while 3.5% underwent emergency coronary artery bypass surgery. In the final analysis, there were 300 patients in the IABP group and 298 in the control group.

76.7.1 The Primary Outcome: 30-Day Mortality

There was no significant difference in the primary outcome, the 30-day mortality, between the IABP and control groups. In the IABP group, 39.7% of patients died, compared with 41.3% in the control group (relative risk: 0.96; 95% CI, 0.79–1.17; $P = 0.69$). On per-protocol analysis, the relative risk of mortality was similar.

The relative risk of mortality remained similar after multivariate modeling, adjusting for variables including non-ST-elevation myocardial infarction, anterior wall myocardial infarction, resuscitation before randomization, and the study site. On subgroup analysis, there was no difference in the 30-day survival based on age, gender, history of hypertension, type of myocardial infarction, previous infarction, the presence of hypothermia, or systolic BP <80 mm Hg.

76.7.2 Secondary Outcomes

Among the secondary outcomes, no significant difference was noted in the time to hemodynamic stabilization, ICU length of stay, serum lactate levels, dose and duration of treatment with catecholamine infusions, and renal function between the two groups. The timing of IABP insertion—whether before or after revascularization did not affect outcomes. The incidence of reinfarction in the hospital and stent thrombosis was also similar in both groups.

Overall, 33 patients (5.5%) received a ventricular assist device. More patients in the control group underwent insertion of a ventricular assist device. Mortality was higher among patients who received a ventricular assist device compared to those who did not.

76.7.3 Safety Outcomes

Safety outcomes, including major bleeding, limb ischemia requiring intervention, stroke (ischemic or hemorrhagic), and sepsis, were similar in both groups. The main study outcomes are summarized in Table 76.1.

Table 76.1 Main study outcomes

Outcomes	IABP group	Control group	Significance
30-day all-cause mortality	39.7%	41.3%	$P = 0.69$
Re-infarction in hospital	3%	1.3%	$P = 0.16$
Stroke in hospital	0.7%	1.7%	$P = 0.40$
Median catecholamine days	3.0	3.0	$P = 0.81$
Median ventilation days	3.0	3.0	$P = 0.44$
Median ICU days	6.0	6.0	$P = 0.34$

Abbreviation: *IABP* intra-aortic balloon pump

76.8 Study Conclusions

Among patients with acute myocardial infarction with cardiogenic shock who were planned for early revascularization, intra-aortic balloon counterpulsation did not lead to improved survival at 30 days. Besides, there was no significant difference in hemodynamic stabilization, use of catecholamine therapy, renal function, and lactate levels compared to the control group. The incidence of major bleeding was also similar in both groups.

76.9 Strengths

The IABP shock trial, in a large RCT, questioned the perceived benefits of IABP in cardiogenic shock following acute myocardial infarction.

The authors carried out an RCT employing a device that was widely considered to be beneficial and recommended by guidelines, over a 3-year period across 37 centers in Germany. This represents a commendable achievement and poses several questions regarding the appropriateness of IABP use in patients with cardiogenic shock. All except two patients were included in the primary outcome analysis with minimal loss to follow-up. This landmark study was a logical culmination of several previous studies, including the IABP-SHOCK trial, that had raised questions regarding the perceived usefulness of IABP. After the publication of this trial, IABP use has been downgraded in guidelines [8] with a decline in clinical use [9]. The use of IABP before coronary revascularization had been proposed as a measure to improve left ventricular unloading, thereby improving outcomes [10]. However, the IABP-SHOCK II trial did not corroborate these findings—the mortality was similar among patients who underwent balloon counterpulsation before and after revascularization.

76.10 Limitations

The study had a few limitations. Blinding was not feasible and could have led to bias. The 40% mortality was slightly lower than expected, which may suggest a less severely ill patient population at baseline. Hence, the question arises whether IABP would be beneficial in patients who are more severely ill. The lack of benefit in the subgroup of patients with a systolic BP of <80 mm Hg makes this conclusion less likely. There were many crossovers from the control to the IABP arm, which could have impacted the results of the study; however, this appears unlikely as borne out by multivariate and per protocol analysis. A type II error from a small sample size also appeared improbable, considering the minimal difference in mortality and no signal of difference in secondary outcomes. The study evaluated outcomes at 30 days; the question remained whether there may be a difference in longer-term outcomes.

76.11 Summary

Over half a century, the IABP evolved as the cornerstone of care in patients with cardiogenic shock following acute myocardial infarction. Conventional wisdom suggested efficacy based on its salutary effects on improved coronary circulation and reduced left ventricular afterload. Limited evidence of efficacy from observational studies also led to guidelines recommending its use. The earlier IABP-SHOCK trial, although of small sample size, had raised questions regarding the impact on clinical outcomes, with no evidence to support improved organ function by balloon counterpulsation. The IABP-SHOCK II trial remains the largest RCT that evaluated the efficacy of balloon counterpulsation in patients with acute myocardial infarction and cardiogenic shock. This well-conducted RCT clearly showed that balloon counterpulsation does not improve survival in this patient population. Besides, it failed to reveal a significant impact on hemodynamic stabilization, catecholamine use, or renal function. Predictably, this landmark trial led to a drastic reduction in the clinical use of what was once considered to be a life-saving mechanical device.

References

1. Kantrowitz A, McKinnon WM. The experimental use of the diaphragm as an auxiliary myocardium. Surg Forum. 1958;9:266–8.
2. Moulopoulos SD, Topaz S, Kolff WJ. Diastolic balloon pumping (with carbon dioxide) in the aorta – a mechanical assistance to the failing circulation. Am Heart J. 1962;63:669–75.
3. Kantrowitz A, Tjonneland S, Freed PS, Phillips SJ, Butner AN, Sherman JL. Initial clinical experience with intraaortic balloon pumping in cardiogenic shock. JAMA. 1968;203(2):113–8.
4. Thiele H, Zeymer U, Thelemann N, Neumann FJ, Hausleiter J, Abdel-Wahab M, et al. Intraaortic balloon pump in cardiogenic shock complicating acute myocardial infarction. Circulation. 2019;139(3):395–403.
5. Prondzinsky R, Lemm H, Swyter M, Wegener N, Unverzagt S, Carter JM, et al. Intra-aortic balloon counterpulsation in patients with acute myocardial infarction complicated by cardiogenic shock: the prospective, randomized IABP SHOCK Trial for attenuation of multiorgan dysfunction syndrome*. Crit Care Med. 2010;38(1):152–60.

6. Thiele H, Allam B, Chatellier G, Schuler G, Lafont A. Shock in acute myocardial infarction: the Cape Horn for trials? Eur Heart J. 2010;31(15):1828–35.
7. Thiele H, Zeymer U, Neumann FJ, Ferenc M, Olbrich HG, Hausleiter J, et al. Intraaortic balloon support for myocardial infarction with cardiogenic shock. N Engl J Med. 2012;367(14):1287–96.
8. Ibanez B, James S, Agewall S, Antunes MJ, Bucciarelli-Ducci C, Bueno H, et al. 2017 ESC Guidelines for the management of acute myocardial infarction in patients presenting with ST-segment elevation: the Task Force for the management of acute myocardial infarction in patients presenting with ST-segment elevation of the European Society of Cardiology (ESC). Eur Heart J. 2018;39(2):119–77.
9. Shah M, Patnaik S, Patel B, Ram P, Garg L, Agarwal M, et al. Trends in mechanical circulatory support use and hospital mortality among patients with acute myocardial infarction and non-infarction related cardiogenic shock in the United States. Clin Res Cardiol. 2018;107(4):287–303.
10. Abdel-Wahab M, Saad M, Kynast J, Geist V, Sherif MA, Richardt G, et al. Comparison of hospital mortality with intra-aortic balloon counterpulsation insertion before versus after primary percutaneous coronary intervention for cardiogenic shock complicating acute myocardial infarction. Am J Cardiol. 2010;105(7):967–71.

77 Pulmonary Artery Catheter in the ICU: The PAC-Man Trial

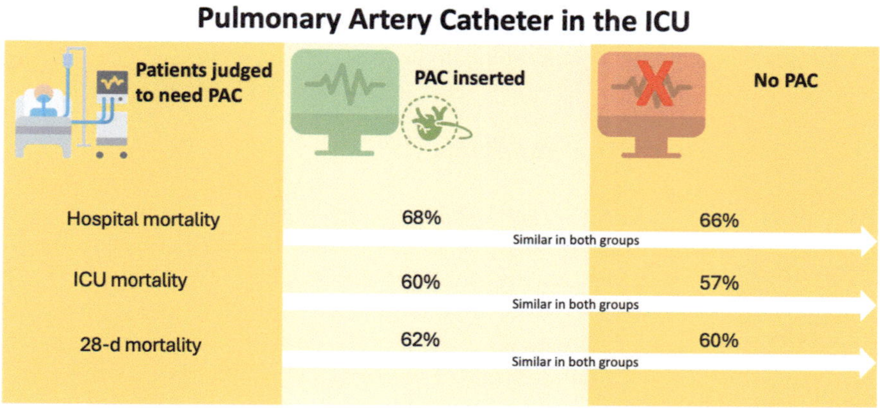

Harvey et al. (Lancet, 2005)

Quick Take

Do pulmonary artery catheters (PACs) improve outcomes in critically ill patients?

The PAC-Man trial assessed whether the use of PACs improves outcomes in critically ill patients compared to standard care without PACs. This multicenter randomized controlled trial enrolled critically ill patients, randomizing them to management with or without PACs. The study found no significant difference in 30-day mortality between the two groups. Additionally, PAC use did not reduce ICU length of stay or complications, raising questions about its routine use in critical care. The

Harvey S, Harrison DA, Singer M, Ashcroft J, Jones CM, Elbourne D, et al. Assessment of the clinical effectiveness of pulmonary artery catheters in management of patients in intensive care (PAC-Man): a randomised controlled trial. Lancet Lond Engl. 2005 Aug 6;366(9484):472–7.

J. Chacko et al., *Landmark Studies in Critical Care*,
https://doi.org/10.1007/978-981-95-0673-6_77

findings suggest that PACs provide limited clinical benefit and emphasize the need for alternative strategies to guide hemodynamic management.

77.1 Introduction and Background

On a bright autumn afternoon of 1967, Jeremy Swan stood by the beach at Santa Monica, watching sailboats pass by. He was a cardiologist at the Cedars of Lebanon Hospital, Los Angeles, and had taken time off following a particularly difficult cardiac catheterization just a few days ago. As the sailboats cruised along, propelled by the wind, an inspirational thought dawned upon him. Could he guide a catheter from the right heart through to the pulmonary artery, driven by the direction of blood flow? A sail or parachute-type appendage attached to the tip of the catheter could enable floatation of the catheter along the direction of flow.

He joined hands with a colleague, William Ganz, to refine the concept and contrived the balloon-tipped pulmonary artery catheter (PAC), creating the eponymous device that turned out to be a milestone in the history of medicine.

77.1.1 The Early Years of the Swan

In the years that followed, the novel device was extensively used in operating rooms and ICUs. Although no controlled trial had evaluated its impact on clinical outcomes, clinicians were swayed by the information on hemodynamic variables offered by the catheter and its ready availability at the bedside. Although the usage of the PAC rose, no tangible outcome benefits were demonstrable during the same period. On the contrary, similar or higher mortality rates and a longer duration of hospital stay were observed among those who underwent PAC-based management [1]. Furthermore, catheter-related complications began to surface; these included thrombosis of the internal jugular vein and the pulmonary artery, pulmonary artery rupture, pulmonary hemorrhage, infective endocarditis, knotting of the catheter, and occasionally, fatal arrhythmias [2, 3].

77.1.2 The SUPPORT Investigators Rock the Boat

A quarter of a century had elapsed since its introduction to clinical practice when Connors et al. designed a prospective cohort study to evaluate clinical outcomes among ICU patients who underwent PAC-based management [4]. A randomized controlled trial (RCT) on the use of the PAC seemed unrealistic in that era—such was the deep-rooted faith clinicians seemed to pin on the device. A previous RCT [5] had to be aborted following the refusal of many treating clinicians to participate as they considered it unethical not to use a PAC!

The SUPPORT study by Connors et al. evaluated 5735 patients who were admitted to the ICU of five hospitals in the USA [4]; of these, 2184 patients underwent

PAC insertion within the first 24 h of ICU admission. On unadjusted analysis, the PAC was associated with a significantly higher mortality at 30, 60, and 180 days. The duration of stay in the ICU and hospital was also longer in patients who underwent pulmonary artery catheterization. In propensity-matched analysis, higher mortality was consistently observed with PAC-based care. Furthermore, the cost of care was higher, the duration of ICU stay longer, and the intensity of care higher in patients who underwent pulmonary artery catheterization compared to those who did not.

The study was limited by its observational design and the likelihood of confounding variables that may have led to bias. It was confined to five hospitals and lacked generalizability to other settings. The study evaluated PAC use within the first 24 h of ICU admission; hence, the possibility of a beneficial effect with later use could not be excluded. The authors recommended an RCT considering the adverse outcomes noted in their retrospective observational study. An accompanying editorial proposed a moratorium on the use of the PAC if an RCT was considered infeasible.

77.1.3 Background to the PAC-Man Trial

Despite the findings of the SUPPORT study, PAC use continued in many ICUs through the late 1990s and into the new millennium. Proponents continued to argue for its merits, including the relative ease of cardiac output monitoring once the catheter was in place and other potentially useful hemodynamic parameters. Detractors raised questions about the accuracy of the measured variables, the lack of evidence supporting improved clinical outcomes, and, most of all, safety concerns. The PAC-Man trial was conceptualized as a pragmatic RCT to test the hypothesis that PAC-based management of critically ill patients leads to reduced hospital mortality.

77.2 Population and Design

The PAC-Man trial was conducted between October 2001 and March 2004 across 65 ICUs in the UK [6]. Adult patients admitted to the ICU who were considered to require pulmonary artery catheterization based on clinician judgment were enrolled. The ICUs included could choose not to use an alternative, less invasive cardiac output monitoring device (stratum A) or retain the option of using such a device (stratum B).

Patients were randomly assigned to PAC-based monitoring or no PAC in a 1:1 ratio. Randomization was stratified by age, the underlying clinical syndrome, and the surgical status.

77.2.1 Excluded

The study excluded patients admitted to the ICU for preoperative optimization and those who already had a PAC in place on ICU admission. Potential organ donors undergoing hemodynamic optimization were also excluded.

77.3 Intervention—The PAC Group

The PAC was inserted as soon as possible post-randomization and was retained for as long as considered appropriate by the treating clinician. Assessment of hemodynamic status and management was entirely at the clinician's discretion. No specific treatment algorithm was followed based on PAC data.

77.4 The Control Group

Patient management was based on clinician judgment. An alternative method of hemodynamic monitoring could be used instead of the PAC among patients in stratum B.

77.5 Sample Size

Assuming a mortality of 50% in patients managed with a PAC, an initial sample size of 5673 patients was calculated to detect a 5% difference in hospital mortality. As the study progressed, the mortality in the control group was noted to be 69%—higher than initially estimated. Hence, the sample size was revised to 1281 patients to allow detection of a 10% mortality difference with 90% power at a 5% level of significance.

77.6 Results

The study randomized a total of 1041 patients—519 to the PAC group and 522 to the control group. In the control group, 24 patients (5%) underwent PAC insertion; 34 patients (7%) in the PAC group did not receive the intervention. PAC insertion was withheld due to a change in the clinical situation (3%) or the potential for complications (1%). Attempts at insertion were unsuccessful in 14 (3%) patients.

Most patients were medical (66%), followed by those who underwent emergency (28%) or elective surgical procedures (6%); there was no significant difference between groups. In most patients, the PAC was considered necessary to guide the titration of vasoactive medication (>70%). Multiorgan dysfunction was present in 65% of patients in the PAC group and 66% of patients in the control group. Patients had a high baseline severity of illness—the mean APACHE II score was 22.1 (6.6) in the PAC group and 22.7 (6.5) in the control group.

A change in the management strategy within 2 h of PAC insertion occurred in 80% of patients—mainly related to additional fluid administration and commencement or increased dosage of vasoactive medication. The median duration of PAC-based management was 3 (2–4) days.

77.7 The Primary Outcome—Hospital Mortality

Among patients managed with a PAC, 346/506 (68%) died in hospital, compared with 333/507 (66%) in the control group; the difference was non-significant.

77.8 Secondary Outcomes

77.8.1 ICU and 28-Day Mortality

The ICU and 28-day mortality were also similar in both groups. The ICU mortality was 60% and 57%, respectively, in the PAC and the control groups. In the PAC group, 62% of patients had died by day 28, compared with 60% in the control group.

77.8.2 Other Outcomes

The in-hospital survival up to 90 days was similar in both groups. The ICU length of stay and the number of days of organ support were also similar.

77.8.3 Subgroup Analysis

On subgroup analysis, there was no significant difference based on the APACHE II scores, the underlying clinical syndrome, and regardless of an alternative method of cardiac output measurement.

77.9 Adverse Events

Complications directly related to PAC insertion occurred in 10% of patients. These included hematoma at the insertion site, arterial puncture, and arrhythmias requiring treatment. Pneumothorax occurred in two patients, while one patient sustained a hemothorax. There were two instances of lost guidewires that had to be retrieved from the femoral vein and the inferior vena cava. The main study outcomes are summarized in Table 77.1.

Table 77.1 Main study outcomes

Outcome	PAC group	Control group	Significance
Hospital mortality	68%	67%	$P = 0.39$
ICU mortality	60%	57%	$P = 0.37$
Hospital LOS, survivors	34%	40%	$P = 0.43$
Median organ support days, survivors	19	19	$P = 0.32$

Abbreviations: *PAC* pulmonary artery catheter, *LOS* length of stay

77.10 Study Conclusions

Among critically ill patients managed with a PAC, there was no difference in hospital mortality compared with those managed without a PAC. Furthermore, the duration of organ support, and the length of stay in the ICU or in the hospital were also similar in both groups.

77.11 Strengths of the Study

The PAC-Man trial was a pragmatic RCT that compared the outcomes of patients who were managed with or without a PAC. No specific treatment strategy was followed based on the information obtained from PAC, reflecting real-world practice. The study was conducted across 65 ICUs in the UK, thus providing external validity. There was high compliance with the assigned treatment strategy, and follow-up was complete. Analysis was by intention to treat, adding further strength to the study.

77.12 Weaknesses

Critics would continue to posit that the utility of any monitoring device would depend on a structured, algorithmic therapeutic approach based on the data that it offers. However, the PAC-Man study adopted a pragmatic methodology and reflected evaluation of real-world practice. Cardiologists and their surgical colleagues continue to aver that among their patient population with heart failure, the PAC provides invaluable information and titration of therapeutic interventions, including the use of inotropes.

The study was conducted in an era when ultrasonography was not widely used to guide catheter insertion. Perhaps some of the complications may have been attributable to the blind approach of catheter insertion.

The ability of ICU staff in identifying waveforms and data from the PAC may also be questionable based on evidence from previous studies [7, 8]. The PAC-Man trial did not assess the adequacy of catheter use or the interpretation of data. However, the level of experience of study centers with the use of the PAC did not appear to influence outcomes.

77.13 Summary

The PAC-Man trial was an eye-opener regarding the role of the PAC in the management of critically ill patients. This large, adequately powered RCT reflected the real-world practice of the time, and conclusively demonstrated no added benefit with the use of the PAC. Needless to say, the lack of a protocolized approach continues to remain a thorn in the flesh in the management of critically ill patients with shock. However, several newer, less-invasive modalities of cardiac output monitoring have been increasingly used in the management of hemodynamically unstable patients, including bedside echocardiography and pulse contour analysis [9, 10].

The once iconic "Yellow Snake" as it is often alluded to, appears to be on the verge of extinction after having lived a charmed life for over half a century.

References

1. Gore JM, Goldberg RJ, Spodick DH, Alpert JS, Dalen JE. A community-wide assessment of the use of pulmonary artery catheters in patients with acute myocardial infarction. Chest. 1987;92(4):721–7.
2. Chastre J, Cornud F, Bouchama A, Viau F, Benacerraf R, Gibert C. Thrombosis as a complication of pulmonary-artery catheterization via the internal jugular vein: prospective evaluation by phlebography. N Engl J Med. 1982;306(5):278–81.
3. Rowley KM, Clubb KS, Smith GJ, Cabin HS. Right-sided infective endocarditis as a consequence of flow-directed pulmonary-artery catheterization. A clinicopathological study of 55 autopsied patients. N Engl J Med. 1984;311(18):1152–6.
4. Connors AF, Speroff T, Dawson NV, Thomas C, Harrell FE, Wagner D, et al. The effectiveness of right heart catheterization in the initial care of critically ill patients. SUPPORT Investigators. JAMA. 1996;276(11):889–97.
5. Guyatt G. A randomized control trial of right-heart catheterization in critically ill patients. Ontario Intensive Care Study Group. J Intensive Care Med. 1991;6(2):91–5.
6. Harvey S, Harrison DA, Singer M, Ashcroft J, Jones CM, Elbourne D, et al. Assessment of the clinical effectiveness of pulmonary artery catheters in management of patients in intensive care (PAC-Man): a randomised controlled trial. Lancet Lond Engl. 2005;366(9484):472–7.
7. Iberti TJ, Daily EK, Leibowitz AB, Schecter CB, Fischer EP, Silverstein JH. Assessment of critical care nurses' knowledge of the pulmonary artery catheter. The Pulmonary Artery Catheter Study Group. Crit Care Med. 1994;22(10):1674–8.
8. Gnaegi A, Feihl F, Perret C. Intensive care physicians' insufficient knowledge of right-heart catheterization at the bedside: time to act? Crit Care Med. 1997;25(2):213–20.
9. Schmidt S, Westhoff TH, Hofmann C, Schaefer JH, Zidek W, Compton F, et al. Effect of the venous catheter site on transpulmonary thermodilution measurement variables. Crit Care Med. 2007;35(3):783–6.
10. Chaney JC, Derdak S. Minimally invasive hemodynamic monitoring for the intensivist: current and emerging technology. Crit Care Med. 2002;30(10):2338–45.

78 Pharmacist Participation on ICU Rounds and Adverse Drug Events: Leape et al.

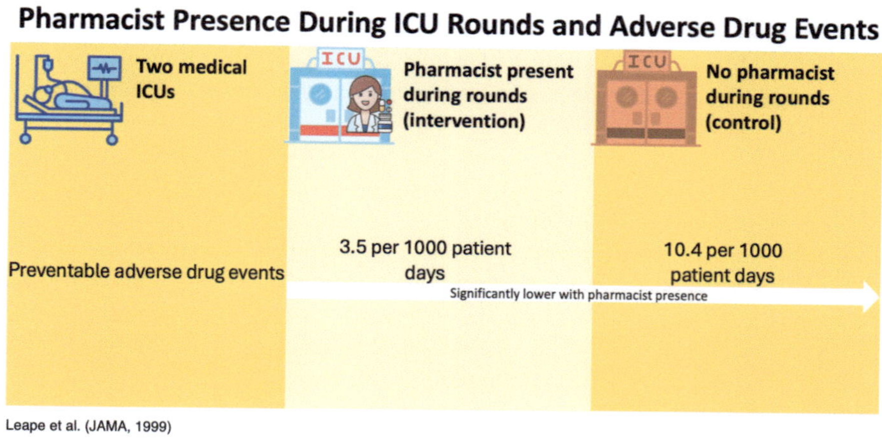

Quick Take

Can pharmacist involvement in ICU rounds reduce adverse drug events?

The study by Leape et al. evaluated the impact of pharmacist participation in physician rounds on the incidence of adverse drug events (ADEs) in the ICU. This prospective, observational study compared ICU patients with and without pharmacist involvement during daily rounds. The results showed a significant reduction in ADEs when pharmacists were included in rounds, particularly in medication errors related to drug interactions, dosing, and administration. The study concluded that active pharmacist participation in the ICU team can substantially improve patient

---

Leape LL, Cullen DJ, Clapp MD, Burdick E, Demonaco HJ, Erickson JI, et al. Pharmacist participation on physician rounds and adverse drug events in the intensive care unit. JAMA. 1999 Jul 21;282(3):267–70.

J. Chacko et al., *Landmark Studies in Critical Care*,
https://doi.org/10.1007/978-981-95-0673-6_78

safety and medication management, advocating for greater integration of pharmacists into critical care settings.

78.1 Introduction

Errors occur during the prescription of drugs in the ICU. Such errors may lead to adverse drug events (ADE) [1]. The incidence of adverse drug events may be twice as high in ICUs compared with non-ICU settings [2]. Adverse drug events may lead to unfavorable clinical outcomes, including an increase in the duration of hospital stay [3]. Pharmacist involvement and review of prescriptions reduce the incidence of errors [4] and may reduce the drug-related cost of care [5]. The pharmacist typically reviews physician orders after the drugs have been prescribed. However, this approach may not be efficacious as the pharmacist may lack clinical information. Pharmacist input may be substantially greater at the time of prescribing—during physician rounds in the ICU.

Leape et al. conducted a clinical study to evaluate the impact of pharmacist participation and input during the medical ICU rounds on the incidence of adverse drug events [6].

78.2 Population and Design

The study was conducted in two medical ICUs—intervention and control units—of the Massachusetts General Hospital and followed a before-after design. Study outcomes were compared before and after implementation of the intervention; besides, outcomes during the post-intervention period were compared with those of the control unit during the same period. Thus, there were three study groups—patients admitted to the study unit during the pre-intervention period, those admitted during the post-intervention period, and those in the control unit during the post-intervention period. Seventy-five patients were selected in each of the three groups by random number generation. The study unit was a 17-bedded medical ICU, while the control unit was a 15-bedded coronary care unit.

The pre-intervention period was between February 1 and July 31, 1993 (phase 1); the post-intervention period extended between October 1, 1994, and July 7, 1995 (phase 2).

78.3 Intervention

A senior pharmacist was assigned to join rounds with the patient care team in the study unit. Following rounds, the pharmacist was present in the unit for consultations all morning and available on call through the rest of the day. This involved a commitment of approximately half of the pharmacist's duty time.

78.4 Control

The usual practice was followed—a pharmacist was available for part of the day but did not join the clinical rounds.

78.5 Outcomes

The authors compared the incidence of adverse drug events in the ordering stage. A preventable adverse drug event was defined as an injury caused by an error associated with the use of a medication. Trained investigators identified medication errors or adverse drug events by reviewing medical records and laboratory investigations. Two physicians reviewed incidents independently and classified them based on whether they constituted adverse drug events. They evaluated the severity and preventability of the event using pre-established criteria. Besides, if an error occurred, they evaluated the type of error and the stage at which it had occurred. Disagreements between reviewers were resolved by consensus, and if required, by arbitration by a third reviewer.

The incidence of preventable adverse drug events related to prescriptions decreased significantly in phase 2 compared with phase 1. The rate of preventable adverse drug events per 1000 patient-days decreased by 66% post intervention [10.4 (95% CI, 7–14) vs. 3.5 (95% CI, 1–5); $P = 0.001$).

The rate of preventable adverse drug events per 1000 patient-days was 72% lower in the intervention unit compared with the control unit in phase 2 [3.5 (95% CI, 1–5) vs. 12.4 (95% CI, 8–17); $P = 0.001$)

In the control unit, the incidence of adverse drug events rose non-significantly from phase 1 to phase 2 [10.9 (95% CI, 6–16) vs. 12.4 (95% CI, 8–17); $P = 0.76$).

During phase 2, a total of 398 pharmacist-initiated interventions occurred. Among these interventions, the large majority (366) were related to ordering; all except four were accepted by physicians (99% acceptance). Prominent among the pharmacist-initiated interventions were clarification or correction of order, provision of information regarding the drug, recommendation of alternate therapy, identification of interactions, identification of allergic reaction, and non-formulary drug use.

The pharmacist offered drug information in 100 instances; these were usually at the time of decision-making regarding a drug order. In 47 instances, the pharmacist recommended alternative therapy with a safer or cheaper, but equally effective therapy. In 22 instances, potential drug interactions or allergies were identified with the recommendation of alternatives. The main study outcomes are summarized in Table 78.1.

Table 78.1 Main study outcomes

Outcomes	Study unit pre-intervention phase	Study unit post-intervention phase	Control unit pre-intervention phase	Control unit post-intervention phase	Significance
Adverse drug events (number)	35	10	16	30	
Adverse drug event rate/1000 patient days	33	11.6	34.7	46.6	$P < 0.001$
Preventable drug events (number)	11	3	5	8	
Preventable adverse event rate related to ordering/1000 patient days	10.4	3.5	10.9	12.4	$P < 0.001$

78.6 Study Conclusion

Pharmacist presence with the patient care team during clinical rounds in the medical ICU was associated with a significantly lower rate of adverse drug events arising from prescription errors. Nearly all the changes suggested by the pharmacist were accepted by the physician doing round.

78.7 Strengths

Conventionally, pharmacist involvement with ICU prescription has been largely retrospective, with review of errors after decision-making. Leape et al. tested the concept of pharmacist review of physician orders at the time of prescribing. They performed a prospective, before-after study that evaluated the impact of a pharmacist joining the ICU team during rounds and offering their input. They evaluated the baseline incidence of adverse drug events and compared it with the incidence of such events post-intervention. The event rate was also compared with a control unit that followed the usual practice of prescribing.

Pharmacist input during rounds was associated with a nearly three-fold decrease in preventable adverse drug events, clearly establishing the efficacy of pharmacist input at the time of prescribing. A high level of acceptance of pharmacist intervention was observed, with physicians accepting 99% of the modifications suggested by the pharmacist.

78.8 Limitations

The study was conducted in a single ICU of a teaching hospital in the USA. The findings may not be generalizable to other centers. Review of records may not represent the true incidence of preventable adverse drug events; potential adverse drug events or "near misses" may not be captured in this type of review. Although an impactful intervention, there may be practical difficulties in ensuring pharmacist participation during multiple clinical rounds carried out by several clinicians at different times during the day. Interpersonal relationships play an important role, especially in the adoption of a new concept involving additional team members. The pharmacist involved may need to establish a sound rapport with the care team to win their confidence and ensure that the system works efficiently.

78.9 Subsequent Studies

A retrospective observational study reviewed pharmacist interventions in five ICUs at the Singapore General Hospital over a 7-month period [7]. A total of 619 interventions were recorded, involving 775 medication-related problems; 91.1% of these were accepted by the intensivist. The most common medication-related problem was an inappropriate drug regimen (49.2%), with anti-infective agents topping the list.

A systematic review with meta-analysis evaluated the impact of critical care pharmacists as part of multidisciplinary ICU teams on clinical outcomes [8]. Fourteen studies were included in the meta-analysis. Critical care pharmacist involvement was significantly associated with reduced mortality compared with no pharmacist involvement (odds ratio, 0.78; 95% CI, 0.73–0.83; $p < 0.00001$). The mean ICU length of stay was also lower when critical care pharmacists were part of the multidisciplinary team. The incidence of adverse drug events was significantly lower with pharmacist intervention.

Alsayed et al. conducted a prospective observational study including patients admitted to a medical ICU in the United Arab Emirates [9]. During the study period, the pharmacist recommended 1004 interventions involving 200 patients. Most of the interventions were accepted (92%) and implemented in full (82%) by the ICU physician. The authors observed 1003 drug-related problems during the study period, most commonly involving antimicrobial agents. The drug-related problems identified involved the choice of drug (61%) or the prescribed dose (22%). On adjusted analysis based on demographic data and the score on the Glasgow Coma Scale, more than 4 interventions reduced the hazard of death within 90 days of ICU stay. The authors concluded that pharmacist intervention improved clinical outcomes in the medical ICU.

78.10 Summary

Conventionally, pharmacist involvement with drug prescription was through retrospective review of charts; however, this strategy may not prevent adverse drug events. Leape et al. evaluated the impact of pharmacist participation and input during ICU physician rounds on clinical outcomes. The before-after study involved a single medical ICU of a teaching hospital; a coronary care unit acted as the control unit in the post-intervention period. During the intervention period, a senior pharmacist joined the ICU team rounds and was available in the ICU all morning and on call thereafter.

The 6-month pre-intervention period was followed by a 9-month post-intervention period. The incidence of preventable adverse drug events decreased by 66% during the post-intervention period. In the control unit, no change was noted in the rate of adverse drug events. Overall, the pharmacist suggested 366 recommendations on drug prescription; 362 (99%) of these were accepted by the physician. The authors concluded that pharmacist presence during ICU clinical rounds led to a substantially lower rate of adverse drug events related to prescription errors. This landmark study established the efficacy of pharmacist input on physician prescriptions during ICU rounds in reducing adverse drug events.

References

1. Bates DW, Cullen DJ, Laird N, Petersen LA, Small SD, Servi D, et al. Incidence of adverse drug events and potential adverse drug events. Implications for prevention. ADE Prevention Study Group. JAMA. 1995;274(1):29–34.
2. Cullen DJ, Sweitzer BJ, Bates DW, Burdick E, Edmondson A, Leape LL. Preventable adverse drug events in hospitalized patients: a comparative study of intensive care and general care units. Crit Care Med. 1997;25(8):1289–97.
3. Vargas E, Terleira A, Hernando F, Perez E, Cordón C, Moreno A, et al. Effect of adverse drug reactions on length of stay in surgical intensive care units. Crit Care Med. 2003;31(3):694–8.
4. Folli HL, Poole RL, Benitz WE, Russo JC. Medication error prevention by clinical pharmacists in two children's hospitals. Pediatrics. 1987;79(5):718–22.
5. Montazeri M, Cook DJ. Impact of a clinical pharmacist in a multidisciplinary intensive care unit. Crit Care Med. 1994;22(6):1044–8.
6. Leape LL, Cullen DJ, Clapp MD, Burdick E, Demonaco HJ, Erickson JI, et al. Pharmacist participation on physician rounds and adverse drug events in the intensive care unit. JAMA. 1999;282(3):267–70.
7. Soong JL, Ang LY, Chan JLE, Lie SA. Clinical impact of pharmacists' interventions in intensive care units in a tertiary institution in Singapore—a retrospective cohort study. Proc Singapore Healthcare. 2023;32:20101058231218527.
8. Lee H, Ryu K, Sohn Y, Kim J, Suh GY, Kim E. Impact on patient outcomes of pharmacist participation in multidisciplinary critical care teams: a systematic review and meta-analysis. Crit Care Med. 2019;47(9):1243–50.
9. Ali Hussain Alsayed H, Saheb Sharif-Askari F, Saheb Sharif-Askari N, Halwani R. Clinical pharmacist interventions in an intensive care unit reduces ICU mortality at a tertiary hospital in Dubai, United Arab Emirates. Explor Res Clin Soc Pharm. 2024;14:100431.

MIX
Papier aus verantwortungsvollen Quellen
Paper from responsible sources
FSC® C105338

If you have any concerns about our products,
you can contact us on
ProductSafety@springernature.com

In case Publisher is established outside the EU,
the EU authorized representative is:
Springer Nature Customer Service Center GmbH
Europaplatz 3, 69115 Heidelberg, Germany

Printed by Libri Plureos GmbH
in Hamburg, Germany